# Me in the Classroom

## The Teacher's Role in Diagnosis and Management

**FOURTH EDITION**

**Edited by**
**Robert H. A. Haslam**
**and**
**Peter J. Valletutti**

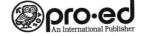

**pro·ed**
An International Publisher

8700 Shoal Creek Boulevard
Austin, Texas 78757-6897
800/897-3202    Fax 800/397-7633
www.proedinc.com

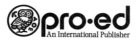
An International Publisher

© 1975, 1985, 1996, 2004 by PRO-ED, Inc.
8700 Shoal Creek Boulevard
Austin, Texas 78757-6897
800/897-3202    Fax 800/397-7633
www.proedinc.com

**Library of Congress Cataloging-in-Publication Data**

Medical problems in the classroom : the teacher's role in diagnosis and management /
    [edited by] Robert A. Haslam & Peter J. Valletutti.—4th ed.
        p. cm.
    Includes bibliographical references and index.
    ISBN 0-89079-923-7
    1. School health services—United States.   2. School children—Health and
hygiene—United States.   3. Children with disabilities—Health and hygiene—
United States.   4. Children—Diseases—Diagnosis.   I. Haslam, Robert H. A., 1936–
II. Valletutti, Peter J.

    LB3409.U5M43    2003
    371.7′1—dc21

                                                                        2003043165

Illustration on dedication page by Morgan Haslam, age 8.

This book is designed in Minion and Gill Sans.

Printed in the United States of America

1   2   3   4   5   6   7   8   9   10      07   06   05   04   03

*To Brendan, Morgan, Thomas, and Matthew,*
*today's students on the lifelong journey of learning.*
—R.H.A.H.

*To my brother Dr. Angelo Valletutti,*
*a brilliant and dedicated physician*
*and a very special human being.*
—P.J.V.

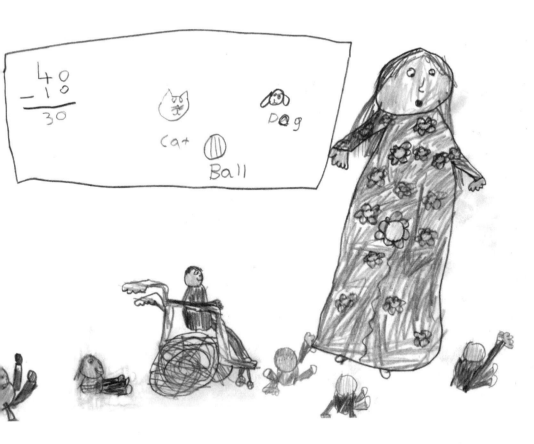

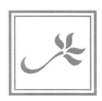

# Contents

# Preface

There has been continuing emphasis on the placement of children with physical and intellectual disabilities within the educational mainstream beginning with the Education for All Handicapped Children Act of 1975 (Public Law [P.L.] 94-142), followed by the Education of the Handicapped Act Amendments in 1986 (P.L. 99-457). These two acts mandated intervention services from infancy to 31 years of age for a diverse population of individuals with a myriad of medical and developmental disorders. These laws were replaced in 1990 by the Individuals with Disabilities Eduation Act (IDEA; P.L. 101-476), which establishes free, appropriate education for all school-age children with disabilities and early intervention services for preschool-age children (3 years and above). IDEA also established federal incentives for individual states to develop programs for infants and toddlers. In addition, the Americans with Disabilities Act of 1990 (P.L. 101-336) outlined provisions that all public accommodations, including existing schools as well as new schools, must meet the accessibility guidelines established by the act and that teachers and administrators make the schools comfortable and safe for students with physical disabilities.

It is relatively common to find a child with cerebral palsy, mental retardation, epilepsy, or a chronic health problem such as an eating disorder in a regular classroom, as well as students with behavioral or psychological disorders and others with such potentially acute medical conditions as asthma or a seizure disorder. Thus, educators must be familiar with the various manifestations of these conditions and how they may affect the students' learning and socialization so that appropriate curriculum planning and classroom adaptation can occur, and meaningful information can be conveyed to parents and health professionals.

The educator can play an important role as a diagnostician and referral source, because of continuous contact with a relatively small group of children over a significant period of time. Furthermore, teachers are becoming increasingly sophisticated in the identification of symptoms and behaviors, such as alterations in thought processes or in general well-being and appearance, that may suggest an underlying illness or disorder in one of their students. It follows that, to be effective, the teacher must keep abreast of new diagnostic techniques and therapeutic developments in the field of child health care.

The third edition of *Medical Problems in the Classroom* provided the educator, psychologist, social worker, speech therapist and audiologist, occupational and physical therapist, physician, and parents with an overview of common medical problems in the school-age population. It stressed the role of the teacher as a facilitator of good health in its broadest sense. The book has also proved useful for students preparing for careers that will focus on interaction with children and youth. In the 7 years since the third edition, ongoing advances have been made in child health care in response to the emergence of new medical, genetic, and social problems, and an increased emphasis on prevention or wellness rather than sickness and illness. The major impetus for this fourth edition continues to be the enthusiastic response and constructive criticism received from the students and professionals who have used previous editions of the book in their workplace or in the classroom.

As in the third edition, it is not feasible to cover all aspects of pediatric medical and related problems, but rather to highlight the conditions that a teacher is most likely to encounter. As in the previous editions, the first chapter, written by an educator, Peter Valletutti, sets the stage by introducing concepts and posing questions about common health problems in children within the classroom as seen through the eyes of a teacher. Valletutti provides many helpful recommendations and suggestions to the educator concerning health-related matters. Authors from the previous edition have significantly updated their chapters on prevention of chronic disabilities and diseases; infectious diseases; growth, development, and endocrine disorders; diabetes; genetic mechanisms; visual disorders; hearing problems; communication disorders; dental disorders; orthopedic problems and sports injuries; neurological disorders; adolescent eating disorders; sexual development; sexually transmitted diseases; and child abuse.

The fourth edition of *Medical Problems in the Classroom* has been significantly revised to include newly written chapters by selected medical experts on chronic illnesses in children, cerebral palsy, attention-deficit/hyperactivity disorder, mental retardation, autistic spectrum disorders, drug and substance abuse, and the science of reading and dyslexia. This edition has been significantly expanded to include contemporary and practical issues and health topics prevalent in today's classroom. The scope of the book has been expanded to include critically important chapters on emotional and behavioral problems in the classroom and school-based violence prevention.

We anticipate that *Medical Problems in the Classroom* will continue to be used as a source of information for many of the common medical disorders in the school setting by a wide variety of professionals. The chapters are presented with the objective of sharing knowledge that may be helpful in understanding basic disease mechanisms. Important symptoms and signs indicative of specific diseases or conditions, modern methods of diagnosis, state-of-the-art technology, therapeutic advances and pitfalls, and a focus on prevention are highlighted with graphic illustrations and tables. Most important, the fourth edition strives to encourage interactive communication on health issues between the parent, health professional, and educator, on behalf of the student.

# REFERENCES

Americans with Disabilities Education Act of 1990, 42 U.S.C. § 12101 *et seq.*

Education for All Handicapped Children Act of 1975, 20 U.S.C. § 1400 *et seq.*

Education of the Handicapped Act Amendments of 1986, 20 U.S.C. § 1400 *et seq.*

Individuals with Disabilities Education Act of 1990, 20 U.S.C. § 1400 *et seq.*

# ACKNOWLEDGMENTS

**W**e would like to extend our sincere appreciation to the contributors of the fourth edition of *Medical Problems in the Classroom.* Many of the original authors continue to share in the production of this book, adding a wealth of experience since their initial contribution to the first edition in 1975, almost 30 years ago. We are particularly grateful to the new authors, whose chapters have significantly added to the scope and depth of the text. All contributors are physicians or educator clinicians in frequent contact with the educational system and the community. They were invited to participate in the fourth edition because of their commitment to children with medical problems. The authors are indebted to the many students and professionals whose suggestions and ideas led to the development of this edition. We also are grateful to the readers of previous editions of *Medical Problems in the Classroom* who recommended new concepts and chapter ideas, which are included in the fourth edition.

*Robert H. A. Haslam*
*Peter J. Valletutti*

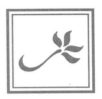

# Contributors

**Pasquale J. Accardo, MD**
    Professor of Developmental Research in Pediatrics
    Virginia Commonwealth University
        at Medical College of Virginia Campus
    Developmental Pediatrician
        Children's Hospital
    Richmond, Virginia

**Patricia M. Blasco**
    Associate Professor
    Department of Education
    Portland State University
    Portland, Oregon

**Peter A. Blasco, MD**
    Associate Professor
    Department of Pediatrics
    Oregon Health and Science University
    Director of Neurodevelopment Programs
    Child Development and Rehabilitation Center
    Portland, Oregon

**George D. Carson, MD, FRCSC, FSOGC**
    Clinical Professor of Obstetrics and Gynecology
        and Reproductive Sciences
    University of Saskatchewan
    Head of Obstetrics and Gynecology
    Regina Health District
    Regina, Saskatchewan

## Sheila L. Carson, RN
Tutor
Nursing Education Program of Saskatchewan
Regina, Saskatchewan

## Denis Daneman, MD
Professor of Pediatrics
University of Toronto
Head Division of Endocrinology
The Hospital for Sick Children
Toronto, Ontario

## Michael H. Epstein, EdD
Professor of Special Education
Director of the Center for At-Risk
    Children's Services
University of Nebraska–Lincoln
Lincoln, Nebraska

## Marcia Frank, MHSc, RN
Clinical Nurse Specialist
Division of Endocrinology
Department of Pediatrics
The Hospital for Sick Children
Toronto, Ontario

## Ronald Gold, MD
Professor Emeritus of Pediatrics
Faculty of Medicine
University of Toronto
Honorary Consultant and Former Chief
Division of Infectious Disease
The Hospital for Sick Children
Toronto, Ontario

## Jorge E. Gonzalez, PhD
Research Assistant Professor
Center for At-Risk Children's Services
University of Nebraska–Lincoln
Lincoln, Nebraska

## James Harder, MD, FRCSC

Associate Professor of Surgery
University of Calgary
Calgary, Alberta

## Robert H. A. Haslam, MD, FAAP, FRCPC

Emeritus Professor and Chair
Department of Pediatrics
Professor of Medicine (Neurology)
University of Toronto
Emeritus Pediatrician-in-Chief
The Hospital for Sick Children
Toronto, Ontario

## Shinya Ito, MD

Head of the Division of Clinical
    Pharmacology and Toxicology
The Hospital for Sick Children
Associate Professor of Pediatrics, Medicine,
    Pharmacology, and Pharmacy
University of Toronto
Toronto, Ontario

## Douglas H. Johnston, DDS

Associate Professor
Faculty of Dentistry
University of Toronto
Dentist-in-Chief
The Hospital for Sick Children
Director of Dental Services
Bloorview MacMillan Children's Centre
Toronto, Ontario

## Dilip J. Karnik, MD

Head of Child Neurology
Seton Medical Center
Adjunct Associate Professor
University of Texas at Austin
Austin, Texas

**Debra K. Katzman, MD, FRCPC**
Associate Professor of Pediatrics
Medical Director
The Eating Disorder Program
The Hospital for Sick Children
and The University of Toronto
Toronto, Ontario

**Thaddeus E. Kelly, MD, PhD**
Professor of Pediatrics
Division of Medical Genetics
University of Virginia School of Medicine
Charlottesville, Virginia

**David J. Kenny, BSc, DDS, PhD**
Professor
Faculty of Dentistry
University of Toronto
Toronto, Ontario

**Susan M. King, MD**
Associate Professor of Pediatrics
University of Toronto
Division of Infectious Diseases
Department of Pediatrics
The Hospital for Sick Children
Toronto, Ontario

**Gideon Koren, MD, FABMT, FRCPC**
Director of The Motherisk Program
Professor of Pediatrics, Pharmacology, Pharmacy,
Medicine, and Medical Genetics
The University of Toronto
Senior Scientist
The Research Institute
The Hospital for Sick Children
Toronto, Ontario

**Alex V. Levin, MD, MHSc, FAAP, FAAO, FRCSC**
Staff Ophthalmologist
Associate Professor
Departments of Pediatrics, Genetics, and Ophthalmology
The Hospital for Sick Children
University of Toronto
Toronto, Ontario

**Marcellina Mian, MD**
Professor of Pediatrics and Public Health Services
Director of Undergraduate Medical Education
Department of Pediatrics
University of Toronto and The Hospital for Sick Children
Toronto, Ontario

**Ron Nelson, PhD**
Research Assistant Professor
Co-Director of the Center for At-Risk Children's Services
Center for At-Risk Children's Services
University of Nebraska–Lincoln
Lincoln, Nebraska

**Vicky Papaioannou, MClSc**
Audiology Practice Leader
Associate Director, Cochlear Implant Program
The Hospital for Sick Children
Instructor
Department of Otolaryngology
University of Toronto
Toronto, Ontario

**Herbert H. Severson, PhD**
Research Scientist
Oregon Research Institute
Principal Investigator
Institute on Violence and Destructive Behavior
College of Education
University of Oregon
Eugene, Oregon

## Bennett A. Shaywitz, MD

Professor of Pediatrics and Neurology
Yale University School of Medicine
Co-Director
NICHD–Yale Center for the Study of
Learning and Attention
New Haven, Connecticut

## Sally E. Shaywitz, MD

Professor of Pediatrics
Department of Pediatrics
Yale University School of Medicine
Co-Director
NICHD–Yale Center for the Study of
Learning and Attention
New Haven, Connecticut

## Michelle Shouldice, MD, FRCPC

Section Head
Pediatric Outpatient Consultation
Division of Pediatric Medicine
The Hospital for Sick Children
Toronto, Ontario

## Jeffrey R. Sprague, PhD

Co-Director
Institute on Violence and Destructive Behavior
College of Education
University of Oregon
Eugene, Oregon

## Margaret Thompson, MD, FRCPC, dABEM, dACMT

Assistant Professor
Departments of Medicine and Pediatrics
University of Toronto
Medical Director, Ontario Regional Poison Information Center
Division of Clinical Pharmacology and Toxicology
The Hospital for Sick Children
Toronto, Ontario

**Peter J. Valletutti, EdD**
Retired Dean of Education and Graduate Studies
Coppin State University
Baltimore, Maryland

**Hill M. Walker, PhD**
Co-Director
Institute on Violence and Destructive Behavior
College of Education
University of Oregon
Eugene, Oregon

**Mary Anne Witzel, PhD**
Speech Pathology Consultant
Kitchener, Ontario

# CHAPTER I

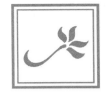

# The Crucial Role
# of the Teacher

Peter J. Valletutti

**T**eachers, especially those who teach at the preschool and elementary levels, have an unparalleled opportunity to assist in the identification and habilitation of children and youth with medical problems. The early identification by a teacher of a potential medical problem is often a critical antecedent to medical diagnosis and thus a crucial precursor to treatment and management of the problem. Furthermore, early identification of a medical problem typically results in the prevention of secondary physical and psychological problems, including impairments in learning and behavior. Teachers are ideally situated to observe student behavior and to make perceptive judgments about the possible existence of an untoward medical condition, and are less likely than parents and other lay caregivers to engage in the denial process. The defense mechanism of denial, although an important stage in a parent's emotional response to his or her child with disabilities, often results in parents' failure to seek needed professional guidance and advice. This predilection, therefore, unfortunately interferes with the early identification and the solution or mitigation of the medical problem (McLoughlin, 1993; Seligman, 2000).

After students enter the school system, teachers interact with children on a sustained basis more often than do many parents and other human service professionals. Many parents, in their efforts to meet their essential financial needs, to attain higher standards of living, or to fulfill their own personal agendas, spend little time with their children. School-age children, as a result, spend much of their time with their teachers, and many spend their out-of-school time in peer interactions or in front of the television screen and various other technological gadgetry and games, away from adult influence or interaction. Restricted time and reduced objectivity limit parents' insightful observations. Teachers thus can play a crucial role in the health care system, especially when the economic limitations and cultural practices of some parents and other lay caregivers reduce the likelihood that the child will receive regular medical evaluations and care. The teacher has a special role in identifying the possible existence of a medical problem, while avoiding the temptation to engage in specific diagnoses or prognoses.

Teachers must be concerned about medical conditions that may affect a student's learning or behavior. They need to be aware of any condition, especially when subtle deviations from the normal are present and are more likely to be overlooked by parents and other caregivers who have limited opportunities to observe the child's behavior (Kirk, Gallagher, & Anastasiow, 1993). In most cases, when a medical problem is severe, it will be observed by parents and diagnosed by physicians early in the child's life. Sometimes this recognition occurs even at birth, when a physical abnormality is obvious, as in the case of Down syndrome and various cranial anomalies. Identification of severe disabilities by parents and physicians also occurs when an apparently normally developing child develops multiple deficits, as in Rett syndrome (Katsiyannis, Ellenburg, Acton, & Torrey, 2001).

Subtle problems, such as the following, are more likely to go undetected:

- Mild mental retardation is typically not identified prior to the school years and is usually recognized when the student fails to meet academic demands.

- A mild orthopedic problem that does not obviously interfere with a student's gross and fine motor facilities necessary to meet the performance demands of school is likely to go undetected (Kirk et al., 1993).

- The early stages of the Duchenne form of muscular dystrophy may go unnoticed until a teacher observes the student begin to fall in class when he seldom did so previously, then to fall more frequently despite being able to get to the standing position with little difficulty, and ultimately to experience great difficulty in getting up.

- A bilateral mild or moderate high-frequency sensorineural hearing loss may not be obvious to the casual observer because the child has sufficient hearing to respond to environmental and speech sounds (but not always with understanding).

- A traumatic brain injury early in a child's life may have no apparent residual damage until learning disabilities and concomitant behavioral problems manifest themselves.

- Deep-seated emotional problems in a child whose charm and apparently conforming behavior masks the problems are unlikely to be identified by teachers.

Teachers, therefore, in both day-to-day observations and more formal evaluations of students, must be alert to the possibility that a specific behavior may be a sign of some untoward medical condition and be especially alert to the more subtle signs that a medical problem exists or is emerging. The problem of identifying the possible existence of a significant medical condition is exacerbated by the fact that teachers of young children, especially during the preschool years and the elementary grades, must be particularly careful not to overreact to behaviors that are developmentally within the normal range. At the same time, they must not disregard signs that point to a possible significant deviation from the normal that requires prompt professional attention. Teachers should not be reluctant to suggest that a problem exists because they feel that it is too soon to know or too risky an observation to be articulated. By avoiding the reporting of a suspected problem in a young child because of the risk of being seen as overly cautious or wrong, a teacher can interfere with the early correction or mitigation of medical problems.

A teacher who is alert to the possible presence of a medical problem always seeks to discover *why* a child's specific behavior or constellation of behaviors exists. A competent teacher always seeks feasible explanations for a behavior that deviates from normal expectations. Each feasible explanation must then be treated as an etiologic hypothesis which the teacher sets out to either accept or reject until the most feasible explanation is arrived at through focused observation and careful deliberation.

Diagnostic hypothesizing concerning the presence of a medical condition from the soft data of teacher observation, however, involves significant risk taking because there are often several feasible explanations for the symptoms and signs demonstrated. For example, the teacher may note the following behaviors:

- Johnny often responds to my questions with such expletives as "Huh?" or "What?"

- He stares closely at my face whenever I speak to him.
- He omits final voiceless consonants in his connected speech.

From these observations, the teacher might hypothesize that Johnny's behavior is the result of a hearing loss. The teacher must then set out to confirm this etiologic hypothesis by observing the student's many interactions and by structuring classroom experiences to elicit behaviors that support this contention while simultaneously attempting to reject the etiologic hypothesis by postulating alternate feasible explanations, such as whether Johnny's behaviors were instead the result of one of the following:

- impaired auditory comprehension
- attention-deficit disorder
- boredom and failure to listen
- petit mal (absence) seizures
- fatigue, malnourishment, or clinical depression

This diagnostic process should continue until one of the explanations has empirical support, either from the teacher's own observations and testing or from diagnostic procedures performed by physicians and other human service professionals.

An awareness of medical problems that may exist in students is one of the essential diagnostic–prescriptive skills required of all teachers, as this awareness and its accompanying knowledge and skills are prerequisite to making judicious decisions about the following (Friend & Cook, 2000; Mostert, 1996; Mueller & Murphy, 2001):

- the need for medical or medically oriented diagnosis or treatment
- appropriate referral sources and procedures
- logical and appropriate individualized instructional goals and objectives
- appropriate and stimulating instructional activities and experiences
- suitable and productive classroom organization practices and procedures
- perceptive behavioral management strategies and techniques
- facilitative methods, materials, and specialized equipment
- productive and insightful teacher–parent interactions

- effective consultation and communication with other teachers, paraeducators, and school personnel

# PREVENTING SECONDARY AND TERTIARY PHYSICAL AND MENTAL DISABILITIES

It is necessary for teachers to maintain an increased sensitivity to those patterns or constellations of behaviors that suggest the presence of a medical problem, especially when that problem can be ameliorated or reversed. *The earlier a disability is identified, the more likely it will be reversed or its debilitating effects minimized.* Secondary prevention involves the early identification of a problem that results in a disability. Tertiary prevention seeks to decrease the severity of the condition through appropriate treatment modalities. Because teachers have prolonged contact with students, they have the singular opportunity to prevent secondary and tertiary physical and mental disabilities by assisting students in obtaining pertinent medical and other health-related therapeutic services.

Teachers infrequently postulate a medical condition as the cause of deviations in student performance. Because teachers usually work with students who are physically able, they are more likely to seek reasons for academic failure or behavioral problems within the student's intellectual, motivational, and affective systems or within his or her social history, than to attribute the problem to an underlying physical impairment. This predilection occurs, perhaps, because typical teacher training emphasizes the behavioral and social sciences and minimizes the biological basis of behavior. Teachers also may be reluctant to suggest a physiological reason for learning and behavioral problems because of fears and anxieties associated with physical anomalies, deviations, and impairments.

Certainly, teachers' tendency to focus on psychological and sociological factors is a realistic orientation, given that the majority of students in general education classes have no significant organic impairments of a chronic or acute nature. Although it is reasonable to seek the cause of a student's learning or behavioral difficulties in the instructional process, in the student's psychological and temperamental makeup, or in social and environmental stress, teachers should not ignore potential medical problems because of their lower degree of occurrence or because of denial or ignorance. In the interest of early identification and preventive medicine, especially when dealing with subtle physical deviations, it perhaps is better for a teacher to suspect a problem and then reject it later than to overlook a significant medical problem.

Thus, teachers can play a major part in preventing learning and behavioral problems that arise from untreated medical problems. Moreover, not only must teachers be cognizant of possible medical problems and their symptomatology, but they must be aware of the child's future need for special education and related services that may be critical to the student's successful acquisition of key cognitive, motor, and affective skills. As the inclusion process continues to place more and more students with severe disabilities in general education classrooms, teachers must be knowledgeable about many syndromes, even those of low incidence (Hardman, Drew, & Egan, 1996; Heward, 2000; Vaughan, Bos, & Schum, 2000).

> Given current trends in special education, along with the Individuals with Disabilities Education Act Amendments of 1997 (IDEA 97), emphasizing the expanded use of placements in the least restrictive environment for students with disabilities, public schools will address the needs of people with rare syndromes such as Rett syndrome in school-based programs. (Katsiyannis et al., 2001, p. 75)

The primary sensory modalities through which learning occurs are hearing and vision. Therefore, teachers must be especially alert to behaviors that suggest that a sensory deficit may be present. It logically follows that students with deficits in auditory or visual acuity, processing, and memory, might have significant difficulty (depending on type, degree, and age of onset) in acquiring key academic, motor, and social–emotional competencies. When one considers the possible effects of a sensory loss on student behavior and learning, one should view that loss from a behavioral perspective—that is, the relationship between the type and severity of loss and its impact on the individual's overall functioning (Hull, 2000).

## Hearing Loss

A student with a moderate bilateral sensorineural loss of hearing (with its characteristic high-frequency loss) hears low-frequency sounds at the normal level (see Chapter 9). This student typically reacts to sounds, including noises and voices, so the student's hearing loss may escape the attention of unsuspecting and unsophisticated listeners and then contribute to the development of learning and behavior problems. A student who has an undetected bilateral congenital loss of hearing in the mild to moderate range and has never experienced normal hearing cannot easily engage in the self-diagnostic process in which he or she recognizes that a discrepancy exists and reports that concern to a parent, teacher, or other significant individual.

The problem of early detection is exacerbated when acuity screenings by school systems are carried out infrequently, are limited to elementary and middle grades, are improperly carried out by poorly trained personnel, and are not routinely conducted on an ad hoc basis. Whenever a student returns to school after having been severely ill with a febrile disease, especially meningitis or encephalitis, audiometric testing must be done to determine whether the recent illness has resulted in a hearing loss. Early detection of hearing loss, for example, can be greatly facilitated by audiometric testing of all students at frequent intervals *throughout* their school career. Students may acquire a hearing loss between routine testing due to infections, toxic substances, or certain antibiotics and other drugs.

Such behaviors as failure to respond to oral directions, confusion in the execution of oral directions, giving wrong answers to simple questions, frequent requests for directions and questions to be repeated, articulation deficits (particularly the distortion of fricative consonants), faulty voice production (including hypernasality, a monotony of inflection, and loudness), mispronunciations, the uttering of inquiring expletives (e.g., "Huh?" or "What?"), behavioral problems, and diminished vocabulary ought to alert the observer to the possibility that the individual has a hearing loss and should be tested. If these behaviors occur together and with a degree of consistency, the existence of an underlying hearing loss is a highly feasible etiologic hypothesis that should be confirmed or rejected through appropriate audiometric tests and otologic examination. Furthermore, attention should be paid to those behaviors that suggest that an ongoing ear infection may be present. Complaints by the student of pain, pressure in his or her ear(s), and dizziness along with the presence of fever should be communicated immediately to the parent or other significant caregiver and steps taken to facilitate medical care and treatment.

## Visual Loss

Possible indicators of visual problems include shifting or covering one eye, stumbling or tripping over small objects, abnormal positioning and distance spacing of the head vis-à-vis reading material, squinting, frequent blinking, excessive sensitivity to light, complaints of poor vision, frequent rubbing of the eyes, and faulty or peculiar eye movements (see also Chapter 8). Several of these signs occurring together strongly point to a possible visual defect. Students with visual impairments are likely to develop problems in perception, sensorimotor skills, and social, preacademic, and academic areas, especially those that require intact visual functioning (Bishop, 1996; Koenig, 1996). Many display emotional concomitants such as irritability and reduced on-task behavior. When a student manifests this constellation of behaviors over time, an appropriate ophthalmologic examination should be conducted.

Teachers who work with students with partial vision must be concerned with the adequacy of classroom illumination, both natural and artificial. They must be aware of the effect that the color of walls and ceilings has on learning among students with partial sight. They need to provide these students with instructional materials pertinent to their specific visual functioning. Teachers need to be cognizant of the need for special materials and equipment such as Braille writers, special pens, paper with bold or raised lines, reading lamps, large-type books and textbooks, optical aids, and technological aids such as specialized computers, microfiche, and microslide viewers. Additional devices that may significantly enhance learning for individuals with visual impairments include the Optacon, a portable electronic device that converts print to vibrating letter images; the Kurzweil Reading machine, which converts printed matter into connected speech; voice-activated computers; and talking calculators (Bishop, 1996; Cox & Dykes, 2001; Hardman et al., 1996; Hill & Snook-Hill, 1996; Koenig, 1996).

# DIAGNOSTIC–PRESCRIPTIVE TEACHING

Teachers are being asked to improve their skills in administering and interpreting the results of standardized tests and to refine their informal diagnostic skills as a necessary foundation to the design of logical educational interventions or prescriptions. Essential professional questions thus become What is educational diagnosis? and How does one diagnose a student? Answering these questions appropriately should result in effective educational programming as well as a heightened awareness of the role of medical, psychological, and sociological factors in the educational decision-making process and in the design and implementation of educational programs. The often championed and legislated but infrequently honored or observed goal of individualizing instruction, elusive as ever, requires the precise and comprehensive appraisal of each student by teachers and a host of other professionals. Comprehensive diagnostic testing cannot be accomplished if attention is directed primarily to performance while ignoring causation and the effect of the specific etiology on behavior. Without a comprehensive evaluation process, a distinctive program of instruction and management cannot be designed or effectively implemented (Kame'enui & Carnine, 1998; Thompson, Quenemoen, Thurlow, & Ysseldyke, 2001).

An educationally relevant diagnostic model has three independent components:

1. educational evaluation for programming purposes and for developing strategies for classroom organization and behavioral management

2. diagnostic awareness of underlying, and perhaps reversible, medical conditions for which medically based diagnosis and treatment should be obtained through a well-designed referral process

3. an appreciation for the special methods of instruction and management needed to meet the education and related needs of students with medical problems

## The Teacher as Evaluator–Programmer

Although agreement often is possible on effective and efficient methods and materials of instruction, consensus on specific educational goals and their priorities is virtually impossible in a pluralistic society such as ours (Kame'enui & Carnine, 1998; Turnbull, Turnbull, Shank, & Leal, 2002). National standards must have built-in flexibility to meet state and local needs, values, and priorities and to meet the needs, interests, and wants of the individual student and his or her family whether or not the student is disabled (Walsh, 2001). Without a clear understanding of what needs to be taught, educators cannot possibly arrive at a precise determination of what needs to be evaluated.

Although school systems, for most of their history, minimized the need to evaluate students for instructional purposes, individual diagnosis and instruction have become the cornerstone of assessment and intervention in special education (Venn, 1994). "A special education teacher uses individual diagnosis and prescription to develop for a student an instructional plan based on observation and testing" (Venn, 1994, p. 10). For the most part, prior to the Education for All Handicapped Children Act of 1975 (P.L. 94-142), the diagnostic approach that occurred for students with special needs was labeling for placement purposes. Adhering to the existing medical model, educators used diagnosis to characteristically identify and label students for the purpose of segregating exceptional students in special schools or even denying them an education at all. Too often those students placed in segregated settings received *no* specialized treatment, as if this administrative arrangement ipso facto was the essential treatment procedure with little else needed (Ysseldyke, Algozzine, & Thurlow, 1992).

The practice of labeling for instructional purposes implies homogeneity of condition that is both a spurious and nonproductive assumption. The assignment of a diagnostic label in the absence of a thorough behavioral analysis, including the impact of a medical condition on the individual student's behavior, is incompatible with the quintessential need to individualize instruction and thus make it meaningful to the student and his or her family and to society in general.

An essential programming skill, then, is to look first at the person with a disability in terms of his or her abilities, interests, needs, and strengths. This diagnostic or evaluative effort should be largely accomplished before exploring the impact of the disability on behavior and learning. The programming challenge, from an educational viewpoint, is to shun the disability model, which focuses on an individual's "diseased" parts or systems rather than on the total individual, with his or her distinct profile of abilities and disabilities. Disabilities must be approached from the vantage point of demonstrated abilities, so that previous knowledge and experiences as well as acquired skills can serve as the basis for remedial and developmental programming. Individualized programs should build on the strengths while remediating the weaknesses.

An understanding of underlying medical problems is needed to put into better perspective the individual's strengths, weaknesses, and treatment needs from both educational and medical perspectives. Such modifications may include the following:

## Teacher Education Programs

- The addition of units of instruction on disabilities and people with disabilities.

- A study of death and dying and the nature and goals of hospitals and clinical settings.

## Classroom Teaching

- The addition of auditory training and speech reading for individuals who are hard of hearing and the introduction of the topic of the deaf culture to students who are hard of hearing (Etting, Johnson, Smith, & Snider, 1994).

- Orientation, mobility, and social competency training, especially to remove the mannerisms and reduce the excessive verbalisms, for young children who are blind (Cox & Dykes, 2001; Hill & Snook-Hill, 1996).

- Training for students with mental retardation in many self-care skills, including toilet training and other social skills generally acquired by most children prior to entry into school programs (Bender, Valletutti, & Baglin, 1996a, 1996b).

- Programming concerned with value and attitude development in students with behavioral disorders, in addition to programming designed to facilitate cognitive development. At first, a great deal of a teacher's time may be devoted to preparing a student to be receptive to learning and to function in a group setting. Time must be spent in dealing with the psychological concomitants of learning problems because a student's self-worth, as well as anxiety about the learning task, may have to be dealt with before learning can take place.

- Teachers must also ask whether a student with a medical problem requires a modification in curriculum and instructional practices. In particular, the modification of the curriculum to meet the life skills or functional needs of students with disabilities should be addressed (Polloway, Patton, Payne, & Payne, 1989; Valletutti, Bender, & Sims-Tucker, 1996; Valletutti, Bender, & Smith Hoffnung, 1996).

Furthermore, a teacher working with students with disabilities must keep in mind that "most disabling conditions have multiple dimensions.

There is no great compensatory 'supermechanism' that counterbalances disabilities with abilities; rather, disabilities cluster together in blatant disregard of providential fairness" (Valletutti, 1984, p. 5). An appreciation for this factor requires that teachers arrive at a comprehensive profile for each student that considers demonstrated abilities and the effect of multiple disabling conditions on student performance and instructional methodology. The critical role of other professionals, including physicians and other medically oriented professionals, in shaping program design must play a vital part in student evaluation and instructional programming whenever a medical condition is present. Effective instructional programming involves the establishment of individualized educational goals and objectives, facilitative instructional methods and materials, and appropriate assessment strategies. Programming decisions must always consider the consequences of a medical problem on all elements of instructional programming. The teacher as a competent evaluator–programmer must continually be alert to the possibility that a medical problem exists and, when appropriate, design his or her educational program, in part, based on medically related findings.

## The Teacher as a Referral Agent

The recognition that a student in one's class may have a medical problem is especially relevant to the teacher's diagnostic role as a referral agent. A teacher who suspects that a medical, sociological, or psychological problem exists often must be the one to initiate the referral process. He or she may be the only adult who is in a position to observe a child over a long period of time and who is objective and distanced enough emotionally to appreciate the need for referral. Furthermore, teachers often have to initiate the referral process even when the proposed services are not available directly within the school system or through the usual referral channels.

   Whenever a student fails to meet an educational goal or instructional objective despite quality instruction, teachers should be alert to the possibility that a medical condition may be among the possible reasons for this failure. Moreover, whenever teachers observe behaviors that appear to be significantly below the range of normal developmental expectations, they need to be concerned that a medical condition might be the cause. They must also wonder, if a medical problem does exist, whether existing medical procedures might improve the student's physical and mental health and at the same time facilitate learning. At this critical juncture, teachers can play a major role in the preventive-medicine process by helping students obtain various medical and allied health diagnostic and therapeutic procedures. This referral process differs from the referral process concerned with determining special education eligibility or placement. The process discussed here is similar to the prereferral intervention process that seeks to identify students who are at risk for school failure and does not necessarily lead to identification of the student as having a disability that requires special education and related services (Blackhurst & Berdine, 1993).

Teachers must understand that an untreated medical problem may affect learning and behavior and may also influence motivation for learning. A thorough understanding of normal and deviant development and the effects of a person's physiological state on learning and behavior is necessary. As the age of entry into school continues downward, the teacher's role in identifying behaviors that signal medical problems increases in importance and in difficulty. Teachers must be knowledgeable and skillful enough to differentiate behaviors that represent normal variations in development during this period of usually rapid growth from those behaviors that are symptomatic of an existing or emerging medical problem. As a case in point, teachers should attempt to determine whether a student's difficulty in fine or gross motor coordination is merely a benign developmental variation within normal limits or suggests a possible neurological or orthopedic disorder that requires the immediate attention of a physician.

The early diagnosis of medical problems is a valuable contribution to preventive medicine whenever it results in prompt treatment and management. This is true whether the treatment directly or indirectly affects learning or simply corrects the medical problem with no impact on the educational program. The prompt securing of medical care and rehabilitation is likely to prevent further deterioration and, perhaps, permanent damage to the involved organs or systems. Untreated medical problems such as ear infections can lead to permanent hearing loss, and untreated metabolic disease (such as phenylketonuria) and drug abuse can lead to irreversible brain damage with resulting mental retardation and possibly psychosis. Early correction of physical problems will likely minimize the effects of such conditions on learning. This is especially true when the problem affects vision and hearing. The longer the student is sensorially disabled, the more difficult it will be to remediate learning problems and facilitate new learning.

The teacher's role in diagnosis and management has also increased in complexity as more and more children with severe and profound disabilities are placed in classroom settings, especially in mainstreamed classes. A diagnostic awareness of possible medical problems assumes greater importance with this population because of the multiplicity of disabilities typically found in students with severe physical disabilities (Perat & Neville, 2001). Students with cerebral palsy may demonstrate multiple disabilities, including hearing loss, visual impairments, seizures, and mental retardation, in addition to the basic neuromuscular disorder (G. Miller & Clark, 1998; see also Chapter 14 in this text). Very often a student's physical status has direct implications for programming purposes. As a case in point, when a student with cerebral palsy has drooling and swallowing problems, speech–language–hearing pathologists, occupational therapists, teachers, and physicians must work collaboratively on a program designed to overcome or minimize the problems. Teachers must always be cognizant of those physical limitations that require task and curriculum modifications as well as collaborative treatment initiatives with other human service professionals and caregivers, whether or not they are members of the school staff (Dormans & Pelligrino, 1998; Friend & Cook, 2000; Hollingsworth, 2001; F. Miller & Bachrach, 1998; Mostert, 1996).

The teacher's role in the identification of medical problems not only includes referral to physicians but also involves assisting in the process of obtaining needed medically related health services such as occupational, physical, and speech–language–hearing therapy. These services sometimes may be obtained without an intervening referral to a physician. When a school employs specialized personnel, such as psychologists, therapists, social workers, and nurses, the referral process has usually been precisely established. Typically, these related service professionals request referrals from teachers and supply them with the appropriate referral forms.

On the other hand, when diagnostic or treatment services are required that are not provided within the school system, the referral process is usually more equivocal. To serve as effective referral agents to outside agencies and professionals, teachers must become familiar with the school's procedure for referring to outside parties. Frequently, however, structured procedures have not been fully developed and articulated, and decisions must be made and processes initiated on an ad hoc basis by the concerned teacher. The teacher then must decide whether to proceed through direct communication with parents or parent surrogates or through an intermediary such as the school principal, nurse, or pupil personnel worker.

At times, teachers may decide that parents should be approached directly. A direct approach is appropriate when it conforms to school policy, when a special rapport with parents exists, and when suggested examinations or consultations are unlikely to be viewed as a threat, interference, or invasion of privacy. Parents, however, may resist advice relevant to medical or medically related diagnosis and treatment. This reluctance may be due to financial worries, fear, guilt, or disinterest, or possibly to value systems, including religious proscriptions. Whenever parents fail to follow through on recommendations, teachers must seek alternate approaches and strategies. When parents heed suggestions, teachers should establish follow-up procedures through which they may be informed of any findings that necessitate modifications in classroom organization, instructional procedures, and behavior management. Teachers should also encourage parents to inform medical personnel that they, the teachers, are willing to incorporate therapeutic goals into their educational program, as long as these elements do not interfere with established instructional priorities for the student or for the class as a whole.

Whenever teachers refer a student for diagnosis and possible treatment, they should compile sufficient anecdotal and other data that support the referral. The best documentation is a written report in which pertinent behaviors of the referred student are described in sufficient detail and in behavioral terms. Included in this report should be the conditions under which the specified behaviors have occurred, the frequency and duration of these behaviors, and their consistency over time. Teachers in their referral process should avoid using ambiguous words, labeling the student, or interpreting the behavior.

On occasion, the referral process may require that referral be made to an outside agency rather than a specific individual practitioner. Teachers must be aware of those community agencies that provide medical and other health-related programs and treatment services. Familiarity with hospital-related programs and those offered by public and private agencies is necessary. Many general hospitals offer a variety of special clinics as part of their comprehensive medical programming. Some of the larger medical centers provide itinerant services. State, county, and city departments of health provide diagnostic and treatment services on a regular, and sometimes itinerant, basis so that all areas of the community, no matter how remote, may receive needed services. Mobile units in specially equipped vans often carry professional services to relatively inaccessible areas of a community to avoid the expense of duplicate costly diagnostic and treatment equipment. Private organizations, usually established by parent advocacy groups, provide diagnostic and treatment programs for individuals with special medical problems. Specialized hospitals, such as children's hospitals and university-affiliated facilities, also provide special diagnostic clinics and treatment facilities. Teachers, as effective referral agents, must know not only the medical services available in their community, but also the type of clients they serve, referral requirements, fee structures, nature of services provided, and approximate waiting time for appointments and treatment.

Whatever referral procedures are followed, teachers should ensure that the results of professional consultations are communicated back to them quickly and directly, except when it might be an invasion of the student's privacy. Teachers, in cooperation with other key professionals, must establish mechanisms through which they receive input and are able to provide future feedback to these professionals concerning the results of their therapeutic regimens on the student's learning and behavior.

The problem of selecting an appropriate professional for referral of a student with a suspected problem may be compounded by the ambiguity of some professional boundaries. To be effective referral agents, teachers must know the professional scope and limitations of such medical specialties as dermatology, endocrinology, internal medicine, neurology, ophthalmology, orthopedics, otolaryngology, pediatrics, and psychiatry. Also, educators should know the nature, scope, and limitations of such therapies as art, dance, music, occupational, physical, and speech–language–hearing. They also should be familiar with the goals, purposes, and functions of child life specialists, dentists, nurses, nutritionists, orthotists, prosthetists, psychologists, rehabilitation counselors, social workers, and therapeutic recreation specialists.

With increased awareness of behavioral clues that point to a possible medical problem, teachers are likely initially to overrefer students with hypothesized medical problems. Considering the devastating impact of undetected pathology, overreferral is preferable to underreferral. It is certainly better to refer too many students who, when formally assessed, are found to be functioning in the normal range, than to overlook a student who needs medical attention. With sufficient experience and training, most teachers improve in their ability to differentiate benign differences from those that require medical interventions.

## Special Programming and Management Needs

When preparing instructional materials, establishing curricular priorities, choosing methodological approaches, organizing the classroom's physical environment, and managing behavior, teachers must always take into consideration the special needs of students with medical problems. The classroom's physical environment or its prosthetic environment is a key element in ensuring the success of instruction and in facilitating appropriate behavior of students with medical problems and students in general. According to Meese (1994), "Clearly, the physical structure or arrangement of the classroom contributes to learning and classroom behavior.... Aspects of physical structure include: (a) teacher proximity and view, (b) separation of space, (c) traffic patterns, (d) extraneous stimuli, and (e) seating arrangements" (pp. 75–76). The type of lighting, window treatments, wall color, classroom size, and position of chalk and bulletin boards all contribute to or interfere with learning and behavior (Blackhurst & Cross, 1993; Woodward & Gersten, 1992).

Whenever a student has a medically related problem, teachers must determine whether special modifications should be made in the physical environment so that students obtain optimum benefits from their school experience. Teachers must examine the accessibility, safety, and specialized equipment features of the school. Among the provisions of the Americans with Disabilities Act of 1990 (ADA; P.L. 101-336) is the provision that all public accommodations, including schools, must be free from architectural barriers. Educators, therefore, must review existing schools as well as plans for new schools to make certain that they meet the accessibility guidelines of the ADA. Teachers must also go beyond and enhance the prescriptions of the law to make schools as safe, comfortable, and comforting as possible for students with physical problems. Among the questions to be asked pertinent to the design of schools are the following:

- Does the school have entrance and exit ramps?

- Does the school have elevators?

- Do the elevators have Braille numbering and sound signals?

- Do the corridors have walking rails?

- Are special railing bars installed at urinals and commodes, and are doorways wide enough for students in wheelchairs to enter cubicles?

- Is a pay telephone available at wheelchair level and for students with short stature?

- Are cushioned floors and padded helmets available for students with seizures and those with unsteady balance?

- Are standing tables and walkers available?

- Is there a place for a student to rest following a seizure or when a student has a migraine or tension headache?

• Do teachers stand so that the light illuminates their face, and do they speak in such a way that they are easy subjects to speech-read?

Appreciation for the programming and management needs of students with medical problems involves a strong knowledge base, special skills, and an empathic, supportive attitude. Superior teachers always inspire and challenge students to greater achievement. However, if the motivating force of success is fully understood, the power of positive thinking must be tempered by realistic expectations. Also, a supportive attitude must not be confused with being overly solicitous and failing to challenge the student to greater achievement within the context of his or her abilities. Infantilizing and overprotecting a student with medical problems and reinforcing dependency will invariably result in reduced achievement. Encouraging and challenging performance, when it is possible and does not cause undue stress in the student, is a critical component of an effective educational program.

Teachers also must consider the energy-depletion impact of the student's participation in diverse therapeutic and educational activities, as well as the possible impact of having to relate during the school day to many different adults with varying personalities, strategies, techniques, and goals. For example, a student with the athetoid form of cerebral palsy with an accompanying moderate to severe hearing loss is likely to require physical and occupational therapy, auditory training, speech reading, speech and language development, and training in the use of augmentative communication and special instruction in the care and use of a hearing aid. He or she may require a relaxed classroom atmosphere and low-intensity instruction to minimize the exacerbation of involuntary movements that characteristically increase when a student with this neurological disability attempts any physical action. Because of the concomitant hearing loss, he or she may require special seating arrangements and the use of special visual cues or signals for the management of behavior (Bauman-Wangler & Bauman-Wangler, 1999; Hull, 2000; Pappas, 1998).

Insufficient emphasis has been given to the stress placed on students when educational programming is inappropriately difficult, fails to consider fatigue factors, or fails to appreciate the pervasive pressures from having a disability. Whenever one is treating a child with a medical problem, attention must be directed to the effects of fatigue and its accompanying depression on the quality of a child's life. Abnormal fatigue is the loss of energy that is out of proportion to effort or tiredness that is not relieved by rest. Many medical conditions are associated with fatigue, including neoplasms, infections, and toxins, including poisoning from environmental agents such as lead. Pressure to read more fluently for a bright student with significant nystagmus, for example, or a lengthy term paper expected from a student with limited motor skills is likely to cause inordinate stress. Being concerned with teacher burnout and stress must not overshadow the arguably greater stress being experienced by the student with disabilities (Farber, 1991). Depressed students and students with anemia, anorexia, anxiety disorders, diabetes, kidney disease, and leukemia may manifest weakness and fatigue as an integral part of the pathology. Programming must consider the energy-depleting effects of classroom activities and other stress factors on these and other medical problems (Crewe & Clarke, 1996).

Teachers must be especially aware of the social and psychological problems that arise from looking and being different. The legendary cruelty of children to those who are clearly different must be dealt with in a direct and forceful manner. Appropriate units of instruction and sensitivity training are required if the barbs and taunts of peers are to be replaced by empathy, support, and companionship. Too many children with problems are lonely, depressed, and friendless (Asher & Gazelle, 1999; Margalit, 1994). Educators must program to prevent avoidance reactions in others and must assist students with disabilities in developing the social competencies required for successful interaction with their peers and adults.

# INVOLVEMENT WITH STUDENTS WITH MEDICAL PROBLEMS

## Students with Orthopedic and Neurological Impairments

Teachers must familiarize themselves with a wide range of assistive devices, including wheelchairs, canes, crutches, walkers, braces, artificial limbs, catheters, voice synthesizers, hearing aids, and a host of other specialized equipment often required by students with medical problems. "The growth of scientific technology, electronics, and computerized equipment has done much to assist the severely physically handicapped population. In the past few years, space age prosthetics, electronic sensory devices, specially equipped vans, and audiovisual equipment have been designed to augment the program needs to such students" (Smith, 1984, pp. 89–90).

Teachers with students who experience seizures must examine their own feelings about seizures and spend classroom time helping classmates understand and deal with their fears and feelings toward a classmate with a convulsive disorder. School systems need to adopt comprehensive health and safety education programs in which sensitivity to the needs of people with disabilities is included. Through participation in these programs, teachers will possess the skills needed to deal with a seizure before, during, and following its occurrence. With epilepsy, as with other chronic conditions, it is important to direct the attention of peers to the needs of the students with medical problems and to describe the condition simply and realistically so that the mystery, mythology, and stigma may be reduced and eventually eliminated (see Chapter 13).

Pain is an important factor in many medical conditions. It is the most frequent complaint encountered in medicine and is a common symptom of a mental disorder. In fact, psychogenic pain syndrome is the most common medical condition that teachers are likely to observe in their students. According to the American Psychiatric Association's (2000) *Diagnostic and Statistical Manual of Mental Disorders–Fourth Edition–Text Revision* (DSM–IV–TR), there are two types of pain disorders, those associated with psychological factors and those associated with both psychological factors and a medical condition in which psychological factors play a major role. Teachers must be knowledgeable about the existence of pain when the student is at rest, during movement, and after movement has occurred. Students with juvenile rheumatoid arthritis, cancer, sports injuries, hemophilia, and depressive disorders experience pain as part of these medical conditions. Teachers, therefore, must realize the debilitating effects of pain on concentration, attention, and motivation. They must consider these factors in educational programming and in the selection of suitable activities (Benz & Berkow, 1999; Hales & Yudofsky, 1999; Magni, 1987, 1991).

## Students with Chronic Health Problems

When working with students with chronic health problems, teachers must provide a school program that takes into consideration reduced energy, strength, and motivation, as well as various personality elements. Teachers have to be sensitive to changes during the progression of illness, and especially responsive to crises and exacerbations. When a student with a chronic health problem has a terminal illness, teachers must examine and resolve their own feelings and attitudes and deal with both the student's and his or her classmates' fears and concerns about death and dying.

## The Hospitalized Child

Whenever students are hospitalized as part of the treatment regimen, teachers must consider the tremendous stress that results from the child's separation from home and family. Also to be considered is the stress engendered by the hospital environment with its different personnel, strange and frightening equipment, and unusual procedures. Curriculum experiences need to be directed toward helping students understand the nature of medical settings, personnel, and equipment. It may also be necessary to assist students to understand their medical condition, the nature of their specific medical interventions, and the role of the interventions in the management of the condition. Discussions should be scheduled that help the hospitalized child deal with the ignorance, fear, and anxiety of others, as well as with his or her own fear, anger, and need for positive attention.

## Students with Attention-Deficit/Hyperactivity Disorder

Teachers need to be cognizant of the effects of medical intervention strategies on learning and behavior. Of special interest to teachers is the ubiquitous use of drug therapy to control the behavior of students who have been diagnosed as having attention deficits or hyperactivity. Advocates of drug therapy believe that abnormal levels of body chemicals cause problems and that drug therapy brings the chemical levels into balance. A number of concerns are related to the use of drug therapy with children with attention-deficit/hyperactivity disorder:

- The paucity of studies that show a positive effect on learning

- The lack of consensus that there is a reduction in inappropriate behavior

- The danger of adverse physiological side effects

- The neglect of alternative and more humanistic behavior management strategies

- The perils of adverse psychological side effects
- The absence of legitimate student-oriented goals (i.e., the underlying purpose is for the teacher's convenience)

Many adverse side effects and toxicity occur when dosages of prescribed medications are inappropriate to the person's age, size, and physical status. Interaction effects of medications must also be considered by physicians and by caregivers, including teachers, to avoid serious synergistic problems (Benz & Berkow, 1999; "Health and Fitness," 2001). Teachers need to know the nature of specific illnesses and be aware of the medications their students are taking in order to be alert to the presence of adverse side effects and toxicity.

Teachers face a number of professional problems when they are expected to aid in dispensing medication to students (see also Chapter 15). Teachers must consider unresolved legal, professional, and ethical ramifications before agreeing to participate in such a program. Schools need to establish written policies relevant to the administration of prescribed medications of any kind as well as to the overall relationship between medical treatment and instructional programs. Specific policies are needed not only for legal reasons, but also to provide a framework for improving teacher feedback. Releases to administer drugs should include data on expected changes in behavior, possible adverse side effects, symptoms of toxic reactions or inadequate dosage, and dates of therapy initiation and review (Stevens & Crook, 2001).

Caution is especially pertinent when dealing with students who have been classified as having attention-deficit/hyperactivity disorder (ADHD) and are receiving stimulants. Because hyperactivity is a subjective phenomenon, teachers may be in diagnostic disagreement with parents, other teachers, and physicians. Some teachers may view the behavior of a student as being within normal limits, whereas others view the same child as having a disability. The use of drugs as a management strategy may conflict with a teacher's approach to behavior modification. If a student is on a drug regimen, does this prevent a teacher from teaching the student how to develop and exercise emotional controls? Does this interference by a medical intervention strategy unfairly disrupt a teacher's professional responsibilities? Does the use of medication reduce student activity, and thus inhibit learning? The answers to these questions are further confounded by the fact that megavitamin therapy, herbal remedies, and special diets continue to be proposed and aggressively marketed as alternate treatment procedures for a variety of medical conditions, including ADHD (Barkley, 1998; Zentall, 1993).

When students are placed on special diets because of ADHD, endocrine problems (such as diabetes mellitus), convulsive disorders (ketogenic diet), or allergies (including allergic reactions to peanuts), it is essential that teachers assist these students in meeting the constraints imposed by their special diets and be prepared to use injectable epinephrine in case of a life-threatening allergic reaction. In the typical classroom, this may be a difficult task in that serving junk food for snacks and at class parties is often a school tradition. Also, parents are not always consistent in sending a properly prescribed lunch.

# COMMUNICATING WITH PHYSICIANS AND OTHER HEALTH PROFESSIONALS

Teachers who for many years have been exhorted to teach the whole child must retain this holistic emphasis as they share "parts" of students who have medical problems with other professionals. Teachers, already confused by medical jargon and the specialized vocabulary of medically oriented professionals, are further bewildered when physicians and other health professionals disagree and when largely unsubstantiated treatments are precipitously accepted by naive educators willing to jump on and off traditional and burgeoning nontraditional medically influenced treatment bandwagons. Teachers who have students with medical problems in their classroom are often faced with a variety of alternate medical approaches, many of which rely on the gullibility and magical thinking of parents and teachers. This is especially true when the medical approaches have a direct impact on instructional practices and classroom management. Teachers with a history of teaching students with special needs have been expected in the past to teach these students, among other things, to crawl in order to recapitulate ontogeny, to help establish left-hemisphere dominance, and to use the largely discredited facilitative communication to reach autistic children (Valletutti, Bender, & Smith Hoffnung, 1996). Parents have asked teachers whether they should subject their child to visual training exercises recommended by their optometrist as an aid to correcting visual problems. Other parents seek the advice of teachers relative to the rapid proliferation of herbal and nontraditional panaceas that flood the market. Teachers are often nonplussed when faced with such alien and esoteric questions and marketing propaganda.

Teachers are not adequately prepared by most schools of education to share "parts" of the whole child with others. Educators must help in clarifying the role that they must play when working with a student who requires related services. For example, oral language is the medium of interchange through which most classroom interactions occur. Oral language development underlies the teaching of reading, writing, arithmetic, and all other subject areas (Merritt & Culatta, 1998; Valletutti, Bender, & Smith Hoffnung, 1996). Educators need to clarify what is the teacher's responsibility, as the supreme generalist, for oral language development and what is the role of the speech–language–hearing pathologist. Furthermore, most teachers accept the responsibility for leisure-time education. Therefore, clarification of their role vis-à-vis the roles of occupational, physical, and recreational therapists is necessary (Auxter, Pyfer, & Huettig, 1997). Occupational therapists are concerned with these functional activities. They must include educational objectives, when needed by students with medical problems, to develop fine motor facility and coordination as well as the use of arms and hands in eating, dressing, grooming, and written communication. A physical therapist is concerned about the mobility training of students with physical disabilities, and so is the teacher of those students. Mobility is not only a physical skill, but also a combination of skills involving the cognition of space, time, and direction.

Teachers frequently are viewed by other human service professionals as carryover agents. This added responsibility might not only tax a teacher's emotional reserve but also deplete the time available to teach skills within his or her own previously established educational priorities. Other human service professionals are not always as receptive as teachers when asked to be carryover agents for educational priorities. Collaboration is replete with obstacles. How does a professional view his or her status in the professional hierarchy relative to that of a teacher? How do the specialists (i.e., the physician and the therapists) view the generalist (i.e., the teacher)? How do the personality and temperament of each member of an interdisciplinary team affect his or her perception of the other responsibilities of the team? Perception of status and personality factors can create a dysfunctional team. Of equal importance is the question of how teachers view their status in the professional hierarchy when they are part of a team that addresses the needs of students with medical problems. To teach students with physiological problems as successfully as possible, teachers must believe that they are equal members of a team with a distinct body of knowledge and skills of coequal value to the physicians and the other human service professionals (Mostert, 1996).

# SUMMARY

The teacher plays a critical role in the identification and management of students with medical problems. This chapter has clarified the three separate areas of professional responsibility involved in diagnostic–prescriptive teaching:

- Educational evaluation for programming purposes and for developing strategies for classroom organization and behavioral management

- A diagnostic awareness of the possibility that a medical problem exists for referral purposes

- An appreciation for the special methods and materials of instruction and management for students with medical problems

Physicians and teachers, in fulfilling their professional responsibilities, must empathize with and examine fully those pertinent and unique factors in the life of their clients and their families that determine requisite treatment practices. Teachers and all other human service professionals working with a child with medical problems must enter the skin of the child and his or her parents. In individual practice and in collaborative efforts, this professional privilege and special empathy must always shape and direct professional practice.

# REFERENCES

American Psychiatric Association. (2000). *Diagnostic and statistical manual of mental disorders–fourth edition–text revision.* Washington, DC: American Psychiatric Association.

Americans with Disabilities Act of 1990, 42 U.S.C. § 12101 *et seq.*

Asher, S. R., & Gazelle, H. (1999). Loneliness, peer relations, and language disorders in childhood. *Topics in Language Disorders, 19,* 16–33.

Auxter, D., Pyfer, J., & Huettig, C. (1997). *Principles and methods of adapted physical education and recreation*. Dubuque, IA: Brown & Benchmark.

Barkley, R. A. (1998). *Attention deficit hyperactivity disorder: A handbook for diagnosis and treatment* (2nd ed.). New York: Guilford Press.

Bauman-Wangler, J. A., & Bauman-Wangler, J. (1999). *Articulatory and phonological impairments: A clinical focus*. Boston: Allyn & Bacon.

Bender, M., Valletutti, P. J., & Baglin, C. A. (1996a). *A functional curriculum for teaching students with disabilities: Self-care, motor skills, and household management and living skills*. Austin, TX: PRO-ED.

Bender, M., Valletutti, P. J., & Baglin, C. A. (1996b). *A functional curriculum for teaching students with disabilities: Interpersonal, competitive job-finding, and leisure time skills*. Austin, TX: PRO-ED.

Benz, M. H., & Berkow, R. (Eds.). (1999). *The Merck manual of diagnosis and treatment* (17th ed.). Whitehouse, NJ: Merck Research Laboratory.

Bishop, V. E. (1996). *Teaching visually impaired children* (2nd ed.). Springfield, IL: Charles C. Thomas.

Blackhurst, A. E., & Berdine, W. H. (1993). Issues in special education. In A. E. Blackhurst & W. H. Blackhurst (Eds.), *An introduction to special education* (3rd ed., pp. 37–75). New York: HarperCollins.

Blackhurst, A. E., & Cross, D. P. (1993). Technology in special education. In A. E. Blackhurst & W. H. Berdine (Eds.), *An introduction to special education* (3rd ed., pp. 77–103). New York: HarperCollins.

Cox, P. R., & Dykes, M. K. (2001). Effective classroom adaptations for students with visual impairments. *Teaching Exceptional Children, 33,* 68–74.

Crewe, N., & Clarke, N. (1996). Stress and women with disabilities. In D. Krotoski & M. Turk (Eds.), *Women with physical disabilities* (pp. 193–202). Baltimore: Brookes.

Dormans, J. P., & Pelligrino, L. (Eds.). (1998). *Caring for children with cerebral palsy: A team based approach*. Baltimore: Brookes.

Education for All Handicapped Children Act of 1975, 20 U.S.C. § 1400 *et seq.*

Etting, C. J., Johnson, R. C., Smith, D. L., & Snider, B. N. (1994). *The deaf way: Perspectives from the International Conference on Deaf Culture*. Washington, DC: Gallaudet University Press.

Farber, B. A. (1991). *Crisis in education: Stress and burnout in the American teacher*. San Francisco: Jossey-Bass.

Friend, M., & Cook, L. (2000). *Interactions: Collaboration skills for school professionals*. New York: Longman.

Hales, R., & Yudofsky, S. C. (Eds.). (1999). *Synopsis of psychiatry*. Washington, DC: American Psychiatric Press.

Hardman, M. L., Drew, C. J., & Egan, M. W. (1996). *Human exceptionality, society, school, and family*. Boston: Allyn & Bacon.

Health and fitness. (2001, August 14). *The New York Times,* p. F10.

Heward, W. L. (2000). *Exceptional children: An introduction to special education*. Upper Saddle River, NJ: Prentice Hall.

Hill, E. W., & Snook-Hill, M. (1996). Orientation and mobility. In M. C. Hollbrook (Ed.), *Children with visual impairments: A parent's guide* (pp. 260–286). Bethesda, MD: Woodbine House.

Hollingsworth, H. L. (2001). We need to talk: Communication strategies for effective collaboration. *Teaching Exceptional Children, 33,* 4–8.

Hull, R. H. (Ed.). (2000). *Aural rehabilitation: Serving children and adults* (4th ed.). San Diego, CA: Singular.

Individuals with Disabilities Education Act Amendments of 1997, 20 U.S.C. § 1400 *eq seq.*

Kame'enui, E., & Carnine, D. (1998). *Effective teaching strategies that accommodate diverse learners.* Upper Saddle River, NJ: Prentice Hall.

Katsiyannis, A., Ellenburg, J. S., Acton, O. M., & Torrey, G. (2001). Addressing the needs of students with Rett syndrome. *Teaching Exceptional Children, 33,* 74–78.

Kirk, S. A., Gallagher, J. J., & Anastasiow, N. J. (1993). *Educating exceptional children.* Boston: Houghton Mifflin.

Koenig, A. J. (1996). Growing into literacy. In M. C. Holbrook (Ed.), *Children with visual impairments: A parent's guide* (pp. 227–257). Bethesda, MD: Woodbine House.

Magni, G. (1987). On the relationship between chronic pain and depression where there is no organic lesion. *Pain, 31,* 1–21.

Magni, G. (1991). The use of antidepressants in the treatment of chronic pain. *Drugs, 42,* 730–748.

Margalit, M. (1994). *Loneliness among children with special needs: Theory, research, coping, and intervention.* New York: Springer-Verlag.

McLoughlin, J. A. (1993). Families of exceptional children. In A. E. Blackhurst & W. H. Berdine (Eds.), *An introduction to special education* (3rd ed., pp. 177–217). New York: HarperCollins.

Meese, R. L. (1994). *Teaching learners with mild disabilities: Integrating research and practice.* Pacific Grove, CA: Brooks/Cole.

Merritt, D., & Culatta, B. (1998). *Language intervention in the classroom.* San Diego, CA: Singular.

Miller, F., & Bachrach, S. J. (1998). *Cerebral palsy: A complete guide for caregivers.* Baltimore: Johns Hopkins University Press.

Miller, G., & Clark, G. D. (Eds.). (1998). *The cerebral palsies: Causes, consequences, and management.* Woburn, MA: Butterworth-Heinemann.

Mostert, M. P. (1996). Interpersonal collaboration in schools: Benefits and barriers in practice. *Preventing School Failure, 40,* 135–138.

Mueller, P. H., & Murphy, F. V. (2001). Determining when a student requires paraeducator support. *Teaching Exceptional Children, 33,* 22–27.

Pappas, D. G. (1998). *Diagnosis and treatment of hearing impairment in children.* San Diego, CA: Singular.

Perat, M. V., & Neville, B. G. R. (Eds.). (2001). *Cerebral palsy.* New York: Elseviers Science.

Polloway, E. W., Patton, J. R., Payne, J. S., & Payne, R. A. (1989). *Strategies for learners with special needs* (4th ed.). Columbus, OH: Merrill.

Seligman, M. (2000). *Conducting effective conferences with parents of children with disabilities.* New York: Guilford Press.

Smith, O. S. (1984). Severely and profoundly physically handicapped students. In P. J. Valletutti & B. Sims-Tucker (Eds.), *Severely and profoundly handicapped students: Their nature and needs* (pp. 85–152). Baltimore: Brookes.

Stevens, L. J., & Crook, W. G. (2001). *12 effective ways to help your ADD/ADHD child: Drug-free alternatives for attention deficit disorder.* Putnam, NY: Avery Penguin Putnam.

Thompson, S. J., Quenemoen, M. L., Thurlow, J., & Ysseldyke, E. (2001). *Alternate assessments for students with disabilities.* Arlington, VA: CEC and Corwin Press.

Turnbull, P., Turnbull, R., Shank, M., & Leal, D. (2002). *Exceptional lives: Special education in today's schools* (3rd ed.). Upper Saddle River, NJ: Merrill.

Valletutti, P. J. (1984). Introduction and overview. In P. J. Valletutti & B. Sims-Tucker (Eds.), *Severely and profoundly handicapped students: Their nature and needs* (pp. 1–10). Baltimore: Brookes.

Valletutti, P. J., Bender, M., & Sims-Tucker, B. (1996). *A functional curriculum for teaching students with disabilities: Functional academics.* Austin, TX: PRO-ED.

Valletutti, P. J., Bender, M., & Smith Hoffnung, A. (1996). *A functional curriculum for teaching students with disabilities: Nonverbal and oral communication skills.* Austin, TX: PRO-ED.

Vaughan, S., Bos, C., & Schum, J. (2000). *Teaching exceptional, diverse, and at-risk students in the general education classroom.* Boston: Allyn & Bacon.

Venn, J. (1994). *Assessment of students with special needs.* New York: Merrill/Macmillan.

Walsh, J. M. (2001). Getting the big picture of IEP goals and state standards. *Teaching Exceptional Children, 33,* 18–26.

Woodward, J., & Gersten, R. (1992). Innovative technology for secondary students with learning disabilities. *Exceptional Children, 59,* 407–421.

Ysseldyke, J. E., Algozzine, B., & Thurlow, M. L. (1992). *Critical issues in special education* (2nd ed.). Boston: Houghton Mifflin.

Zentall, S. S. (1993). Research on the educational implications of attention deficit hyperactivity disorder. *Exceptional Children, 60,* 143–153.

# CHAPTER 2

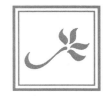

# Prevention of Chronic Disabilities and Diseases

Robert H. A. Haslam

**P**revention is generally defined as "keeping from happening by precautionary measures" or "acting ahead." Through the medium of education, the teacher is well placed to assist in the prevention of disabilities that may have their onset during early childhood or adolescence. Prevention of disabilities is an ongoing process that may be implemented at various stages of growth and development. Primary prevention implies that the condition producing the disability can be eliminated, thereby reducing its occurrence in the population. Secondary prevention is directed toward early identification of a problem that results in a disability so that, with suitable intervention, the disability may be ameliorated or lessened. Tertiary prevention attempts to reduce the severity of the disability through the use of specific medical, educational, and behavioral techniques.

Unfortunately, what is known about prevention is not always attended to by the physician, educator, and parent. Furthermore, the medical profession traditionally has deemphasized the concept of prevention and concentrated on the diagnosis, management, and follow-up of acute illnesses in children and adults. The overriding challenge to the health educator is not the discovery of new prevention methods or techniques, but the application of current knowledge to the population at risk (Haslam, 1983). This chapter is a summary of some conditions that can be prevented if suitable measures are adopted before conception, during embryonic and fetal development, at the time of birth and the neonatal period, or during the growth and development of the infant, child, and adolescent.

# IMMUNIZATION

Immunization of infants and children, an example of primary prevention, is a highly effective method of preventing life-threatening illnesses or severe disabling conditions. For example, only a few decades ago poliomyelitis claimed the lives of countless children. For those who survived, significant motor disabilities were common. Since the advent of the polio vaccine, this dreaded disease has been eliminated in the Western Hemisphere. The immunization schedule for normal infants, children, and adolescents as recommended by the American Academy of Pediatrics (2003) is shown in Figure 2.1. Unfortunately, not all children receive this protection because some parents and health care providers have become complacent in the administration of recommended immunization practices.

Until recently, *Haemophilus influenzae* type b (Hib) was the most common cause of bacterial meningitis in infants and children between 3 months and 3 years of age, causing death in about 5% of cases. Significant lifelong sequelae, including deafness, epilepsy, mental retardation, hydrocephalus, learning disorders, and behavioral problems, occur in approximately 20% of survivors. Hib is also a common cause of pneumonia, acute epiglottitis, septic arthritis, cellulitis, and bacteremia (presence of bacteria in the blood). Hib meningitis is more likely to occur in children attending day care. Prior to the introduction of Hib conjugate vaccination in the United States, there were approximately 15,000 cases of Hib meningitis annually. Since the introduction of Hib conjugate vaccines in 1988, the incidence of invasive disease caused by Hib has declined by 99% (Centers for Disease Control and Prevention [CDC], 1999). Invasive disease presently occurs primarily in underimmunized children and among infants too young to have completed the primary immunization series. Because of the success of Hib immunization, the U.S. Public Health Service has targeted Hib disease for elimination in children younger than 5 years of age (Booy, Moxon, MacFarlane, Mayon-White, & Slack, 1992; Eskola, Takala, Kaynty, Peltola, & Makelä, 1991).

The hepatitis B virus (HBV) can be mild with few symptoms, or it can result in hepatitis with jaundice and, in some cases, lead to sudden death. Chronic HBV infection, with persistence of the hepatitis B antigen, can produce chronic liver disease or cancer of the liver. Transmission of the virus from an infected mother to the infant may occur during the perinatal period; without intervention, as many as 80% to 90% of these children will become chronically infected. Furthermore, chronically infected infants

## Recommended Childhood and Adolescent Immunization Schedule—United States, 2003

| Vaccine | Birth | 1 mo | 2 mos | 4 mos | 6 mos | 12 mos | 15 mos | 18 mos | 24 mos | 4–6 yrs | 11–12 yrs | 13–18 yrs |
|---|---|---|---|---|---|---|---|---|---|---|---|---|
| Hepatitis B | | HepB #1[a] | HepB #2 | | | HepB #3 | | | | | HepB series | |
| Diphtheria, Tetanus, Pertussis | | | DTaP | DTaP | DTaP | | DTaP | DTaP | | DTaP | Td[b] | |
| Haemophilus influenzae type b | | | Hib | Hib | Hib | Hib | | | | | | |
| Polio | | | IPV | IPV | | IPV | | | | IPV | | |
| Measles, Mumps, Rubella | | | | | | MMR #1 | | | | MMR #2 | MMR #2 | MMR #2 |
| Varicella | | | | | | Varicella | | | | Varicella | | |
| Pneumococcal | | | PCV | PCV | PCV | PCV | PCV | | PCV | | | |
| Hepatitis A | | | | | | | | | | HepA series | | |
| Influenza | | | | | | | Influenza (yearly) | | | | | |

Vaccines below this line are for selected populations

☐ = range of recommended ages for immunization.
▨ = vaccines to be given if previously recommended doses were missed or given earlier than the recommended minimum.

**FIGURE 2.1.** Recommended childhood and adolescent immunization schedule—United States, 2003. *Note.* [a] Only if mother is HBsAg–negative. [b] Tetanus and dihtheria toxoids. From "Recommended Childhood and Adolescent Immunization Schedule—United States, 2003," by Advisory Committee on Immunization Practices, American Academy of Pediatrics, and American Academy of Family Physicians, 2003 (January), *AAP News*, p. 22. Additional information is available on the American Academy of Pediatrics Web site: http://www.aap.org

are at greater risk of dying from liver disease than infected adults. To reduce transmission of HBV, hepatitis B vaccination is recommended as a component of the immunization schedule for children.

Another example of a severe disabling disorder that results from incomplete immunization is the rubella syndrome (congenital rubella). The rubella syndrome results from the transfer of the rubella (German measles) virus from the mother to the fetus across the placenta. Although rubella is a mild illness in the child or adult, it may be devastating to the fetus, particularly if the pregnant mother develops rubella during the first trimester. The clinical features of congenital rubella include low birth weight, congenital heart disease, cataracts, bleeding into the skin, and liver disease in the newborn period, as well as microcephaly, mental retardation, and sensorineural hearing loss.

Although there has been a marked reduction in the incidence of German measles since the introduction of the rubella vaccine in 1969, the rubella syndrome still occurs because of poor vaccination practices in susceptible women of childbearing age. Rubella is difficult to diagnose and often is confused with other viral illnesses. Thus, a woman of childbearing age who is not certain of her rubella status should have her blood titers determined before she becomes pregnant. If the titers are low, she should be immunized with rubella vaccine prior to conception. Rubella control has been most successful in those states that have a comprehensive vaccination program aimed at the postpubertal female. Eventual elimination of rubella, however, will be achieved only when all children are immunized during infancy.

The varicella (chicken pox) vaccine was introduced in the United States in 1995 and is recommended for use in healthy children 12 months of age or older who have not had varicella. In the past, varicella was regarded as a benign infection, and parents often held "chicken pox parties" so that their child could contact the infection and "get it out of the way." However, varicella is associated with many potentially life-threatening conditions, including serious skin infections, pneumonia, glomerulonephritis, and neurological complications including strokes and spinal cord and nerve inflammation (Guillain-Barré syndrome). The side effects from varicella immunization are minimal and the benefit is significant (see also Chapter 3).

Beginning in the early 1970s and especially during the past decade, there has been a significant increase in immunization rates in children (see Table 2.1). Childhood vaccination has prevented millions of illnesses and tens of thousands of deaths (CDC, 1999). National coverage with routinely recommended childhood vaccines increased substantially after the

**TABLE 2.1**

Vaccination Levels of U.S. Children Ages 19 to 35 Months,
by Selected Vaccines, in 1992 and 2000

| Vaccine | Percentage Vaccinated | | Vaccine | Percentage Vaccinated | |
|---|---|---|---|---|---|
| | 1992[a] | 2000[b] | | 1992[a] | 2000[b] |
| DTaP3 | 83.0 | 94.1 | Hib3 | 28.2 | 93.4 |
| DTaP4 | 59.0 | 81.7 | 1MMR | 82.5 | 90.5 |
| OPV3 | 72.4 | 89.5 | HepB3 | — | 90.3 |

DTaP3 or DTaP4 = diphtheria, tetanus toxoids and acellular pertussis, 3 or 4 doses; OPV3 = orally administered polio vaccine, 3 doses; Hib3 = Haemophilus influenzae Type b, 3 doses; 1MMR = measles–mumps–rubella vaccine, 1 dose; HepB3 = hepatitis Type b, 3 doses.

[a] Data from "Vaccination Coverage of 2-Year-Old Children: United States, 1992–1993," 1994, *Morbidity and Mortality Weekly Report, 43,* pp. 282–283.

[b] Data from "National, State, and Urban Area Vaccination Coverage Levels Among Children Aged 19–35 Months—United States, 2000," 2001, *Morbidity and Mortality Weekly Report, 50*(30), p. 638.

Childhood Immunization Initiative was implemented in 1993 (CDC, 1994). For these health benefits to continue, high levels of vaccination coverage must be attained for each new birth cohort and must be monitored to ensure protection from disease, to characterize unvaccinated populations, and to evaluate efforts to increase coverage.

# DISABILITIES RESULTING FROM DRUGS

It is well known that certain drugs consumed during pregnancy may have an adverse effect on the fetus, resulting in significant disabilities. For example, heavy cigarette smoking is associated with prematurity (Rush, 1974). The premature infant is at much greater risk for cerebral palsy, mental retardation, learning disorders, and related conditions because of an immature central nervous system. In the early 1960s, the teratogenic drug thalidomide was given to many pregnant women as a sleeping pill, particularly in Europe. Thalidomide subsequently was found to produce serious defects in the formation of the musculoskeletal system, especially the arms, if taken during the first 20 to 35 days of pregnancy, when many mothers are unaware that they are pregnant. Another important example of a drug producing a teratogenic effect on the developing embryo is alcohol, which can cause the fetal alcohol syndrome.

## Fetal Alcohol Syndrome

Fetal alcohol syndrome (FAS) is a common disorder that is estimated to occur at the rate of 5.2 per 10,000 live births in the United States, making it one of the most common causes of identifiable mental retardation (CDC, 1997). FAS is characterized by prenatal and postnatal growth retardation; congenital heart disease; skeletal anomalies; genital abnormalities in the male; facial malformation, particularly a thin upper lip, poorly developed philtrum (groove from tip of nose to upper lip), short nose, and ptosis (droopy eyelids); mental retardation; feeding difficulties; and microcephaly (see Figure 2.2). The severity of FAS seems to be directly related to the duration, quantity, and frequency of alcohol consumption by the pregnant mother (Smith, Jones, & Hanson, 1976). There does not seem to be a safe level of alcohol consumption during pregnancy. Mills, Granbard, Harley, Rhoads, and Berendes (1984) showed that consumption of one or more drinks was associated with an increased risk of growth retardation in the newborn infant. It is not known how alcohol damages the fetus, but there is some evidence that the drug causes constriction of the placental vessels, producing a significant reduction in blood flow and hence reduced levels of oxygen and nutrients to the fetus.

Some children born to women who consumed alcohol during pregnancy do not have congenital anomalies or growth retardation but display hyperactivity, attention-deficit disorder, learning problems, speech disorders, abnormalities of motor coordination, and behavioral disturbances. These symptoms have been termed *fetal alcohol effects* (FAE) and have an estimated incidence of 1 per 300 live births (Olegard et al., 1979).

In 1996, the Institute of Medicine published a report that clarified the terminology for conditions in which there is a history of maternal alcohol exposure (substantial regular intake or heavy episodic drinking), proposing the terms *alcohol-related neurodevelopmental disorder* (ARND) and *alcohol-related birth defects* (ARBD) (Stratton, Howe, & Battaglia, 1996). These terms provide a pathophysiologic basis to describe the facial anomalies, growth retardation, central nervous system abnormalities, cognitive deficits, and birth

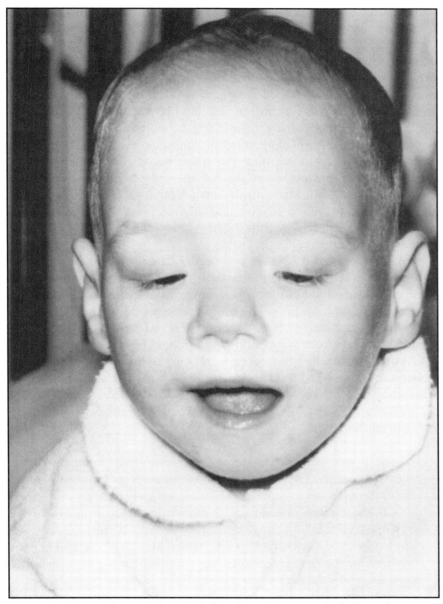

**FIGURE 2.2.** An infant with fetal alcohol syndrome born to an alcoholic mother. Note the droopy eyelids (ptosis) and small mouth and jaw. The ptosis was subsequently corrected by plastic surgery. Feeding problems were prominent during the first year of life, necessitating prolonged hospitalizations. The child's developmental milestones have been delayed.

defects that result from confirmed maternal exposure to alcohol and allow for a more precise definition and classification of alcohol-related neurodevelopmental disorders that were previously placed under the rubric of FAE.

Unfortunately, the manifestations of FAS, ARND, and ARBD persist into the adult years and remain lifelong disabilities. Aside from behavioral problems and conduct disorders (e.g., lying, stealing, oppositional behaviors), these individuals continue to manifest hyperactivity and impulsivity. Memory deficits, poor abstract reasoning, subnormal cognitive functioning, and difficulty with mathematical computation, especially difficulty with abstraction, including time and space, become particularly evident during adulthood. Most never achieve age-appropriate socialization or communication skills. Many display maladaptive social functioning with social withdrawal, mood lability, and anxiety, typically associated with mental health disorders, chemical dependency, and inappropriate sexual behavior (Streissguth et al., 1991).

FAS, ARND, and ARBD are preventable causes of mental retardation and associated cognitive disabilities. Early diagnosis is important to reduce the secondary disabilities mentioned above (Streissguth & Kanter, 1997). The economic costs for providing comprehensive care for individuals with FAS, ARND, and ARBD are staggering. Annual cost estimates for the United States vary from $75 million to $9.7 billion (Hanwood & Napolitano, 1985), and the total lifetime cost for caring for an individual with FAS has been estimated to be $1.4 million (Streissguth et al., 1991). Clearly, greater effort must be placed on the prevention of FAS and related conditions. The following recommendations have been proposed by the American Academy of Pediatrics (2000):

1. Because there is no known safe amount of alcohol consumption during pregnancy, The Academy recommends abstinence from alcohol for women who are pregnant or who are planning a pregnancy.

2. Major efforts should be made at all levels of society to develop high-quality educational programs about the deleterious consequences of alcohol for the unborn child. This information should be integrated into a comprehensive drug prevention education curriculum for all elementary, junior high, and high school students. It also should be a part of similar education efforts in all postsecondary and adult centers of learning.

3. Pediatricians and other health care professionals who provide care for women and their newborns should increase their own awareness and that of their patients about FAS, ARND, and ARBD and their prevention. Pediatricians should increase their awareness of the prevalence

of alcohol use by pregnant women in their communities and advocate for programs that identify the users and offer them treatment. When a child with problems related to maternal alcohol consumption is identified, alcohol treatment and prevention resources should be offered to the family and affected child.

4. Infants and children with a suspected diagnosis of FAS, ARND, or ARBD should be evaluated by a pediatrician who is knowledgeable and competent in the evaluation of neurodevelopmental and psychosocial problems associated with the diagnoses. The need for a skilled evaluation at an early age necessitates referral to a pediatric medical specialist as well as referral to early intervention and education agencies providing services under the provisions of the Individuals With Disabilities Education Act.

5. Parents of children given a diagnosis of FAS, ARBD, or ARND should receive appropriate support services for themselves and their child, including careful anticipatory guidance directed toward preventing similar problems in the future.

6. The Academy supports federal legislation that would require the inclusion of health and safety measures in all print and broadcast alcohol advertisements based on the U.S. Surgeon General's warning: "Drinking during pregnancy may cause mental retardation and other birth defects. Avoid alcohol during pregnancy."

7. The Academy supports the development of state legislation that makes information about FAS, ARND, and ARBD available at marriage-licensing bureaus and other appropriate public places, including points of alcohol sale.

8. Pediatricians are encouraged to assume a leadership role in public education campaigns aimed at decreasing the incidence of FAS through reduction in alcohol use by pregnant women. (American Academy of Pediatrics, 2000, p. 358)

## Cocaine

Although the use of cocaine has declined in recent years, it remains one of the most common illicit drugs, especially during pregnancy. Debate continues as to the consequences of cocaine exposure during pregnancy, but recent studies consistently show that "heavy" maternal cocaine use can cause significant long-lasting neurobehavioral changes (heavy use is defined by the concentration of cocaine in the fetal hair and meconium). It has been difficult to determine the precise deleterious effect of cocaine on the developing fetus and newborn as most users also smoke cigarettes, use other drugs including alcohol, have poor nutrition, and attend antenatal clinics irregularly, all of which are known risk factors for an abnormal infant. Furthermore, the determination of the amount and duration of cocaine use during pregnancy has been inaccurate. Interviews with the mother are generally unreliable, and measurement of the newborn's urine only provides information on the quantity of cocaine consumed for a short period prior to delivery. The most accurate indicator of measuring maternal use of cocaine during the third trimester utilizes a technique that determines the concentration of cocaine from a sample of the infant's hair at the time of birth. Combined with measurement of the concentration of cocaine in the infant's meconium and direct questioning of the mother as to her cocaine and additional drug consumption, reasonably accurate data concerning the amount of cocaine exposure to the fetus can be determined (Graham, Koren, Klein, Schneiderman, & Greenwald, 1989).

Cocaine is a prominent cause of intrauterine growth retardation, prematurity, and microcephaly, possibly due to vasoconstriction of the placental blood vessels, which causes decreased fetal perfusion and hypoxemia, as well as the drug's effect on neural circuitry, especially the monoaminergic systems. There is also mounting evidence that cocaine causes abnormalities of neuronal migration that lead to structural abnormalities of the brain, including absence of the corpus callosum. Animal studies have shown that cocaine adversely affects the central nervous system neurotransmitter function in that changes in the dopaminergic and serotoninergic pathways in the developing rat brain are induced by cocaine (Frick & Dow-Edwards, 1995). Alteration of fetal neurotransmitters may decrease the speed of processing of auditory information, which can directly impact language development. Cocaine also may alter arousal and memory mechanisms that directly influence language and cognitive skills. In addition, fetal exposure to cocaine results in brain infarction and hemorrhages. Ultrasound studies of newborns whose mothers were classified as heavy users of cocaine showed vascular injuries of the central nervous system (subependymal hemorrhage in the caudothalamic groove), particularly in the basal ganglia and brain stem, that potentially can result in cognitive and behavioral abnormalities (Frank et al., 1999).

Occasionally, a newborn infant exposed to maternal cocaine use develops significant irritability, altered sleep–awake states, poor feeding, and in some cases, seizures on the second or third day of life. This complication is usually self-limiting and tends to disappear spontaneously. Some studies have found an increased incidence of the sudden infant death syndrome in these infants, possibly related to the drug's action on the respiratory control centers.

The long-term cognitive and behavioral effects of cocaine on the developing nervous system have not been clearly identified. Tests used previously to determine the infant's development, such as the *Bayley Scales of Infant Development* (Bayley, 1969), were incapable of accurately reflecting the impact of the central nervous system lesions discussed above. However, studies are now emerging that show a strong association between heavy maternal use of cocaine and the infant's auditory comprehension skills. Using the *Preschool Language Scale–Third Edition* (Zimmerman, Steiner, & Pond, 1992), Singer et al. (2001) performed a longitudinal study of the sequelae of fetal cocaine exposure in a cohort of 134 cocaine-exposed and 134 nonexposed newborn infants. At 1 year of age, the more heavily exposed infants had poorer auditory comprehension scores and significantly lower total language scores. Although the debate continues, it now seems clear that heavy use of cocaine during pregnancy is a powerful teratogen and that the infant is likely to have significant long-standing neurological and behavioral consequences (Volpe, 1992). The next step is to develop reliable screening tools to identify cocaine-exposed infants at risk in order to provide appropriate remediation and educational assistance.

## Other Drugs During Pregnancy

As a rule, the pregnant mother should refrain from taking drugs, particularly during the first trimester or at the onset of labor. Drugs that may have a detrimental effect on the fetus in addition to cigarettes and alcohol include cannabis, tranquilizers and sedatives, and excessive quantities of Vitamins A and D. Severe congenital anomalies may result in the fetus of a mother using retinoic acid (brand name, Accutane), an analogue of Vitamin A used to treat acne, particularly if the mother is taking the drug during the first trimester. The possible malformations include hydrocephalus, microcephaly, abnormalities of neuronal migration, and malformations of the posterior fossa. Additional abnormalities include cleft palate, congenital heart defects, and defects of the retina and optic nerve (Lammer et al., 1985). Cold remedies should be checked carefully, and excessive aspirin use should be discouraged, particularly near term, as the drug may enhance bleeding. Large amounts of antacids can alter the electrolyte composition in the fetus, which can lead to serious consequences, including abnormalities in heart function and a tendency to hemorrhage in vital organs. Some anticonvulsant drugs, particularly phenytoin, also can produce abnormalities in the fetus. Maternal use of the anticonvulsant valproic acid causes neural tube defects in the developing fetus in approximately 1% of cases (Omtzigt et al., 1992). It is important to remember that virtually every drug ingested by the mother is capable of crossing the placenta and affecting the fetus. If there is any question about the safety of the drug, the expectant mother should consult her physician or pharmacist.

# ACCIDENTS

Accidents are the leading cause of mortality and morbidity in children and adolescents. Accidents causing death in this age group are more common than the next five causes combined, which are congenital abnormalities, cancer, diseases of the heart, homicide, and suicide (National Safety Council, 1980). Although motor-vehicle accidents are the major cause of accidental deaths and morbidity in children and adolescents, poisoning, burns, motorcycle and bicycle accidents, and playground injuries are also important. Effective accident prevention includes education, protection, and legislation mandating the use of seat belts and sports helmets.

## Motor-Vehicle Accidents

Several factors can influence the severity of injury in a motor-vehicle accident. A study in the state of Washington showed that deaths in infants could be decreased by 91% and in older children by 81% with the appropriate use of seat belts and restraints (Scherz, 1976; also see Halman, Chipman, Parkin, & Wright, 2002). This study documented a similarly impressive decrease in morbidity as well. Unfortunately, many adults and children do not use seat belts, and without legislation these frightening statistics will persist. There is some evidence that education of expectant parents during prenatal classes is a potentially effective means of promoting the use of infant seat restraints following the birth of their baby.

Other factors that have contributed to a lower mortality rate in automobile accidents include airbags, padded dashboards, collapsible steering wheels, shatterproof glass, and protective bumpers. Infants and children should never sit in the front seat of an automobile with airbags, as they may seriously injure or suffocate the child if released at contact during an accident. Drivers' education programs in many high schools are designed to reduce the frequency and severity of accidents by specific educational methods. However, there are no studies that support the efficacy of student driver education programs; the fatality rate in adolescents 16 and 17 years of age with and without training remains approximately the same (Robertson, 1980).

## Bicycle Accidents

Bicycle accidents cause relatively few deaths but are responsible for many injuries, including severe trauma to the central nervous system. Approximately 1,200 deaths are related to bicycle accidents each year in the United States, and in 1997, an estimated 111,300 children attended an emergency department for the management of a bicycle-related head, facial, or ear injury (Miller & Spicer, 1998). Approximately 150 children died in 1997 following a head injury. Most fatal bicycle accidents involve an automobile and usually occur during the passing of a cyclist. Children on bicycles who are involved in a motor-vehicle accident frequently are at fault because of riding on the wrong side of the road, failing to signal a turn, or making careless and unpredictable maneuvers. The frequency of serious bicycle accidents can be reduced by providing a bike path for cyclists and by encouraging children to use proper lights and reflectors and to wear bright clothing and a helmet at all times.

There is strong evidence that the proper use of bicycle helmets significantly reduces the probability and severity of head injury in bicycle accidents. In a study in Seattle of 99 patients with head injuries as a result of bicycle accidents, only 4 had been wearing helmets at the time of their accidents. It was determined that bicycle helmets reduced the risk of head injury by 85% (Thompson, Rivara, & Thompson, 1989). In a more recent review of five case-control studies, it was found that helmets reduced the risk by 63% to 88% for head, brain, and severe brain injury among cyclists of all ages (Rivara, Thompson, & Thompson, 2000). As helmet use has increased, hospital admissions and deaths from bicycle-related injuries have decreased (Cook & Sheikh, 2000). Pediatricians and other health care professionals, including teachers, can enhance the use of bicycle helmets by counseling and educational sessions in the office and classroom. One report indicated that a pediatrician was much more likely to provide bicycle helmet counseling to his or her patients if another patient had experienced a head injury or died as the result of a cycling accident (Ruch-Ross & O'Connor, 1993). Another approach to encourage the use of bicycle helmets is police enforcement. A rural community in Georgia provided free helmets, with fitting instructions and safety education, to children in kindergarten through Grade 7. Police then began impounding bicycles of unhelmeted children. Prior to the initiation of the program, none of the 97 observed cyclists wore a helmet. Two years after the program had been in place, 54% were observed wearing a helmet (Gilchrist et al., 2000). Passage of bicycle helmet legislation in all 50 states is a national objective promoted in the Healthy People 2000 initiative; at the time of writing, 16 states have helmet laws for children (Alabama, California, Connecticut, Delaware, Florida, Georgia, Maine, Maryland, Massachusetts, New Jersey, New York, Oregon, Pennsylvania, Rhode Island, Tennessee, and West Virginia). Thus, experience would suggest that the most effective methods to encourage helmet use include a combination of giveaway, educational, and enforcement programs.

## Playground Accidents

Accidents at school are likely to occur during physical education or on the playground. In 1988 the Centers for Disease Control reported that playgrounds accounted for about 200,000 accidents treated in hospitals annually in the United States, and accident frequency has not declined significantly in recent years (Phelan, Khoury, Kalkwarf, & Lanphear, 2001). Many injuries result from falls off playground climbing equipment (Reichelderfer, Overbach, & Greensher, 1979; Tinsworth & Kramer, 1990). Head injuries are particularly common and are more likely to be severe if a child falls onto asphalt, cement, or hard-packed ground. Many severe injuries can be prevented if playground equipment is placed over an impact-absorbing surface, such as grass, wood shavings, or rubber-lined insulation (Bond & Peck, 1993; Sosin, Keller, Sacks, Kresnow, & van Dyck, 1993). The older the student, the greater the likelihood that injury on the playground will result from contact sports such as football.

It is important to design new playgrounds that conform to contemporary safety standards (Ramsey & Preston, 1990). Playgrounds that are outdated or have been unattended must be upgraded to include appropriate and safe surfacing material. The educator can play a critical role in ensuring that the school's playgrounds are safe and perhaps in influencing state and local health departments to interact with the school boards to provide healthy playgrounds that will help prevent serious injuries in the school-age population.

## Poison Prevention

Toddlers are notoriously curious. Thus, it is not surprising that many ingest potentially lethal medications and household substances. Unfortunately, children die every day from poisoning. If they do survive, a chronic disability may result. The most frequent and serious substances that are ingested include salicylates (aspirin), iron compounds (used to treat anemia), psychotherapeutic drugs (sedatives, antidepressants), hydrocarbons (kerosene, gasoline, furniture cleaners), drainpipe cleaners, and pesticides (organophosphates).

The most important aspect in the management of accidental poisoning is prevention. The dispensing of medications should be supervised by an adult, and the child should not be persuaded to take the drug as if it were candy. Parents should be encouraged to place all drugs and harmful substances in a locked cabinet. Outdated drugs or those remaining after completion of a specific treatment protocol should be discarded. Syrup of ipecac, which induces vomiting, should be available in every household and used if necessary following consultation with a poison control center or physician. The use of child-resistant containers for drugs and safety-closure containers for dangerous household substances has had an impressive impact on decreasing mortality and morbidity in toddlers (Harriss, 1969; Scherz, 1970). Unfortunately, the use of child-resistant containers is not universal.

# SCREENING PROGRAMS
# FOR SPECIFIC DISEASES

Screening for specific diseases or conditions in the whole population or in special at-risk groups can prevent serious disabilities by the implementation of therapy prior to the development of irreversible biological or psychological changes (i.e., secondary prevention). Screening for phenylketonuria, hypothyroidism, and learning disabilities will be examined briefly here as a method of preventing disabilities.

## Phenylketonuria

Phenylketonuria (PKU) occurs in approximately 1 per 15,000 live births. In the untreated infant, it is characterized by mental retardation, seizures, a musty odor, blond hair, blue eyes, and eczema. A special diet consisting of minimal amounts of phenylalanine, an amino acid, is effective in preventing mental retardation if it is introduced soon after birth in the child with classical PKU.

Screening for PKU, done by a blood test performed before the infant is discharged from the newborn nursery, and the early implementation of treatment have been remarkably successful. But with every success, a new problem is likely to be created. As children with PKU treated with a low-phenylalanine diet approach adolescence and adulthood, they are likely to discontinue the unsavory diet. As a result, their blood phenylalanine levels will rise to very high values. If such an individual then becomes pregnant, the fetus will be exposed to toxic maternal levels of phenylalanine, resulting in congenital malformations and mental retardation. If, on the other hand, the PKU mother is once again placed on a low-phenylalanine diet prior to conception and throughout the pregnancy, the child will be born without disabilities.

## Congenital Hypothyroidism

Congenital hypothyroidism, which occurs with a frequency of 1 per 5,000 live births, is difficult to diagnose in the newborn because its symptoms are subtle. The infant may be listless and have feeding problems, there may be difficulty in maintaining the body temperature, and the infant may have severe constipation and prolonged jaundice. In time, more characteristic signs become apparent, including a large tongue, a protuberant abdomen with an umbilical hernia, cool and mottled skin, and a hoarse cry.

To screen for congenital hypothyroidism, a sample of blood is obtained at birth at the same time as the PKU test, and the level of thyroid hormone is determined in a laboratory. If the diagnosis is made prior to 6 weeks of age, mental retardation can be prevented by the introduction of lifelong thyroid hormone replacement therapy. However, severe mental retardation can result if treatment is delayed.

## Learning Disabilities

Learning disabilities are prominent in school-age children. The screening of preschool children through tests of motor and visual function, memory, comprehension, and language skills has not proven to be a reliable predictor of academic and social failure upon entry into school. Newer testing procedures that encompass measures of maturation, selective attention, and task attainment hold greater promise (Meltzer, Levine, Palfrey, Aufseeser, & Oberklaid, 1981; Wu, Anderson, & Castiello, 2002). Certainly, those children with severe deficits in language and cognitive function are likely to benefit from early intervention, including speech and language therapy. It is not clear whether the child with cerebral palsy or mental retardation benefits in a similar fashion (Russman, 1983).

# CHILDHOOD ANTECEDENTS OF ADULT DISEASE

Several adult diseases originate during fetal development or in childhood. Some of the common disorders of this type are described briefly in this section.

## Obesity

Obesity is a common problem and is reaching epidemic proportions in our society, in spite of the increasing emphasis on diet and exercise. Obesity is defined as a body mass index at or above the 85th percentile for age and gender. Body mass index is equal to the weight in kilograms divided by the square of the height in meters. From 1982 to 1997, the prevalence of obesity increased from 5% to 8% in children ages 4 to 5 years, 4% to 11% in the 6- to 11-year age group, and to 23% in adults (Whitaker, Wright, Pepe, Seidel, & Dietz, 1997).

The hypothalamus controls energy metabolism by regulating energy intake, fat metabolism, and energy expenditure. Fat cells (*adipocytes*) are the sole source of leptin, which binds to a leptin receptor. Leptin decreases energy intake and increases energy expenditure. Mutated leptin can result in obesity. Initially there was considerable enthusiasm following the discovery of leptin as a potential new treatment for obesity. Unfortunately, mutated leptin is an uncommon cause of obesity, as most cases result from environmental factors. Although there is evidence that environmental factors interact with genetic determinants, the increasing prevalence of obesity is not primarily explained by genetic factors. An individual who is obese has an increase in the number and size of adipocytes. It is not clear whether the increased adipocyte population results from obesity or plays a role in its etiology. Adults who are obese have an enhanced risk of diabetes mellitus, coronary heart disease, hypertension, respiratory difficulties, and a shortened life span. The medical illnesses associated with obesity usually occur in adulthood, but adults rarely achieve sustained weight loss. Therefore, prevention of obesity in childhood and effective treatment of overweight children is essential. Children who are obese have increased respiratory infections and are more likely to develop slipped capital femoral epiphysis (a softening or weakening of the bone that allows the head of the femur to slip off the neck of the femur). The greatest disability a child who is obese suffers is ridicule and rejection by schoolmates.

A fairly recent study has shed some light on the pathogenesis of obesity in the pediatric population (Whitaker et al., 1997). It showed that a child's risk of developing obesity as an adult is much greater if either the mother or father is obese. At every age interval, both obese and nonobese children are at greater risk for obesity as adults if at least one parent is obese. It is likely that obesity in one or both parents probably influences the risk of obesity in their offspring because of shared genes or environmental factors within families.

The treatment and prevention of obesity are difficult and prolonged processes and must take into account several factors. For example, low-income mothers do not perceive their child as overweight, whereas well-educated mothers are aware that their child is overweight. Maternal educational levels, interestingly enough, do not have much impact on the mothers' overweightness (Whitaker et al., 1997). Ultimate failure in sustained weight reduction is frequent. Obesity may have its onset during infancy by overfeeding, introducing solids too early, allowing frequent snacks, or pacifying the child with a bottle. Caution should be used in treating overweight children less than 3 years of age who do not have obese parents; few will become obese adults. In contrast, any 1- to 2-year-old child who has an obese parent, and especially two obese parents, is susceptible to obesity in young adulthood (Whitaker et al., 1997). Later, the child who is obese may eat when upset or depressed, thereby entering a vicious cycle. Prevention must begin during infancy with a nutritious diet and proper feeding practice.

The management of a child or adolescent who is obese involves diet control, attention to psychological factors, consistent exercise, and the use of behavior modification techniques (Epstein, Valoski, Wing, & McCurley, 1990). There is absolutely no role for the use of medication or fad diets in the treatment of children who are obese. Successful therapeutic results are more likely to occur if the entire family is involved and the child can be convinced that the process of sustained weight reduction is a long-term commitment.

## Hypertension

High blood pressure (hypertension) is an extremely common health problem. A 1960–1962 survey in the United States found 17 million adults with significant hypertension (Paul & Ostfeld, 1965). More recently Dekkers, Snieder, Van Den Ord, and Treiber (2000) performed a 10-year longitudinal study of blood pressure from childhood to adulthood. The detection and prevention of sustained high blood pressure in adults recently has received a great deal of publicity because of the known association between hypertension and congestive heart failure, cerebrovascular accidents (strokes), and coronary heart disease.

The prevalence of hypertension in childhood is quite low (1% to 3%), and the majority of these children have only mild elevations of blood pressure (Jung & Ingelfinger, 1993). Hypertension may be primary (essential) or secondary. Primary hypertension accounts for the majority (90%) of hypertension in children and results from both genetic and environmental factors. Studies have shown a positive correlation between blood pressure (BP) readings of parents and their children. Environmental factors that directly influence BP levels include obesity, lower socioeconomic status, and high salt intake. The major causes of secondary hypertension in children include kidney diseases, adrenal conditions, and heart abnormalities such as coarctation of the aorta. Primary hypertension is much more prevalent in the adolescent, whereas secondary hypertension due to underlying organic abnormalities is more common in the infant. BP recordings must be determined in a quiet room with the student supine. A BP cuff of the proper size must be used, covering approximately two thirds of the upper arm. Even with appropriate techniques, an inaccurate recording may be determined in the child or adolescent because their BP levels are characteristically unstable and the child may be anxious or frightened. Repeated recordings may show that the student does not have high blood pressure.

Figure 2.3 gives the age-specific percentile values of BP measurements for boys and girls. Normal BP, using the tables in Figure 2.3, is defined as systolic and diastolic BPs less than the 90th percentile for age and gender. Hypertension is present when the average systolic or diastolic BP measurement is equal to or greater than the 95th percentile for age and gender on at least three occasions (National Heart, Lung, and Blood Institute, 1987). The majority of adolescent males with hypertension have primary (essential) hypertension, and approximately 30% to 40% of this group will continue to have hypertension as adults. Black males are particularly at risk during adolescence. Most individuals with essential hypertension are asymptomatic. On occasion, frontal headaches, nosebleeds, dizziness, nervousness, lethargy, and a poor appetite may accompany essential hypertension. The physician usually can separate primary from secondary hypertension by a careful history, a physical examination, and a few laboratory tests, including a urinalysis. The examinations are always normal in the adolescent with primary hypertension.

The long-term outlook for children and adolescents with elevated BP levels is uncertain. However, because at least one third of these individuals continue to have elevated recordings as adults, it would seem prudent to take measures to reduce the BP level. The adolescent with hypertension should have a reduced salt intake (5 to 6 g of salt daily). Foods that have an excessive salt content include TV dinners, pickles, salted crackers and nuts, potato chips, salted cottage cheese, canned soups, pizza, hot dogs, ketchup, and cold cereals. Asymptomatic adolescents with essential hypertension should be encouraged to participate in a weight-reduction program if obese (obesity occurs in 50% of the cases), discontinue smoking, reduce stress, and engage in a recreational program. Certain drugs, including diuretic agents, may be necessary in some adolescents.

The most difficult component of a preventive program for hypertension, however, is alteration of the adolescent's eating habits (Lieberman, 1982). As in the management of obesity, a program must be devised that

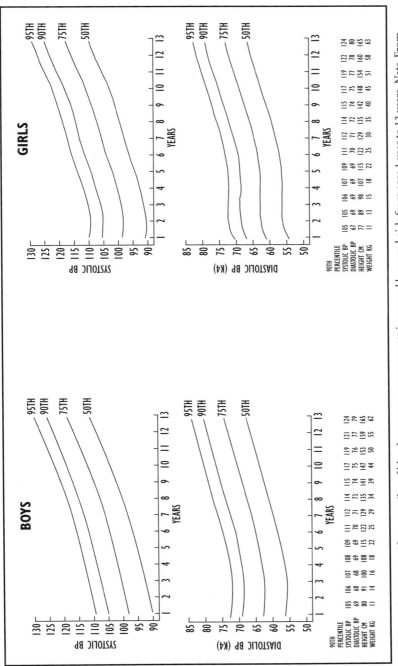

**FIGURE 2.3.** Age-specific percentiles of blood pressure measurements in normal boys and girls from ages 1 year to 13 years. *Note.* From "Report of the Second Task Force on Blood Pressure Control in Children," by the National Heart, Lung and Blood Institute, 1987, *Pediatrics, 79,* pp. 6–7. Reprinted with permission.

will consider the cultural and economic needs of the patient and family while providing an understanding and resourceful health care worker as the team leader. For weight reduction to be effective, the entire family must be involved in the dietary program (Epstein, Valoski, Wing, & McCurley, 1990). A National Heart, Lung, and Blood Institute Task Force (1977) on BP control in children published these recommendations:

1. Children 3 years old and above should have their blood pressure measured annually as part of their total health care.

2. Isolated screening programs for hypertension should be discouraged.

3. Blood pressure measurement techniques should be appropriate for the size and age of the child.

4. Blood pressure measurements should be plotted on grids like those shown in Figure 2.3.

5. Caution should be exerted in labeling children as hypertensive; the term *high normal blood pressure* should be used instead during evaluation and follow-up.

6. Children whose sustained blood pressure levels exceed the 95th percentile on the grids are considered abnormal and should be evaluated by history, physical examination, and selected laboratory tests.

7. Children with sustained elevated blood pressure should receive a systematic follow-up program that includes general health counseling and specific antihypertensive drugs when needed.

8. Children at risk of developing elevated blood pressure should be evaluated for other atherosclerotic risk factors.

The strategies for preventing hypertension in childhood may include an active educational approach or a passive environmental design. The most successful strategy incorporates the building of social skills and health-related behavior into the school health education program. Some school programs have concentrated on reducing students' salt intake and increasing physical activity. The "Know Your Body" program, a school-based program focusing on hypertension, has resulted in lower blood pressures in students enrolled in the program than in students in control schools in New York and Washington, D.C. (Bush et al., 1989; Walter, Hofman, Vaughan, & Wynder, 1988). In these programs, special attention has been directed to increasing exercise among all students rather than concentrating on building skills in competitive sports for selected elite athletes. Environmental programs designed to reduce hypertension in school-age children do not require active participation by the student. For example, two boarding schools in New England performed a study in which one modified the sodium content of food prepared in the school's dining hall through changes in food purchasing. In the school that did not lower the sodium content, blood pressure values of its students continued to rise compared with those of students in the "treatment" school (Witschi et al., 1985). These studies suggest that modest changes in the nutrient composition (especially sodium content) of food products consumed by students, including products in fast food chains, could have a major impact on hypertension in the pediatric population.

## Arteriosclerotic Heart Disease

Hyperlipidemia (elevated plasma cholesterol or triglycerides) in infants, children, and adolescents is a precursor to arteriosclerotic heart disease during adulthood. The first study that proved that elevated plasma cholesterol was a risk factor in the development of atherosclerosis in children was done by the Bogalusa Heart Study (Newman et al., 1986). Postmortem studies of young and otherwise normal individuals who die accidentally show evidence of early arteriosclerotic changes in the blood vessels consisting of fat-laden plaques. This process appears to be significantly accelerated in those patients with hyperlipidemia associated with very high levels of low-density lipoprotein cholesterol. Cholesterol is the primary blood lipid related to the development of heart disease.

The risk factors for arteriosclerotic heart disease include smoking, hypertension, obesity, and an elevated cholesterol level (Kannel & Dawber, 1972). There are several types of hyperlipidemia, which are classified according to the family history, age of onset, symptoms and signs, plasma cholesterol and triglyceride level, and the lipoprotein electrophoretic pattern. The most common form of hyperlipidemia identified in children is one in which the plasma cholesterol is elevated but the triglyceride level is normal.

Screening for hyperlipidemia in children should be reserved for high-risk populations, including families with a history of premature vascular disease in a parent or grandparent. Vascular disease is considered premature if it occurs in a male prior to 50 years of age and in a female before

60 years of age. Approximately one third of children in such families are found to have hyperlipidemia.

Diet is the most important component of therapy once hyperlipidemia has been established in the child. A major goal of dietary management is reducing the total fat content, principally by increasing the intake of vegetables and decreasing the portions of beef and dairy products consumed, which increases the polyunsaturated to saturated fat ratio. In general, the diet should consist of less than 30% of total calories as fat (less than 10% saturated fat, up to 10% polyunsaturated fat, and the remaining 10% to 15% monounsaturated fat), 50% to 60% of total calories as carbohydrates, and from 10% to 20% of total calories as protein. Cholesterol intake should be approximately 100 mg of cholesterol per 1,000 calories. If a child is obese, caloric restriction should be followed. As with other forms of dietary management in children, it is imperative that the entire family become involved in the program. Certain drugs, particularly cholestyramine, are very effective in lowering plasma cholesterol by binding it within the gastrointestinal tract (West, Lloyd, & Leonard, 1980). The treatment of hyperlipidemia in children is a lifelong commitment consisting of dietary control in conjunction with a drug such as cholestyramine, with the hope that arteriosclerotic heart disease can be prevented (Cortner, Coates, Liacouras, & Jarvik, 1993).

# PREVENTION OF SELECTED GENETIC DISEASES

An increasing number of genetic diseases can be prevented through counseling or through detection during early pregnancy. Three genetic disorders associated with disabilities—Down syndrome, fragile X syndrome, and neural tube defects—are considered here.

## Down Syndrome

Down syndrome is the most common chromosomal abnormality resulting in mental retardation (see Chapter 7 for the clinical features of Down syndrome). It has an incidence of approximately 1 per 900 live births. Although Down syndrome can occur in any family, there is an increased risk with advanced maternal age: The incidence at 35 years is 1 per 350; at the age of 40, the risk rises to 1 per 100; and at the age of 45, the risk is 1 per 25 births (Morris, Mutton, & Alberman, 2002). Recent studies have shown that determination of the levels of three substances—alpha-fetoprotein, beta-human chorionic gonadotropin, and unconjugated estriol—in maternal blood between 16 and 18 weeks of gestation can be predictive of a fetus with Down syndrome or a neural tube defect. If the screening study is positive, an abdominal ultrasound and amniocentesis are recommended to confirm the diagnosis.

Amniocentesis provides a practical, relatively safe, and reliable method of identifying chromosomal abnormalities in the fetus at risk. The procedure should be discussed with parents if they are known to have an abnormal chromosome pattern, if they have had a previous child with chromosomal abnormalities, or if the mother is 35 years of age or older at the time of conception. Following detailed counseling, the couple may elect to undergo amniocentesis and, possibly, therapeutic abortion if a fetus with disabilities is identified.

Individuals with Down syndrome are at an increased risk for atlantoaxial instability due to laxity of the ligaments supporting the upper cervical vertebrae. (The atlas and axis are the first two cervical vertebrae.) Slippage of the cervical vertebrae can result in compression of the cervical spinal cord, causing neck pain, gait abnormalities, urinary and fecal incontinence, and head tilt. These symptoms require immediate investigation and possible surgical intervention to stabilize the vertebrae. It is recommended that lateral X-ray films of the neck in the neutral, flexion, and extension positions be obtained at 3 to 5 years, 10 to 12 years, and 18 years and older in individuals with Down syndrome who are interested in sports participation, and that those found to have radiographic evidence of atlantoaxial instability be advised not to participate in sports that might place undue pressure on the neck, such as football, tumbling, and diving (Haslam, 1995).

## Fragile X Syndrome

Fragile X syndrome is a disorder of males characterized by mental retardation and macroorchidism (large testes). There may be associated anomalies, including a prominent jaw, broad forehead, large ears, macrocephaly (large head), and pale blue eyes (Hagerman, McBogg, & Hagerman, 1983; Turner, Daniel, & Frost, 1980), and many autistic features, including marked language delay, echolalia, and hand flapping. Chromosomal analyses typically show that affected males have a constriction of the X chromosome at the tip of the long arm, forming a thin filament that is prone to breakage when special culture techniques are used. A highly accurate DNA molecular diagnostic test has been developed to confirm the diagnosis of the fragile X syndrome (VerKerk, Eussen, Van Hemel, & Oostra, 1992).

It is becoming evident that the fragile X syndrome is an important single-gene disorder, producing mental retardation second in frequency only to Down syndrome. Some clinicians suggest that the investigation of mental retardation in the male is incomplete until the fragile X has been excluded. Once an individual with the fragile X syndrome has been diagnosed, a thorough study of the family should be initiated so that carrier females may be identified and information as to the risk of more affected males may be imparted by genetic counseling. As greater numbers of families are studied, it is evident that the carrier female is often also abnormal, but to a lesser degree than the male. These individuals may have mild mental retardation and significant learning and behavioral abnormalities.

## Neural Tube Defects

Neural tube defects, including anencephaly, encephalocele, and spina bifida, have a variable incidence in different ethnic groups, but the overall incidence is approximately 3 or 4 per 1,000 live births. A couple that has produced one child with a neural tube defect has a 2% to 5% risk of another occurrence in subsequent pregnancies, and, if they are unfortunate enough to have had two affected children, the risk for future abnormal children approximately doubles. Neural tube defects are thought to result from many factors, including genetic and environmental influences, particularly poor nutrition during pregnancy.

Anencephaly and large encephaloceles can be detected in utero by ultrasound. The combination of an abnormal ultrasound and the finding of elevated levels of alphafetoprotein and acetylcholinesterase in the amniotic fluid between 14 and 16 weeks of pregnancy is a reliable method of confirming an open–neural-tube defect in the fetus at risk.

During the past 10 years, studies have provided confirmation that maternal periconceptional administration of folic acid significantly reduces the incidence of neural tube defects in pregnancies at risk (MRC Vitamin Study Research Group, 1991; Smithells et al., 1981). To be effective, folic acid supplementation should be initiated prior to conception and continued until at least the 12th week of gestation, when the process of neurulation is completed. The U.S. Public Health Service recommends that all women of childbearing age take 0.4 mg of folic acid daily and that women who have previously had a child with a neural tube defect take 4 mg of folic acid daily beginning 1 month prior to conception, under the supervision of a physician who can provide counseling and follow-up. The modern diet provides about half the daily requirement of folic acid. To increase the folic acid intake, fortification of flour, pasta, rice, and cornmeal with 0.15 mg folic acid per 100 g was mandated by the United States and Canada in 1998 (Quinlivam & Gregory, 2003). Unfortunately, the added folic acid is insufficient to meet the minimal requirements to prevent neural tube defects (4 mg daily). Therefore, informative educational programs remain essential for those women planning to become pregnant.

# THE TEACHER'S ROLE

The teacher can play an important role in the primary, secondary, and tertiary prevention for a variety of conditions common to school-age children. The teacher may use the success of immunization to demonstrate how good public health measures may eliminate devastating diseases such as smallpox, poliomyelitis, and *Haemophilus influenzae* infections. Many school programs have introduced well-developed educational programs to discuss the serious consequences of drugs such as alcohol, cocaine, and other illicit drugs, and the deleterious effects that they can have on the user as well as the fetus. Some teachers will be responsible for the education of children with fetal alcohol syndrome and alcohol-related neurodevelopmental and birth defects. In the classroom, the teacher will be practicing tertiary prevention to reduce the burden of the significant cognitive and social consequences of these devastating conditions. The teacher may also play an important role in accident prevention by encouraging the use of bicycle helmets and safe play at home and school, including the proper installation and use of playground equipment. Finally, the educator can encourage good health by teaching the importance of regular exercise and good nutrition, which will ultimately have a positive impact on the prevention of obesity and hypertension. Many teachers are powerful role models for their students and the messages that they impart can have a lifelong influence on their pupils. Thus, teachers are an important component of the health care team and in the future could play an even greater role in the prevention of many childhood disorders.

# SUMMARY

Many conditions that produce disabilities continuing throughout life can be prevented by using simple techniques. Complications that can be corrected and phenomena that may injure the fetus should be sought by the physician during the antenatal period. Mothers at risk for an abnormal pregnancy should be referred to a major medical center for assessment, delivery, and management of the newborn. It is important to determine the susceptibility to rubella of all females in the childbearing age and to recommend immunization for those found to be unprotected.

Physicians and teachers could play a more active role in the prevention of head injuries resulting from motor-vehicle, bicycle, and playground accidents by providing information to children and their parents. Children and families at risk for the complications of obesity, hypertension, and arteriosclerotic heart disease would benefit from a thorough evaluation by the pediatrician and by follow-up in a clinic setting.

More can and must be done to prevent chronic disabilities that have their onset during infancy or childhood. Society at large must be educated and then convinced that specific lifestyle changes, including abstention from drugs during pregnancy (particularly cigarettes, cocaine, and alcohol); proper immunization practices; use of infant restraints, bicycle helmets, and seat belts; and protection of infants from accidental poisoning by the use of containers with a safety closure, can have a significant impact on the future of our children.

# REFERENCES

Advisory Committee on Immunization Practices, American Academy of Pediatrics, & American Academy of Family Physicians. (2003, January). Recommended childhood and adolescent immunization schedule—United States, 2003. *AAP News*, p. 22.

American Academy of Pediatrics. (2000). Fetal alcohol syndrome and alcohol-related neurodevelopmental disorders. *Pediatrics, 106*, 358–361.

Bayley, N. (1969). *Bayley Scales of Infant Development.* San Antonio: The Psychological Corporation.

Bond, M. T., & Peck, M. G. (1993). The risk of childhood injury on Boston's playground equipment and surfaces. *American Journal of Public Health, 83,* 731–733.

Booy, R., Moxon, E. R., MacFarlane, J. A., Mayon-White, R. T., & Slack, M. P. E. (1992). Efficacy of Haemophilus influenzae type b conjugate vaccine in Oxford region. *Lancet, 340,* 847.

Bush, P. J., Zuckerman, A. E., Taggart, V. S., Theiss, P. K., Peleg, E. D., & Smith, S. A. (1989). Cardiovascular risk factor prevention in Black school children: The "Know Your Body" evaluation project. *Health Education Quarterly, 16,* 215.

Centers for Disease Control. (1988). Playground related injuries in preschool aged children: United States, 1983–1987. *Morbidity and Mortality Weekly Report, 37,* 629–632.

Centers for Disease Control and Prevention. (1994). Reported vaccine-preventable disease —United States, 1993, and the Childhood Immunization Initiative. *Morbidity and Mortality Weekly Report, 43,* 57–60.

Centers for Disease Control and Prevention. (1997). Surveillance for fetal alcohol syndrome using multiple sources, Atlanta, GA, 1981–1989. *Morbidity and Mortality Weekly Report, 46,* 1118–1120.

Centers for Disease Control and Prevention. (1999). Ten great public achievements— United States, 1990–1999. *Morbidity and Mortality Weekly Report, 48,* 241–243.

Cook, A., & Sheikh, A. (2000). Trends in serious head injuries among cyclists in England: Analysis of routinely controlled data. *British Medical Journal, 321,* 1055.

Cortner, J. A., Coates, P. M., Liacouras, C. A., & Jarvik, G. P. (1993). Familial combined hyperlipidemia in children: Clinical expression, metabolic defects and management. *Journal of Pediatrics, 123*(2), 177–184.

Dekkers, J. C., Snieder, H., Van Den Oord, E. J., & Treiber, F. A. (2002). Moderators of blood pressure development from childhood to adulthood: A 10-year longitudinal study. *Journal of Pediatrics, 141,* 770–779.

Epstein, L. H., Valoski, A., Wing, R. R., & McCurley, J. (1990). Ten year follow-up of behavioral, family-based treatment for obese children. *Journal of the American Medical Association, 264,* 2519–2523.

Eskola, J., Takala, A., Kaynty, H., Peltola, H., & Makelä, P. H. (1991). Experience in Finland with Haemophilus influenzae type b vaccines. *Vaccine, 9,* 514–516.

Frank, D. A., McCarten, K. M., Robson, C. D., Mirochnick, M., Cabral, H., Park, H., & Zuckerman, B. (1999). Level of in utero cocaine exposure and neonatal ultrasound findings. *Pediatrics, 104,* 1101–1105.

Frick, G. S., & Dow-Edwards, D. L. (1995). The effects of cocaine on cerebral metabolic function in periweanling rats: The roles of serotonergic and dopaminergic uptake blockade. *Brain Research, 88,* 158–170.

Gilchrist, J., Schieber, R. A., Leadbetter, S., & Davidson, S. C. (2000). Police enforcement as a comprehensive bicycle helmet program. *Pediatrics, 106,* 6–99.

Graham, K., Koren, G., Klein, J., Schneiderman, J., & Greenwald, M. (1989). Determination of gestational cocaine exposure by hair analysis. *Journal of the American Medical Association, 262,* 3328–3330.

Hagerman, R. J., McBogg, P., & Hagerman, P. J. (1983). The fragile X syndrome: History, diagnosis and treatment. *Journal of Developmental and Behavioral Pediatrics, 4,* 122–130.

Halman, S. I., Chipman, M., Parkin, P. C., & Wright, J. C. (2002). Are seat belt restraints as effective in school age children as in adults? A prospective crash study. *British Medical Journal, 324,* 1108–1109.

Hanwood, H. J., & Napolitano, D. M. (1985). Economic implications of the fetal alcohol synrome. *Alchohol Health Research World, 10,* 38–43.

Harriss, W. E. (1969). Safety cap closures on drug bottles: A neglected approach to prevention of childhood poisoning. *Clinical Pediatrics, 8,* 735–737.

Haslam, R. H. A. (1983). Preventable causes of mental retardation. *Annals of the Royal College of Physicians and Surgeons of Canada, 16,* 121–124.

Haslam, R. H. A. (2003). The nervous system. In R. E. Behrman, R. Kliegman, & A. M. Arvin (Eds.), *Nelson textbook of pediatrics* (17th ed.). Philadelphia: Saunders.

Jung, F. F., & Ingelfinger, J. R. (1993). Hypertension in childhood and adolescence. *Pediatrics in Review, 14*(5), 169–179.

Kannel, W. B., & Dawber, T. R. (1972). Atherosclerosis as a pediatric problem. *Journal of Pediatrics, 80,* 544–554.

Lammer, E. J., Chen, D. T., Hoar, R. M., Agnish, N. D., Benke, P. J., Braun, J. T., Curry, C. J., Fernhoff, P. M., Grix, A. W., Lott, I. T., Richard, J. M., & Sun, S. C. (1985). Retinoic acid embryopathy. *New England Journal of Medicine, 313,* 837–841.

Lieberman, E. (1982). Hypertension in childhood and adolescence. *Cibia Symposium, 34,* 3–43.

Meltzer, L. J., Levine, M. D., Palfrey, J. S., Aufseeser, C. L., & Oberklaid, F. (1981). Evaluation of a multidimensional assessment procedure for preschool children. *Journal of Developmental and Behavioral Pediatrics, 2,* 67–73.

Miller, T., & Spicer, R. (1998). How safe are our schools? *American Journal of Public Health, 88,* 413–418.

Mills, J. L., Granbard, B. I., Harley, E. E., Rhoads, G. G., & Berendes, H. W. (1984). Maternal alcohol consumption and birth weight: How much drinking in pregnancy is safe? *Journal of the American Medical Association, 252,* 1875–1879.

Morris, J. K., Mutton, D. E., & Alberman, E. (2002). Revised estimates of the maternal specific live birth prevalence of Down's syndrome. *Journal of Medical Screening, 9,* 2–6.

MRC Vitamin Study Research Group. (1991). Prevention of neural tube defects: Results of the Medical Research Council Vitamin Study. *Lancet, 338,* 131–137.

National Heart, Lung, and Blood Institute. (1977). Report of the Task Force on Blood Pressure Control in Children. *Pediatrics, 59*(Suppl.), 797–820.

National Heart, Lung, and Blood Institute. (1987). Report of the Second Task Force on Blood Pressure Control in Children. *Pediatrics, 79*(1), 1–25.

National Safety Council. (1980). *Accidents facts, 1979.* Chicago: Author.

Newman, W. P., Freedman, D. S., Voors, A. W., Gard, P. D., Srinivasan, S. R., Cresanta, J. L., Williamson, G. D., Webber, L. S., & Berenson, G. S. (1986). Relation of serum lipoprotein levels and systolic blood pressure to early atherosclerosis: The Bogalusa Heart Study. *New England Journal of Medicine, 314,* 138–144.

National, state, and urban area vaccination coverage levels among children aged 19–35 months—United States, 2000. (2001). *Morbidity and Mortality Weekly Report, 50*(30), 638.

Olegard, R., Sabel, K. G., Aronsson, M., Sandin, B., Johansson, P. R., Carlsson, C., Kyllerman, M., Iverson, K., & Hrbek, A. (1979). Effects on the child of alcohol abuse during pregnancy. *Acta Paediatrica Scandinavia, 275*(Suppl.), 112–121.

Omtzigt, J. G., Los, F. J., Grobbee, D. E., Pijbers, L., Jahoda, M. G., Brandenberg, H., Stewart, P. A., Gaillard, H. L., Sachs, E. S., & Wladimiroff, J. W. (1992). The role of spina bifida aperta after first-trimester exposure to valproate in a prenatal cohort. *Neurology, 42*(4, Suppl. 5), 119–125.

Paul, O., & Ostfeld, A. M. (1965). Epidemiology of hypertension. *Progress in Cardiovascular Diseases, 8,* 106–116.

Phelan, K. J., Khoury, J., Kalkwarf, H. J., & Lanphear, B. P. (2001). Trends and patterns of playground injuries in United States children and adolescents. *Ambulatory Pediatrics, 1,* 227–233.

Quinlivan, E. P., & Gregory, J. F., III. (2003). Effect of food fortification on folic acid intake in the United States. *American Journal of Clinical Nutrition, 77,* 221–225.

Ramsey, L. F., & Preston, J. D. (1990). *Impact attenuation performance of playground surfacing materials.* Washington, DC: Consumer Products Safety Commission.

Reichelderfer, T. E., Overbach, A., & Greensher, J. (1979). Unsafe playground. *Pediatrics, 64,* 962–963.

Rivara, F. P., Thompson, D. C., & Thompson, R. S. (2000). Bicycle helmets: It's time to use them. *British Medical Journal, 321,* 1035–1036.

Robertson, L. S. (1980). Crash involvement of teenaged drivers when driver education is eliminated from high school. *American Journal of Public Health, 70,* 599–603.

Ruch-Ross, H. S., & O'Connor, K. G. (1993). Pediatricians: A random national survey. *Americal Journal of Public Health, 85,* 728–730.

Rush, D. (1974). Examination of the relationship between birth weight, cigarette smoking during pregnancy, and maternal weight gain. *Journal of Obstetrics and Gynecology of the British Commonwealth, 81,* 746–752.

Russman, B. S. (1983). Early intervention for the biologically handicapped infant and young child: Is it of value? *Pediatrics in Review, 5,* 51–55.

Scherz, R. G. (1970). Prevention of childhood poisoning: A community project. *Pediatric Clinics of North America, 17,* 713–727.

Scherz, R. G. (1976). Restraint systems for the prevention of injury to children in automobile accidents. *American Journal of Public Health, 66,* 451–456.

Singer, L. T., Arendt, R., Minnes, S., Salvator, A., Siegel, A. C., & Lewis, B. A. (2001). Developing language skills of cocaine-exposed infants. *Pediatrics, 107,* 1057–1064.

Smith, D. W., Jones, K. L., & Hanson, J. W. (1976). Perspectives on the cause and frequency of the fetal alcohol syndrome. *Annals of the New York Academy of Science, 273,* 138–139.

Smithells, R. W., Sheppard, S., Schorah, C. J., Seller, M. J., Nevin, N. C., Harris, R., Reed, A. P., & Fielding, D. W. (1981). Apparent prevention of neural tube defects by periconceptional vitamin supplementation. *Archives of Disease in Childhood, 56,* 911–918.

Sosin, D. M., Keller, P., Sacks, J. J., Kresnow, M. J., & van Dyck, P. C. (1993). Surface-specific fall injury rates on Utah school playgrounds. *American Journal of Public Health, 83,* 733–735.

Stratton, K., Howe, C., & Battaglia, F. (Eds.). (1996). *Fetal alcohol syndrome: Diagnosis, epidemiology, prevention and treatment.* Washington, DC: National Academy Press.

Streissguth, A. P., Aase, J. M., Clarren, S. K., Randels, S. P., LaDue, R. A., & Smith, D. F. (1991). Fetal alcohol syndrome in adolescents and adults. *Journal of the American Medical Association, 265,* 1961–1967.

Streissguth, A., & Kanter, J. (Eds.). (1997). *The challenge of fetal alcohol syndrome: Overcoming secondary disabilities.* Seattle, WA: Washington Press.

Thompson, R. S., Rivara, F. P., & Thompson, D. C. (1989). A case-control study of the effectiveness of bicycle safety helmets. *New England Journal of Medicine, 320,* 1361–1367.

Tinsworth, D. K., & Kramer, J. T. (1990). *Playground equipment: Related injuries and deaths.* Washington, DC: Consumer Products Safety Commission.

Turner, G., Daniel, A., & Frost, M. (1980). X-linked mental retardation, macroorchidism, and the Xq27 fragile site. *Journal of Pediatrics, 96,* 837–841.

Vaccination coverage of 2-year-old children: United States, 1992–1993. (1994). *Morbidity and Mortality Weekly Report, 43,* 282–283.

VanKerk, A. J., Eussen, B. H., Van Hemel, J., & Oostra, B. A. (1992). Limited size of the fragile X site shown by fluorescence in situ hybridization. *American Journal of Medical Genetics, 43,* 187–191.

Volpe, J. J. (1992). Effect of cocaine use on the fetus. *New England Journal of Medicine, 327,* 399–406.

Walter, H. J., Hofman, A., Vaughan, R. D., & Wynder, E. L. (1988). Modification of risk factors for coronary heart disease: Five year results of a school-based intervention trial. *New England Journal of Medicine, 318,* 1093–1100.

West, R. J., Lloyd, J. K., & Leonard, J. V. (1980). Long term follow-up of children with familial hypercholesterolaemia treated with cholestyramine. *Lancet, 2,* 873–875.

Whitaker, R. C., Wright, J. A., Pepe, M. S., Seidel, K. D., & Dietz, W. H. (1997). Predicting obesity in young adulthood from childhood and parental obesity. *New England Journal of Medicine, 337,* 869–873.

Witschi, J. C., Ellison, R. C., Doane, D. D., Vorlein, G. L., Slack, W. V., & Stare, F. J. (1985). Dietary sodium reduction among students: Feasibility and acceptance. *Journal of the American Dietetic Association, 85,* 816–821.

Wu, K. K., Anderson, V., & Castiello, U. (2002). Neuropsychological evaluation of deficits in executive functioning for ADHD children with or without learning disabilities. *Developmental Neuropsychology, 22,* 501–531.

Zimmerman, I. L., Steiner, V. G., & Pond, R. E. (1992) *Preschool Language Scale–Third Edition.* San Antonio, TX: The Psychological Corporation.

# CHAPTER 3

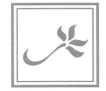

# What Every Teacher Should Know About Infectious Diseases

Ronald Gold

The most common cause of acute illness in schoolchildren is infection. Infections are a hazard not only to students, but also to their teachers. Understanding something of the nature of infectious diseases, how they are spread, and how they can be prevented is essential if teachers are to minimize the impact of infections on their students and themselves.

Managing illness in children requires the coordinated efforts of children, parents, teachers, physicians, and public health professionals. The purpose of this chapter is to provide information to help teachers manage infections in the classroom. Although this chapter provides guidelines, it is not meant to make teachers into doctors or nurses. A list of suggested reading materials is included at the end of the chapter for teachers who wish to read more about infectious diseases and their prevention.

## SIGNS AND SYMPTOMS OF INFECTION

Most infections begin with one or more of the following features:

- change in behavior
- runny nose, cough, wheezing, or rapid or labored breathing
- loss of appetite, vomiting, or diarrhea
- rash
- headache or muscle aches
- fever

Three of these symptoms that are common with many infections are discussed in the following sections.

## Change in Behavior

Assessment of behavior is the key to determining how serious any illness is. A child who is alert, responsive, and active is not likely to have a serious illness. Changes in behavior such as lethargy or unusual sleepiness, irritability, and difficulty breathing are signs suggesting a more serious illness and the need to be seen by a physician as soon as possible.

## Rash

Because there are many causes of rashes, identification often requires an examination by a physician. Children who develop a rash in association with fever or a change in behavior should be seen by a nurse or physician.

## Fever

Body temperature varies during the day, cycling from a low in the early morning (2:00 to 4:00 A.M.) to a peak in the late afternoon (4:00 to 6:00 P.M.). The difference between the minimum and maximum temperature is usually 1°F (0.5°C) or more. Body temperature increases as a result of overdressing, exercise, or infection.

*Fever* is a body temperature above normal. Fever is present when an oral temperature is equal to or greater than 100.4°F (38.0°C) or a rectal temperature is equal to or greater than 101.3°F (38.5°C). The height of the fever does *not* correlate well with the severity of infection. The behavior of a child with an infection tells much more about the severity of illness than the amount of fever.

Fever is rarely dangerous. Fever is actually part of the body's defense against infection. Fever is a warning sign that infection may be present and it helps fight the infection. Fever must be extremely high (greater than 106.7°F or 41.5°C) to cause direct damage to the body.

Some children may develop a convulsion or seizure when their body temperature rises rapidly. One or more febrile convulsions occur in approximately 3% of normal children, almost always between 6 months and 6 years of age. Such convulsions do not cause brain damage or lead to epilepsy in later childhood.

# RESPIRATORY INFECTIONS

## Common Cold

Most children have several colds every year. A healthy child may have 8 to 10 colds per year between 1 and 10 years of age. The frequency of colds decreases slowly during adolescence to the adult average of 4 to 5 per year. Almost all colds are caused by viruses. One reason that colds are so common is that over 200 different viruses have been identified that are capable of causing colds in humans. Moreover, many cold viruses do not stimulate long-lasting immunity, so reinfections can occur many times with the same virus.

A viral cold may produce one or more of the following signs of damage to the respiratory tract: runny nose, sore throat, hoarseness, coughing, and sneezing. More general symptoms are often present, including fever, loss of appetite, aches in the muscles, and headache. In a viral infection, the nasal discharge usually is clear and colorless at first, but often becomes yellow or green within a day or two. The color change is not a sign of a more serious infection, but reflects the changes caused by the viral damage to the lining of the nose. A runny nose due to a cold should clear within 5 to 7 days. If it lasts more than 7 days, the child should be seen by a doctor to check for a sinus infection.

Although a cough is often thought to indicate infection or other disease of the lungs, coughing can result from irritation anywhere in the respiratory tract, from the nose to the lungs. Causes of coughing include infection, allergy, asthma, chemical irritation (especially cigarette smoke), a variety of chronic diseases of the lungs (e.g., cystic fibrosis), and habit. Children learn at an early age that coughing is an excellent attention-getting device.

Antibiotics should not be used to treat colds. Antibiotics do not help the child to get better sooner and do not prevent complications. Excessive use of antibiotics, especially to treat viral colds, has resulted in marked increases in the occurrence of bacteria that are resistant to common antibiotics. Most viral colds get better without any treatment within a week or less. Complications of colds include bacterial infections of the ears (otitis), sinuses (sinusitis), or lungs (pneumonia). Antibiotics are used to treat these complications.

Colds are common not only because of the large number of viruses, but also because the viruses spread easily from person to person. During a cold, the virus is present in nasal secretions and saliva and is released into the air when people cough, sneeze, or blow their noses. If the droplets land in the nose or eye of or are inhaled by a nearby person, a new infection may occur. The virus can also be spread when someone wipes a runny nose, gets nasal secretions on the fingers, and touches someone or something else. Although viruses do not multiply outside the body, they may survive for several hours on toys or furniture and infect another person who touches the contaminated object.

It is almost impossible to stop the spread of cold viruses. Children may have very mild or no symptoms but still may be contagious. The virus is often present and transmissible before the child becomes ill. Because children in school are in close contact with each other, colds spread very easily.

## Influenza

*Influenza* is the term used for infections caused by the influenza virus. Influenza occurs as an epidemic every year some time between November and March. The size of the outbreaks varies widely from year to year, depending on the proportion of people who have developed immunity to the strains of virus in circulation, and on whether new strains have appeared that are able to evade immune defenses.

The typical case of influenza begins very abruptly with fever, sore throat, headache, pain in all muscles, and cough. The illness lasts for 3 to 7 days. The spectrum of illness caused by influenza viruses ranges from asymptomatic infection to an ordinary cold to full-blown flu to fatal pneumonia. At particularly high risk of severe illness and complications are persons over 65 years of age and anyone, regardless of age, with chronic heart or lung disease.

Influenza is highly contagious. The virus spreads rapidly because the incubation period is very short, 1 to 2 days, and because infected persons excrete large quantities of virus whenever they cough or sneeze, symptoms that are very common in this infection. Most outbreaks begin among schoolchildren, who spread it to the rest of the community. A sure sign of an influenza epidemic is a sudden increase in school absentee rates to over 10%.

Influenza vaccine is very effective in reducing the severity of illness in the elderly and others at increased risk of complications. Because its protection does not last much more than 1 year, annual boosters are required to maintain immunity. Because the influenza virus has the ability to change over time, new strains must be identified rapidly, so that the strains used to make the vaccine match those that are causing infections.

Because of the short duration of immunity and the need for annual boosters, routine immunization of children and healthy adults is not recommended. Although such vaccination programs might reduce the number of illnesses caused by influenza, they would not have a significant impact on the total number of respiratory infections in schoolchildren, due to the many other viruses that cause illnesses similar to influenza.

## Strep Throat

Strep throat is an infection of the throat, tonsils, and lymph nodes in the neck caused by a bacteria called Group A *Streptococcus pyogenes*. These infections are more common in primary schoolchildren than at any other age.

The illness associated with Group A strep occurs in a wide range of severity, from asymptomatic infection to sore throat without fever to sore throat with high fever, enlarged tonsils, and swollen tender lymph nodes in the neck. Some strains of strep produce a toxin during the course of infection that damages small blood vessels in the skin, resulting in the rash of scarlet fever. Although very rare, strains of strep also can produce toxins that cause more severe damage throughout the body, resulting in a very severe, rapidly fatal illness with shock and failure of multiple organs. Two complications of Group A strep infections may occur a week or more after the acute illness: acute rheumatic fever (a disease affecting the heart and joints) and acute glomerulonephritis (acute inflammation of the kidneys). Group A strep also can cause infections of the skin (impetigo, cellulitis), ears, blood stream (bacteremia), and lungs (pneumonia).

It is not possible to make a diagnosis of strep throat by looking at the throat. A swab of the throat must be taken to detect Group A strep either by a rapid test or an overnight culture. Treatment of strep throats and other strep infections with penicillin, an antibiotic, shortens the duration of the illness and prevents rheumatic fever. Such treatment, however, is not effective in preventing acute glomerulonephritis. For treatment to be effective, the antibiotic must be taken orally for 10 days.

## Bronchitis and Pneumonia

Bronchitis is an infection of the large airways (bronchi) which carry air from the windpipe (trachea) to the airspaces (alveoli). Bronchitis is characterized by symptoms of a cold, complicated with more severe or frequent coughing and often with fever. Pneumonia is an infection of the airways and small airspaces of the lung. It is more severe than bronchitis. Because of the inflammation of the airways and airspaces, it becomes more difficult for the person to move air in and out of the lungs, so that the person breathes more rapidly and must work harder to breathe.

Both bronchitis and pneumonia are most common in the first 2 years of life, but they can occur at any age. Both infections are most frequently caused by viruses. Cigarette smoke, however, greatly increases the risk of bronchitis or pneumonia as a complication of a cold in infants and children whose parents smoke in the home, as well as in smokers of all ages.

Pneumonia may also be caused by bacteria, especially the pneumococcus (*Streptococcus pneumoniae*) and mycoplasma (*Mycoplasma pneumoniae* and *Chlamydia pneumoniae*). Bacterial pneumonia is treated with antibiotics. Hospitalization may be required, especially if the child is so sick that he or she requires oxygen and medication by intravenous injection. The pathogens causing pneumonia are spread in the same way as those causing the common cold. Fortunately, pneumonia is not a common complication of a cold.

## Pertussis (Whooping Cough)

Pertussis, or whooping cough, is a bacterial infection of the nose and bronchi (large airways). It is commonly thought of as a disease of infants and young children, but in fact it occurs quite frequently in schoolchildren, adolescents, and young adults. Outbreaks of pertussis occasionally occur in schools, especially in the 12- to 18-year age group. It is most severe and most likely to cause complications, including brain damage and death, in infants younger than 6 months.

Pertussis begins as a profuse runny nose and cough. The attacks of coughing become increasingly more frequent and severe. During the paroxysm of coughing, the child cannot take a breath and often gets blue in the face. The illness lasts for 6 to 10 weeks. In older children and adults, complications are extremely rare, but the cough is very troublesome because of its paroxysmal nature and prolonged duration. Antibiotic treatment may shorten the duration of coughing, but only if treatment is started in the first week of illness.

Pertussis vaccine, which is recommended for all children, is given in the form of a combined vaccine containing diphtheria toxoid (D), acellular pertussis vaccine (aP), and tetanus toxoid (T). DaPT vaccine is administered at 2, 4, 6, and 18 months and at 4 to 6 years of age. The new acellular pertussis vaccine is composed of five different proteins isolated in purified form from the pertussis bacteria. Unlike the original pertussis vaccine made from killed whole bacteria, the new acellular pertussis vaccine can be given to adolescents and adults because severe reactions are rare at all ages. The vaccine is much more effective in reducing the severity of illness than in preventing infection. It reduces the risk of infection with pertussis bacteria by about 85%, and reduces the risk of severe illness by over 90%. Some authorities have recommended routine boosters in adolescents with the new vaccine to reduce outbreaks in schools and to prevent spread to young infants less than 6 months of age who may not have been fully immunized.

Pertussis is very contagious because the infected child releases a large number of bacteria into the surrounding air through coughing. The contagious period lasts from the start of the runny nose until 3 weeks after the start of coughing spells. Antibiotic treatment eradicates the pertussis bacteria and renders the child noncontagious, even if it does not relieve the coughing.

## Pinkeye (Conjunctivitis)

Pinkeye, or conjunctivitis, is an infection of the covering of the eye (conjunctiva) and eyelids. It is most often caused by a virus (one of the many cold viruses), but may be caused by bacteria. It also may be caused by exposure to chemicals, smoke, or injury. Symptoms of pinkeye include a scratchy sensation or pain in the eye and excessive tears. The conjunctiva of the eye and eyelids appears red because the blood vessels are inflamed and dilated. If the infection is caused by bacteria, pus or yellow discharge will be present. Conjunctivitis is easily spread from person to person, especially when caused by a virus. The infection spreads in the same way as a common cold.

# INFECTIONS OF THE GASTROINTESTINAL TRACT

Diarrhea is the second most frequent infection of childhood after the common cold and other respiratory infections. Diarrhea means an increase above normal in the frequency of bowel movements or a change in consistency of stool to unformed or watery. Infection is only one of many causes of diarrhea. Diarrhea can be dangerous if the loss of fluid in the stool exceeds the amount the child drinks, resulting in dehydration and shock.

Most infectious diarrheas are caused by viruses, such as rotavirus, torovirus, adenovirus, and many others. Such infections are very contagious because enormous numbers of viral particles are excreted in the watery stool. Many of the viruses are extremely stable and survive for long periods in the environment.

Other infectious diarrheas are caused by bacteria such as *Campylobacter, Salmonella, Shigella,* and *Escherichia coli* (*E. coli*). Bacterial diarrheas tend to be more severe than viral diarrheas, producing fever, abdominal pain, cramps, and sufficient damage to the lining of the intestines to cause blood in the stool. One strain of *E. coli* (designated 0157H7) produces a toxin that can cause damage to blood vessels throughout the body, especially in the kidneys. This illness, called the hemolytic uremic syndrome, is much more common in children than in adults.

Diarrhea spreads in two ways: directly from person to person, especially if personal hygiene is poor (as in toddlers still in diapers), and indirectly when food or water is contaminated with stool containing the pathogens. Proper hand washing before eating or preparing food and after going to the toilet is an essential barrier to the spread of pathogens causing diarrhea. In addition, proper cooking of chicken, turkey, eggs, beef, and pork is essential, because many animals are infected with strains of bacteria that can cause disease in humans.

# INFECTIONS OF THE SKIN
# AND SCALP

## Herpes Simplex (Cold Sores)

There are two types of Herpes simplex virus (HSV): HSV 1 and HSV 2. Infections with HSV 1 usually involve the mouth and lips and are spread from person to person by direct contact with saliva containing the virus or by contact with the lesions. Infections with HSV 2 usually involve the genital tract and are spread through sexual contact.

The first infection with HSV 1 usually takes place in childhood and often occurs without any symptoms. A few children will suffer a more severe illness, with many painful ulcers throughout the mouth and high fever. Because of the pain, the child may not be able to eat or drink. Treatment with a medicine called acyclovir appears to shorten the duration of such infections.

Once HSV enters the body, it produces a lifelong infection. The virus survives in nerve cells near the spinal cord and may become active again at any time. Some people get recurrent attacks of cold sores (vesicles or blisters) on and around the lips with HSV 1 or in the genital area with HSV 2. The frequency of attacks, number of lesions, and intensity of pain vary greatly from person to person.

Because transmission of HSV 1 and HSV 2 requires close physical contact, spread of the virus is not very common in the school setting. Children or staff with cold sores do not have to be excluded, but should use good personal hygiene.

## Head Lice

Head lice cause panic, alarm, and uproar among parents, teachers, and health departments, but rarely bother the child infested with them. Head lice are common in children and are not caused by lack of hygiene or cleanliness. Head lice are not a medical problem, as they do not spread any disease.

Head lice are insects that live on the scalp. Their eggs (nits) are tightly attached to the hair shaft. The nits are whitish-gray or tan specks about the size of a grain of sand. They are so firmly glued to the hair that it is difficult to remove them. Most children with lice have no symptoms. Some may have itching because of an allergic reaction to the bites. Head lice spread from person to person by direct contact between children, or through contaminated objects such as hats, combs, or hairbrushes. Head lice cannot fly or jump. The most effective treatment of head lice is a cream rinse containing a synthetic insecticide called permethrin. It is very safe and effective because it kills both the lice and the eggs.

# GENERALIZED INFECTIONS WITH RASH

## Chicken Pox (Varicella)

Chicken pox is a very common childhood infection. Approximately 95% of children have had it by 18 years of age. It is caused by the varicella-zoster virus.

Chicken pox is often mild in young children. It usually begins with fever and mild aches and pains for 1 to 2 days, followed by the rash. The rash begins as small red spots, which quickly become fluid-filled blisters. New spots appear for 2 to 3 days. Within a few days, the fluid becomes cloudy and the blisters dry up and form a crust. The rash may be very itchy, the symptom that causes the most distress to the child.

Chicken pox is more severe in adolescents and adults than in younger children. In adults, the rash is more extensive, the fever is higher, and the illness lasts longer. Complications of chicken pox include pneumonia, secondary bacterial skin infections, and encephalitis (inflammation of the brain). These complications are rare, but are more common in adults than in children.

Varicella-zoster virus, like herpes simplex virus, survives in the body in an inactive or latent form within nerve cells. Reactivation of the latent virus results in an attack of shingles or zoster, a rash similar in appearance to that of chicken pox, but occurring only in a localized area of skin.

Chicken pox is highly contagious and is spread very easily from person to person. A child with chicken pox is contagious 1 to 2 days before the onset of rash. Once the rash appears, contagiousness decreases rapidly, so the child is no longer contagious 5 days after the appearance of the rash. Because the spread of chicken pox usually occurs during the 1 to 2 days before the rash appears, excluding children from school after the rash develops is not very effective in preventing the spread of chicken pox. Both the American Academy of Pediatrics (1994) and the Canadian Pediatric Society (1992) recommend that if a child has a mild illness and feels well enough to take part in normal activities, the child can continue to attend school rather than be excluded.

A chicken pox vaccine has been available for several years. It is very safe in infants, children, and adults and very effective in preventing chicken pox. The vaccine's effectiveness is between 71% and 100% against disease of any severity and 95% and 100% against moderate and severe cases (Galil et al., 2002). It is recommended for all children on or shortly after their first birthday. Older children and adults who have never had chicken pox should also be vaccinated, because chicken pox is much more severe in adolescents and adults than in young children.

## Fifth Disease (Erythema Infectiosum)

Fifth disease, also known as *Erythema infectiosum,* is an infection caused by parvovirus B19. Many children do not develop any illness after infection with this virus, although some have mild fever, aches and pains, and a distinctive rash. Outbreaks of Fifth disease occur in primary school-age children. The rash starts as a bright red rash on the cheeks that looks as if the child's cheeks have been slapped. After 1 to 4 days, a lacelike rash appears on the arms and body. This rash may come and go over the next few weeks. If a child with sickle cell disease or certain other forms of chronic anemia is infected with parvovirus B19, the anemia may suddenly get much worse.

As with many viruses, parvovirus infection is more severe in adults than in children, causing more prolonged fever and joint pain. If a pregnant woman becomes infected with parvovirus B19, there is a small risk that the fetus may also become infected. The virus does not cause malformations, but may produce a severe anemia in the fetus, which may cause death of the baby.

Most adults were infected with this virus in childhood. Immunity is lifelong; thus, adults will not be infected again if exposed to a child with Fifth disease. A blood test is now available to determine whether one is immune to the infection.

Parvovirus spreads from person to person like other respiratory viruses. Contagiousness occurs during the mild illness before the rash appears. Once the rash develops, it indicates that immunity to the virus has developed.

Children with the rash are no longer contagious and do not have to be excluded from school.

## Measles

Measles is now uncommon due to the success of routine immunization. The measles virus causes a serious illness, with high fever, runny nose, conjunctivitis, and cough for a few days before onset of the rash. The illness lasts for 7 to 10 days, even without complications. The most common complications, occurring in 10% to 15% of cases, are bacterial infections such as ear infections or pneumonia. The most serious complication is encephalitis (inflammation of the brain), which affects 1 out of every 1,000 cases. Approximately one third of children with encephalitis die and another one third sustain permanent brain damage. As with many viral infections, the disease is more severe in adults than in children.

Measles is the most contagious of all childhood infections. It spreads very readily from person to person because large amounts of virus are shed into the air by coughing and sneezing. The virus can survive in the air for several hours. Because the person with measles is contagious for 3 to 5 days before the rash starts and the disease is recognized, it is difficult to prevent its spread.

The measles vaccine is usually administered as a combined vaccine containing measles, mumps, and rubella (MMR) vaccines to all children between 12 to 15 months of age and again before school entry at 4 to 6 years of age. The success of the two-dose measles vaccine program has led to the halt of transmission of measles in most of Canada and the United States. Most cases occurring in these countries are the result of travelers bringing measles back with them after being infected during a trip. Because measles is so contagious and because the vaccine is not 100% effective, it is extremely important to notify public health authorities whenever a case of measles is suspected so that the diagnosis can be confirmed and control measures instituted.

## Rubella (German Measles)

Rubella, like measles, has also become rare due to routine immunization with MMR. Unlike measles, the rubella virus usually causes only a mild illness in children. Indeed, many children are infected without having any symptoms. The illness most often consists of a low fever, swelling of the lymph glands, and a rash with small red spots. Complications are uncommon in children. Rubella spreads from person to person through airborne droplets containing the virus. Infected persons are contagious from a few days before until 5 to 7 days after the rash appears.

Rubella causes a more severe illness in adults, with fever, sore throat, headache, and muscle pain. Almost one half of adult women develop joint pain or arthritis after rubella, which, in rare cases, may progress to chronic arthritis.

The rubella virus causes very severe problems if it occurs in a pregnant woman during the first 3 months of pregnancy. The virus crosses the placenta and infects the fetus, causing serious damage in most babies, including malformations of the brain, eyes, ears, heart, and other organs. More than three fourths of infected fetuses are seriously damaged, and many die before birth.

The major purpose of routine vaccination of all children with rubella vaccine is to prevent spread of the virus in the community so that pregnant women are not exposed. All women should be tested for immunity to rubella before becoming pregnant and be vaccinated if susceptible. The rubella vaccine is very safe in childhood, but can cause joint pain and, rarely, chronic arthritis in adult women, but it does so much less frequently than the natural infection.

# INFECTIONS SPREAD BY CONTACT WITH BLOOD

## Hepatitis B

The hepatitis B virus (HBV) infects the liver. During the infection, the virus is present in the liver, blood, and certain body fluids such as semen, cervical secretions, breast milk, and saliva. Infection with HBV can result in illnesses with a wide range of severity. Many people have no symptoms after infection, whereas others have sufficient damage to the liver that they develop fever, nausea, vomiting, loss of appetite, fatigue, and jaundice (yellow color in skin). Most people recover completely from the acute infection and are immune for life. Others develop chronic infection of the liver, which may lead to chronic liver disease (chronic hepatitis), scarring of the liver (cirrhosis), or cancer of the liver.

The risk of chronic infection varies with age. Newborn infants born to mothers infected with HBV have the greatest risk; about 90% of infected newborns develop chronic infection. The risk of chronic infection falls to about 30% if the virus is acquired at 3 years of age and to approximately 10% in older children and adults.

HBV is spread by direct contact with blood or bloody body fluids containing the virus. HBV is rarely spread by transfusion of blood or blood products any longer because all blood is now tested before it is used. HBV is not spread by air, food, or water and it is not present in urine or stool. The major means of spread are the following:

1. Directly from one person to another
   • by sexual intercourse
   • from an infected mother to baby before or during delivery
   • through direct, intimate physical contact with infected infant or young child

2. Indirectly by exposure to infected blood or bloody body fluids
   • by sharing needles used for intravenous drug abuse
   • by penetrating injuries such as bites

The major routes of HBV spread in the United States and Canada are through sexual intercourse and through sharing of needles during illicit drug use. Spread from infants and young children to persons in close contact with them can occur, but is uncommon. Transmission of HBV from teachers to children has never been documented in a school setting; however, transmission from an infected child to other students or teachers can occur, although it is uncommon. Spread of HBV from an infected child to another person requires three conditions to be present: high infectivity of the child; release of virus from the child as a result of bleeding, trauma, or biting; and a means of entry into another person by injury or through an open skin lesion.

Hepatitis B infection can be prevented. A very safe and effective vaccine is available. Routine vaccination of all children is recommended in the United States and Canada because it is the only way to prevent the severe consequences of chronic hepatitis B. The economic costs of chronic hepatitis B disease are so great that large savings will result by vaccinating all children.

In addition to vaccination, all pregnant women should have a blood test to determine if they have chronic infection with hepatitis B. If a mother is infected, then the newborn infant can be protected by administration of special immunoglobulin immediately after birth and by vaccination started in the first week after birth. Such a program protects at least 95% of such infants against acquiring hepatitis B from their mothers.

## HIV and AIDS

Human immunodeficiency virus (HIV) is the cause of acquired immune deficiency syndrome (AIDS), a condition in which the immune system is destroyed as a result of the viral infection. The infected person becomes unusually susceptible to infections; may develop certain forms of cancer; and may suffer direct damage to the brain, lungs, and other organs from HIV itself (see Chapter 22).

HIV is *not* very contagious. It does not spread as a result of ordinary contact in the home or school. Spread of HIV occurs in the following ways:

- through intimate physical contact such as sexual intercourse

- from direct contact with contaminated blood by sharing needles while taking illegal drugs

- from an infected pregnant mother to her baby before or during birth or by breast feeding

HIV does not penetrate the intact skin. Because all blood donors are now screened for infection with HIV, the risk of acquiring HIV infection from transfusions of blood or blood products in the United States is extremely small. HIV is much less contagious than hepatitis B; spread between persons requires direct, intimate physical contact. No infections with HIV have been documented to have occurred as a result of ordinary contacts at school. Even within families with a member infected with HIV, spread by means other than sexual intercourse has been extremely rare.

# SEXUALLY TRANSMITTED DISEASES

In addition to hepatitis B and HIV, discussed in the previous section, several other infections are spread by sexual activity, especially unprotected sex. Some of these infections are becoming increasingly more frequent among sexually active adolescents, including gonorrhea, chlamydia infections, genital herpes, and genital warts caused by human papillomavirus. Although the school is usually not the location where such infections are transmitted, the school can play a vital role in the prevention of sexually transmitted diseases, if effective sex education programs are made part of the curriculum.

# INFECTIONS AS POTENTIAL OCCUPATIONAL HAZARDS TO TEACHERS

## Colds and Other Viral Respiratory Infections

Teachers cannot avoid frequent exposure to respiratory viruses because of the high rate of colds and similar infections in school-age children. Moreover, other than influenza, no vaccines are available for these viruses. Therefore, teachers probably suffer more colds than other adults. Fortunately, these infections tend to be milder in adults than in children. The only means to reduce the risk of acquiring a cold from a child is thorough careful hand washing after direct contact with nasal secretions, such as after wiping a child's nose.

## Pertussis

Adults do get pertussis or whooping cough. The protection afforded by the pertussis vaccine administered to infants and young children wears off after 3 to 5 years. Therefore, whenever there is an outbreak of pertussis in schoolchildren, teachers are frequently infected. Although pertussis can cause a prolonged cough, lasting for weeks, complications are rare in adults. The new acellular pertussis vaccine is safe and produces high concentrations of protective antibodies when given as a booster to adults. Teachers may want to consider receiving a booster to be protected against pertussis.

## Chicken Pox

More than 90% of adults are immune to chicken pox as a result of infection during childhood. This is fortunate, because chicken pox is much more severe in adults than in children: The rash is more extensive, fever is higher and longer lasting, and complications are more common. A history of having had chicken pox is a reliable predictor of immunity. Most adults who do not know whether they had chicken pox are also likely to be immune, because chicken pox can be so mild in early childhood that it is not recognized. Susceptibility to chicken pox can be determined by a blood test to detect antibodies against chicken pox.

The peak attack rate of chicken pox is in children 5 to 9 years of age. Chicken pox is very contagious, so that up to 50% of susceptible children in a classroom will be infected. Chicken pox is an occupational hazard only for those teachers who did not have chicken pox in childhood.

Chicken pox is a potentially serious problem if it occurs in a pregnant woman. If the infection occurs during the first 20 weeks of pregnancy, there is about a 2% risk of serious damage to the fetus, including low birth weight, skin scars, impaired growth of limbs, eye damage, and brain damage. If the fetus is infected after 20 weeks of pregnancy, there is no increased risk of damage, but the baby may develop shingles during infancy or early childhood.

If a pregnant woman develops chicken pox from 5 days before to 2 days after delivery, there is a risk of very severe chicken pox in the newborn. It is standard practice under such circumstances to administer varicella zoster immunoglobulin (VZIG) to the newborn as soon as possible after birth. VZIG, a preparation of immune globulin containing large amounts of antibody against chicken pox, is very effective in reducing the severity of the illness in newborns.

If a pregnant teacher is exposed to chicken pox, she should check with her physician immediately. If she had chicken pox in childhood, she is immune and there is no risk to the fetus. If uncertain about her history of chicken pox, a blood test should be drawn right away to determine whether she is susceptible. If she is susceptible, VZIG can be administered to reduce the risk of severe disease in the mother. It is not known whether VZIG will protect the fetus. All teachers who have never had chicken pox should receive the chicken pox vaccine to reduce their risk of illness when exposed to children with chicken pox.

## Parvovirus B19

Children with parvovirus infection are contagious during the mild illness before the rash appears. Therefore, children with rash do not have to be excluded from school. Approximately 50% of adults are immune to parvovirus because of prior infection. During school outbreaks, the risk of a teacher becoming infected is about 20%. If the teacher is susceptible and pregnant, there is approximately a 10% risk of the fetus becoming infected and developing severe anemia. Therefore, the overall risk of a fetus having a problem as a result of exposure of the mother (a pregnant teacher) to parvovirus during a school outbreak is equal to the product of the probability of susceptibility times the probability of infection times the probability of fetal illness, or 1% (50% × 20% × 10%).

Blood tests are available to determine immunity to parvovirus and to detect recent infection. If a pregnant teacher is exposed to a child with parvovirus infection, such tests should be performed. Evidence of anemia in the fetus can be detected by ultrasound examinations. If such anemia does occur and is severe, blood transfusions can be administered to the fetus in the uterus.

## Measles, Mumps, and Rubella

Even though measles, mumps, and rubella are now uncommon in school children because of the success of the vaccine programs, all teachers should be protected against these infections. If immune status is not known, blood tests can be performed to test susceptibility and the vaccine can be administered if the teacher is found to be susceptible.

## Hepatitis B and HIV

Transmission of hepatitis B virus in the school setting from a child to another child or to a teacher has occurred, but the risk is very small. Transmission of HIV in the school setting has never been reported in North America. Nevertheless, because of the potential severity of infection with these viruses, it is appropriate for all teachers to follow recommended infection control practices whenever there is the possibility of exposure to blood. Hepatitis B virus and HIV do not penetrate through normal skin.

Nevertheless, whenever dealing with a child who is bleeding, it is appropriate to use disposable plastic or latex gloves to minimize direct exposure to blood. When the situation is under control, the teacher should remove the gloves and wash his or her hands carefully.

Because the risk of spread in the school setting is so small, vaccination of teachers with hepatitis B vaccine is not routinely recommended. Universal vaccination of all children is recommended in both the United States and Canada. Once vaccination programs have been fully implemented, the possibility of spread of hepatitis B virus in schools will be reduced below the already very low risk.

## SUGGESTED READING

American Academy of Pediatrics. (1994). *School health: Policy and practice* (5th ed.). Elk Grove, IL: American Academy of Pediatrics.

American Academy of Pediatrics & American Public Health Association. (1992). *Caring for our children: National health and safety performance standards—Guidelines for out-of-home child care programs*. Elk Grove, IL: American Academy of Pediatrics.

Canadian Paediatric Society. (1992). How to prevent illness. In *Well beings* (pp. 45–114). Toronto, Ontario, Canada: Creative Premises.

Canadian Paediatric Society. (1992). Managing illness. In *Well beings* (pp. 119–201). Toronto, Ontario, Canada: Creative Premises.

Canadian Paediatric Society. (1997). *Your child's best shot—A parent's guide to vaccination.* Ottawa, Ontario: Canadian Paediatric Society.

Galil, K., Lee, B., Strine, T., Carraher, C., Baughman, A. L., Eaton, M., Montero, J., & Seward, J. (2002). Outbreak of varicella at a day-care despite vaccination. *New England Journal of Medicine, 347,* 1909–1915.

Offit, P. A., & Bell, L. M. (1999). *Vaccines: What every parent should know* (rev. ed.). New York: IDG Books.

# CHAPTER 4

# Growth, Development, and Endocrine Disorders

Denis Daneman

**G**rowth is a complex process that involves the interrelated effects of genetic, environmental, nutritional, hormonal, and psychological factors. Physical growth encompasses changes in the size and function of the organism and begins in utero. Both intellectual and emotional growth begin at birth and are dependent on normal neurological and behavioral maturation and on healthy family and peer relationships. From conception to adolescence, growth proceeds in biologically determined cycles that fall into five distinct periods:

1. Intrauterine growth, including organ development and function

2. Early infancy—rapid growth from birth to 2 years of age

3. Childhood—slower growth from 2 years of age to the onset of puberty

4. The rapid pubertal growth spurt up to ages 14 to 16 (earlier in girls than boys)

5. A sharp deceleration to maturity

These periods of physical growth are intertwined with predictable cycles of social and developmental growth in such a way that problems in one may have a profound effect on the other. (Figure 4.1 depicts the normal postnatal growth patterns in boys and girls from birth to age 19.)

Problems in growth and development can be a major cause of concern and anxiety to children, adolescents, parents, and teachers. This chapter reviews the normal events of growth and development and indicates the common problems that may interfere with these. Other more common disorders

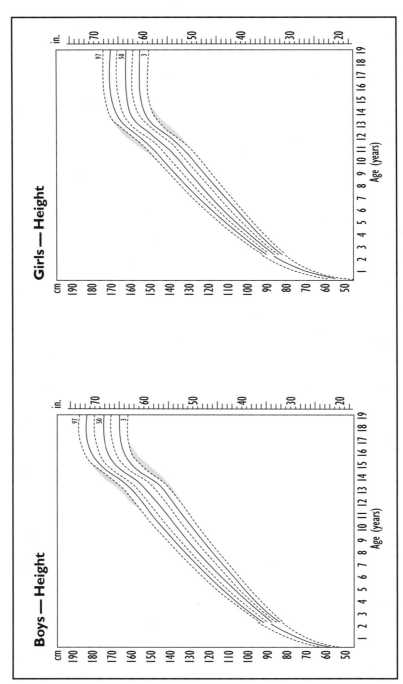

**FIGURE 4.1.** Growth charts for boys (left) and girls (right) from birth to age 19 years. *Note.* Adapted from "Clinical Longitudinal Standards for Height, Weight, Height Velocity, Weight Velocity and Stages of Puberty," by J. M. Tanner and R. H. Whitehouse, 1976, *Archives of Diseases of Children,* 51(3), pp. 170–179. Copyright 1976 by Castlemead Publications. Adapted with permission.

of the endocrine system are also discussed. A Suggested Reading list is provided at the end of the chapter for teachers who want to read more on the subject.

# PHYSICAL GROWTH

## The Fetus

Growth begins with the implantation of the fertilized egg in the mother's uterus and subsequent development of the placenta. Normal fetal growth depends on four primary factors:

1. the health and nutrition of the mother
2. the functional integrity of the placenta, the baby's lifeline
3. the size of the mother's uterus and pelvis
4. the potential for normal growth of the fertilized egg

Problems occurring during pregnancy in the mother (infections, chronic diseases, alcohol or drug abuse or use), in the placenta (e.g., vascular insufficiency), in the uterus or pelvis (e.g., small size, multiple pregnancies), or in the fetus itself (e.g., chromosomal abnormalities or malformation syndromes) can result in impaired intrauterine growth involving various body tissues and organs, including the brain. This, in turn, can lead to retarded physical, emotional, or intellectual growth both in utero and following birth. Birth injury (e.g., birth trauma, lack of oxygen to the baby's brain) can also result in permanent damage to physical or mental growth.

Just as the hypothalamus and pituitary gland, both located in the brain, act as the master control system in the hormonal regulation of growth in the child and adolescent, so does the placenta control growth in the fetus. Its function is dependent on a healthy nutrient supply from the mother. The placenta secretes a series of messenger hormones, such as placental lactogen, that are capable of stimulating the production of growth-promoting factors in the fetus. These factors, released from organs such as the liver, along with insulin from the fetal pancreas, play a major role in overall fetal cell division and cell growth and differentiation. Interestingly, fetal pituitary growth hormone and thyroid hormone do not exert major influences on intrauterine growth. These hormones, however, become extremely important for normal growth after birth. Disturbances in early pregnancy will interfere with cell division, limiting the number of cells that develop and the potential for catch-up growth after birth. On the other hand, problems occurring later in pregnancy may interfere with cell size rather than cell number. These later children, although small at birth, are likely to show catch-up growth after birth once the problem has been removed.

## Extrauterine Growth

### Genes

It has long been recognized that growth is closely linked to heredity. This is seen not only in families, where children tend to show patterns of growth similar to their parents, but also in ethnic, tribal, or racial groups, such as in the African pygmies, whose short stature is genetically determined.

Genes are biological units contained within the chromosomes that have the capacity to direct the synthesis of specific proteins. Thus, certain genes are important in the production of growth-promoting hormones; other genes govern the growth of the receptor tissue to which these hormones are directed. Thus, growth is determined not by a single gene, but rather by many genes working in concert (*polygenic inheritance*).

Both genetic errors that result in abnormal or decreased formation of growth-promoting hormones and those that interfere with receptor tissue growth can cause retarded development. Many types of growth failure, including hormonal disorders such as certain types of hypopituitarism (underactivity of the pituitary gland) and receptor problems such as achondroplasia, are due to genetic errors. Conversely, tall stature may be related to increased production of these hormones either on a genetic basis as occurs in certain races or, rarely, in an abnormal fashion (e.g., a growth hormone–producing tumor of the pituitary gland).

### Hormones

The term *hormone* is derived from the Greek *hormaein,* meaning "to set in motion." Hormones are chemical messengers produced in the endocrine glands of the body (e.g., pituitary gland, thyroid, pancreas, adrenal glands, ovaries, testes) that are secreted into the bloodstream and exert their influence by altering selected metabolic processes in their specific target organs. Hormones thus are key regulators of cell function.

The master endocrine gland is the pituitary, located in the brain just behind the eyes. It is regulated by the hypothalamus and neural influences and by blood levels of the circulating hormones such as thyroid hormone, estrogen, testosterone, insulin-like growth factor-1 (IGF-1), and cortisol. The pituitary secretes hormones that stimulate other endocrine glands such as the thyroid (located at the front of the neck), adrenal glands (which sit on top of each kidney), and ovaries in the female and testes in the male. In response to specific pituitary hormones, the thyroid gland secretes its hormone, thyroxine; the adrenal glands, cortisol; and the ovaries and testes, estrogen and testosterone, respectively. The adrenal glands also produce small amounts of androgens and estrogens. These hormones, in turn, exert their effects on specific target tissues throughout the body. The hormones important for growth include growth hormone; thyroid hormone; and the steroid hormones, including cortisol, androgens (male hormones), and estrogens (female hormones).

Growth hormone produced by the pituitary stimulates the liver and other tissues to produce insulin-like growth factor-1 (IGF-1), which stimulates growth of the long bones of the body. The pituitary also produces a hormone, antidiuretic hormone, important in maintaining water balance in the body. Indirectly, this hormone may also influence growth.

Two other endocrine glands are also important in growth: The pancreas, located next to the stomach, secretes insulin, a major regulator of energy metabolism, and the parathyroid glands, embedded in the back part of the thyroid, secrete parathormone, which is essential for calcium metabolism. Insulin, which is chemically similar to IGF-1, is an essential hormone for fetal growth but also plays a role postnatally. Calcium is critically important in bone growth and strength, factors controlled in part by parathormone.

Growth occurs by both cell division and cell enlargement. Growth hormone is an important regulator of cell division. Of the other growth-promoting hormones, thyroid hormone increases cell size, insulin increases cytoplasmic growth, and both, in concert with growth hormone and IGF-1, have an effect on cell division.

Long (e.g., arm and leg) bone growth requires cartilage formation and subsequent replacement of cartilage with calcified bone. IGF-1 is particularly important in cartilage formation, whereas thyroid hormone is more important in the replacement of cartilage with calcified bone. The sex hormones (androgens and estrogens) exert their influence on both processes.

Growth occurs mainly at the ends of the long bones, although some growth does occur in the spine. The child between the age of 3 and the onset of puberty should grow no less than 2 in. (4 to 5 cm) per year. During puberty, growth rates may increase to 3 to 5 in. (6 to 12 cm) per year. This increased growth rate is due to the combined effects of growth hormone, IGF-l, and the sex hormones.

## Puberty

Puberty is the stage of development during which sexual maturation occurs, leading to reproductive capability. Puberty is accompanied by changes in both physical growth and psychological perspective. The terms *puberty* and *adolescence* are used interchangeably.

At puberty, increased production of the hypothalamic hormone, luteinizing hormone-releasing hormone (LHRH), begins. LHRH stimulates production by the anterior pituitary of the two gonadotrophins, luteinizing hormone (LH) and follicle-stimulating hormone (FSH), which together control function of the gonads (ovaries in the females, testes in the male). FSH is important in ovulation in the female and sperm production in the male, whereas LH stimulates estrogen production in the female and testosterone production in the male. Through a feedback mechanism, the hormones produced from the ovaries and testes regulate production of LHRH, LH, and FSH (see Figure 4.2). Small amounts of male hormones, called androgens, are normally produced from the adrenal glands and ovaries of the female, whereas small amounts of the female hormone, estrogen, are produced in the adrenal glands and testes of the male.

In the adolescent female, ovarian estrogens stimulate growth of the uterus, its endometrial lining, and the vagina; influence fat deposition; and accelerate linear growth and skeletal maturation. Their secretion is important in reaching menarche (onset of menstrual periods). Androgens stimulate the growth of pubic and axillary hair and contribute to linear growth increase and advanced skeletal maturation. Androgens are also important in the development of the labia majora and clitoris. The mechanism by which adrenal androgens increase at puberty (called adrenarche) is unknown.

In the adolescent male, testosterone and other androgens stimulate growth of the penis and pubic, axillary, and body hair; accelerate growth rate and skeletal maturation; and increase the size and number of muscle cells. Increased amounts of estrogen in the pubertal male may cause transient en-

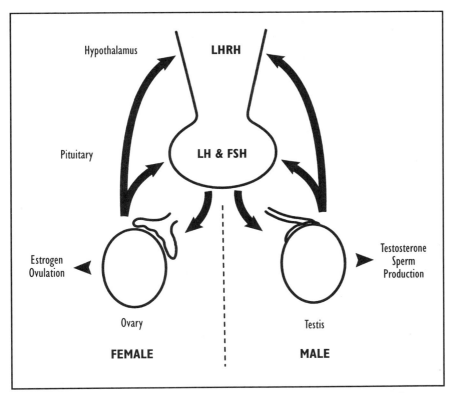

**FIGURE 4.2.** Diagrammatic representation of integrated function of the hypothalamic–pituitary–gonadal axis. At puberty, increasing amounts of luteinizing hormone-releasing hormone (LHRH) from the hypothalamus stimulates release from the pituitary of the gonadotrophins, luteinizing hormone (LH), and follicle-stimulating hormone (FSH). These, in turn, lead to release of the sex hormones—estrogen from the ovaries and testosterone from the testes—and production of the ova and sperm, respectively.

largement and tenderness of the breasts (*gynecomastia*). This occurs to some degree in the majority of pubertal males and generally regresses with time. If the breasts remain large or are slow to regress, it may cause considerable embarrassment to the teen, occasionally necessitating surgical reduction.

Androgens appear to exert a permanent organizing influence on the brain both before and during puberty in boys. Males deficient in androgen may have serious defects involving spatial ability and other specific cognitive skills.

The wide age range of the onset and progression of normal pubertal development often arouses fears of abnormality, self-consciousness, and anxiety about body image (see Figure 4.3). In girls, pubertal changes (usually starting with breast development) begin between ages 6 and 13½ years, with menarche on average about 2 years later (ages 8 to 15). A recent study in the United States found that the definition of early (precocious) puberty in girls needs to be revised given that changes are normal in African American girls as young as 6 and in White American girls as young as 7 years of age (Kaplowitz & Oberfield, 1999). In general, boys start 1 to 2 years after girls, with testicular enlargement beginning at ages 10 to 14. The growth spurt in boys occurs later in the pubertal process than that in girls. The earlier onset of puberty and more rapid growth spurt in females accounts for their taller stature in early adolescence but shorter adult height than in males. This leads to an average adult height in males (5 ft 9 in.) 5 in. taller than in females (5 ft 4 in.).

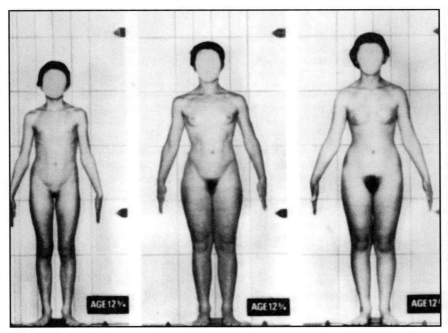

**FIGURE 4.3.** This picture illustrates the variation in normal sexual development in three girls of the same age (12¾ years). *Note.* From *Endocrine and Genetic Diseases of Childhood and Adolescence* (2nd ed., p. 28) by L. I. Gardner, 1975, Philadelphia: Saunders. Copyright 1975 by W. B. Saunders Co. Reprinted with permission.

# FACTORS AFFECTING GROWTH

## Nutrition and Disease

Nutrition has a major influence on both intrauterine and extrauterine growth. Poor nutrition can result in impairments in both physical and mental development. In fact, on a worldwide basis, malnutrition is the single most common cause of growth failure and short stature. Malnutrition, and specifically decreased protein intake, may be associated with very low IGF-1 levels and high growth hormone levels, suggesting that proper nutrition is an integral component of normal endocrine control. The growth failure associated with many chronic diseases may be the result of poor nutrition.

In females, one of the determining factors in the onset of puberty and achievement of menarche is the attainment of a critical body weight. Females who exercise excessively, such as long-distance runners, gymnasts, and ballerinas, may lose body fat and experience a cessation of menstrual function. Such events underscore the importance of good nutrition.

## Psychosocial Factors

Growth retardation; disturbances of intellectual, motor, and emotional development; and bizarre behavior have been observed in infants and children living in severely abnormal environments, particularly those devoid of parental love and support. In severe cases, these children may manifest retardation in height, weight, and skeletal maturation comparable to that seen in growth hormone deficiency (*hypopituitarism*). Motor and intellectual development may also be delayed, and these children may have a range of emotional responses from depressed and withdrawn to inappropriately affectionate. Abnormal feeding behaviors such as rumination, increased thirst, and obtaining food and drink from bizarre sources may also be observed.

The cause of the growth failure is uncertain but may relate to either malnutrition or disturbed growth hormone secretion. This condition, called psychosocial or emotional deprivation, emphasizes the importance of emotional stability in the process of normal growth and development. With removal from the depriving environment, catch-up growth will be observed. This may require removal of these children from their homes and placement in foster or group homes.

## Environmental Factors

Socioeconomic factors, such as poverty and poor hygiene, may be associated with poor nutrition and frequent acute or chronic infections, and consequent poor growth. Seasonal variations in growth rates have been observed in certain areas, with the greatest increases in height being seen in the spring and the lowest in the fall. Exercise promotes growth and strength of both muscle and bone. The prolonged use of drugs such as corticosteroids and stimulant medications for attention-deficit/hyperactivity disorder (e.g., methylphenidate, better known as Ritalin) may also result in growth failure.

# CAUSES FOR CONCERN

Linear growth, weight gain, and the onset and progression of puberty are good indicators of the general health and well-being of the child or teenager. All family physicians and pediatricians should maintain growth charts on the children they evaluate in their offices (see Figure 4.1). In this way, they will be able to detect more quickly the subtle changes in growth characteristics that may not otherwise be obvious.

In relation to delayed growth, teachers should become concerned about the child whose height shows any of the following characteristics:

- is increasing by less than 1½ to 2 in. (4 to 5 cm) a year

- is more that two standard deviations from the mean for age (i.e., below the lowest line on the growth charts)

- is "falling off" the percentile the height previously had been following

- is considerably shorter than would be expected based on the parents' heights

Problems of weight loss, or a weight that is disproportionately lower than height, should also be investigated.

With respect to puberty, girls should be evaluated if breast development occurs before age 6 years in African American girls and 7 in White American girls (a condition called precocious puberty) or if there is very rapid progression of pubertal development, and if there is no breast development by age 13½ (delayed adolescence), or if menstrual function has not begun by age 15 (primary amenorrhea). In boys, development of secondary sexual characteristics before age 9 or 10 or lack of development by age 14 should trigger an evaluation. In general, early puberty is more common in girls than boys, and delayed adolescence is more common in boys. In all of these growth disorders, the presence of other symptoms and signs (e.g., headaches, recent onset of visual disturbance, excessive weight gain with growth failure) should alert the physician, parents, and perhaps also school personnel to the possibility of a significant pathological problem.

# COMMON CAUSES
# OF GROWTH DELAY

## Normal Variants

Figure 4.4 depicts the numerous factors that may interfere with growth and physical development. The most frequent causes fall into the category of "normal variants":

- *Familial short stature:* In general, short parents tend to have short children.

- *Constitutional delay of growth or adolescence:* Some children, often called "late bloomers," will have a delay in their maturation, reaching their adolescence at a later than average age (see Figure 4.5). There is often a family predisposition to this pattern of growth, and it is much more common in boys than in girls.

These two situations are quite distinct. Children with familial short stature are healthy in all respects, and puberty is not delayed, leading to a short final adult height. In children who are constitutionally delayed, general health is also normal, but the onset of puberty is significantly delayed. These individuals will have a normal pubertal growth spurt and reach an adult height well within the normal range. In the prepubertal child, the way to distinguish between these two conditions is by performing a wrist X-ray to determine "bone age." In a child with familial short stature, bony

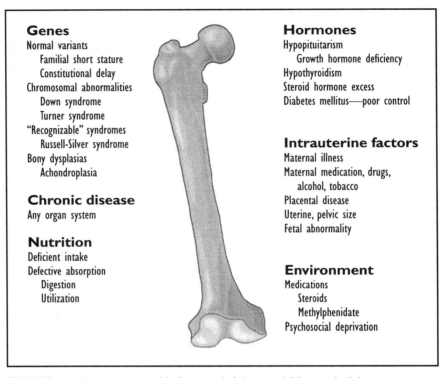

**Genes**
Normal variants
    Familial short stature
    Constitutional delay
Chromosomal abnormalities
    Down syndrome
    Turner syndrome
"Recognizable" syndromes
    Russell-Silver syndrome
Bony dysplasias
    Achondroplasia

**Chronic disease**
Any organ system

**Nutrition**
Deficient intake
Defective absorption
    Digestion
    Utilization

**Hormones**
Hypopituitarism
    Growth hormone deficiency
Hypothyroidism
Steroid hormone excess
Diabetes mellitus—poor control

**Intrauterine factors**
Maternal illness
Maternal medication, drugs,
    alcohol, tobacco
Placental disease
Uterine, pelvic size
Fetal abnormality

**Environment**
Medications
    Steroids
    Methylphenidate
Psychosocial deprivation

**FIGURE 4.4.** Factors responsible for growth failure in children and adolescents.

maturation is age appropriate, whereas in a child who is constitutionally delayed, the bone age is less than chronological age (see Figure 4.6). Thus, at any age, the child with constitutional delay will have greater remaining growth potential. These two conditions account for more than 80% of cases of short stature presented to the pediatrician or family physician. The remaining 20% or less will fall into one of the other categories described in the following section.

## Other Causes of Short Stature

Figure 4.7 illustrates some of the clinical characteristics of the less common causes of short stature. Many of these conditions are distinguished from the normal variants by a growth rate that is less than normal for age.

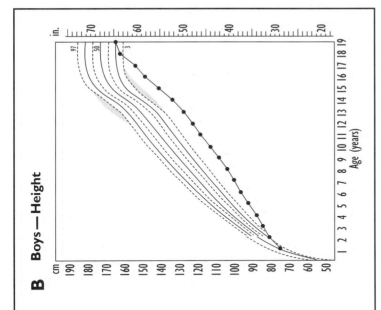

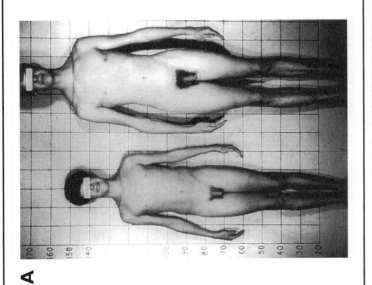

**FIGURE 4.5.** Constitutional delay of growth and adolescence in one of a fraternal twin pair. (A) At age 16 years, the brother on the left is shorter and has delayed puberty compared to his twin on the right. (B) Growth change of brother with delayed growth shows falloff in growth before age 3 years, followed by a normal growth rate throughout childhood and a delay in the onset of the pubertal growth spurt until after 16 years. Note that he does achieve a final adult height within the normal percentiles. *Note.* Growth chart adapted from "Clinical Longitudinal Standards for Height, Weight, Height Velocity, Weight Velocity and Stages of Puberty," by J. M. Tanner and R. H. Whitehouse, 1976, *Archives of Diseases of Children, 51*(3), pp. 170–179. Copyright 1976 by Castlemead Publications. Adapted with permission.

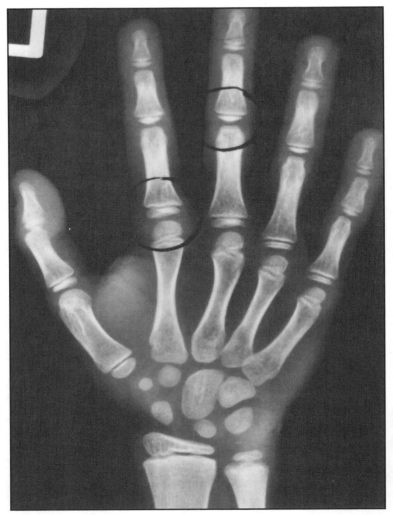

**FIGURE 4.6.** X-ray of the right hand. Circles outline growth centers (*epiphyses*), which are studied to determine bone age, here measured to be 7 years in a boy who is 11 years old.

## Intrauterine Growth Retardation

Any condition that interferes with the well-being of the developing fetus has the potential to limit intrauterine growth and diminish postnatal growth potential. The earlier in pregnancy that the insult occurs, the more

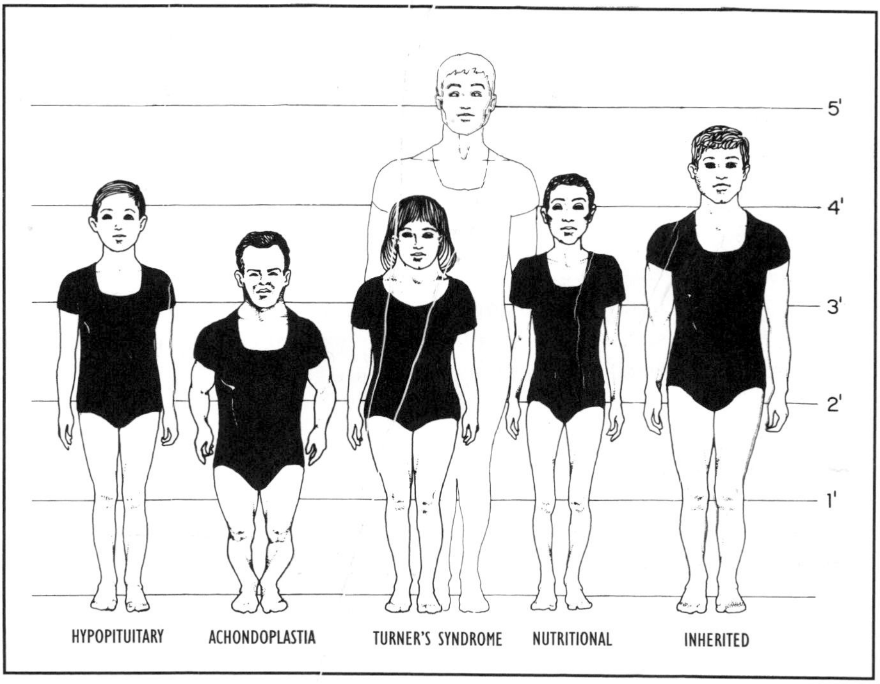

**FIGURE 4.7.** Several causes of short stature, illustrating the characteristic features and body proportions associated with each. All children are the same chronological age.

likely that the growth will be permanently diminished. Causes of intrauterine growth retardation include the following:

- maternal infection (e.g., toxoplasmosis, syphilis, rubella, cytomegalovirus, HIV, herpes virus)
- maternal illness (e.g., cardiac or renal disease, hypertension)
- maternal ingestion of medication that is teratogenic (e.g., phenytoin [Dilantin], thalidomide)
- maternal use of alcohol, tobacco, or illicit drugs during pregnancy
- small uterine or pelvic size
- a chromosomal abnormality (e.g., Down syndrome or Turner syndrome) or malformation syndrome (e.g., Russell-Silver syndrome)

Children with intrauterine growth retardation are distinguished by a birth weight more than two standard deviations below the mean for the gestational age (e.g., less than 2.5 kg at birth in a term infant). By age 2, the infant will usually have caught up to his or her ultimate growth curve. Those that remain low on the percentile charts at age 2 will likely have a permanent decrease in growth potential.

Chromosomal conditions may account for intrauterine growth retardation. Some children are born with either an extra chromosome (a condition called *trisomy*, such as Down syndrome) or a missing chromosome (*monosomy*, such as Turner syndrome). These conditions are inevitably associated with moderate to severe growth failure of uncertain cause. The growth failure generally starts in utero and is accentuated after birth. In addition to short stature, these children may exhibit other physical features that clue the physician to their diagnosis (see Chapter 7).

## Bony Dysplasias

Hereditary conditions that affect the growth of the long bones and spine will lead to disproportionate lack of growth of these bones (bony dysplasias). One of the most severe forms of bony dysplasia is achondroplasia, but less severe variants also occur. In these conditions, the trunk (chest and abdomen) is often normal in size, but the arms and legs are disproportionately short. In general, these conditions do not respond to hormonal therapy; however, techniques have been developed to lengthen the long bones and have successfully resulted in marked height increases in some of these children.

## Chronic Diseases

Any systemic disease of sufficient severity can interfere with physical growth and development. For example, diseases of the cardiovascular, respiratory, gastrointestinal, genitourinary, and neurological systems all have the potential to affect growth. Most of these disorders are fairly obvious by the time growth impairment becomes evident; however, a few disorders may be quite occult and yet interfere significantly with growth. These include malabsorption conditions of the small bowel, such as celiac disease or inflammatory bowel disease, or kidney conditions, such as undiagnosed kidney infections. Management of the underlying disorder will improve the growth potential, particularly if this occurs before the onset of puberty. In those chronic conditions that cannot be cured, such as chronic renal failure leading to dialysis, kidney transplantation, or both, final adult height may be significantly impaired.

Certain medications, such as glucocorticoids, steroids, or stimulant medications used for attention-deficit/hyperactivity disorder (ADHD), may also interfere with growth potential. It is best to maintain these medications at the lowest effective dose to control the underlying condition, hopefully thereby limiting the growth-retarding side effects.

## Malnutrition

Worldwide, malnutrition is far and away the most common cause of short stature. Reversal of the malnutrition at an early stage will allow normal growth potential; however, the later the malnourished state is corrected, the less likely the genetic height potential will be attained. In developed countries, malnutrition is often the result of abuse or neglect, other serious chronic illness, or occasionally fad or exclusion diets imposed on these children. Self-imposed malnutrition is an integral part of eating disorders such as anorexia nervosa. If this condition begins before puberty, it has the potential to impair growth (see Chapter 19). Some cases of growth failure have been reported in children, particularly boys, whose restricted caloric intake was due to the fear of obesity.

## Psychosocial Deprivation Syndrome

In some children, short stature is the result of severe psychosocial deprivation, a serious form of child abuse or neglect. This is an extremely difficult diagnosis to make, as the children often look similar to those with growth hormone deficiency. In fact, their growth hormone levels may be low at the time of initial assessment. They may also exhibit bizarre eating habits and behavior. In fact, many have been noted to drink from toilet bowls, eat dirt, and drink from puddles on the street (Powell, Brasel, & Blizzard, 1967). Removal of these children from the depriving environment usually leads to spectacular catch-up growth.

## Endocrine Disorders Leading to Growth Failure

Although hormones such as growth hormone, thyroid hormones, and steroid hormones play an essential role in growth and development, less than 10% of children with growth failure have a hormonal deficiency or excess. The more common hormonal conditions that interfere with growth are discussed here.

1. *Growth hormone deficiency:* Some children have isolated growth hormone deficiency or deficiency of multiple pituitary hormones (e.g., those that control the thyroid gland, pubertal development, and the adrenal gland). Although growth hormone deficiency may be an inherited or sporadic (*idiopathic*) disorder, it also may result from damage to the pituitary gland from tumors in this region or from irradiation of the head for treatment of malignant diseases (e.g., leukemia). These conditions require specialized testing and can be managed with replacement of the missing hormones. Growth hormone itself is given as a subcutaneous injection 6 to 7 days a week.

2. *Thyroid hormone deficiency:* Lack of sufficient production of the principal thyroid hormone, thyroxine, will lead to a multitude of symptoms (see the "Other Endocrine Disorders" section, later in this chapter), including growth failure. Hypothyroidism is most commonly a result of chronic thyroid inflammation (Hashimoto's thyroiditis) and can be managed by replacement doses of the missing hormone.

3. *Steroid hormone excess syndromes:* Growth will be impaired if the body is exposed to excessive amounts of the glucocorticoid hormones, either produced by the adrenal glands or used as medications (e.g., hydrocortisone, prednisone, dexamethasone) to control a number of systemic medical conditions (e.g., after organ transplantation to prevent rejection, for lupus erythematosus, and for other arthritides). These steroids may also have an impact on growth, although likely to a lesser degree, when used in the inhaled form for severe asthma or in the topical form for severe skin conditions. In all of these situations, physicians must carefully weigh the benefits of treatment with these agents against their potential side effects.

4. *Very poorly controlled diabetes mellitus:* In children with long-standing, poorly controlled diabetes mellitus, growth impairment may be seen. Improved metabolic control will invariably improve growth velocity.

# INVESTIGATION OF THE CHILD WITH SHORT STATURE

All short children deserve evaluation by their physician and referral to a specialist if necessary. The reasons for evaluation are twofold: (a) reassurance and counseling for those whose short stature is due to one of the normal variants or genetic syndromes and (b) management of those conditions amenable to hormonal or other therapy. Investigation will be more urgent in the slow-growing child than in one who is short but showing normal annual height increments (greater than 2 in. a year).

Short stature may have important social implications for children in the classroom. They may be singled out as different and have unpleasant epithets (e.g., "shrimp," "dwarf," "midget") hurled at them by their classmates. In addition, the child who is severely short may face additional difficulties in opening doors, reaching water fountains, and fighting the hustle and bustle around the school. Teachers may inadvertently stigmatize the short child by asking the class to line up according to size or by always choosing these children to do certain tasks or play certain roles (e.g., the baby) in class activities. Singling out these children may produce emotional disturbance, including withdrawal, aggression, or other acting-out behaviors. Although research suggests that short stature is not uniformly damaging emotionally, there may be significant psychological distress in some children (Voss, 2001).

The strongest source of support for these children will be the guidance and encouragement of their parents, but teachers can also play an important role by encouraging participation in all school activities and avoiding stigmatizing comments or actions. Short children should always be treated according to their mental and chronological age and *not* according to their size. Occasionally, school personnel may be tempted to hold the short child back a year so he or she will be with children of more equivalent size in the classroom. This practice is to be avoided at all costs, unless the child has a learning difficulty that makes holding back appropriate. Special education may be required for certain short children with specific learning disabilities. For example, mental retardation is common in Down syndrome, and specific deficits, such as spatial and math deficiencies, are common in Turner syndrome.

These problems also hold true for taller than average children, who may be singled out in exactly the opposite way by being expected to perform at an age-inappropriate higher level because of their size.

Treatment of children with disorders of growth and sexual development should not only take into account the obvious medical concerns, but also be sensitive to the educational, social, psychological, and vocational needs of these children and adolescents. Medical treatment is not required for all short children. For many, counseling and reassurance with careful follow-up represent the most appropriate therapy.

Some families are willing to "do anything" to enhance the growth potential of their short child. Growth hormone has been shown to be highly effective in increasing height potential in children with growth hormone deficiency, as well as in those with chronic renal (kidney) failure and Turner syndrome. Its effectiveness in other conditions is much more uncertain. In those children who do not have one of the growth hormone–responsive conditions, use of growth hormone should be contemplated only after careful consultation with a pediatric endocrinologist.

# OTHER ENDOCRINE DISORDERS

## The Thyroid Gland

Thyroxine, the major hormone secreted by the thyroid gland, is one of the most important hormones controlling the metabolic rate of the body. As such, it also affects growth and physical development. The teacher may occasionally be faced with students with either underactivity (*hypothyroidism*) or overactivity (*hyperthyroidism*) of the thyroid gland. Either condition may have implications for behavior and performance in the classroom.

Hauser et al. (1993) identified a group of children with an association between a variant of ADHD and generalized resistance to thyroid hormone action. Clinically, these children had nonspecific symptoms and signs of thyroid dysfunction (both hypothyroidism and hyperthyroidism) in addition to the learning disability. However, screening of large groups of children with classical ADHD has failed to reveal an increased incidence of thyroid dysfunction and is likely an unnecessary added investigation in these children.

### Hypothyroidism

Thyroid hormone is critically important for early postnatal brain development, and its lack during this period may produce severe mental retardation (*cretinism*). Newborn thyroid-screening programs have been developed over the past 20 to 25 years to detect the 1 in 3,500 to 4,000 newborns with congenital hypothyroidism. Treatment in the first week or two of life has been remarkably effective in eliminating the associated retardation.

Hypothyroidism that develops after the first few years of life will not interfere with intellectual development but may have a major impact in delaying growth and physical development (see Figure 4.8). These children may have a goiter (enlargement of the thyroid gland at the front of the

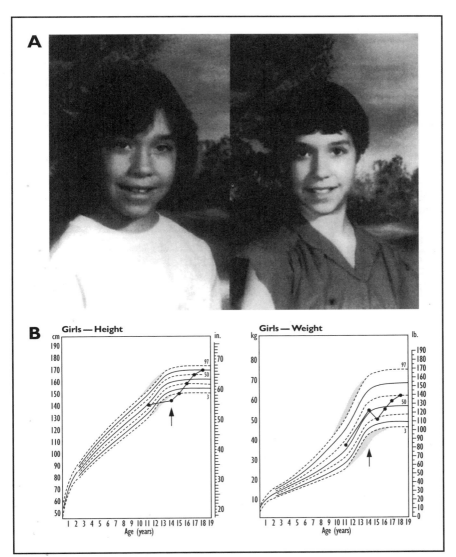

**FIGURE 4.8.** Severe acquired hypothyroidism presenting as growth failure in a 14-year-old girl showing (A) facial appearance before (left) and 1 year after (right) initiation of thyroid replacement therapy, and (B) growth chart for both height (left panel) and weight (right). The arrow denotes the time of diagnosis, with a remarkable increase in height and leveling off of weight gain after starting treatment. *Note.* Growth charts adapted from "Clinical Longitudinal Standards for Height, Weight, Height Velocity, Weight Velocity and Stages of Puberty," by J. M. Tanner and R. H. Whitehouse, 1976, *Archives of Diseases of Children,* *51*(3), pp. 170–179. Copyright 1976 by Castlemead Publications. Adapted with permission.

neck), evidence of growth failure and eventual short stature, weight gain, dry hair and skin, muscle weakness, and poor energy level. They may also become severely constipated and complain of abdominal pains. While hypothyroid, they often perform well at school with little distraction from outside activities. The cause of the hypothyroidism is most often Hashimoto's thyroiditis, a chronic inflammatory (autoimmune) condition in which the gland may eventually "burn out." This condition is 10 times more common in girls than boys.

Investigation of hypothyroidism includes measurement of the thyroid hormone levels, with management consisting of replacement treatment with the synthetic hormone, L-thyroxine. This invariably leads to excellent catch-up growth and development and reversal of the symptoms described. However, in the early treatment phase, there may be poor concentration and deteriorating school performance as the body readjusts to a normal thyroid state. Teachers should be informed when one of their students is starting on treatment and should be sensitive to changes in the student's performance and attention. Any marked changes should be communicated to the parents because the dose of medication may need adjustment.

## Hyperthyroidism

Hyperthyroidism, like acquired hypothyroidism, is most frequently the result of chronic inflammation in the thyroid gland (Graves disease). In some cases, underactivity of the gland ensues; in others, overactivity results. Although growth is usually not affected by hyperthyroidism, virtually every other system may be involved. In addition to the presence of a goiter, these children may show emotional lability, hyperactivity and short attention span, restlessness and nervousness, increased appetite but weight loss, disturbed sleeping habits, heat intolerance and increased sweating, increased heart rate, tremor of the hands, and diarrhea. These symptoms may lead to deteriorating school performance. In addition, some hyperthyroid children may show prominence of their eyes (*proptosis*).

Diagnosis requires demonstration of elevated levels of thyroid hormones, and treatment consists of thyroid-suppressive medication. In some, failure to respond to oral medications or side effects of these medications may necessitate the use of either radioactive iodine or surgery to ablate the gland. Normal behavior and school performance would be expected to return once the thyroid condition is under control, although noncompliance with medications may lead to a relapse of symptoms and signs. During the period of hyperthyroidism, these students should refrain from vigorous physical activities.

## Effects of Excess Cortisone Medication

Cortisone and other glucocorticoid medications may be prescribed for a variety of medical conditions. In addition to impairment of physical growth and development, these medications may cause significant weight gain and change in body habitus, with truncal obesity and thinning of the arms and legs (see Figure 4.9). They may also produce marked acne, face reddening, stretch marks (*striae*), easy bruising, and a tendency to acquire infections more easily. Because treatment with cortisone diminishes or abolishes the body's ability to secrete more of its own cortisone in response to stress, any intercurrent illness or accident in children receiving these medications may pose a serious threat. Teachers should be aware of this and inform the parents immediately should the child develop a serious intercurrent illness at school. Vomiting is particularly dangerous, as it will prevent absorption of the oral medication. Cortisone will then need to be administered by injection.

## Disorders of Puberty

Any of the conditions that cause short stature may also be associated with a delay in the onset or progression of the secondary sexual characteristics at the time of puberty. This is called delayed adolescence or delayed puberty and can be diagnosed in a girl who has failed to show any breast development by age 13 to 13½ years or in a boy who shows no enlargement of the testicles by age 14 years. Conversely, early sexual development (before age 6 to 7 in girls and 9 to 10 in boys) is called precocious puberty. Both delayed adolescence and precocious puberty can have serious psychosocial implications for students.

## Delayed Adolescence

Delayed adolescence is much more common in boys than in girls. In boys with such a delay, there is often a family history of late bloomers and, in the

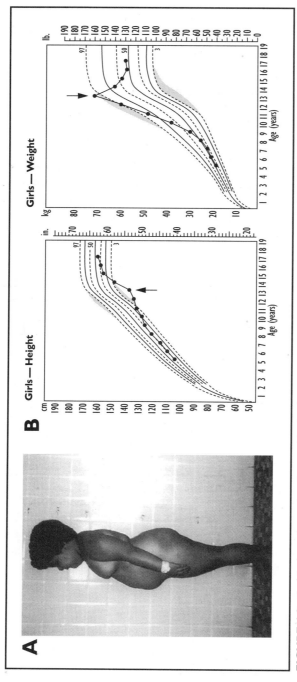

**FIGURE 4.9.** Cushing's syndrome (corticosteroid excess) presenting as growth failure and obesity in a 13-year-old girl. (A) The typical truncal obesity and short stature. (B) Height falloff (left panel) and excessive weight gain (right) before diagnosis (arrow). Removal of her pituitary tumor led to catchup in height and marked weight loss. *Note.* Growth charts adapted from "Clinical Longitudinal Standards for Height, Weight, Height Velocity, Weight Velocity and Stages of Puberty," by J. M. Tanner and R. H. Whitehouse, 1976, *Archives of Diseases of Children, 51*(3), pp. 170–179. Copyright 1976 by Castlemead Publications. Adapted with permission.

absence of obvious chronic disease, it is usually considered a benign condition (normal variant) in that a pathological cause is rarely found. Treatment depends on the degree of delay and the psychosocial impact on the particular boy. The most commonly employed therapy is a short course of testosterone injections, which will initiate puberty. This may rapidly enhance self-esteem and ego development.

In girls, late onset of puberty is more likely the result of a pathological condition such as anorexia nervosa or other eating disorder or an absence of the ovaries or uterus. Poor ovarian development is a feature of Turner syndrome. In these girls, short stature and characteristic physical features will be associated with the delay. Delayed adolescence in girls, therefore, warrants a more vigorous investigation than it does in boys.

## Precocious Puberty

Early sexual development is more common in girls and is almost invariably a benign condition. The earlier the onset and the more rapid the progression of puberty, the more likely there will be a pathological explanation for the precocity. Conversely, sexual precocity is uncommon in boys and, when it occurs, warrants full investigation to exclude the possibility of pituitary, testicular, or adrenal conditions that may require therapy.

Treatment of precocious puberty is warranted for one of two reasons: First, early and rapid sexual development will be associated with the pubertal growth spurt. The earlier the growth spurt, the earlier the attainment of final adult height will occur. Thus, children with sexual precocity will show rapid growth and be tall in comparison to other children early in life. However, by reaching final adult height earlier, they may be quite short as adults. Therapy that delays puberty may also increase final height potential. Second, early sexual development may cause significant anxiety and social discomfort among these children and their families. These children may be singled out by others and treated as though they were older by teachers, peers, and the population at large. Whereas girls with early development rarely, if ever, show promiscuous sexual behavior, boys with this condition may show aggression, masturbate in public, and generally be disruptive.

The treatment available for precocious puberty consists of monthly injections of a hormone analog called LHRH analog or agonist. This medication overstimulates the pituitary, thereby shutting off its production of the two hormones, LH and FSH, that control ovarian function in the female and testicular function in the male. Discontinuation of these agents at an appropriate age will allow normal progression of pubertal development.

## THE TEACHER'S ROLE

Disorders of growth or of other components of the endocrine system may have a wide variety of presentations, including significant implications for healthy personal development and learning. Teachers should be aware of these possibilities and inform parents of students whose growth appears to fall outside of the normal range. Teachers are in a unique position to detect variations in normal growth and pubertal development because they have a readily available group of classmates as a normal reference. By informing parents of these concerns, teachers will help to initiate appropriate investigation and management, where necessary, earlier rather than later. Furthermore, teachers should deal sensitively with children with disordered growth, preventing their stigmatization either by their classmates or school personnel.

## SUGGESTED READING

Kelnar, C. J. H., Savage, M. O., Stirling, H. F., & Saenger, P. (1998). *Growth disorders: Pathophysiology and treatment.* Philadelphia: Chapman and Hall Medical Publishers.

Lee, P. A. (1999). Central precocious puberty. An overview of diagnosis, treatment, and outcome. *Endocrinology and Metabolic Clinics of North America, 28*(4), 901–918.

## REFERENCES

Gardner, L. I. (1975). *Endocrine and genetic diseases of childhood and adolescence* (2nd ed.). Philadelphia: Saunders.

Hauser, P., Zametkin, A. J., Martinez, P., Vitiello, B., Matochik, J. A., Mixson, A. J., & Weintraub, B. D. (1993). Attention deficit-hyperactivity disorder in people with generalized resistance to thyroid hormone. *New England Journal of Medicine, 328*, 997–1001.

Kaplowitz, P. B., & Oberfield, S. E. (1999). Reexamination of the age limit for defining when puberty is precocious in girls in the United States: Implications for evaluation and treatment. *Pediatrics, 104,* 936–941.

Powell, G. F., Brasel, J. A., & Blizzard, R. M. (1967). Emotional deprivation and growth retardation simulating idiopathic hypopituitarism: I. Clinical evaluation of the syndrome. *New England Journal of Medicine, 276,* 1271–1278.

Turner, J. M., & Whitehouse, R. H. (1976). Clinical longitudinal standards for height, weight, height velocity, weight velocity and stages of puberty. *Archives of Diseases of Children, 51*(3), 170–179.

Voss, L. D. (2001). Short normal stature and psychosocial disadvantage: A critical review of the evidence. *Journal of Pediatric Endocrinology and Metabolism, 14*(6), 701–711.

# CHAPTER 5

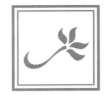

# The Student with Diabetes Mellitus

### Denis Daneman and Marcia Frank

Type 1 diabetes (previously called insulin-dependent diabetes mellitus or IDDM, or juvenile onset diabetes) is one of the most common chronic disorders of childhood. In fact, it is second in prevalence only to asthma. In Canada and the United States, the incidence of this type of diabetes is 10 to 20 or more new cases per 100,000 youth under the age of 20 each year. Although type 1 diabetes can present at any time in childhood, the peaks of incidence are in the early school-age and early adolescent years. By the end of high school, approximately 1 in 400 to 500 individuals has developed this condition.

Type 2 diabetes (previously called non–insulin-dependent diabetes mellitus or maturity onset diabetes) has begun to increase rapidly in particular high-risk population groups in North America, including Native Americans and Canadians, African Americans, and Hispanics. This type of diabetes is often associated with a strong family history of diabetes and a propensity to obesity.

Diabetes cannot be cured. However, children and adolescents with well-controlled diabetes can expect to enjoy healthy school years, participate in the same kinds of activities as their nondiabetic siblings and friends, and look forward to a healthy future. For young people with diabetes, good health over the short and long term is hard work, an achievement resulting from careful attention to a rigorous program of self-management (Daneman, Frank, & Perlman, 1999; Haire-Joshu, 1992). More specifically, these individuals, with the help and support of their families, take multiple (2–5) insulin injections each day or use continuous subcutaneous insulin infusion pumps, frequently monitor their blood sugar (glucose) levels, attend to their diet, plan for their activities, and respond to acute emergencies of high and low blood sugar concentrations. Clearly, the demands of such a regimen cannot help but have an impact on the school life of these children.

Teachers and other school personnel need to be aware of the student with diabetes in the classroom. By understanding the essential features of diabetes management, the teacher can facilitate healthy adjustment of the student to the classroom situation and in peer relationships. Teachers also have an important role in ensuring the ongoing safety of these students in the classroom, on the playground, and on school trips; in alleviating parental anxiety; and in preventing minor crises from getting out of hand.

The teacher's ability to provide the student with the appropriate level of support is contingent on a sound understanding of diabetes and its implications. A number of studies have documented the relatively inadequate knowledge base that most teachers have concerning diabetes (Anderson, Hess, & Hiss, 1989). Given the incredibly large number of disorders teachers may encounter among their students, this is not surprising; health care providers and parents should not be critical about this seeming lack of preparedness. Furthermore, in a study evaluating the effectiveness of mass education of 244 teachers in the Salt Lake Valley, Gesteland and Lindsay (1989) concluded that this approach was largely ineffective. The conclusion to be drawn from this and other studies is that diabetes education for teachers should be targeted to those who presently have or will have in the next year a student with diabetes in their classrooms (Anderson et al., 1989; Bradbury & Smith, 1983; Gesteland & Lindsay, 1989; Henderson, 1993). By virtue of having completed a diabetes education program and having taken care of their child's diabetes at home, the parents should be considered experts in diabetes management and the major source of information for their child's teachers.

In this chapter, we provide teachers with an overview of diabetes and principles of management; describe the impact of diabetes on lifestyle and daily activities; outline expectations for general health, school attendance, and performance; define the teacher's role in relation to that of the student and his or her family; and offer helpful hints in dealing with special situations such as school activities, trips, and party days. Although we focus on type 1 diabetes, many of the same principles apply to the management of type 2 diabetes. Where differences exist, these will be highlighted. For additional information, teachers might wish to contact the organizations or refer to the Web sites listed in the Other Resources section at the end of this chapter.

# OVERVIEW OF DIABETES

Type 1 diabetes is caused by a lack of insulin in the body. Insulin is a hormone produced by the pancreas. More specifically, the beta cells, which are housed in the islets of Langerhans, secrete insulin in response to increasing blood glucose concentrations. Insulin circulates in the blood, binds to its target cells, and stimulates a series of events that lead to glucose uptake by the cell. Without insulin, glucose cannot be used as the energy source of the cells and life cannot be sustained.

Children with type 1 diabetes develop a complete lack of insulin secretion from the pancreas and, as a result, require insulin replacement, by injection, for life. This situation is quite different from the more common type 2 diabetes, which occurs with increasing prevalence in older individuals and accounts for about 85% of all cases of diabetes. Type 2 diabetes often presents in overweight adults and teens at high risk (due to strong family history, obesity, ethnicity); insulin secretion is present but inadequate to meet the demands of the aging and enlarging body. The symptoms are usually much less severe, and the condition can often be managed by either diet alone or diet in combination with pills that increase insulin secretion or action. Because most people know adults with type 2 diabetes, teachers should take care to avoid extrapolating from their experiences with such individuals to the care of their students in the classroom.

## Causes of Diabetes in Children

The cause of type 1 diabetes is not well understood. It is probably the result of a combination of factors leading to chronic inflammation and destruction of the islet cells that produce insulin (Atkinson & Eisenbarth, 2001). That there is a genetic or hereditary component to type 1 diabetes is beyond doubt; however, it is the predisposition to the condition and not the diabetes itself that appears to be inherited. Unidentified environmental influences appear to be important in converting this predisposition into disease. A couple of myths need to be exploded for the classmates of the student with newly diagnosed diabetes: (a) Diabetes is *not* an infectious disease, and (b) it is *not* the result of eating too much sugar. Type 2 diabetes tends to have a stronger inherited component and to be closely related to the development of obesity and a sedentary lifestyle in high-risk individuals.

## Signs and Symptoms of Untreated or Uncontrolled Diabetes

Without insulin, children are unable to use sugar from the food they eat as a source of energy. Instead, the unused sugar builds up in the blood (*hyperglycemia*) and is "dumped" out in the urine, dragging with it large amounts of water. This increased urination, day and night and often associated with enuresis (bed-wetting), may be the first sign of the onset of diabetes in a previously well child; in someone with diagnosed diabetes, it may signal that the level of control is less than optimal. The increased urination and water loss creates an increase in thirst. Because glucose loss in the urine represents energy loss, there will often also be associated hunger, weight loss, and increasing fatigue or lethargy. Finally, fat breakdown will occur in an effort to replace glucose as the energy source. Eventually this results in a buildup of acid in the blood, severe dehydration, and a potentially life-threatening condition called diabetic ketoacidosis.

These symptoms and signs—increased urination, increased thirst, increased *or* decreased appetite, weight loss, and poor energy level—will clue the family and physician to the diagnosis of diabetes in an otherwise well child. At school, the teacher may notice that the child leaves the class frequently to urinate, has a poor energy level, and generally appears unwell. These same symptoms and signs may occur after the diagnosis of diabetes during periods of intercurrent illness or if insulin dosages are inadequate or omitted. Well-controlled diabetes should eliminate all of these symptoms.

Of note, a study in Italy showed that when teachers and other school personnel were made aware of these symptoms of diabetes, they were often able to facilitate an early diagnosis in students before ketoacidosis developed (Vanelli et al., 1999). The awareness of school personnel was accomplished by the strategic placement of colorful posters that reminded teachers of the symptoms of diabetes.

# PRINCIPLES OF
# DIABETES MANAGEMENT

## Concept of Balance

In nondiabetic individuals, insulin secretion is so finely regulated that blood glucose concentrations are maintained in an extremely narrow range: 60 to 110 mg/dl (3.3–6.0 mmol/L) before meals and below 180 mg/dl (10 mmol/L) after eating. In children with diabetes, the internal regulation of glucose levels is lost. Therefore, diabetes management entails the reestablishment of blood glucose balance through a multicomponent treatment program:

1. Insulin is replaced either by multiple (2–5) daily injections of short- and longer acting insulin preparations or by continuous infusion using a portable pump.

2. Meals and snacks are taken at consistent times and in consistent amounts to provide some predictability to the action of the injected insulin.

3. Regular monitoring of blood glucose (and urine ketones when indicated) provides feedback regarding the effectiveness of the treatment program.

This approach can mimic only to a degree the functioning of the non-diabetic (normal) pancreas. Despite their very best efforts, students with type 1 diabetes and their families will not always be able to achieve perfect blood sugar control. At times, the blood glucose may be high (hyperglycemia), whereas at other times it may drop precipitously low (hypoglycemia). Achieving the balance can be difficult and frustrating, especially early on after diagnosis. Teachers need to maintain a nonjudgmental attitude as these families adjust to their new reality. The challenge for children and adolescents is to learn as much as possible about their diabetes and to incorporate the treatment measures into their daily lives so as to minimize the risks of both hyperglycemia and hypoglycemia and to maintain good health over both the short and long terms (Haire-Joshu, 1992).

## Diabetes Education for Families

Successful diabetes management depends on the child's and family's mastery of the necessary cognitive and technical skills, as well as their healthy adjustment to the disorder. From the time of initial diagnosis, these children and their families should have the opportunity to participate in a developmentally appropriate program of diabetes care, education, and support. In most centers, this comprehensive program is provided by a multidisciplinary team of health care providers with expertise in childhood diabetes. Members of such a team include a physician, diabetes nurse, dietitian, and social worker or psychologist (Haire-Joshu, 1992).

In general, parents are highly motivated and quickly learn about the pathophysiology and management of diabetes. They learn to monitor the effectiveness of the treatment program and make the adjustments necessary to maintain good diabetes control. They are taught strategies to detect, treat, and prevent diabetes-related emergencies and are informed about the long-term complications of the disease. The level of involvement of the child will depend on his or her age and cognitive maturity. Younger children are not able to comprehend the intricate details of diabetes care, whereas most older children and adolescents can be active participants in the program. Ongoing education of the child and family will serve two purposes: reinforcing present skills and knowledge, and keeping the child's understanding consistent with his or her developmental stage.

Contact between school teachers and members of the health care team should be encouraged for the cooperative dissemination of information and assistance in problem solving (Henderson, 1993). The parents' agreement is obviously required to allow such interchange to occur. In a number of centers, a member of the diabetes team attends the child's school after diagnosis to help school personnel understand the crucial aspects of diabetes care, to answer their questions and those of the student's classmates, and to establish a line of communication between the school and the health care team. Unfortunately, this is a luxury most diabetes teams cannot easily afford.

## Goals of Therapy

Current treatment regimens for type 1 diabetes are based on the need to achieve and maintain blood sugar levels as close to those in nondiabetic individuals as possible, while at the same time minimizing the risks of hypoglycemia (low blood sugar). These goals are determined by the results of the landmark Diabetes Control and Complications Trial Research Group (1993) from 1982 to 1993 that demonstrated a close relationship between the level of blood sugars and the risk of the long-term complications of diabetes, such as damage to the eyes, kidneys, and nerves. These goals translate into the attempt to achieve premeal blood sugar levels in the 70 to 145 mg/dl (~4–8 mmol/L) range in teens and older children, 70 to 180 mg/dl (4–10 mmol/L) range in younger school-age children, and 110 to 220 mg/dl (~6–12 mmol/L) range in infants and toddlers.

## Insulin Replacement

Insulin was discovered at the University of Toronto in 1921 by the Canadian physician Frederick Banting and his student Charles Best. Prior to the discovery of insulin, children with type 1 diabetes died. The only way to replace insulin is by injection; taken by mouth, insulin, which is a protein hormone, would be digested in the stomach and rendered ineffective.

Usually a syringe with a short, fine needle or a pen injection device is used to inject the insulin into the subcutaneous tissue (fatty tissue under the skin) of the upper arms, thighs, abdomen, or buttocks. Injected insulin enables the individual with type 1 diabetes to use glucose for his or her energy supply. Its effect is to lower the blood glucose concentration, but, unlike naturally secreted insulin, there is no internal regulation. In other words, the effect of the injected insulin does not wear off until it has all been absorbed from the subcutaneous site and used in the body. Thus, injected insulin may lower the blood glucose too much if there is an inadequate supply of glucose from food to balance its action.

At present, most children with type 1 diabetes take insulin injections multiple times each day. Most diabetes experts prescribe three or four injections a day for children and teens with diabetes. There is also a rapidly increasing trend toward the use of insulin pumps in children and teens with type 1 diabetes. These pumps deliver insulin through a rubber tube (catheter) which is placed under the skin. Insulin is delivered constantly at a low (basal) rate throughout the day and night, with extra doses (boluses) given at each meal (and snack) time. There is no doubt that increasingly intensified approaches to diabetes management place greater demands on the student during the school day. As a result, the role of teachers and other school personnel in supporting these children and teens has also increased.

In general, insulin injections are administered by the parents of young children, with self-administration under supervision being encouraged as the child reaches about age 10. Wide individual differences exist in the age at which children begin self-injection. As parents transfer the technical responsibility of insulin injection to their children, they should supervise the activity closely until the child reaches a high level of maturity and demonstrated skill (Daneman, 1991).

With intensive treatment approaches, teachers and other school personnel are being called on more frequently to participate in the diabetes routines (e.g., supervising or performing injections of blood sugar tests). Policies differ in various jurisdictions as to the role teachers may or may not play in such management.

## Diet

Maintenance of the appropriate balance between food and insulin is essential to good blood glucose (diabetic) control. When the parents or health care providers decide on an insulin dose for the child with type 1 diabetes, they assume that the food intake will be kept relatively consistent. Although teachers do not need to know all the details of a student's meal plan, they should understand that the diet for people with diabetes is based on the following principles:

1. The child should eat a similar quantity of food each day.

2. The child should eat meals and snacks at the same times each day.

3. The child should avoid foods containing excess amounts of concentrated sugars (e.g., candies, regular soft drinks).

These principles should be followed not only on a regular day-to-day basis at school, but also during field trips, other school trips, and even detentions. It is almost always possible to integrate the child's meal plan into the daily school schedule. For example, snacks can be taken at recess or during snack time. Only occasionally will it be necessary for the student to eat his or her snack during class. Every effort should be taken to avoid criticizing or singling out these students. Many students find that low-noise foods, such as cheese or dried fruit, minimize classroom disruption.

Younger children with diabetes will likely require extra supervision in both the classroom and the lunchroom to ensure that they eat most of what has been provided for each meal or snack. Overeating or eating candies will not cause an immediate problem but is cause for concern if done regularly, in which case school personnel should inform parents of such behavior. A far more serious problem may arise if the student misses a meal or snack or has much too little food at such time. Lower food intake may precipitate a medical emergency by causing the blood glucose to drop too low. This condition is called an insulin or hypoglycemic reaction. The appropriate treatment for such a reaction is to have the student ingest a quickly absorbable form of sugar (for details see the "Hypoglycemia" section later in this chapter).

With a little planning, students with diabetes can eat most of the foods that their classmates eat. Parents of younger children should be notified ahead of time of parties, hotdog or pizza days, or other special events involving food. Suitable treats include popcorn, fruit, cookies, potato chips, and pizza.

Increasingly, children and teens with type 1 diabetes are learning to adjust insulin dosages according to the amount of carbohydrate-containing food to be ingested at the next meal or snack, an approach called carbohydrate counting. However, in most cases, teachers and other school personnel cannot be expected to participate in this process.

## Monitoring

To assess the effectiveness of their treatment regimens, and to prevent hypoglycemia and hyperglycemia, every student with diabetes should have a system for monitoring blood glucose concentrations on a regular basis. Blood glucose testing is performed by pricking a finger with a spring-loaded device and then applying a drop of blood to a strip, which is read by a blood glucose meter. In addition, children and teens should use urine testing strips to detect the presence of ketones, a product of fat breakdown. Usually they are encouraged to test blood sugar levels three or more times a day, usually before the main meals and at bedtime, but specific protocols vary with different treatment centers. Urine ketones should be monitored during periods of illness or poor metabolic control.

With older children and adolescents, school personnel usually are not requested to participate in testing routines unless the student is having significant problems with control and requires assistance in performing the test at school. However, with increased efforts to achieve tight glucose control in most treatment centers, teacher involvement in testing routines is often required. Teachers and other school personnel involved in such testing require instruction regarding technique, method of recording, and interpretation of test results. Furthermore, they must observe universal precautions to prevent potential transfer of blood-borne diseases. Also, if teachers are involved in monitoring at school, they should have very clear, and preferably written, guidelines about what actions should be taken in response to the result of the test.

One problem that can occur when students monitor under the guidance of school personnel is the tendency for school staff to become overinvolved in a student's diabetes care and overconcerned that every nuance of behavior is a result of changes in blood glucose. Teachers caught in such a situation should request help from the parents and health care team to clarify and redefine their role in the child's diabetes care at school.

# SPECIAL SITUATIONS

## Hypoglycemia

Hypoglycemia, insulin reaction, and insulin shock are different names for the same thing: an emergency situation caused by a low blood sugar level. Because the normal pancreas is able to turn insulin secretion on and off as required, the risk of low blood glucose levels in individuals without diabetes is essentially nonexistent. In those with type 1 diabetes, however, hypoglycemia is an ever-present risk and can develop within minutes of the child's appearing healthy and normal.

The causes of hypoglycemia include the following:

- too much insulin (this is usually inadvertent, but occasionally intentional)

- not enough food, due to a delayed or missed meal or snack

- too much unplanned, vigorous activity (i.e., inadequate provision of extra food for additional physical activities)

For many episodes of hypoglycemia, however, the cause cannot be determined.

The symptoms of hypoglycemia can be divided into the early warning symptoms, caused by increased secretion of the counterregulatory or stress hormones of the body (glucagon, adrenaline/epinephrine, cortisol, and growth hormone), and those caused by poor glucose supply to the brain, termed *neuroglycopenia*. The early warning symptoms include a feeling of shakiness or jitteriness, hunger, cold, clammy or sweaty skin, tiredness or drowsiness, blurring of vision, anxiety or nervousness, headache, abdominal pain or nausea, and looking quite pale ("white as a ghost"). In younger children, the main features may be behavioral change, with irritability, hostility, or mood swings. The neuroglycopenia will present as increasing confusion and clumsiness or staggering gait, with progression to a decreasing level of consciousness, coma, and a seizure or convulsion if left untreated. Mild, occasional hypoglycemic episodes that can be easily identified and treated are quite commonplace. Most people with type 1 diabetes report at least one a week. More severe episodes that require outside assistance are quite uncommon in the school setting. Every effort should be made to avoid these by careful planning, regular monitoring, and the establishment of realistic goals for blood glucose control.

Treatment of mild hypoglycemia requires ingestion of simple sugar, such as juice, regular soft drinks, or glucose tablets. At home, children are encouraged to test their blood sugar to confirm the presence of hypoglycemia, then to take a modest amount of simple sugar (e.g., 4 ounces of juice or regular soda, or 2 to 4 glucose tablets). At school, if the student does not have testing equipment easily available, treatment should be initiated without testing. The student should be treated in the classroom, so sugar should be readily available for emergencies. It may take some encouragement to get these children to drink or eat, but the teacher must insist they do. If there is no noticeable improvement in about 10 to 15 minutes, the treatment should be repeated. When the condition has improved, the child should have some solid food, usually in the form of the next regular meal or a snack. The child should not be left unsupervised until fully recovered. To facilitate treatment of hypoglycemic episodes, the parents should provide the teacher or other school personnel with a handy supply of juice, soda, or glucose tablets. This should be replenished after each episode.

If the hypoglycemic episode is more severe—that is, confusion or beyond—the school should call the local ambulance service and have the child treated by qualified health professionals. The teacher must not give anything by mouth if the child is unconscious, as the child may aspirate the food into his or her lungs.

For home management of severe hypoglycemia, all families have learned to give glucagon. When injected during severe hypoglycemia, this medication quickly raises the blood glucose level and the child recovers. It is rarely necessary for school personnel to learn how to administer glucagon. If, however, the parents and health care team consider it appropriate for school personnel to know how to give glucagon, instruction can be accomplished with the help of the parents, school nurse, or health care team.

Prevention of hypoglycemia is an important component of diabetes management. Careful attention to the total treatment package, with rational adjustment of insulin, an appropriate nutritional plan, regular monitoring, and exercise planning, will help to prevent many, but not all, hypoglycemic episodes. Parents should be informed of all hypoglycemic episodes that occur at school, because these may signal a need to alter the treatment regimen and thus prevent further and potentially more severe events from developing.

If the teacher is unsure as to whether the child is having a low blood sugar reaction, the safest course of action is to give sugar. A temporary excess of sugar will not harm the child, but a low blood glucose reaction is potentially very serious.

## Intercurrent Illness

More myths to be exploded: Students with diabetes do *not* acquire more frequent or more severe illnesses than their nondiabetic peers, and they are *not* poor healers. However, when children with diabetes become ill with the usual fevers and other childhood illnesses, the blood glucose balance is likely to be upset (Daneman & Frank, 1984). Careful monitoring with blood glucose and urine ketone tests, a clear fluid diet, and extra (or less) insulin may be required. This is the responsibility of the parents, not the school personnel.

When a child with diabetes becomes ill at school, the parents should be notified immediately so they can take appropriate steps to prevent the development of either hypoglycemia or ketoacidosis. Vomiting or the inability to retain food or fluids is a potentially serious situation that requires prompt attention. If the child vomits, the teacher should inform the parents immediately; if they cannot be reached, the child should be taken directly to the nearest hospital.

Virtually all episodes of hypoglycemia and ketoacidosis during illness should be preventable. Recurrent episodes of ketoacidosis requiring repeated hospitalization are the result of insulin omission and signal significant family dysfunction and distress in the student.

## Exercise and Special Events

Children with diabetes should be encouraged to participate in as many school activities as they choose, and they should be included in school trips. For students who participate in vigorous physical activity, good planning is essential to maintain good diabetes control. Physical activity requires extra energy and thus an increased need for glucose. In a child with diabetes, involvement in physical activities will likely lead to a decrease in blood glucose levels and the possibility of developing hypoglycemia. This may occur during the activity or for several hours afterward. In general, students with diabetes are encouraged to take extra food when embarking on physical activities that are beyond those they do on a daily basis (e.g., gym at school, sports events). Some students will decrease their insulin dose in anticipation of such activities. Teachers should be aware of the particular student's exercise-related food habits and, at least for younger children, provide appropriate supervision. As part of the information provided by the parents (see Figure 5.1), common practices around exercise should be included in Special Instructions.

Ensuring safety in the classroom and on the playground on a day-to-day basis is the major focus for a teacher who has students with diabetes. However, the teacher must be prepared for special events that might occur during the school year, including day and overnight trips, special sporting events, and classroom celebrations such as birthdays and public or religious holidays. Careful preparation for such events helps to prevent unnecessary problems. Consultation with the family and, where applicable, the health care team is indicated before taking a child with diabetes on any significant trips away from the school. If the trip involves an overnight stay or absence from the home at the time of an insulin injection or blood glucose test, an individual (teacher, other school personnel, or parent) must be identified who will take responsibility for either performing or supervising the specific task. Furthermore, the school personnel should have

## PERSONAL INFORMATION
## TO BE PROVIDED BY PARENTS

Name _____ Age _____ Grade _____

Parent's name _____

Address _____

Home phone _____ Business phone _____

Alternate person to call in an emergency _____

Are there other siblings in school? _____

Name _____ Grade _____

Doctor's name _____ Phone _____

Health insurance number _____

Time of day when low blood glucose is most likely to occur _____

Symptoms commonly experienced _____

_____

What has been provided to treat hypoglycemia? _____

_____

Where is it located? _____

Alternatives: 4 oz fruit juice / 4 oz pop (not diet)

Type of morning snack _____

Type of afternoon snack _____

Suggested treats for in-school parties _____

_____

Special Instructions

_____    **PHOTO**

_____

_____

_____

_____

**FIGURE 5.1.** Example of information sheet that parents should provide to school to assist with management of a child's diabetes. Reprinted with permission of the Canadian Diabetes Association.

available simple sugars for treating mild hypoglycemia, perhaps glucagon for injection for severe reactions, as well as phone numbers to call in case of an emergency.

Being aware of the child's specific dietary needs and general diabetes routines will provide the teacher with a sense of comfort in dealing with the child without too much fuss or bother. Similarly, when special occasions arise at school, the informed teacher will be able to provide additional food before unplanned extra exercise and assess the likely impact of classroom treats brought in by other students.

## THE TEACHER'S ROLE

The general health care of the student with diabetes is the responsibility of the family in conjunction with members of their health care team. Teachers and other school personnel (excluding the school nurse) are not health care professionals, but they do have an important role in ensuring the safety and comfort of the student. In addition, they have a unique opportunity to contribute to the healthy adjustment of the child to his or her diabetes and the school situation. It is unrealistic to expect teachers to maintain adequate knowledge and skills based on the possibility of having a student with diabetes in the classroom at some time. Nevertheless, when such a student is in a class, it becomes essential for that teacher and other select school personnel to exhibit appropriate attitudes and to acquire the necessary know-how (Henderson, 1993). The poorly informed or misinformed teacher who has great anxiety about having a student with diabetes in the classroom can add to the adjustment and management difficulties encountered by these children and their families.

Once the family has informed the school of the child's diabetes, a meeting should be organized that includes the teacher, other key school personnel, the parents, and the student to discuss the diabetes and the student's individual needs and characteristics (see Figure 5.1 for the kinds of information to be ascertained at the meeting). Such a meeting should be held soon after diagnosis and at the beginning of each school year. Written information is helpful but does not replace personal contact. When the teacher recognizes the expertise of the parent and student and when the expectations of the teacher match those of the family from the outset, the child has the best possible head start for a healthy, happy, productive school year.

The teacher and other school personnel can contribute enormously to the well-being of the student by developmentally appropriate support of their activities at school. The child's age and cognitive maturity, as well as other individual and family issues, will have a major impact on the management of the child's diabetes. In younger children, care is parent oriented, whereas in late childhood and early adolescence, there is a steady transition toward self-care. By late adolescence, the expectation is that the teens will have assumed virtually all the responsibility for the day-to-day management of their diabetes. To achieve a smooth transition from parent- to self-oriented care, management of diabetes requires a developmental approach with expectations for self-care balanced against age, maturity, and demonstrated competence. The expectations of and demands placed on teachers to participate in this care will vary greatly according to the child's age and stage of development, parents' expectations and demands, and the nature of the treatment regimen established for the particular student.

Sometimes problems may arise when the expectations of teachers, parents, and students with diabetes do not balance. For example, parents may expect a high level of independence at a young age, such as expecting a child of 8 years to perform tests, administer insulin, and adjust diet without supervision (Daneman & Frank, 1984). Conversely, the parents may expect school personnel to take responsibility for tasks about which they have inadequate knowledge and skills. As mentioned before, these problems can generally be alleviated by advance planning.

That teachers of students of all ages need to be able to recognize and respond to hypoglycemia (low blood glucose/insulin reactions) is not disputed. However, the role of the teacher in prevention of such episodes is also important. For teachers of older students, this entails awareness of and attention to the special needs of the student at school (e.g., regular meal and snack times, planning for gym classes) so that food, insulin, and monitoring requirements can be incorporated safely and unobtrusively into the school schedule, not only on regular school days, but also during examinations and other special events. Younger children, of course, require direct supervision during school activities. Teachers may need to remind young children of snack and meal times, ensure adequate lunchroom and playground supervision, and provide extra food for extra activity as instructed by the parents. In addition, teachers need to collaborate with the parents to develop a sensitive system for handling special occasions involving food.

Also, the teacher should be aware of the symptoms of hyperglycemia (high blood sugar), such as increased urination and thirst, and decreased energy level. Rather than criticize the student for frequent trips to the bathroom during class, the teacher should inquire as to the level of metabolic control and inform parents of these types of symptoms. The sudden appearance of these symptoms together with another illness (e.g., influenza), especially if the child is vomiting, should trigger an immediate phone call to the parents to allow them to intervene before more serious problems arise. Because viral illnesses are much more common in younger children than in adolescents, it is the teachers of these children who need to be most alert to changes that may occur during the school day.

An increasing number of parents of students with diabetes, particularly younger children, have been making increased demands on school personnel not only to supervise meals and snacks and treat minor hypoglycemic events, but also to perform blood glucose testing and administer insulin and glucagon (the latter for severe hypoglycemic events). Although these medical acts are not the usual responsibility of teachers, many are willing to become proficient in these techniques in an attempt to best integrate the student into everyday activities with minimal risk. In fact, in the United States, Public Law (P.L.) 94-142, the Education for All Handicapped Children Act of 1975, entitles all "physically, developmentally, emotionally, and other health-impaired children to free appropriate public education" (Gray, Golden, & Reiswerg, 1991). Type 1 diabetes is identified in the regulations as an eligible condition, implying that schools, in the United States at least, are obligated to provide for specific health-related needs that would otherwise interfere with normal school participation. This means that all of the components of diabetes care should be provided by school personnel where indicated.

The identification of children and adolescents with type 1 diabetes as students with "special needs" ought to be done with the utmost caution. Diabetes should not be seen as a label that accompanies the child throughout his or her school years and into adult life. Educators' continuous efforts should be to help these students function in as normal a manner as possible. Because the stigmatizing effect of labeling may be long-lasting, labeling should only be used insofar as it serves to identify children with special needs and allows the particular school system to mobilize the necessary resources on their behalf.

Adequate knowledge of diabetes and its management will allow teachers to integrate their students with diabetes into all school activities without the unnecessary stigmatizing or labeling that may have a serious negative effect on a child's self-esteem and classroom adjustment. A well-informed teacher will be able to offset the negative comments of other students and quickly and efficiently deal with contingencies that may arise. It is also ideal for classmates to have appropriate information about the student's diabetes. However, the teacher should not involve the class in a discussion about diabetes without the student's permission to do so. The student is often the best one to lead such a discussion, even at a relatively young age. Teachers can encourage students to share their expertise with classmates through projects, speeches, and so forth. Not only is the information helpful for other students, but it may also serve to boost the self-esteem of the student with diabetes.

## Type 1 Diabetes

Studies have shown that children with chronic diseases have greater school absenteeism than their healthy peers. Although type 1 diabetes is one of the most common chronic disorders of childhood, most children with this condition are otherwise healthy. Research suggests that school performance of children with diabetes is similar to that of their nondiabetic peers. Furthermore, although a pilot study showed that children with diabetes do miss, on average, about 1 week more of school per year than their nondiabetic siblings, most of the difference can be accounted for by visits to health care professionals rather than the result of intercurrent illness (Vetiska, Glaab, Perlman, & Daneman, 2000). Parental overprotection or lack of trust in the ability or willingness of school personnel to provide appropriate supervision may be reasons for greater absenteeism in some children with chronic disorders.

The teacher should be alerted when the student with diabetes has poor school attendance, frequent hospitalizations, or recurrent diabetes-related events at school. Communication with parents should be escalated at these times, and the advice of the child's health care team should be sought. These episodes may be related to a poor understanding of diabetes and its management on the part of the child and parents. They may also result from family dysfunction where the diabetes bears the brunt of the fallout. Regardless, interventions are required to restore or maintain the child's health and end the disruption to his or her school experience.

## Type 2 Diabetes

Although considerably less common than type 1 diabetes, type 2 diabetes is seen with increasing frequency in teens at high risk (strong family history, obesity, member of high-risk ethnic group). Many can be managed with careful attention to diet and exercise; however, oral hypoglycemic agents, medications that help lower blood sugar levels, or insulin injections may be required in a significant number. Schools should promote physical fitness and healthy eating as part of their mandate. In teens with type 2 diabetes, school personnel should provide support for their treatment regimen in much the same way as for those with type 1 diabetes.

# CONCLUSION

Abraham Lincoln once said, "If I had 8 hours to chop down a tree, I'd spend 6 sharpening my axe," underscoring the need for adequate preparation when embarking on a new and unfamiliar task. Such ought to be the case when teachers are faced with the prospect of having a student with diabetes in their classroom. We believe that it is the primary responsibility of the parents to inform the school about their child's diabetes and to provide general literature for key school personnel through personal contact. They should also provide specific information regarding their child's diabetes (e.g., diet issues, testing requirements, specific symptoms when hypoglycemia occurs). Teachers should acknowledge and respect the expertise of the parents and student. Wherever possible, the parents should encourage contact between the school and members of the child's diabetes health care team. Sometimes a visit to the school by a member of the team or someone from the local branch of the volunteer diabetes organization (e.g., the American or Canadian Diabetes Associations) can be arranged to bring more information for both the school personnel and the other students in the child's classroom.

Despite the fact that diabetes is a serious, lifelong disorder with potentially dangerous acute and chronic complications, our experience is similar to that of many others: The vast majority of students with diabetes adjust well to their disorder and attend and perform normally in school. Teachers have an important role to play in early detection of diabetes, in ensuring the safety of the student, and in promoting a healthy adjustment to diabetes in the school setting.

# OTHER RESOURCES

1. An excellent listing of diabetes-related materials can be obtained from:

   National Diabetes Information Clearing House
   Bethesda, MD 20892
   Phone 301/468-2162

2. Support can be obtained through the local branches of the American and Canadian Diabetes Associations. The addresses of the national offices of these two organizations are as follows:

   American Diabetes Association
   1660 Duke Street
   Alexandria, VA 22314
   Phone 800/342-2383
   http://www.diabetes.org

   Canadian Diabetes Association
   15 Toronto Street, Suite 1001
   Toronto, ON M5C 2E3
   Canada
   Phone 800/226-8464
   http://www.diabetes.ca

3. The following highly informative Web site is available in addition to those of the American and Canadian Diabetes Associations:

   http://www.childrenwithdiabetes.com

# REFERENCES

Anderson, R. M., Hess, G. E., & Hiss, R. G. (1989). The knowledge and attitudes of elementary and high school teachers regarding diabetes. *The Diabetes Educator, 15,* 314–318.

Atkinson, M. A., & Eisenbarth, G. S. (2001, July 21). Type 1 diabetes: New perspectives on disease pathogenesis and treatment. *Lancet, 358,* 221–229.

Bradbury, A. J., & Smith, C. S. (1983). An assessment of diabetic knowledge of school teachers. *Archives of Diseases of Children, 58,* 692–696.

Daneman, D. (1991). When should your child take charge? In *Diabetes Forecast* [pamphlet], pp. 61–66.

Daneman, D., & Frank, M. (1984). Managing intercurrent illness in the child with diabetes. *Clinical Diabetes, 2,* 1–7.

Daneman, D., Frank, M., & Perlman, K. (1999). *When a child has diabetes.* Toronto, Ontario, Canada: Key Porter Books.

Diabetes Control and Complications Trial Research Group. (1993). The effect of intensive treatment of diabetes on the development and progression of long-term complications in insulin-dependent diabetes mellitus. *New England Journal of Medicine, 329,* 977–986.

Education for All Handicapped Children Act of 1975, 20 U.S.C. § 1400 *et seq.*

Gesteland, H. M., & Lindsay, R. N. (1989). Evaluation of two approaches to educating elementary schoolteachers about insulin-dependent diabetes mellitus. *The Diabetes Educator, 15,* 510–513.

Gray, D. L., Golden, M. P., & Reiswerg, J. (1991). Diabetes care in schools: Benefits and pitfalls of US Public Law #94-142. *The Diabetes Educator, 17,* 33–36.

Haire-Joshu, D. (Ed.). (1992). *Management of diabetes mellitus: Perspectives of care across the life span.* St. Louis, MO: Mosby-Yearbook.

Henderson, G. (1993). A diabetes education service for school personnel: Safety and health for the student with diabetes. *Beta Release, 17,* 20–24.

Vanelli, M., Chiari, G., Ghizzoni, L., Costi, G., Giacalone, T., & Chiarelli, F. (1999). Effectiveness of a prevention program for diabetic ketoacidosis in children: An 8-year study in schools and private practices. *Diabetes Care, 22*(1), 7–9.

Vetiska, J., Glaab, L., Perlman, K., & Daneman, D. (2000). School attendance of children with type 1 diabetes. *Diabetes Care, 23,* 1706–1707.

# CHAPTER 6

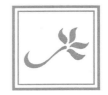

# Chronic Illness in Children

Michelle Shouldice

hronic illness in children refers to medical conditions that affect children for extended periods of time, generally years. The disorders that lead to chronic illness in children include common conditions, such as asthma and allergies, and a range of rare conditions, including arthritis, cystic fibrosis, and sickle cell disease. Due to advances in medical treatments, 80% of children with long-term illness survive to adulthood in developed countries. Therefore, these children are likely to be present within classrooms.

Although chronic illness is relatively common in childhood, the majority of children with chronic illness have few serious symptoms and the potential to function completely normally in all aspects of their lives. An estimated 6% to 10% of school-age children have a chronic illness, amounting to 3.3 to 4.8 million children in the United States (Gortmaker & Sappenfield, 1984). The majority of children with common chronic conditions, such as asthma and allergies, experience minimal impact from the direct effects of the disorder on daily functioning because effective medical management is readily available. Only 2% to 4% of children (approximately 1 million children in the United States) have a severe health condition that directly impacts daily activities on a regular basis. What is more important than identification of the presence of a chronic illness in a child is determination of the severity of the illness and its impact on the child's daily functioning.

Although most chronic illness is mild and symptoms do not directly interrupt daily functioning, the burden of disability may be much more significant than predicted by the severity of the underlying disease. School attendance and achievement are often used as measures of general adjustment to illness. Surprisingly, it is estimated that 40% of children with chronic illness experience school-related problems. The goal of those involved with children with chronic disease should be to minimize this impact of illness and prevent short- and long-term dysfunction. It is essential that communication between the school, family, and health care provider is open and effective to ensure that the child's needs are understood and management is appropriate, and to prevent a chronic childhood illness from resulting unnecessarily in a disability or handicap.

In this chapter, the chronic diseases of childhood that are not dealt with in other chapters are described. Topics covered include impact of chronic illness, and specific common and uncommon disorders that cause chronic illness. A Suggested Reading list is included at the end of the chapter for individuals wishing to read more on the topic of chronic childhood disorders.

# IMPACT OF CHRONIC ILLNESS

The impact of chronic illness is dependent on a number of variables. Identification of risk and protective factors may help those involved with children with these disorders minimize the impact and resulting dysfunction. Features of the illness itself may have an important effect on outcome for the child. The age of onset of the illness may affect outcome and adjustment to illness. The course of the illness is important, including severity and predictability of illness exacerbations. The disease itself may have a direct impact on mobility and cognitive abilities. Visibility of the effects of the illness may influence coping and adjustment.

A number of factors may protect children and reduce the effects of chronic illness. Children probably cope better if they have an understanding of their disease and its treatment. In addition to a positive temperament in the child with the illness, positive parental temperament and positive, appropriate, and attainable parental values and aspirations have a significantly beneficial effect on adjustment to illness. Parental encouragement and reinforcement of self-help abilities are also protective in preventing long-term disability. External supports, supportive teachers and school administrators, and a positive, supportive peer group also may help in the prevention of negative consequences of chronic illness. Success in school is very important to children with chronic illness.

## School Performance

Although the majority of children with chronic illness have normal intelligence, 25% to 33% achieve less successfully than their peers, even when absenteeism is taken into account. Although some chronic illnesses involve the brain and nervous system, intellectual impairment due to the disorder itself is uncommon. Preexisting learning disorders and attention problems may be exacerbated by the illness, however. Anxiety related to the illness and resulting school absence may significantly impact school performance. Fatigue, chronic pain, and side effects of medications may contribute to decreased academic performance. The majority of the effect on school performance, however, is likely not due to direct effects of the illness itself or its treatment, but rather to the adoption of the "sick role" and altered expectations of parents and teachers due to the underlying illness.

## School Attendance

Although some children with chronic illness have normal school attendance, children with chronic illness typically miss more school than the average. Generally, the absences are frequent and short. School absenteeism is related less to the specific diagnosis than to the child's and family's response to the illness and the ability of the child to participate in physical activities.

## Family Functioning

The presence of chronic illness in a child may have a significant impact on family functioning. Some illnesses require family members to provide expensive and time-consuming treatments at home, which may significantly increase day-to-day work for the family. For example, physiotherapy exercises may be required on a regular basis, or medications requiring the use of specialized equipment, such as aerosolized treatments for cystic fibrosis or severe asthma, may be required. Specialized care requirements may limit the ability of parents to work outside the home, resulting in financial strain and loss of benefits. Family leisure time may be significantly reduced or eliminated. Respite and babysitters may be unavailable. The strain resulting from these factors may lead to a higher risk of divorce, family violence, and substance abuse. As a result, siblings may receive less attention from their parents.

## Psychological Impact

The majority of children with chronic illness have no apparent problems with psychological adjustment. Children with chronic illness, however, may be at greater risk of significant behavioral problems, perhaps due to overprotectiveness.

# COMMON DISORDERS CAUSING CHRONIC ILLNESS IN CHILDREN

## Asthma

Asthma is one of the most common chronic diseases of childhood. This disorder affects approximately 5% of children. Two thirds of children with asthma have mild disease with little impact on daily functioning, and one third have moderate to severe disease. Even in severe disease, symptoms and hospitalizations can usually be prevented or decreased with effective medical management.

Asthma is a disorder characterized by recurrent episodes of airway obstruction, which results in wheezing and difficulty breathing. The lungs consist of a series of airways, which are tubes surrounded by muscle and lined by mucous membranes similar to the lining of the nose. Two factors contribute to the symptoms of asthma: (a) narrowing of the airways, which results from tightening of the muscles surrounding the airway tubes in an exaggerated response to specific triggers, and (b) inflammation of the airways, which causes swelling of the lining of the airway tubes and mucus production, much like the swelling of the tissues lining the nose during a common cold. The resulting narrowing of the airways results in difficulty moving air in and out of the lungs, causing wheezing and coughing. With increasing severity of symptoms, children may demonstrate reduced exercise endurance, poorer performance in sports, and decreased school performance. In mild asthma, wheezing occurs less often than once per week and symptoms during sleep rarely occur. Moderate to severe asthma results in more frequent symptoms, which may be more serious and require hospitalizations. Treating the underlying inflammation, avoiding known triggers of symptoms, and managing exacerbations early and effectively may prevent most of the symptoms of asthma.

The cause of the airway problems leading to asthma is unknown, although there is clearly a genetic component. Asthma tends to run in families and is more common in children whose parents have a history of asthma. Allergies and eczema are more common in children with asthma and their families.

A number of factors may trigger airway inflammation and airway muscle constriction. Children with asthma commonly have symptoms at the time of viral infections, such as the common cold. Environmental factors such as pollens from trees, grasses, or ragweed may lead to seasonal exacerbations. Exposure to animal dander, dust, tobacco or wood-burning smoke, and chemicals such as cleaning agents may trigger wheezing or coughing. For some children, symptoms may be induced by cold air or exercise. Elimination of avoidable triggers is important for children with asthma. Avoidance of exposure to tobacco smoke in enclosed environments is recommended. Exposures in the classroom—for example, to a visiting rabbit—may trigger asthma symptoms. Recognition and planning for situations that are likely to trigger asthma symptoms, such as outdoor activities in the cold with a child who has exercise- or cold-induced asthma, or a school trip to a farm in a child whose asthma is triggered by animal dander or hay, may prevent severe symptoms. Management strategies may include limiting duration and extent of exposure, premedicating with bronchodilators or increasing the dosage of anti-inflammatory medication under the guidance of a physician, and close monitoring of symptoms.

Two forms of medication are used to treat asthma. Medications that relax the muscles surrounding the airway tubes (bronchodilator medications) act immediately and may provide some immediate, short-term relief of symptoms. More important, treatment should include a medication to prevent or decrease airway inflammation (anti-inflammatory medication). Although anti-inflammatory medications do not provide immediate relief of symptoms, when used regularly, they provide effective control of the underlying disease and prevent daily symptoms. An increasing requirement for bronchodilator medication in a child with asthma signals (a) worsening disease or problems with compliance with anti-inflammatory medication and (b) the need for closer observation and more aggressive medical management to reduce airway inflammation.

Bronchodilator and anti-inflammatory medications are typically administered with an inhaler, which the child uses regularly, typically twice a day. In younger children, a spacer device called an aerochamber may be recommended to improve delivery of the medication to the lungs. At the time of symptom exacerbation, such as when the child has a cold, an increase in the dose and frequency of anti-inflammatory medication or a switch to a more potent tablet form may be recommended.

These medications tend to improve performance in school and physical activity by decreasing asthma symptoms. Side effects from these medications are few and unlikely to have an impact on school performance when asthma is well controlled. Frequent use of bronchodilators (the most common being Ventolin) may result in shakiness and difficulty maintaining attention and concentration and, as indicated above, may signal the need for medical assessment.

It is important for school personnel to have a clear understanding of the severity of disease, recognize common symptom triggers and symptoms, know the medications required, and have a plan for treatment of asthma exacerbation in a child with asthma. Because ready and available access to medications is essential, the medications should not be stored in a locked cupboard in the school nurse's office. The classroom teacher may be in a good position to recognize and alert parents to worsening of a child's asthma. Children's symptoms may be more obvious during the day when they are more active, and less obvious when they are at home. Communication between the school, family, and health care provider is important in early recognition of worsening symptoms that require a change in medication management or indicate issues with compliance with recommended treatment.

## Environmental Allergies

The most common form of allergy involves nasal and eye symptoms resulting from environmental allergens. This form of allergy may involve 5% to 10% of school-age children, although many experience only mild discomfort. Allergies commonly run in families and may be associated with other chronic medical problems, such as eczema or asthma.

Environmental allergies result from inflammation of the mucous membranes lining the eyes, nose, and throat in response to specific triggers. The most common triggers of environmental allergies are pollens and animal dander. Symptoms include itchy, red, watery eyes; nasal congestion; runny nose; itching of the throat; and sneezing. Symptoms in children who suffer pollen allergies tend to be seasonal, often most severe in the spring and fall. Seasonal allergies are commonly referred to as hay fever. When symptoms are severe and chronic, children tend to breathe through their mouths due to chronic nasal congestion, and may have dark circles under their eyes ("allergic shiners"). Specific triggers may be identified by medical personnel, using skin tests, although the results of these tests may not correlate with clinical symptoms.

Treatment with anti-inflammatory nasal sprays may be recommended for severe, seasonal symptoms, to decrease nasal congestion. Many families use over-the-counter nasal decongestants or antihistamines, taken in the form of oral medications, nasal sprays, or eye drops to treat symptoms, although these medications likely have minimal effect. "Allergy shots" are graduated doses of the allergen given by injection, meant to desensitize the patient to the specific trigger, and are available for a small range of specific allergies, such as ragweed.

Although severe symptoms may be distracting and result in decreased school performance, medications also may affect performance. Some oral antihistamines have a significant sedative effect and may result in sleepiness and poor attention in the classroom. Other, nonsedating antihistamines may interfere with sleep and result in daytime fatigue. However, significant medication side effects are few.

## Allergies to Food and Insect Stings

*Anaphylaxis* refers to potentially life-threatening allergy, which occurs most commonly in response to foods, insect stings, and medications. Of the general population (adults and children), only 1% to 2% experience anaphylaxis in response to insect stings and foods, with a lower reported prevalence for drugs and latex. The foods most commonly associated with allergies include peanuts, eggs, and shellfish. Symptoms of anaphylaxis include hives; swelling of the tongue, lips, and throat; breathing problems (wheezing); a drop in blood pressure leading to paleness of the skin, sweating, and dizziness; abdominal cramping; and diarrhea. Milder allergic reactions may include a rash (hives) alone. Allergies to insect stings and foods tend to be lifelong, and the severity of previous exposures to the allergen does not predict severity of future symptoms. Children with coexisting asthma and allergies are at increased risk of severe reaction.

Avoidance of the trigger is the most effective management strategy. Due to the severity and rapidity of progression of symptoms of severe allergies, prompt recognition and immediate treatment are essential. Treatment of severe allergy or anaphylaxis must include immediate administration of epinephrine (adrenaline) by injection and rapid transportation to a hospital. The school should identify children with significant allergies, so that all teachers are aware. A child with a known allergy should have an EpiPen (injectable form of epinephrine that can be administered by an untrained individual), labeled with the child's name and the medication expiration date, and the EpiPen should be readily accessible at all times (i.e., not locked in a cupboard in the nurse's or principal's office). The child should wear a Medic Alert bracelet to identify the presence of an allergy. School personnel should review identification of symptoms and administration of the EpiPen each school year and before school trips.

Much attention has been paid recently to elimination of peanut exposure in schools to prevent symptoms in susceptible children. Strategies to reduce peanut exposure in schools where there are children known to have peanut allergy may include elimination of trading or sharing of foods, utensils, or containers; ensuring that food-allergic children eat only foods that are prepared at home; promptly and thoroughly washing surfaces exposed to foods; and clearly labeling contents of foods served in school cafeterias. It may be advisable to instruct parents of young children to eliminate peanuts and peanut butter from packed lunches to avoid accidental exposure of a classmate.

A promising new therapy for children with peanut allergy has recently been published (Leung et al., 2003). TNX-901 is a monoclonal antibody that inhibits the binding of IgE (a class of immunoglobulins) to mast cells and basophils, a phenomenon responsible for allergic reactions. In clinical trials, TNX-901 given by injection subcutaneously every 4 weeks for four doses substantially increased the threshold of sensitivity to peanut ingestion, a finding that should significantly protect allergic children against the unintended ingestion of peanuts. Additional studies are required before treatment with TNX-901 becomes universally available.

Strategies to prevent insect stings include elimination of beehives, containment of garbage in closed containers, and ensuring that all food is consumed indoors.

# Eczema

Eczema is a common skin rash that affects up to 3% of children. The rash is due to inflammation of the skin, resulting in redness, dryness, and itching. The skin may become thickened and abraded as children scratch repeatedly. In school-age children, the rash is typically most severe around the creases of the elbows and knees, and behind the ears.

The cause of eczema is unknown, although it tends to run in families. Asthma and allergies are more common in children with eczema. Although it is commonly believed that certain foods trigger exacerbations of eczema, there is no good evidence for this in the scientific literature.

There is no cure for eczema, although most children outgrow it or at least have significant reduction in symptoms with increasing age. Symptoms tend to relapse and remit. Treatment consists of lubricating the skin with ointments or creams and reducing the inflammation with cortisone creams. These treatments provide temporary control of symptoms only. When symptoms improve, medications may be discontinued but will need to be restarted at the time of the next flare-up. Oral antihistamines may be recommended if itchiness is a significant problem.

School performance may be affected if itchiness is distracting the child or interfering with sleep. Antihistamines used to treat itchiness may have a sedative effect, resulting in sleepiness and poor concentration.

# Recurrent Abdominal Pain

An estimated 15% of schoolchildren have recurrent abdominal pain, defined as intermittent episodes of pain severe enough to interfere with normal activities (i.e., at least three episodes occurring within a 3-month period). Fewer than 1% of these children have serious underlying disease.

In the majority of cases when children complain of intermittent pain localized around the umbilicus (navel), no medical cause is found and the cause is thought to be psychological. It is interesting that identification of stressors or psychological factors resulting in this recurrent pain rarely occurs. The exception to this is a subgroup of children who experience pain during the school week but not on weekends. This may be part of a school refusal syndrome or school phobia. Constipation or lactose intolerance may be a factor in some children with recurrent abdominal pain. Features that may indicate underlying medical illness include diminished appetite, weight loss or poor growth, vomiting, diarrhea, blood in the stool, and pain that awakens the child during the night. Most often, however, these features are not present and no identifiable underlying medical condition is found.

Symptoms typically include episodes of midabdominal pain that interferes with activities. Despite a normal physical examination and no evidence of underlying medical illness, children may be extremely debilitated by the recurrent pain, partly due to the reaction of worried parents and exposure to unnecessary medical investigations.

It is important that parents, school staff, and medical professionals work together to identify underlying stressors, promote the child's coping capacity, and prevent prolonged or recurrent school absenteeism. School absenteeism may lead to increased stress, more pain, and further school avoidance, as well as interference with normal, healthy peer interactions. In severe cases, psychological or psychiatric consultation and intervention may be necessary.

## Involuntary Soiling

Incontinence of stool beyond age 4 is seen in up to 3% of children attending a pediatric clinic. In young children with a long history of soiling, the cause is frequently related to chronic constipation. Accumulation of stool results in distention of the bowel and rectum and loss of the sensation of fullness and of elasticity of the bowel. In long-standing chronic constipation, a large mass of hard stool frequently occupies much of the large bowel. Soft or liquid stool flows around the hard mass and leaks out into the underpants. Due to chronic overstretching and subsequent reduction in sensation of the rectum, frequently children are unaware of the leakage of stool until enough is present to be sensed by the skin of the buttocks. In older children with recent onset of soiling, psychological factors may be involved, including traumatic experiences.

The psychological impact of the soiling is significant, with children frequently ostracized by their peers due to odor resulting from stool leakage and resultant feelings of guilt and shame. Parents may become frustrated with the ongoing problem, which they feel the child is doing deliberately or should be able to control.

Treatment includes laxatives to clean out the bowel, regular use of stool softeners, and a high-fiber diet including plenty of fluids, to prevent reaccumulation of stool in the large bowel. Often this treatment requires weeks of careful adherence to result in improvement. Compliance with regular use of stool softeners may be a problem. Behavioral intervention including regular sitting on the toilet and a positive reinforcement program for having a bowel movement in the toilet and clean days is also important. For children with underlying psychological factors contributing to the soiling (a small minority of cases), psychological or psychiatric assessment and intervention may be required.

It is important that the child, parents, and teachers recognize that soiling is typically not intentional or under the child's control, and that the child receives the message that this is not the child's fault. A sensitive teacher who recognizes the child's shame and anxiety about accidents at school and works discreetly with parents so that clean clothes are available if required can prevent significant distress in the child. Managing teasing by peers while maintaining the child's self-esteem and providing quiet reminders to clean and change at the time of accidents may also be necessary.

# UNCOMMON DISORDERS CAUSING CHRONIC ILLNESS IN CHILDREN

## Arthritis

The most common form of childhood chronic arthritis is juvenile rheumatoid arthritis (JRA), which occurs in 1 per 1,000 children. Childhood arthritis is an autoimmune condition resulting in inflammation of the joints. The cause of chronic arthritis in children is not well understood, although genetic factors likely play a role.

There are different types of JRA, and inflammation may be limited to one joint or joints, or may involve other areas of the body, such as the eyes. In one type of JRA, systemic JRA, symptoms at the onset of disease include persistent fever, rash, general malaise, and possible involvement of other organs. Like other autoimmune conditions, some forms of JRA may relapse and remit, resulting in recurrent symptom episodes.

Inflammation of the joints results in pain, redness and swelling, and reduced mobility. Long-term effects of the inflammation may include damage to the joints, resulting in contractures (scar tissue) and subsequent permanent limitation of movement of the joint. Other long-term effects may include failure of growth of the adjacent bone due to damage to the growth plate, resulting in shortening of a limb.

Treatment consists of anti-inflammatory medication taken by mouth and sometimes injections of anti-inflammatory medication into the joints. Physiotherapy is important in maintaining and maximizing mobility. Occupational therapy may be recommended in children who have long-term effects on mobility. Early recognition and monitoring for involvement of other organ systems, particularly the eyes, is essential to prevent outcomes such as vision loss.

Communication between the family, school, and medical professionals is important to maximize function and prevent long-term disability. Exercise is generally recommended to maintain joint mobility after treatment is begun and pain subsides, although modifications may be suggested. A clear understanding of the recommended limitations is important to avoid overprotecting the child or exacerbating disease. Pain and school absences may interfere with school performance. For the most part, medications used to treat JRA are unlikely to affect academic functioning.

## Heart Problems

Serious heart disease involving limitations to the school-age child is rare, occurring in 1 in 1,000 to 2,000 children. A higher number of children are born with heart problems, but most problems are repaired prior to school age or resolve spontaneously, with no residual effects.

Twenty-five to 50% of children are diagnosed with an innocent heart murmur. A heart murmur is a sound that a physician hears with the aid of a stethoscope during examination of the heart. A heart murmur refers simply to the sound of blood rushing through the heart. The majority of heart murmurs in children are "innocent," meaning they indicate no underlying heart disorder, result in no symptoms in the child, and require no treatment or limitation of activity. A minority of heart murmurs in children indicate underlying disease, which is typically diagnosed with the aid of an echocardiogram (ultrasound of the heart).

When confronted with a child whose parents report a heart problem or heart murmur, school personnel need to clarify whether a child truly has heart disease or simply has an innocent heart murmur. It is essential that children with innocent heart murmurs be treated as normal children, which they are, and that imposition of the sick role and unnecessary restriction of activities be avoided.

Children with true heart disease may have an underlying heart valve abnormality, abnormal holes between chambers of the heart, or irregularities of the heart rhythm that may require medications or, in rare cases, a pacemaker. Limitation of activities is infrequently recommended. It is important that parents, school personnel, and medical personnel communicate recommendations regarding limitation of activities, treatment, and recognition of signs of illness if relevant.

## Sickle Cell Disease

Sickle cell disease occurs in approximately 1 to 3 per 1,000 children of African ancestry and also occurs in Latin and Mediterranean populations. Sickle cell disease is caused by an abnormal gene, which results in a defect of hemoglobin, the oxygen carrier within red blood cells. This abnormality causes a change in shape of the red blood cells from the normal donutlike shape to a crescent or sickle shape when the red blood cell is exposed to certain stresses. This abnormal shape causes the red blood cells to break down too quickly, resulting in anemia, and the misshapen cells may obstruct the flow of blood within small blood vessels.

Anemia and reduced oxygen-carrying capacity in the blood may result in fatigue and decreased exercise tolerance in children with sickle cell disease. Triggers of sickling (change in shape) of the red blood cells include low oxygen, cold, dehydration, and infection, particularly of the lung, as this results in further reduction of oxygenation. Obstruction of the small blood vessels that provide oxygen to the bones during sickling events, known as sickle cell crises, leads to severe pain. Chest infections may be very serious in children with sickle cell disease because reduction in oxygenation of the blood leads to increased sickling, which obstructs small blood vessels to the lungs, resulting in reduced oxygenation of the blood and a cycle of worsening disease, known as a chest crisis. Between sickle cell crises, children with sickle cell disease are typically well, apart from possible reduction in exercise tolerance due to chronic anemia. Puberty may be delayed, particularly in boys.

Sickle cell disease is an inherited condition. Both parents of a child with sickle cell disease are sickle cell carriers; that is, they both have one abnormal hemoglobin gene and one normal one, and both are unaffected themselves. Parents who are both carriers of an abnormal gene, such as the sickle cell gene, have a 1 in 4 chance of having a child with sickle cell disease. (Chapter 7 provides a more complete explanation of the genetic mechanism underlying sickle cell disease.)

During a sickle cell crisis, children may require hospitalization for intravenous fluids, antibiotics, and pain control, frequently with morphine. Prompt treatment for infections is particularly important in children with sickle cell disease. Regular monitoring between crises, frequently by a specialized clinic, may cause disruptions in school attendance. New medications are now being used in some children with frequent sickle cell crises to promote the oxygen-carrying capacity of the blood and to prevent sickling of the red blood cells.

Good communication between the parents, school, and medical professionals is essential to understanding the severity of illness and for promoting appropriate recommendations for school attendance and participation in activities. Prevention of the sick role is important, including avoidance of excessively long hospitalizations and school absences and promotion of normal socialization and appropriate participation in regular activities.

## Thalassemia

Thalassemia is an inherited blood disorder. Beta thalassemia is most common in children of Mediterranean descent. Alpha thalassemia is most common in children of Southeast Asian background.

Children with thalassemia are born with a defective gene responsible for production of hemoglobin, the oxygen carrier within red blood cells. Due to the gene defect, insufficient hemoglobin chains are made, resulting in anemia. There are different types of thalassemia, which are classified by the part of the hemoglobin chain that is defective. Children may inherit one abnormal gene, resulting in the carrier state, and demonstrate only mild anemia. Children whose parents are both carriers of the defective gene may inherit both copies of this gene, resulting in thalassemia major and severe disease.

Children with thalassemia major have severe anemia, frequently requiring regular blood transfusions. Other areas of the body may try to compensate for the reduced oxygen-carrying capacity of the blood by enlarging in an attempt to increase blood production, resulting in coarsening of the facial features due to growth of the facial bones and enlargement of the liver and spleen. Severe anemia may result in fatigue and exercise intolerance and, when untreated, failure of the heart to pump sufficient blood to meet the body's needs, resulting in backup of blood and accumulation of fluid in the lungs.

Treatment consists of close medical monitoring and regular blood transfusions for severe anemia. Unfortunately, recurrent blood transfusions may result in accumulation of excess iron in various body organs, interrupting their function.

## Cystic Fibrosis

Cystic fibrosis is estimated to occur in 1 in 2,500 children. It most commonly occurs in children of Anglo-Saxon background and is rarely seen in African and Asian populations.

Cystic fibrosis is an inherited condition, caused by a defect in a gene that affects secretions of the lungs and pancreas. Thick secretions produced in the lungs lead to obstruction of the smaller airways by mucus and predispose the individual to lung infections. Inflammation causes further damage. With aggressive therapy and medical supervision, individuals with cystic fibrosis may now live into mid-adulthood.

Children with cystic fibrosis commonly have significant lung disease, with symptoms of cough and wheeze, by adolescence. They typically require intensive treatment with antibiotics, anti-inflammatory medication, and physiotherapy. They experience progressive fatigue and exercise intolerance. Abnormalities of secretions from the pancreas result in malabsorption of fat and protein, as well as vitamin deficiencies. If untreated, weight loss and frequent passage of large stools result. Diabetes may occur as the pancreatic disease progresses. Lung disease is progressive and eventually lung failure occurs. Heart–lung transplants may be performed during adolescence or early adulthood for terminal disease.

Lung disease and frequent hospitalizations may interfere with school attendance as the disease progresses in children with cystic fibrosis. Compliance with aerosolized lung treatments, antibiotics, and physiotherapy is important as the disease worsens. The psychological impact of a terminal illness that may result in death during early adulthood may be significant.

# THE TEACHER'S ROLE

Chronic illness may have a significant impact during childhood. The role of school personnel in supporting school attendance, promoting healthy social interaction, and encouraging participation in activities appropriate to the medical condition, is vital in supporting a child's adjustment to chronic illness and minimizing the disabling impact of the illness. Open and effective communication between parents, school professionals, and medical care providers is essential to maximizing the well-being of the child.

## SUGGESTED READING

Canadian Pediatric Society. (1995). *Anaphylaxis in schools and other child care settings* (Position Statement). Ottawa, Ontario, Canada: Author.

Perrin, J. M., & MacLean, W. E. (1988). Children with chronic illness. *Pediatric Clinics of North America, 35,* 1325–1337.

Sexson, S. B., & Madan-Swain, A. (1993). School reentry for the child with chronic illness. *Journal of Learning Disabilities, 26,* 115–125.

## REFERENCES

Gortmaker, S. L., & Sappenfield, W. (1984). Chronic childhood disorders: Prevalence and impact. *Pediatric Clinics of North America, 31,* 3–18.

Leung, D. Y. M., Sampson, H. A., Yunginger, I. W., Burks, A. W., Schneider, L. C., Wortel, C. H., Davis, F. M., Hyun, J. D., & Shanahan, W. R., for the TNX-901 Peanut Allergy Study Group. (2003). Effect of anti-IgE therapy in patients with peanut allergy. *New England Journal of Medicine, 348,* 986–993.

# CHAPTER 7

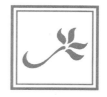

# The Role
# of Genetic Mechanisms
# in Childhood Disabilities

Thaddeus E. Kelly

**G**enetic disorders often involve conditions that result in childhood disabilities; thus, an understanding of these conditions is of major importance in the development of educational programs that seek to minimize the impact of a disability on a child. The functional consequences of these disabilities may be any combination of physical, emotional, social, and educational disabilities. There are literally thousands of genetic conditions, each with specific consequences; however, it is possible to consider them from their functional consequences in such a way as to allow teachers and allied educational professionals to deal with each child individually and knowledgeably. Because the educational setting is an important part of any child's life, a full understanding of the social, psychological, physical, and educational limitations imposed on a child by a genetic disorder is crucial for proper placement and support.

Genetic disorders can be considered by the nature of the genetic alteration responsible for the disability or by the nature of the functional consequence that they impose. This chapter attempts to provide insight into genetic disorders from both perspectives.

## CHROMOSOMES AND
## CHROMOSOMAL ABNORMALITIES

Chromosomes are structures that can be identified and analyzed in detail under the microscope. The nucleus of each human cell contains 46 chromosomes. Chromosomes occur in pairs, with each parent contributing one of each pair, or 23, to each of their children. There are 22 pairs of autosomes and one pair of sex chromosomes, the X and Y chromosomes. A female, whose chromosome constitution is 46,XX, produces eggs with 23 chromosomes, one of which is an X chromosome. A male, whose chromosome constitution is 46,XY, produces sperm with 23 chromosomes, one of which is either an X or a Y chromosome. If an X-bearing sperm fertilizes an egg, this produces a 46,XX karyotype, that of a normal female. If a Y-bearing sperm fertilizes an egg, the result is 46,XY, or a normal male. A female may give either of her two X chromosomes to a son or a daughter. A male gives his single X chromosome to all of his daughters and his Y chromosome to all of his sons (see Figure 7.1).

Chromosomes are packages of genes. The 23 chromosomes given to a child by each parent contain about 30,000 to 40,000 specific genes. Each autosome contains a set of genes specific for that chromosome arranged in a specific linear sequence. The X chromosome contains genes much like that of an autosome, whereas the Y chromosome essentially contains genes that deal with male sex determination and fertility. At the time of conception, the genetic makeup of the fertilized egg serves as a blueprint, containing all the information necessary for the growth and development of an infant from the single fertilized egg cell. An alteration in the chromosomal makeup of a fertilized egg results in an alteration in the blueprint that determines the organization, growth, and development of the resulting child. Chromosomal abnormalities are common at the time of conception. As many as 10% to 15% of all conceptions have a chromosomal abnormality. Most of the time, the resultant effect on growth and development of the embryo is so severe that an early spontaneous abortion occurs. It is only those chromosomal abnormalities that have a less severe consequence that allow for fetal development and delivery of a live-born infant.

Chromosomal abnormalities consist of either a change in the number of chromosomes (i.e., an aneuploidy) or a loss or gain in a portion of a chromosome and the set of genes carried by the involved segment of that chromosome (i.e., a deletion or duplication of part of a chromosome). When such a numerical or structural change involves an autosome, there will be three predictable consequences: abnormal growth (short stature), abnormal physical development (birth defects), and abnormal mental development (mental retardation). With each specific chromosomal change, whether it is numerical or structural, there is a recurring pattern of abnormalities that collectively constitute a recognizable syndrome.

Down syndrome results from a chromosomal aneuploidy in which there are three number 21 chromosomes rather than the normal two, a

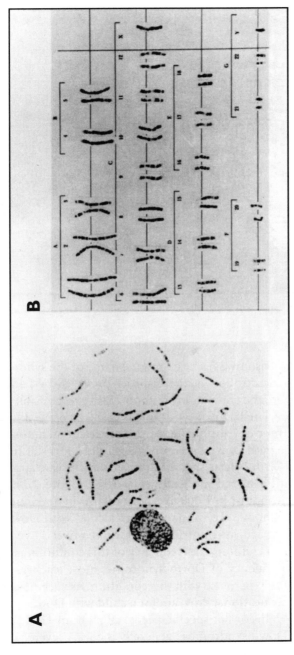

**FIGURE 7.1.** (A) Chromosomes of a normal male as viewed under the microscope. (B) Chromosomes of a normal male as arranged in a karyotype.

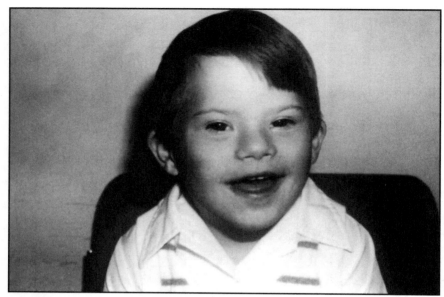

**FIGURE 7.2.** A 5-year-old boy with Down syndrome.

condition called trisomy 21. The eponymic name of the syndrome is based on a published description of the disorder provided by Langdon Down many years before the chromosomal abnormality responsible for the condition was appreciated. Down syndrome is easily recognizable clinically as a result of the three developmental consequences of an autosomal abnormality. Children with Down syndrome have mild short stature, numerous minor physical birth defects that result in a characteristic appearance, and mental retardation in the moderate range (see Figure 7.2). Down syndrome occurs in about 1 in 1,000 live-born infants in developed countries. Because the likelihood of a woman having a child with Down syndrome increases with her age, in countries where women over 35 years of age are commonly having children, the frequency of this condition is higher.

Given the frequency of Down syndrome, most teachers and schools have considerable experience with this condition. As such, it is usually possible to plan an educational program for a child with Down syndrome that is well tailored to his or her specific needs. Of all numerical abnormalities of autosomes, Down syndrome is generally the least severe. This is due to the fact that chromosome 21 is the smallest autosome and the abnormality involves triple doses of genes on chromosome 21 rather than abnormal genes. The presence of a single chromosome 21 at conception is incompatible with fetal life.

Two other aneuploidies involving autosomes are trisomy 13 and trisomy 18. These involve larger chromosomes than number 21 and produce far more severe birth defects. Most infants with trisomy 13 or 18 die in the first year of life, but some survive into childhood. Such children have severe mental retardation and disabilities from their birth defects, including severe congenital heart disease.

The more common a specific chromosomal abnormality is, the more likely it is that it has an eponymic designation as a syndrome and that specific information about the degree of consequences is available. For example, the Wolff-Hirschhorn syndrome involves the loss of a very small amount of chromosomal material from the tip of the short arm of a number 4 chromosome. The amount of material loss may be so small as to make it difficult to recognize the loss under the microscope unless high-quality cytogenetic studies are performed. Nonetheless, the functional consequences of this loss of material are much more severe than those in Down syndrome. Affected children are severely retarded in growth and mental ability and are more likely to have major birth defects.

# CHROMOSOMAL TRANSLOCATIONS

An aneuploidy rarely occurs more than once among the offspring of a couple. Structural abnormalities of chromosomes resulting in a loss or excess of genetic material are more likely to have a high recurrence risk. The risk can be determined by analysis of the chromosomes of the parents. One of them may be a carrier of a balanced chromosomal rearrangement that predisposes the parents to a recurrence of an unbalanced chromosomal state in future offspring. The carrier parent has the appropriate genetic content of each chromosome, but the chromosomes are rearranged. Down syndrome secondary to trisomy 21 implies that either the sperm or, more often, the egg had 24 chromosomes with two, rather than one, number 21 chromosomes. There is a quite small increase in recurrence risk for such a couple. However, Down syndrome may be a familial disorder in some families as the result of a structural abnormality for which many normal family members are carriers. As seen in Figure 7.3, a single chromosome may be composed of the genetic content of a number 14 and a number 21

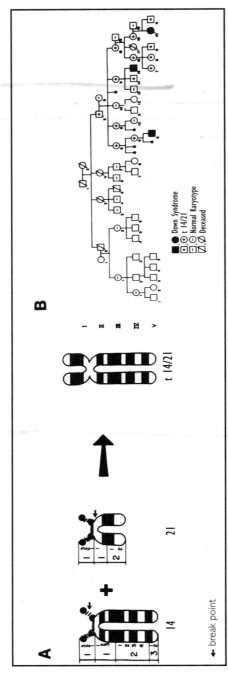

**FIGURE 7.3.** (A) Breakage and fusion of number 14 and number 21 chromosomes to form a translocation chromosome. (B) Familial Down syndrome in a family with a 14/21 translocation.

chromosome, a balanced translocation. The carrier of such a translocation has 45 chromosomes but is normal, as the translocation carries the essential genetic material of two chromosomes. Figure 7.3 shows that such an individual may have children with normal chromosomes, a normal translocation carrier like them, or a child with translocation Down syndrome. The consequences for the child with translocation Down syndrome are no different from those for the child with trisomy 21; however, each normal carrier of a 14/21 translocation has a 5% to 10% chance of having a child with Down syndrome with each pregnancy. Rarely will a child with Down syndrome have 46 chromosomes with one chromosome composed of the components of two number 21 chromosomes. Were a parent to have 45 chromosomes and this 21/21 translocation, the risks for recurrence are virtually 100%. For these reasons, it is prudent to determine the specific chromosomal change responsible for Down syndrome in all affected children.

# SEX CHROMOSOME ABNORMALITIES

Sex chromosome aneuploidies are different from autosomal aneuploidies in that these conditions have a different pattern of consequences. Several syndromes are discussed in the following sections.

## Turner Syndrome

Turner syndrome occurs most commonly with the karyotype 45,X in unambiguous females. The features of the syndrome include the following:

1. *Short stature.* The average height of an untreated woman with Turner syndrome is about 55 to 58 in. Various combinations of hormone therapy, including human growth hormone, usually result in an adult height around 60 in.
2. *Gonadal dysgenesis.* The oocytes, or developing eggs, in the ovary of individuals with Turner syndrome are unable to properly enter the special cell division, meiosis, of germ cells. As a result, the oocytes are rapidly lost in late fetal and early infant life. Without oocytes, the ovaries involute into scar tissue and the female experiences menopause before she has ever achieved menarche. At puberty, without ovarian function, the child has no secondary sexual development or adolescent

growth spurt. Cyclic hormone replacement therapy with estrogen and progesterone promotes normal sexual development with regular menses. Although the lack of oocytes precludes conception, women with Turner syndrome have become pregnant using in vitro fertilization with a donor egg.

3. *Birth defects.* The pattern of birth defects seen with Turner syndrome is the consequence of generalized edema of the body during fetal development. At birth, these female infants have edema of their hands and feet, redundant tissue about their neck, and puffiness about their eyes and ears. The edema generally resolves by 18 to 24 months of age, leaving minor cosmetic consequences. Coarctation, a constriction, of the aorta represents a common and serious birth defect.

4. *Learning disability.* Mental retardation is not a feature of Turner syndrome, but a significant number of these females experience some degree of learning disability. Most commonly this is manifested as difficulty with spatial orientation; mathematics is usually their most difficult subject. It should be emphasized that many of these women have achieved meaningful professional careers in a number of fields and enjoy normal social and family lives.

The diagnosis of the various forms of Turner syndrome may be made at different ages: (a) before birth by abnormalities noted on ultrasonography or chromosomal testing by amniocentesis, (b) at birth by the presence of the typical physical features of Turner syndrome, (c) during childhood because of short stature, and (d) during adolescence or later because of the lack of secondary sexual development, amenorrhea, and infertility.

## Variations on Turner Syndrome

Of females with an X chromosome abnormality and gonadal dysgenesis, about half have a 45,X karyotype and typical Turner syndrome. The remaining half have a wide range of structural abnormalities of the X chromosome involving loss of various portions, but not all, of one X chromosome. Three general phenotypes are observed: (a) gonadal dysgenesis with no other manifestations, (b) gonadal dysgenesis with short stature but not the pattern of birth defects seen in Turner syndrome, or (c) all of the typical Turner syndrome features. Note that the common feature is gonadal dysgenesis.

## Triple X Females

About 1 in 1,000 live-born female infants have 47 chromosomes with three X chromosomes (47,XXX). Most of them will go undetected during their lifetime, as 47,XXX often produces no outward manifestations. However, analysis of a large group of 47,XXX females suggests that as a group there is a 10- to 15-point IQ shift to the left. Thus, females with triple X are found more often than expected among females with learning disabilities or mild mental retardation. There is no gonadal dysgenesis or short stature, and fertility is normal, with no increased risk of a sex chromosome aneuploidy in their offspring.

## Klinefelter Syndrome

Klinefelter syndrome occurs as a result of a 47,XXY karyotype and has a frequency of about 1 in 1,000 live-born, unambiguous males. Usually, these males go undetected until they fail to undergo pubertal sex development along with their peers. Untreated teenage males often develop gynecomastia, male breast development, which is particularly distressing socially. Much like Turner syndrome, the sex chromosome aneuploidy produces gonadal dysgenesis that results in failure of sexual development and infertility. These males tend to be taller than their male relatives and have small testes (see Figure 7.4). With proper diagnosis and hormone replacement treatment with testosterone, normal sexual development will proceed. For males with gynecomastia, a simple, cosmetic mastectomy will alleviate the associated psychosocial problems. Unilateral gynecomastia of a mild degree is not uncommon among normal teenage males. Not unlike 47,XXX females, these males as a group have an IQ shift to the left such that Klinefelter syndrome is encountered more often than would have been expected otherwise among males with learning disabilities and mild mental retardation.

Klinefelter syndrome and 47,XXX are like trisomy 21 in that the frequency of these 47-chromosome states increases with advancing maternal age. There is no association between the frequency of 45,X Turner syndrome and maternal age. DNA (deoxyribonucleic acid) studies have shown that the majority of these three conditions with 47 chromosomes result

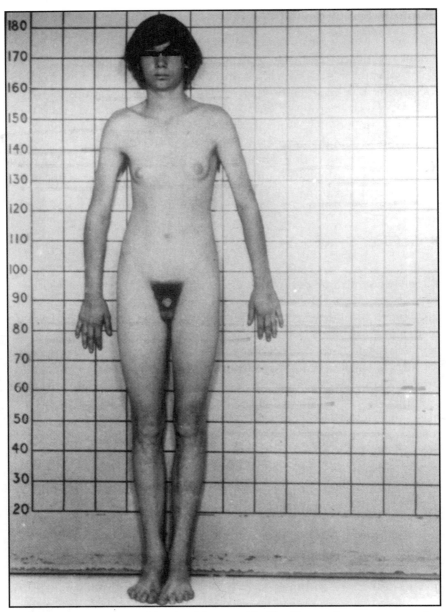

**FIGURE 7.4.** An 18-year-old male adolescent with Klinefelter syndrome.

from the presence of an extra maternal chromosome, whereas in Turner syndrome there is usually the loss of a paternal sex chromosome.

## 47,XYY

The aneuploidy 47,XYY is as common among newborn male infants as is 47,XXY. Following its discovery in the 1960s, there was the suggestion that this aneuploidy might be associated with antisocial or criminal behavior. At present, the bulk of available information strongly suggests that the overwhelming majority of males with an extra Y chromosome have no significant consequences that can be directly attributed to this chromosomal abnormality.

With the widespread use of ultrasound and amniocentesis, sex chromosome aneuploidies are often detected through testing done as a result of the increased risk of an autosomal abnormality in an older mother. When detected, the psychosocial, behavioral, and educational issues, rather than any serious physical disability, create difficult genetic counseling and stressful decision making for couples.

# SINGLE-GENE INHERITANCE

Genes are chemical structures that represent the smallest functional unit of inheritance. The chemical structure of a gene uses four chemicals (nucleotides)—adenine (A), guanine (G), thymidine (T), and cytosine (C)—arranged in units of three (codons) to specify the amino acid sequence of a protein (see Figure 7.5). The genetic code consists of all the triplet combinations of the four nucleotides (64), with each codon specifying a particular amino acid or processing signal. The codons are linearly arranged like beads on a string. A change in the nucleotide sequence of a gene (mutation) may have no effect on the amino sequence of the product protein, and no effect on function, or it may result in a functionally altered protein or the complete lack of production of that protein. The manifestations (phenotype) of a single-gene inherited disorder are based on the degree of abnormality in the protein gene product and its effect on the function normally carried out by that protein. Although chromosomal abnormalities have widespread effects on the developing fetus, single-gene

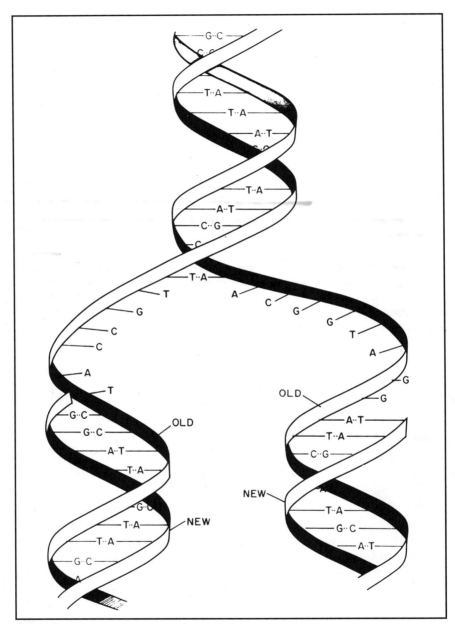

**FIGURE 7.5.** Double-stranded DNA being copied prior to cell division.

abnormalities have more narrow consequences that can be related to the changes in the single-gene product. Inherited mutations of single genes have a wide range of functional consequences. These vary from essentially cosmetic concerns to disorders incompatible with life. The patterns of inheritance of single-gene disorders in humans are the same as the pattern described in garden peas by Gregor Mendel in 1866 (i.e., mendelian inheritance) (Thompson, McInnes, & Willard, 1991).

## Autosomal Dominant Inheritance

When inheritance of a mutation at only one copy of a pair of genes is required for expression of a trait, that trait is said to be dominantly inherited. The trait can be transmitted from one parent to a child, and there is a 50% chance that any offspring of a parent with such a trait will have the same trait. Expression of the trait is independent of inheritance from the unaffected parent. Dominantly inherited traits may vary widely among affected individuals even within the same family. There are a large number of dominantly inherited disorders that have important implications for school-age children (see Figure 7.6).

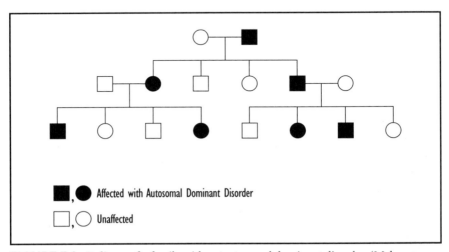

**FIGURE 7.6.** Pedigree of a family with an autosomal dominant disorder. (Males are represented as squares and females as circles.)

## Achondroplasia

Achondroplasia is a dominantly inherited disorder that is the most common form of a skeletal dysplasia producing dwarfism. All of the manifestations of the condition are attributable to defective growth of bones at the site where cartilage is converted to bone in the growth centers of the skeleton. Cell division and growth are controlled by the balancing effects of genes that stimulate growth and those that inhibit growth. The specific mutation producing achondroplasia results in overexpression of a gene that inhibits skeletal growth. Affected children not only are quite short (adult height averages 48 in.), but they have a disproportionate shortening of their arms and legs relative to their trunk (see Figure 7.7). Their sitting height is closer to average than their standing height. Poor growth of the facial bones increases the frequency of ear infections in early childhood and may lead to a permanent hearing loss.

Most children with achondroplasia are healthy and bright; their major problem in school years is the psychosocial consequences of their height and appearance. They often have problems getting on and off the school bus, getting their lunch in a cafeteria line, reaching a water fountain, or using an adult-size toilet. Some may have problems cleaning themselves after a bowel movement because of short arms. In early grades, classmates often consider the age of a child with achondroplasia to be reflected by his or her height; thus, there is a tendency to treat such children as though they were younger than their real age. Such children may assume or be assigned a mascot role, which over the long run may impede their social development.

Although achondroplasia is an autosomal dominantly inherited disorder, only about 10% to 15% of affected children have an affected parent. In most instances, the affected child receives a new mutation from a parent that arose in the germ cell giving rise to that child. The affected child has a 50% chance of transmitting the achondroplasia gene to his or her offspring, but the unaffected parents have no increased risk for a second affected child (see Figure 7.8).

In general, the more severe the physical consequences of a dominantly inherited disorder, the more likely it is that an affected child will represent a new mutation. For a dominantly inherited disorder that prevents the individual from being able to reach adulthood and reproduce, all cases must represent a new mutation. New mutations resulting in dominantly inherited disorders are associated with an increased age of

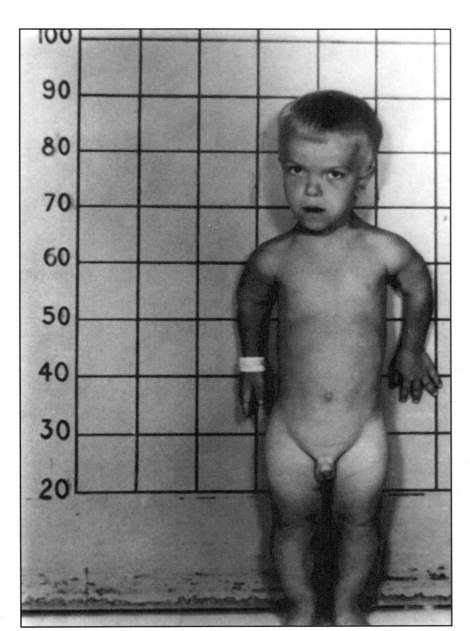

**FIGURE 7.7.** A 6-year-old boy with achondroplasia.

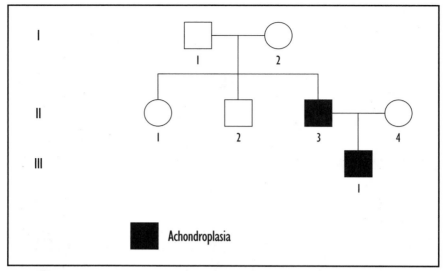

**FIGURE 7.8.** Individual II-3 represents a new mutation for achondroplasia, which was transmitted to III-1.

fathers, as opposed to increased maternal age as is seen with chromosomal aneuploidies.

The Little People of America (LPA) is a support group that maintains a Web site with helpful information about numerous forms of dwarfism.

## Neurofibromatosis

Neurofibromatosis type 1 (NF1), a common dominantly inherited disorder, has as its usual manifestations brown skin spots (café au lait spots) and lumpy skin growths (neurofibromas). The affected gene in this disorder is a tumor suppressor factor. Mutations allow for tumor growth involving tissue of the nervous system. The café au lait spots are usually present in early childhood, whereas the skin growths commonly appear at puberty. The more serious consequence, however, is the development of nerve tumors (neurofibromas) anywhere within the body. These can involve the optic nerve, causing severe visual problems; the acoustic nerve, causing deafness; and nerves along the spine or any part of the brain. Scoliosis (curvature of the spine) occurs commonly in children with neurofibromatosis and is often more difficult to treat than other forms of scoliosis. About 30% to 40% of children with NF1 display a specific pattern of learning disability that is characterized by poor language and reading skills without impaired math skills. They also exhibit deficits in visuospatial and neuromotor skills.

The skin manifestations, spots and lumps, may be the only manifestations of NF1, but can represent a real emotional concern for a school-age child, depending on the size and location of these lesions. The size and number may preclude cosmetic surgery for their removal.

A completely different dominantly inherited disorder with brain tumors but without café au lait spots is called neurofibromatosis type 2. Tumors usually do not occur until young adult years.

## Osteogenesis Imperfecta

A better term for osteogenesis imperfecta, a dominantly inherited disorder, is *brittle bone disease*. The defect resides in collagen, the protein that forms the filamentous network upon which bone is mineralized. The most common form of this disorder usually does not result in spontaneous fractures in affected children, but only minimal trauma might be needed to result in a fracture. This form is called osteogenesis imperfecta type 1 (OI1). The fractures heal normally, but recurring fractures may produce skeletal deformity and body asymmetry. Associated features include blue sclerae (the whites of eyes in this condition are robin-egg blue) and joint laxity, with possible early delays in motor milestones. Loss of movement of the bones of the inner ear (otosclerosis) frequently produces a significant hearing loss in young adults. Although children with OI1 will need limitations in their physical activities consistent with the frequency of their fractures, no cognitive problems are associated with this condition. Indeed, as these children's physical limitations may decrease their occupational opportunities, they should be encouraged to maximally use their intellectual resources to open vocational opportunities.

OI3 is a more severe form of this condition that results in frequent fractures with secondary deformity and poor skeletal growth. Severely affected children are usually confined to a wheelchair. OI2, the most severe form, is incompatible with life and results in stillborn infants or early neonatal death. The degree of severity is usually consistent within a family but varies widely across families.

## Autosomal Recessive Inheritance

The best known example of autosomal recessive inheritance is eye color. Only one copy of the gene for brown eyes is required for a person to have brown eyes. On the other hand, both copies of the gene must code for blue eyes for the person to have blue eyes; thus, blue eyes is a recessively inherited trait whereas brown eyes is a dominantly inherited trait. Once a brown-eyed couple has had a blue-eyed child, they have shown that they are carriers of the gene for blue eyes.

Currently, as with many recessively inherited diseases, having an affected child is the most common means by which carriers for a recessive disorder are recognized (see Figure 7.9). Some autosomal recessive conditions

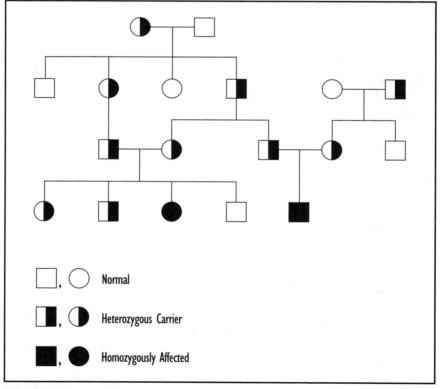

**FIGURE 7.9.** An idealized pedigree of a family with an autosomal recessive trait. Inbreeding increases the risk for autosomal recessive disorders.

**TABLE 7.1**

Some Recessively Inherited Disorders Occurring with High Frequency
in Specific Ethnic Groups

| Disease | Population | Carrier Test |
| --- | --- | --- |
| Tay-Sachs disease | Ashkenazic Jews | Blood hexosaminidase |
| Gaucher disease | Ashkenazic Jews | Blood glucosidase |
| Sickle cell disease | African | Hemoglobin electrophoresis |
| Thalassemia | Mediterranean | Red blood cell volume |
| Cystic fibrosis (CF) | Western European | DNA test of CF gene |

occur more frequently in specific ethnic groups, and carrier testing for these conditions may be available and practical (see Table 7.1). Because a couple with a common set of grandparents (first cousins) may both inherit a mutation from one of the grandparents, rendering both carriers, inbreeding or consanguinity increases the risk of an autosomal recessive disorder.

## Sickle Cell Disease

Sickle cell disease is one of the few recessively inherited diseases that is known to provide carriers with a biological advantage over noncarriers. In equatorial Africa, where sickle cell disease is most common, carriers of the disorder are less likely to die from malaria than are noncarriers. This advantage accounts for the high frequency of the disease within that population. The price for that advantage, however, is the severe consequences for children who inherit two copies of the sickle cell gene from their carrier parents. The carriers for sickle cell disease themselves have no adverse medical consequences as a result of being carriers. Being a carrier is often referred to as having the sickle cell trait. Lack of understanding about the differences between being a carrier and being affected has led to various forms of unjustified discrimination against carriers.

Generally, among recessively inherited disorders, the same mutation occurring in a double dose results in little variability in the severity of the disorder among affected children. Children with sickle cell disease, however, display a surprisingly wide degree of variation in the severity of their disease. Many states screen newborn infants for sickle cell disease because overwhelming infections are a major concern in early childhood. Following the diagnosis in a newborn infant, oral penicillin is given prophylactically.

This is continued into and through school-age years. During school years, such children are prone to episodes of bone infarction, which produce painful crises. This is the most common cause for a high rate of absenteeism. Chronic anemia results in easy fatigability, and the anemia may be sufficiently severe as to require chronic blood transfusion therapy. Despite many years of research, there is no specific therapy for sickle cell disease and treatment is directed at complications of the disease.

## Phenylketonuria

Since the 1960s, virtually all states have screened newborn infants for phenylketonuria (PKU), an inborn error of metabolism, because of its frequency and because dietary therapy started in early infancy can prevent the otherwise inevitable mental retardation. Untreated, this recessively inherited defect in the metabolism of the amino acid phenylalanine results in severe mental retardation without imposing any physical abnormalities. The primary role of the special diet is to restrict dietary intake of phenylalanine, which requires use of a special milk formula with restricted intake of dietary protein. Affected children will not be able to participate in the customary eating habits of their peers and will need to bring lunch from home. Planning is necessary to allow affected children to participate in school parties by having foods available that they can eat. Families usually learn to prepare a wide variety of foods that are low in phenylalanine. Without the dietary restrictions, successfully treated children with PKU would not be otherwise recognized as affected in their school.

Although dietary therapy is most important in the first 2 years of life, discontinuance of the diet when the child enters school has been shown to result in increased behavioral problems and poorer school performance. In most treatment programs, children with PKU continue on some form of dietary therapy throughout their school years. If a female with PKU were successfully treated as a child but went off her diet before starting a family of her own, her PKU essentially places the developing fetus in a PKU environment. Even though the fetus does not have PKU, the result is impaired brain growth and prenatal development. Thus, children born of untreated PKU mothers are severely disabled. Failure to maintain good dietary control in young women could wipe out all the benefits of mental retardation prevention that have been accomplished by treating affected children.

Because of the favorable cost–benefit ratio and the lobbying efforts of family support groups, newborn screening for PKU was widespread in the

**TABLE 7.2**
Disorders Detected Through Newborn Screening Tests

| Disorder | Test[a] |
|---|---|
| Phenylketonuria | Phenylalanine level |
| Maple syrup urine disease | Leucine level |
| Galactosemia | Enzyme and galactose levels |
| Hypothyroidism | Thyroid hormones |
| Biotinidase deficiency | Enzyme level |
| Sickle cell disease | Hemoglobin electrophoresis |
| Congenital adrenal hyperplasia | 17-hydroxy-progesterone |
| Duchenne muscular dystrophy | Muscle enzymes level |
| MCAD | Mass spectroscopy |
| Cystic fibrosis | Trypsinogen level |
| Homocystinuria | Methionine level |

MCAD = medium chain acyl-carnitine dehydrogenase deficiency.
[a] All tests are conducted on blood spots collected on filter paper in the newborn nursery.

United States by the mid-1960s. Once systems were in place for newborn screening, programs were expanded to screen for additional genetic disorders. The primary prerequisites for screening were that the disorder could be detected while the infant was presymptomatic by an inexpensive test and that early treatment would have a major impact on the prognosis. With advancing technology, the number of disorders screened for has grown. For some disorders, screening is based on efforts to provide genetic counseling against recurrence of the disorder rather than preventive treatment. Table 7.2 lists some of the disorders detected through newborn screening tests. Not all states screen for all the disorders listed.

## Cystic Fibrosis

Cystic fibrosis (CF), which is most common among western Europeans, results from a defect in the membrane transport of chloride in and out of cells. As a result, the secretions in the respiratory tract are thick and tenacious, which cause repeated pulmonary infections and progressive respiratory failure. The pancreas, which produces enzymes needed for the intestinal digestion of foods, also is affected. Deficiency in these pancreatic enzymes results in malabsorption of food, creating impaired nutrition. The deficiency can be largely overcome by the use of orally administered enzymes with each meal. School absenteeism is high due to repeated hospitalizations for intensive respiratory therapy. Current therapy requires adherence to a diet, proper use of replacement pancreatic enzymes, frequent antibiotic use, and vigorous chest physical therapy. As each of these aspects of therapy has improved, there has been a continued increase in the life expectancy of individuals with CF. As a result, almost all children with CF are able to participate in school programs from kindergarten through 12th grade. New and exciting experimental forms of therapy currently are being tested.

## Storage Diseases

Storage diseases result from the recessively inherited deficiency of enzymes involved in the degradation of normal, large chemical compounds. Without the necessary catabolism of these large compounds, they accumulate in tissues. The resulting disease depends on the specific tissues in which the involved compounds accumulate. The degree of enzyme deficiency determines the rate of accumulation and, therefore, the rate of progression of the disorder.

The Sanfilippo syndrome (mucopolysaccharidosis III) involves defective degradation of large compounds called mucopolysaccharides, or glycosaminoglycans, which accumulate primarily in the brain. Affected children usually are healthy, but delays in their cognitive development become apparent between 2 and 3 years of age. They develop a striking degree of hyperactivity, which greatly interferes with their participation in school programs and tries their parents' and teachers' patience. This form of attention-deficit/hyperactivity disorder is usually not amenable to drug therapy. After about 6 years of age, there is slow but unremitting loss of cognitive skills, with a life expectancy into the late teens or 20s.

Two other forms of mucopolysaccharidosis, the Morquio syndrome (MPS IV) and the Maroteaux-Lamy syndrome (MPS VI), result in severe skeletal problems with dwarfism, but affected children are not cognitively impaired.

## Defective Carbohydrate Metabolism

Diabetes mellitus is the most common disorder of carbohydrate (sugar) metabolism. It occurs in two distinct forms: insulin-dependent diabetes (type 1) and non–insulin-dependent diabetes (type 2). Insulin-dependent diabetes affects younger individuals and produces more severe complications. There is good evidence that it results from a genetic predisposition wherein individuals respond to some viral infections by producing antibodies that destroy the insulin-producing cells of the pancreas. Because of the insulin deficiency, the body attempts to burn fat as a source of energy. Incomplete burning of fats generates compounds (ketones) that lead to excess acids in the body. The combination of impaired sugar metabolism and excess acids (ketoacidosis) chronically results in poor growth, easy fatigability, and increased susceptibility to infection. Acutely, these changes can produce life-threatening chemical imbalances. A combination of proper insulin dosage and diet are required. Insulin administration without proper dietary intake can lead to episodes of confusion and irritability, even coma, because of hypoglycemia (low blood sugar). This can usually be quickly corrected with a sugar snack (see Chapter 5).

Non–insulin-dependent diabetes is a disorder of adults that segregates in families as an autosomal dominantly inherited disorder. Proper diet and exercise can usually control it. As the frequency of obesity in children has increased dramatically over recent years, there has been an increased incidence of non–insulin-dependent diabetes in school-age children.

Medium chain acyl-carnitine dehydrogenase (MCAD) deficiency produces a defect in the metabolism of fatty acids. Affected children are prone to hypoglycemia, especially with fasting. Glycogen storage disease, of several types, results from an inability of the liver to burn glycogen, the stored form of carbohydrate used for energy production. With both conditions, children require a diet high in complex carbohydrates and low in fat to meet their daily energy requirements without recurring episodes of hypoglycemia. With proper diet, most affected children can participate fully in all school activities, and most have normal cognitive function. Both disorders are recessively inherited.

# X-LINKED INHERITANCE

As discussed earlier, females have two X chromosomes whereas males have a single X and a Y chromosome. The X chromosome carries a large number of genes similar to those located on autosomes, and the Y chromosome essentially carries a gene responsible for male sexual development. As a result, a female may be a carrier for, but unaffected by, a mutation on one

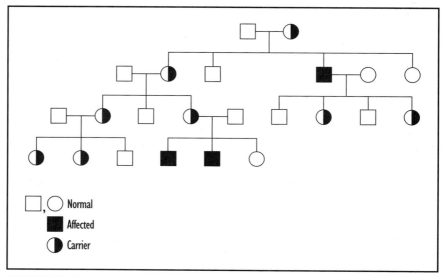

**FIGURE 7.10.** Pedigree for an X-linked recessive trait. Note that female carriers may have affected sons or carrier daughters; affected males have carrier daughters and no affected sons.

of her two X chromosomes. A male, having only one X chromosome, will manifest any mutation that he receives from his mother. Given this pattern of inheritance of sex chromosomes, a woman may transmit a mutant-bearing X chromosome to a son or a daughter. However, a man will always transmit his X to his daughters and his Y to his sons. As a result, X-linked diseases are not transmitted from fathers to sons. However, all the daughters of an affected man will be carriers (see Figure 7.10).

## Color Blindness

Color blindness is the best known form of an X-linked disorder wherein females are carriers and their sons may be color blind. Each son of a carrier woman has a 50% chance of being color blind, and each daughter has a 50% chance of being a carrier. As having color blindness does not significantly affect one's health or ability to reproduce, females may be color blind as a result of inheriting the mutation from both a carrier mother and a color-blind father.

## Hemophilia

Two forms of X-linked hemophilia can occur: a severe A form (Factor VIII deficiency) and a less severe B form (Factor IX deficiency). Having hemophilia, or being a "bleeder," is a result of deficiency of a factor required for the normal clotting of blood. The severity of both forms varies across different families, ranging from frequent nosebleeds and easy bruising to spontaneous internal hemorrhages. The propensity to bleed with minor trauma leads to restricted activity of affected boys.

Cloning of the Factor VIII gene has allowed commercial production of Factor VIII to be used for treatment of boys with hemophilia A. Severely affected boys may require the regular administration of Factor VIII to prevent bleeding, whereas less severely affected boys may only require Factor VIII at times of bleeding. Prior to the use of genetically prepared Factor VIII, the factor was obtained from pooled plasma of donors, some of whom were intravenous drug users infected with the HIV virus who were selling their blood. As a result, many boys with hemophilia who required Factor VIII replacement became infected with HIV and died of AIDS as a result of their therapy. This is no longer a concern for boys with hemophilia who are treated with the genetically prepared product.

## Lesch-Nyhan Syndrome

Lesch-Nyhan syndrome is an inborn error of metabolism that affects the part of the brain, the cerebellum, that controls coordinated speech and muscle activity. Affected boys are dysarthric (garbled speech) and ataxic (poor sense of balance and coordination). They maintain reasonably good receptive language skills, however, and with communication devices can participate in special education classes. The disorder is progressive; one of the most disturbing complications is the development between the ages of 4 and 6 of self-mutilating behavior. This can be managed to some extent by a controlled, structured environment, as heightened anxiety tends to set off episodes of finger and tongue biting. Life expectancy is into the late teens or 20s.

## Duchenne Muscular Dystrophy

Duchenne muscular dystrophy is a common, progressive disorder of muscle that is usually first apparent at 18 to 24 months when motor skills are delayed. The muscles, particularly those of the legs, may appear large and well developed in the face of striking muscle weakness. A large defective gene carries the code for the protein dystrophin, which is defective in muscular dystrophy. A large variety of mutations are known to occur, with resulting wide variability in severity. In the most severe forms of muscular dystrophy (e.g., Duchenne muscular dystrophy), the muscle weakness leads to increasing respiratory difficulty, which may be further complicated by cardiac disease, and eventually leads to death in the late teens or early 20s. Less severe forms (e.g., Becker muscular dystrophy) may allow survival well into adult years, with muscle weakness as the only childhood manifestation. Affected boys usually require wheelchairs during their school years. As with many physically disabling conditions, it is often wise to have two sets of books for these boys, one set kept at home and one set kept at school.

There are a number of less common forms of progressive muscular dystrophy, most of which are recessively inherited. Cognitive problems are uncommon, and the range of disability varies widely in these disorders.

# MULTIFACTORIAL INHERITANCE

It is readily apparent that tall parents tend to have tall children and smart parents tend to have smart children. Although these and many other traits are familial, they are not inherited in families as a result of mutation at a single gene or a chromosomal abnormality. Rather, such traits are determined by a number of genes acting together. In addition to genetic factors, environmental factors play a role in the expression of many of these traits, thus the term *multifactorial causation*. Most common birth defects have multifactorial causes and, as such, have several characteristics in common:

1. The defects are isolated structural birth defects.

2. The impact on the child is the result of the physical disabilities imposed by the birth defect.

3. The defect itself is not physically different from that which occurs as part of single-gene or chromosomally inherited syndromes. The distinction is a clinical one; that is, the defects are isolated or part of a wider series of birth defects.

4. The likelihood of recurrence in a family is on the order of 3% to 5%, but the risk increases with the severity of the birth defect and the number of family members affected.

This mechanism of inheritance is sometimes referred to as "genetic predisposition" when it is applied to familial adult disorders such as arthritis, coronary artery disease, hypertension, and others.

## Cleft Lip and Palate

Cleft lip with or without a cleft palate results from a failure of midfacial structures to fuse in the midline during early embryonic life. There are numerous single-gene and chromosomal disorders in which clefting occurs as one of numerous birth defects clustered as a distinct syndrome. More commonly, however, clefting occurs as an isolated birth defect under multifactorial causation. When an infant is born with a cleft, it is important to distinguish between an isolated cleft and one associated with other malformations, as the prognosis for growth and development, as well as the risk for recurrence within the family, for the two situations is quite different (see also Chapter 10).

Isolated clefting is not associated with growth or cognitive disabilities. The major issue for such children is often the psychosocial problems associated with their appearance and any speech pathology. The prognosis for a child with clefting that is part of a single-gene or chromosomal syndrome is dependent on the nature of the syndrome rather than just the clefting. Isolated cleft lip or cleft lip and cleft palate are most often multifactorially caused. Cleft palate with a normal lip is more often part of a wider syndrome of birth defects.

Cleft lip repair is usually undertaken at about 6 to 10 weeks of age and repair of the cleft palate at about 10 to 15 months of age. Clefting may produce feeding problems for the infant, such as regurgitation of milk into the nasopharynx with associated repeated ear infections. Cleft palate may cause poor closure of the upper airway, giving rise to speech problems that may be aggravated by a hearing loss from repeated infections.

Sometimes, further surgery may be indicated prior to entry into school to achieve a better cosmetic result of the repaired cleft lip or to improve the child's speech. Speech therapy often is required for these children in early school years.

## Congenital Heart Disease

Like clefting, congenital heart disease is a common component of many single-gene and chromosomal syndromes; only as an isolated defect is it multifactorially caused. Congenital heart disease produces problems for a child by one of three physiological consequences:

1. Blood is rerouted through the heart such that it is not passed adequately through the lungs for oxygenation. This is the basis for "blue babies" with cyanotic heart disease (e.g., tetralogy of Fallot).

2. The structure of the heart is such that it cannot work efficiently as a pump, and congestive heart failure results (e.g., ventricular septal defect).

3. There is an obstruction in the pathway by which oxygenated blood from the lungs is delivered to body tissues (e.g., coarctation of the aorta).

Any of these three problems may be partially or completely corrected by heart surgery. Like clefting, heart defects occur in many syndromes, and a realistic prognosis for a child with congenital heart disease must take into account whether or not the defect is isolated and, if not, what are the consequences of the associated problems. For example, roughly 30% of children with Down syndrome have congenital heart disease.

The very thought of heart disease in a child is enough to frighten a parent. It is not uncommon for children with functionally insignificant heart disease or surgically corrected heart disease to be unnecessarily restricted by a well-meaning but overbearing parent. After a while, even the child begins to view him- or herself as disabled. Teachers who are not fully informed about the child's condition may add to the child's psychological burden.

## Neural Tube Defects

The neural tube consists of the bony encasement of the brain (skull) and the spinal cord (vertebral column). Embryologically, both begin as a flat membrane that folds onto itself and fuses to form a protective tube. At any point, there may be incomplete closure of the tube, ranging from anencephaly (no skull and virtually no brain tissue) to a small skin-covered cyst at the base of the spine that may have no functional consequence. A variety of screening techniques have been developed for the early recognition of neural tube defects during pregnancy.

Anencephaly is incompatible with survival beyond a few days after birth. The severity of spina bifida (meningomyelocele) depends on the location along the spine where incomplete closure of the neural tube occurs and the degree of damage sustained by the spinal cord. Spina bifida with survival most commonly involves the lower spine with the following consequences:

1. The spinal cord at the site of the open defect is damaged, with resulting paralysis from that point down. The child may later be wheelchair bound or walk with braces and crutches. The nerves supplying the bladder and lower bowel often are damaged, resulting in incontinence. This predisposes such children to repeated urinary tract infections.

2. The spinal cord is firmly attached to the vertebral column at the site of the defect. As a result, it pulls downward on the brain, creating an obstruction leading to hydrocephalus. Hydrocephalus that begins to develop before birth often later results in poor intellectual development. Most often hydrocephalus is not significant at birth. Shortly after birth, a shunt around the blockage usually is installed surgically at the same time the defect in the back is closed. Repeated blockages in the shunt may require numerous surgical revisions. However, as long as infection within the fluid system of the brain (ventricles) is prevented, there is usually good cognitive development (see Figure 7.11).

A variety of research projects have strongly implicated dietary deficiencies as a causative factor of neural tube defects. In the early 20th century, there was a high incidence of neural tube defects in Ireland. However, as Irish immigrants came to the United States, the incidence in this population dropped dramatically over several generations. Such a change was too rapid to be genetically based. There is a good correlation worldwide between the frequency of spina bifida and the living standards of the

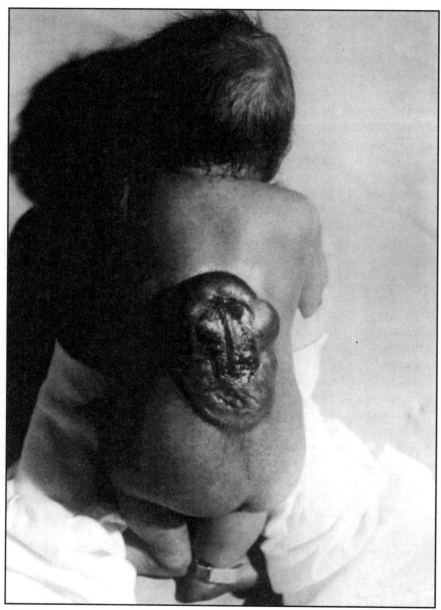

**FIGURE 7.11.** Newborn infant with a large thoraco-lumbar meningomyelocele.

population. The Centers for Disease Control has implemented efforts to increase the folic acid intake of the U.S. population as a measure to prevent neural tube defects (see Chapter 2).

# MITOCHONDRIAL INHERITANCE

Mitochondria are organelles within the cytoplasm of cells that function as a cellular furnace, generating and regulating chemical energy production. The mitochondria also contain a small circular chromosome whose DNA codes for some of the proteins involved in mitochondrial energy production. Most of the genes coding for mitochondrial proteins are carried on the 46 nuclear chromosomes.

Spermatozoa are designed to travel to the site of conception and penetrate the egg in order to deliver a nucleus, the paternal genetic contribution. All of the cytoplasm present after fertilization is supplied by the egg, including the mitochondria and the mitochondrial DNA. (Recognizing the genetic importance of the X chromosome compared to the Y chromosome and of mitochondrial DNA, a boy would benefit most by choosing his mother rather than his father.) Disorders due to mutations of mitochondrial DNA are transmitted only from the mother to her offspring. Most mitochondrial disorders involving nuclear genes are autosomal recessively inherited.

Mitochondrial disorders, whether due to mutations of mitochondrial or nuclear DNA, are characterized by slowly progressive muscle weakness, often associated with visual impairment, seizures, hearing loss, and some degree of intellectual impairment. No specific therapy is available, but supportive care can significantly improve the quality of life.

# RECENT ADVANCES IN MEDICAL GENETICS

## Deletion Syndromes

A number of syndromes have been described in children that have several features in common. These include short stature, some degree of mental retardation, and behavioral features and physical findings of a highly specific and diagnostic nature. Affected children are quite similar in their manifestations, and yet the overwhelming majority of cases occur sporadically within families. There have been occasional case reports of an affected parent and child. Therefore, previously it was assumed that, although there was the potential for parent-to-child transmission, this was consistent with autosomal dominant inheritance. The disorder was thought to usually arise as a new mutation of a single gene and transmission did not occur largely because the condition greatly reduced the individual's potential for reproduction.

In rare instances, a given case has been associated with a visible chromosomal change. These cases have directed research into a more careful examination of these syndromes, using a variety of laboratory techniques. As a result, a number of these syndromes have been recognized to occur as a result of a small, often microscopically invisible deletion of chromosomal material. Small pieces of DNA whose precise chromosomal location are known are tagged with a fluorescent dye and used as probes. By comparing the DNA pattern at these locations in DNA from an affected child and from the parents, it is possible to demonstrate that a portion of the chromosome, a change too small to see under the microscope, was lost in transmission of that chromosome from parent to child. Rather than mutation of a single gene, the deletions involve a number of contiguous genes. Some of the better known syndromes in which deletions have been demonstrated are listed in Table 7.3.

## Imprinting

The term *imprinting* originally was used biologically to refer to the innate ability of turtles and other animals to return to the site of their birth for breeding years later. More recently, it has been used in genetics with an entirely different meaning. Geneticists long have assumed that a mutation inherited from a father had the same biological consequences as the same mutation inherited from a mother. Evidence from lower animals and humans now shows clearly that as some genes are copied in making sperm or eggs, they are modified to function differently depending on the sex of the parent. This process, called imprinting, apparently involves single genes or several genes over a small chromosomal segment. The following two syndromes, Angelman syndrome and Prader-Willi syndrome, are examples of imprinting in that they demonstrate different patterns of modification of DNA inherited from mothers and fathers.

**TABLE 7.3**

Deletion or Contiguous Gene Syndromes

| Eponym | Chromosomal Band Deleted | Typical Clinical Features |
|---|---|---|
| Angelman syndrome | 15q11–12 | Fair complexion, nonverbal, seizures, inappropriate laughter, ataxia |
| Prader-Willi syndrome | 15q11–12 | Truncal obesity, insatiable appetite, low muscle tone, fair complexion, small hands |
| DiGeorge syndrome | 22q11 | Immune deficiency, left-sided congenital heart disease, short stature, mental retardation, hypocalcemia |
| Sprintzen syndrome | 22q11 | Congenital heart disease, elongated midface, velopalatal incompetence, mental illness |
| Smith-Magenis syndrome | 17p11.2 | Sleep disorder, hoarse voice, self-destructive behavior, prognathism, tendency to put objects in the ears |
| Williams syndrome | 7q11.23 | Hyperactivity, good verbal skills, "cocktail party" personality, music skills, poor academic skills |
| Miller-Dieker syndrome | 17p13.3 | Lissencephaly (major brain development defect), seizures, forehead furrowing |
| Beckwith-Wiedemann syndrome | 11p15.5 | Large birth weight, omphalocele, newborn hypoglycemia, mild to moderate retardation, newborn macroglossia |

Angelman syndrome is characterized by severe mental retardation in which affected children are nonverbal. They have a light complexion compared to family members, an unsteady gait, and a seizure disorder. They also appear quite happy, with inappropriate laughter. Although several different types of mutational events in a small area of chromosome 15 are responsible for the syndrome, it occurs only when the mutational event involves loss of function of genetic material from the mother. (This disorder exemplifies an interesting feature of TV talk shows. Support groups for specific genetic diseases often seek to have an affected individual appear on a talk show as a means of publicizing their efforts and educating the public about the condition. Following the interview of a family with a child with Angelman syndrome several years ago on a popular talk show, our clinic received three self-referrals from families who thought their child might have Angelman syndrome. The children had been followed by various physicians for a number of years, given their multiple problems. In each case, the family was right and we were able to confirm the diagnosis of Angelman syndrome.)

Prader-Willi syndrome is characterized by striking muscle weakness in infants, who appear quite delayed in all developmental parameters. By age 2, the children have gained considerable muscle strength and made striking motor developmental strides. As older children they demonstrate mild to moderate mental retardation, good social and verbal skills, short stature, small hands, and an insatiable appetite. At school lunch they will clean not only their plates but also those of children sitting nearby. As a result, they develop marked exogenous obesity. Families often will resort to locking refrigerators and pantries. The basis for this syndrome is the loss of the same genetic function as Angelman syndrome, but it occurs when the origin of the loss is from the father (see Figure 7.12).

## Anticipation

In some genetic conditions, the disorder becomes more severe as it is transmitted over generations within a family. With each generation, the disorder starts at a younger age and progresses faster, a process called anticipation. Previously, the explanation was that the disorder was highly variable in families and it was only by chance that it seemed to be getting worse. However, several genetic disorders are now recognized to increase in severity over generations in a family, and the molecular basis for these changes is partially understood. Furthermore, the increase in severity is related to the gender of the parent transmitting the mutation. Examples of conditions in which anticipation occurs include myotonic dystrophy, Huntington disease, and fragile X syndrome.

Myotonic dystrophy is the most common form of muscular dystrophy among adults. It has its usual onset in the 20s, with progression thereafter leading to death in the 40s or 50s. The myotonia may be recognized when an individual grasps a door handle and has difficulty releasing his or her

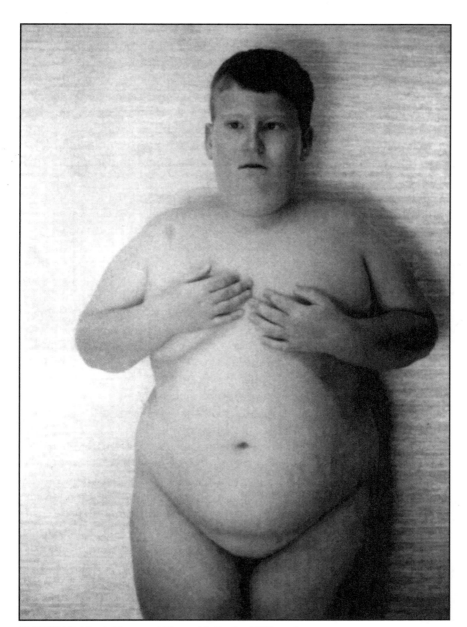

**FIGURE 7.12.** A 10-year-old boy with Prader-Willi syndrome.

grip. It long has been recognized that when the disorder is inherited from the father, the course usually will follow that seen in the father. However, when the condition is inherited from the mother, it often results in a congenital form of muscular dystrophy. If the affected infant does not die from respiratory compromise because of the muscle weakness, he or she will later demonstrate mental retardation and a slowly progressive muscular dystrophy. Anticipation is exemplified by a family in which the grandmother had cataracts but no overt muscle disease; her daughter had typical onset of myotonic dystrophy in her 20s; and the grandchild had congenital myotonic dystrophy.

Huntington disease (HD) is a progressive form of dementia with involuntary movements, usually affecting individuals 45 years of age and older. Occasionally, the disorder may be recognized in children as young as 2 to 3 years of age. In contrast to myotonic dystrophy, when HD is inherited from the mother it usually follows her age of onset and progression. When HD is inherited from the father, there is usually a younger age of onset. One may observe a grandfather with onset at 50 years of age, a son with onset at 25 years of age, and a grandchild with onset at 4 to 6 years of age.

The fragile X syndrome is the most common form of mental retardation caused by a single-gene mutation. Its incidence is roughly 1 in 1,000 in males, and it accounts for a significant percentage of learning disability in females. Males function in the range of moderate mental retardation but display no behavioral problems and usually have good social and interpersonal skills. On entering school, they often display a short attention span and immaturity. There are no significant health problems, and life expectancy is not shortened. The responsible gene is on the X chromosome and inheritance follows an X-linked pattern. As males give their Y chromosome to their sons, male-to-male transmission is not observed. Males with fragile X syndrome are fully fertile. A man or a woman may be a carrier for a premutation, a change in the gene toward a full mutation but one that does not result in mental retardation. This premutation may develop into a full mutation when transmitted by females but not when transmitted by males. Originally, the diagnosis of this disorder was based on the cytogenetic appearance of the X chromosome in affected males; it appeared to have a fragile end on the long arm of the X chromosome (see Figure 7.13). Currently, the diagnosis is made by direct DNA analysis of the mutation.

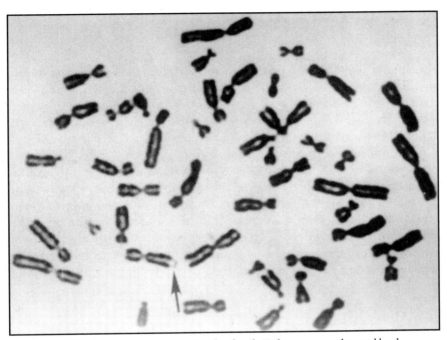

**FIGURE 7.13.** A chromosome spread with a fragile X chromosome denoted by the arrow.

These three conditions, as well as several disorders that are less well known, have been recognized to result from a relatively new class of mutations. Within or around the DNA of specific genes, a segment of DNA, often a three-nucleotide repeat (e.g., CAG), normally may be repeated several times. For reasons currently unknown, in the production of sperm or eggs, these repeated segments may increase in size such that, at a critical level of expansion, the function of the gene is lost or altered. As with imprinting, there is a difference in which genes are expanded depending on the gender of the transmitting individual.

In myotonic dystrophy and fragile X syndrome, the expansion occurs in oogenesis; thus, the severity of the disorder increases when the mutation is transmitted by mothers. In Huntington disease, the expansion occurs in spermatogenesis; thus, increasing severity is recognized when the disease is transmitted by the father.

# PSYCHOSOCIAL ISSUES

For children, any situation that sets them apart from their peers can produce significant psychosocial problems that often are of greater consequence than the physical differences. Genetic disorders set children apart from their peers in many ways that often are unrelated to the child's native abilities and skills. Clearly, conditions that result in an obvious and strikingly different physical appearance create considerable emotional stress for children.

The ability of children with disabilities to take advantage of the educational opportunities open to them is often seriously impeded by associated behavioral problems. Although these behavioral problems may originate with the inability of the parents or the child to deal with the disability, some genetic disorders have specific behavioral problems as an integral part of the disorder. Table 7.4 lists some examples of genetic disorders in which specific and reproducible patterns of psychological and educational problems arise.

# SUPPORT GROUPS

Most genetic disorders occur sufficiently infrequently that a primary care physician may have had no prior experience with a certain disorder. Not only is most medical literature regarding these disorders unintelligible to most laypersons, it often does not contain the kinds of information about life experiences and effective management schemes that families seek. There has been an amazing proliferation of family support groups in recent years; support groups now exist for virtually all genetic disorders. These support groups provide an invaluable service to families through several mechanisms:

1. The groups usually have prepared pamphlets providing the general kind of information the family seeks about a particular genetic disorder present in their child.

2. They produce a periodic newsletter with updates on research, conferences, and family stories.

**TABLE 7.4**
Psychological and Educational Problems
Associated with Some Common Genetic Disorders

| Disorder | Educational Problems | Psychological Problems |
|---|---|---|
| Achondroplasia | None | Dwarfism |
| Neurofibromatosis | LD | Cosmetic |
| Fragile X syndrome | Mild to moderate MR | Hyperactivity, immaturity |
| Lesch-Nyhan syndrome | Ataxia, dysarthria | Self-mutilation |
| Angelman syndrome | Severe MR | Seizures, inappropriate laughter |
| Prader-Willi syndrome | Mild to moderate MR | Obesity, pleasant personality |
| Down syndrome | Moderate MR | Stigmatization |
| Turner syndrome | Mild LD | Short stature, delayed sexual maturation |
| Klinefelter syndrome | Mild MR to LD | Social and physical immaturity |
| Williams syndrome | Moderate MR | Hyperactivity, fearless behavior, gregariousness |
| Osteogenesis imperfecta | None | Limited physical activity |
| Phenylketonuria | None, if properly treated | Severe dietary restrictions |
| Sickle cell disease | None | Pain crises, absenteeism |

Note. LD = learning disabilities; MR = mental retardation.

3. They sponsor conferences on regional and national levels, which combine research updates with practical information for families and opportunities to meet and socialize with other families.

4. They can provide information about resources needed for the child's care in the family's geographic area. They also can put the family in contact with other families in their geographic area.

It is beyond the scope of this chapter to attempt a listing of all the genetic support groups. Most groups have Web sites and can be accessed on the Internet by simply conducting a search for the name of the condition.

The following organization is able to put families and teachers in contact with specific support groups:

Alliance of Genetic Support Groups
35 Wisconsin Circle, Suite 440
Chevy Chase, MD 20815
800/336-GENE
Fax 301/654-0171

# REFERENCE

Thompson, M. W., McInnes, R. R., & Willard, H. F. (1991). *Genetics in medicine* (5th ed.). Philadelphia: Saunders.

# CHAPTER 8

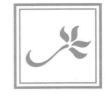

# Common Visual Problems in the Classroom

Alex V. Levin

**V**ision is one of the most important physical traits required for learning in traditional educational systems. Today's mainstreaming projects allow children with low vision or blindness to be educated in the same setting as their normally sighted peers. This chapter deals mostly with the common visual difficulties that most teachers will encounter with sighted individuals who do not fit the definition for legal blindness. In addition, there are many problems, symptoms, and signs that teachers might attribute to a possible visual disorder or that may prompt a referral for a visual evaluation but in fact are of nonocular origin. A Suggested Reading list is provided at the end of the chapter for individuals who want more information on visual problems.

## GLASSES AND CONTACT LENSES

Normal vision is arbitrarily designated as 20/20 (6/6 in the metric system). This means that a person with normal vision can see letters of a universally standard size on a chart 20 ft away. The 20/20 eye takes an image and focuses it without any assistance from glasses or contact lenses. The image enters the eye through the front crystalline domed surface (cornea), passes through the pupil, and then through the lens, which is behind the pupil. The cornea and lens act just like the lens on a camera, focusing the image onto the film, which in the case of an eyeball is the retina (the inner lining of the inside of the back of the eyeball). If you were to open a tennis ball, you would find that it has a pink inner lining. Likewise, the eye has an inner lining, which is the retina.

In the normal 20/20 eye, this system works perfectly, in that the image is focused by the cornea and lens in such a way that it falls precisely on the retina. However, just as some people are shorter or taller but still normal, many individuals have eyes that are microscopically longer or shorter, but otherwise perfectly healthy. Because all corneas and lenses have about the same focusing power, if an eye is too short or too long, thus placing the retina at a different distance behind the cornea and lens, then the focused image no longer falls exactly on the retina. The cornea and lens do their jobs perfectly, but because the eye is a bit too short (farsighted) or long (nearsighted), the focused image falls behind or in front of the retina, creating a blurred image.

If the eyeball is a bit shorter or longer than the normal 20/20 eye, glasses simply assist the cornea and lens of the eye to direct the image to be focused on the retina. However, because these eyes are otherwise *perfectly healthy*, once the image gets to its proper destination (the retina), it will be in perfect focus and the patient will see 20/20. Therefore, it is wrong to say that a person who is farsighted or nearsighted has bad eyes, even if the glasses they wear are very thick and their vision without them is very blurry. Actually, these individuals have absolutely healthy eyes that simply need some assistance in bending the light to achieve the 20/20 image that they are perfectly capable of obtaining once the image of the world is focused on their healthy retinas. In fact, measuring a person's vision without his or her glasses does not provide important information. It would be like taking a perfectly normal camera and trying to take a picture without a lens screwed on the front. The camera is not broken and the film is perfectly good, yet the pictures would be very blurry. One would not throw that camera out or send it to a repair shop. Rather, one would simply screw on the appropriate lens, a situation analogous to putting on the appropriate pair of glasses and then measuring the vision.

Nearsightedness and farsightedness are called *refractive errors*, that is, variations from the ability of an eye of average length to focus images with the assistance of glasses. *Astigmatism* is another kind of refractive error. Although the eye may be of perfectly normal (average) length, the front surface of the eye is not perfectly round. This microscopic alteration in the contour of the eye surface (cornea) causes some distortion in vision, which can also be corrected by wearing glasses to aid the eye in focusing the light properly. Once again, the eyeball is perfectly healthy and capable of seeing 20/20 with the assistance of glasses.

Contact lenses are the same as glasses, with the exception of their position relative to the eye. Today, people usually wear either soft contact lenses or gas-permeable lenses (often referred to as *semisoft* or *semihard*). Some people are unable to wear contact lenses because of dryness in their eyes, allergies to contact lens cleaning solutions, or unusually high amounts of astigmatism. Most individuals, however, can successfully wear contact lenses if they desire. Children also can wear contact lenses; no age is too young. For some eye conditions, contact lenses are prescribed in infancy. In these situations, parents learn to insert and remove the lenses daily. Other contact lenses can be worn for more extended periods of time. The youngest age at which children may be able to insert and remove their contact lenses unassisted is approximately 7 years. More often children start at about 9 years of age. A general guideline is that children are able to manage their own contact lenses when they are old enough to manage their own person: cleaning their room, cleaning themselves, and caring for their personal belongings. Although contact lenses do afford clearer vision, particularly for children who must wear very thick glasses, older children wear them for cosmetic reasons or to avoid the inconvenience of glasses.

It is important for the school teacher to realize a few facts about contact lenses.

1. Any child who wears contact lenses and develops a red eye should receive urgent care. In particular, the contact lens should be removed by the child, the school nurse, or the child's parent. Prompt evaluation by an eye doctor is suggested within 24 hours.

2. If a contact lens comes out accidentally in the classroom, the first thing to do is have everyone "freeze." Many contact lenses that fall out are lost or damaged. Contact lenses tend to be sticky and therefore adhere to surfaces on their way to the ground. Look carefully for the concave clear lens sticking to a piece of clothing or tabletop or lying on the floor. They usually do not travel very far. Although all children should carry a spare contact lens case, in the absence of this device, a contact lens can be submersed in liquid in any container. If the lens is a gas-permeable lens, only a drop or two of liquid is necessary to store the lens. Although it is preferable to use contact lens solutions, in an emergency situation, the lens can be placed in tap water. Children should not reinsert their contact lens after it has fallen onto a dirty surface, or after it is in tap water, unless the lens is sterilized according to the protocol instructed by the child's eye doctor. If a child is dependent on his or her contact lens to a degree that the loss of that lens will result in poor vision (this would only be true

if the other eye does not see well), then it is advisable for the child to have a spare pair of glasses in his or her desk at school, should a lens be lost.

3. Wearing of contact lenses should not prevent any child from engaging in activities, including contact sports.

4. Contact lenses do not improve learning any more than the equivalent pair of glasses.

There are many myths about glasses and contact lenses. For example, once a child is beyond the age of visual development (see the later section on amblyopia), the failure to wear glasses will not make vision permanently worse. Children above these ages (7 to 9 years old) should be allowed to wear their glasses when they feel that glasses are helpful. Most teachers write large enough on the blackboard that vision of 20/20 is not necessary. Therefore, a child can perform quite normally in a classroom even though his or her vision is not 20/20. If the child's vision without glasses is a bit less than 20/20, the child will still function perfectly well without any undue strain or stress on the eyes. Certainly, one would hope that children would wear their glasses to optimize their vision so that they may learn more readily; however, peer pressures are sometimes so strong that a child would rather sit in the front of a classroom to see the board more clearly than wear glasses that cause him or her to be taunted by peers. Doing so will not cause any harm to the eyes.

Another myth surrounds the use of reading glasses in children. Children do not need reading glasses except in the extraordinary instance of certain unusual neurological diseases, which would be obvious even to the medically untrained observer. In fact, children have an unusually strong focusing ability. A typical child can read a newspaper attached to the end of the nose. Many children, especially those in the first few years of school, place their heads very close to their reading material as a form of concentration. As long as the child can see the blackboard normally, one does not have to worry about his or her near vision. Many children will even take their glasses off to read, particularly if they are nearsighted. This should not be discouraged as it is not harmful.

Wearing glasses does not make a person "addicted" to them, which is another common myth. People who wear glasses often tend to wear them more when they first get them. This is simply because they see better and, consciously or unconsciously, like seeing better. With the start of eyeglass treatment, they now better appreciate how poorly they saw before and therefore use the glasses more often. Again, however, if they are in a situation where they do not need to see as clearly as their glasses allow them to (such as viewing the blackboard), then going without glasses will do no harm.

It should be stressed that children under the age of 6 or 7 years are still in the developing years of visual growth. In these age groups, it is important that children wear their glasses, especially when they have a strong prescription, to encourage the visual system to develop and to avoid the onset of amblyopia. If an educator has a question about the recommended wearing schedule for any child, the educator should ask the child's parent for consent to speak with the child's ophthalmologist or optometrist to determine what schedule was recommended. Likewise, if a teacher suspects that a child is having trouble with vision, appropriate referral is indicated. Signs that a child is having visual difficulty might include squinting, always holding things very close, and needing to sit in the front row, with difficulties in identifying letters or pictures from afar. Sometimes glasses are prescribed not to improve vision but to help straighten the eyes (see the later section on strabismus).

# LASER EYE SURGERY

Much is found today in the media and lay discussions about laser eye surgery, also known as photo-refractive surgery and Lasik surgery. An older form of surgery to correct refractive errors was radial keratotomy. All of these procedures are designed to cut the cornea, either with a laser beam or a knife (radial keratotomy), so that it takes on a new shape. As a result of this reshaping, the cornea can focus images directly on the retina without the help of glasses or contact lenses.

It must be remembered that these procedures are not designed to "fix" an abnormal eye. The eye is healthy but needs the help of glasses or contact lenses to focus images on its retina. If a person is so unhappy with glasses or contact lenses that he or she is willing to take the risks of the surgery, then the person can be quite satisfied with the result of eliminating the inconvenience, expense, and troubles of glasses or contact lenses. The procedures, however, may actually make the eye *less* healthy. Complications, which rarely occur, include loss of vision or chronic problems such as glare or blurring at night. The long-term effect of these procedures is not well known. This is one of the many reasons that these procedures are not usually available for children.

# AMBLYOPIA

The term *lazy eye* is often used by the lay public to refer to an eye with either amblyopia or strabismus. *Amblyopia* refers to the failure of the brain to develop the vision normally in an eyeball. Anything that causes the brain to prefer one eye over the other may result in amblyopia. For example, if one eye is extremely nearsighted and the other eye is not, then the brain will favor the non-nearsighted eye and ignore the development of vision in the very nearsighted eye, even though the nearsighted eye would have been capable of 20/20 vision if appropriate glasses had been placed in front of it at an early age. In addition to unequal refractive errors, other abnormalities can lead to amblyopia. If a patient has eyes that are not pointing in the same direction (e.g., crossed eyes), then the brain may prefer to keep one eye straight for viewing while the other eye turns away. The turned eye is then ignored and visual development does not proceed correctly.

Correction of amblyopia must begin before the age of 7 to 9 years, when visual development comes to an end. By intervening at a time when the visual development is still proceeding, the brain is still flexible (or "plastic") in its ability to redevelop vision in an ignored eye. Treatment simply consists of correcting any underlying problem in the unpreferred eye and then forcing the brain to use that eye by patching the good eye (see Figure 8.1). A child with unilateral nearsightedness might be given glasses or contact lenses to correct the nearsightedness in the affected eye, while the good eye is patched. Sometimes the patching is done for just part of the day, and at other times it is done around the clock. This decision is made by the eye doctor. As patching sometimes is a source of ridicule among peers, attempts might be made to do most of the patching when the child is not in school.

Another treatment of amblyopia is the instillation of eye drops in one eye to blur the vision in the good eye, allowing the brain to use the unpreferred eye. The eye drops cause the pupil to be dilated compared with the other. The dilated pupil does not constrict to bright light. Yet another alternative to patching is the placement of a suction cup occluder on the back of the child's glasses, to act as a patch over the good eye (see Figure 8.2).

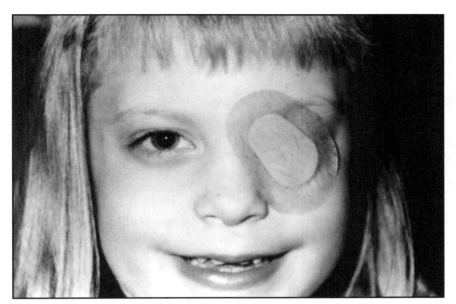

**FIGURE 8.1.** Patch commonly used in the treatment of amblyopia. The good left eye is patched to treat the amblyopia in the right eye.

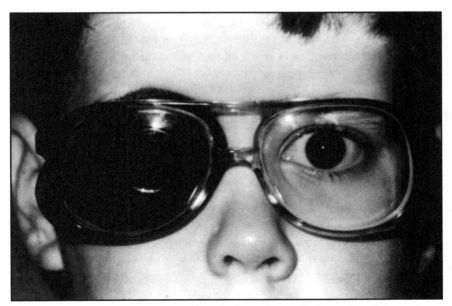

**FIGURE 8.2.** The suction cup occluder, which attaches to the inner side of glasses, is an alternative to patching in the treatment of amblyopia.

In rare cases, the brain can fail to develop vision adequately in both eyes (bilateral amblyopia). This might occur if both eyes have severe near-sightedness, farsightedness, or astigmatism that goes uncorrected for many years. Fortunately, this usually is detected in school screening programs or through the simple observation that the child is having trouble with his or her vision. Once again, early intervention by the correction of such problems as refractive errors (with glasses) can lead to 20/20 vision in each eye.

Once a child reaches the age of 7 to 9 years, the failure of visual development may be irreversible. Even if the good eye is patched and the brain is forced to begin using the weaker eye, the vision cannot be improved to the 20/20 level. This fact emphasizes the need for early screening by schools, pediatricians, and family physicians to identify children who have poor vision in one eye at an early age when intervention can correct the deficiency.

Unfortunately, most children who have poor vision in one eye are unaware that they have a problem. A child's brain is "wired" in such a way that the brain automatically uses the better eye without any undue strain. Because children with one eye function normally (see the section "The Monocular Child" below), there is no way to detect a child with poor vision in one eye unless formal visual testing is performed. This is particularly true of children who are born with a problem in one eye, as they never come to know that it is abnormal for one eye to see less clearly than the other. However, the educator is wise to take seriously a child's complaint that all of a sudden the vision in one eye is worse than the other. This can be confirmed simply by having the child cover the bad eye and then asking him or her to read the blackboard. The child could then cover the good eye to perform the same task. Should there be a discrepancy between the two eyes, prompt referral to an eye doctor is indicated.

# STRABISMUS

*Strabismus* refers to any kind of misalignment of the eyeballs; that is, the eyes are not pointing in the same direction. The eyes may be crossed (*esotropia;* one or both eyes pointing toward the nose), turned out (*exotropia* or "wall eyes"; one or both eyes pointing out toward the ears), or vertically misaligned (one eye pointing straight ahead and the other eye pointing up or down; see Figures 8.3 and 8.4).

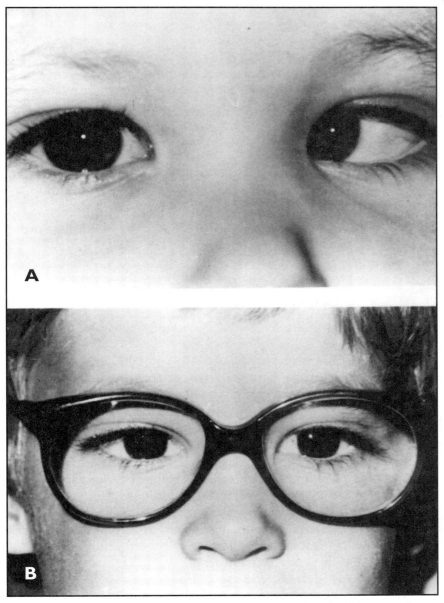

**FIGURE 8.3.** (A) Left esotropia (crossed left eye). (B) With farsighted glasses on, the crossed eye is now straightened.

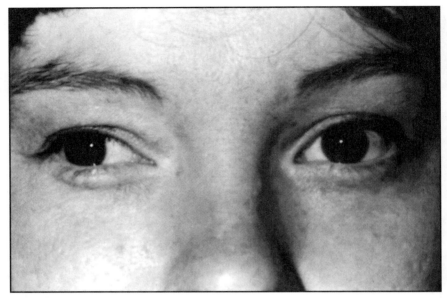

**FIGURE 8.4.** Right exotropia (turned-out right eye).

Strabismus does not mean that a child sees poorly. In fact, many children with misaligned eyes either have one good eye that can see 20/20 while the other eye is misaligned, or have the ability to sometimes keep one eye straight and at other times keep the opposite eye straight, thus retaining good vision in each eye due to equal stimulation of the brain's visual development in each eye. Although misaligned eyes can be quite unsightly and the cause of peer ridicule, as long as the vision in at least one eye is perfectly normal, strabismus by itself does not interfere with school or athletic performance. In fact, many athletes and surgeons have misaligned eyes. Straightening of the eyes is undertaken, however, to ensure normal visual development in both eyes and to restore a child's facial appearance to normalcy.

There are three reasons why children might develop strabismus. Sometimes it is simply the result of an uncorrected refractive error. A child with farsightedness may develop crossed eyes (see Figure 8.3), whereas a child with nearsightedness may develop turned-out eyes (see Figure 8.4). By wearing glasses, the eyes will be straightened. However, when these children take their glasses off, the eyes will become misaligned; this is of no concern. An analogy might be individuals with diabetes who take insulin: When they take their medication, they feel well, but when they do not take their medication, they are quite ill. In some forms of strabismus, glasses are the medication for the problem.

Children have powerful focusing muscles inside their eyes that can correct for farsightedness. This can allow them to see 20/20 without glasses despite farsightedness. However, in some children, this focusing effort also results in crossing of the eyes. If glasses are prescribed to do the focusing, instead of allowing the child to use the internal eye muscles, then the eyes do not cross. When the glasses are removed and the eyes attempt to focus unaided, the crossing recurs. The vision is the same with or without glasses. Over time (measured in years of glasses wear), the eyes may eventually be able to remain straight without glasses. At that point the glasses will no longer be needed.

The second cause of strabismus is eye muscle imbalance. Doctors do not know why this occurs in many cases. However, because these children do not need glasses to straighten their eyes, surgery is often recommended. This surgery is almost always an outpatient procedure, and the child can return to school in 1 or 2 days with few, if any, restrictions. The eyes may look "bloody red" for many days, but most children are not particularly sore and can perform all educational and athletic tasks normally. Sometimes a child may have double vision for 1 or 2 weeks after surgery, which is usually no cause for alarm. Approximately 15% of children require two operations to get their eyes straight. Occasionally, three or more operations are necessary. If a child wears glasses before surgery, then he or she typically needs to wear glasses following surgery, as the operation only repositions the eyeballs, and cannot change the focusing ability or length of the eye, which causes the refractive error.

The third cause of strabismus is poor vision in one eye. If the poor vision is simply due to amblyopia, then patching of the good eye, designed to correct the vision in the weak eye, might result in the straightening of the alignment. However, strabismus may result from an abnormality in the eyeball, such as a cataract. Therefore, all children with strabismus must be evaluated by an ophthalmologist to ensure that no serious abnormalities of the eyeball structure are present. The new development of strabismus in a child who has not previously shown any misalignment is a particular concern and should result in a prompt referral to an eye physician.

Some myths surround strabismus. First, an eye cannot "get stuck" in a misaligned position. Most strabismus occurs in eyes that can move normally. But if one eye is preferred for vision, the other eye will appear to be always turned. Correction of the underlying cause of the strabismus by glasses, surgery, or other means will return the turned eye to the normal position. Second, children with crossed eyes are not less intelligent. Although they sometimes look like they are not focusing on their work, they should be able to learn perfectly well, provided that the vision in the nonturned eye is normal. Finally, children rarely turn their eyes out of position on purpose. Although this behavior certainly does occur, one should not ignore the presence of strabismus by attributing turned eyes to child misbehavior.

## THE MONOCULAR CHILD

Some children will have permanent loss of vision in one eye but normal vision in the other eye. These children are referred to as monocular. The poor vision can be the result of a number of abnormalities, including untreated amblyopia, cataract, injury, and other conditions that cause the eye to see poorly. Children with one eye function entirely normally in the school setting and in athletic activities, particularly when the unilateral poor vision develops at birth or in the very early years of visual development. Many famous athletes, entertainers, scientists, and surgeons have poor vision in one eye.

Children with one functional eye have fantastic adaptive mechanisms. They develop unconscious strategies to give them virtually normal function in a wide range of peripheral vision (usually by turning their head) and use many monocular clues to give them remarkably good functional depth perception. Many people falsely say that people with one eye have no depth perception. If you cover one eye and look across the room in which you are sitting, you can easily recognize which objects are in front of other objects. Although at first, as an adult, you may experience some trouble with fine depth perception tasks (e.g., hammering a nail), you would quickly learn to adapt so that you can perform these tasks almost normally. Therefore, a child with one normal eye should learn normally and require no special seating or educational interventions.

Some children have had an eye removed, most often as a result of trauma or tumor. Like all monocular children, if the remaining good eye sees normally, they function normally. However, the eye on the affected side is an artificial (prosthetic) eye. This is not a glass eye; rather, it is a porcelain shell that fits over the tissues that are left to fill the eye socket (see Figure 8.5). If this shell is removed, there is no excavated hole where the previous eye existed. Rather, there is pink tissue that covers the eye

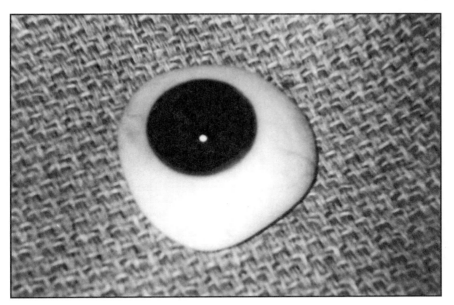

**FIGURE 8.5.** Prosthetic eye (artificial eye).

socket. Sometimes, a prosthetic shell is placed over a blind eye that is cosmetically unacceptable. The eye may be shrunken or badly scarred and is only visible when the prosthesis is removed.

If the prosthetic eye were to come out during a classroom session, there is no need to be alarmed or to be concerned about harm. Most children, even at a young age, can insert their prosthetic shell themselves. If a child is unable to do so, there is no harm in continuing the session with the shell wrapped in a tissue and placed in the child's pocket. The parent can then reinsert the prosthesis when the child returns home. However, if the child is concerned about appearance or is otherwise uncomfortable with his or her prosthetic eye out, the teacher should discharge the child to the care of the school nurse or parent, who can either reinsert the prosthesis or patch the eye socket for the remainder of the day's session. Patching should be done with the upper eyelid closed under the patch. If the shell repetitively falls out during class, the teacher might ask the parent to return to the oculist who made the prosthesis to determine if the fit is correct. Some children have been known to remove their eye as a source of entertainment (positively or negatively) for their peers. If this becomes a problem, the parents should be consulted.

The most important point in the management and care of the monocular child is protection of the good eye from accidental injury. All children who have only one functional eye should be wearing glasses with lenses made out of breakproof polycarbonate plastic, or equivalent, to prevent the good eye from becoming injured accidentally. Even if the child has no refractive error and therefore sees 20/20 from the good eye without glasses, these protective glasses should still be worn, albeit without any prescription for refractive error. Likewise, all monocular children should wear appropriate protective eyewear for sports, particularly for sports that involve physical contact, balls, or racquets. Monocular children need not be restricted from sports provided they wear appropriate protective eyewear. A number of styles are available, usually through consultation with a local optician. Specific sport goggles are adequate for most sports, although visors (football), face masks (hockey, lacrosse), and chin guards (baseball batting helmets) are used in particular circumstances.

# LOW VISION

Legal blindness is defined in most jurisdictions as vision that is 20/200 or worse in the better eye or a severe constriction of peripheral vision (less than 20 degrees) such that the child is left with tunnel vision in the better eye. Having vision of 20/200 means that the individual needs to stand at 20 feet to see what a normal person can see from 200 feet away. Remember that visual acuity refers to the best corrected vision, that is, the vision with glasses or contact lenses on. If a person sees 20/200 with glasses off, but 20/20 with glasses on, then he or she has no ocular problem. The eyeball is healthy. Children who are legally blind have vision in their better eye of 20/200 even after the best glasses have been prescribed.

Of course, there is a whole range of vision between 20/20 and legal blindness (20/40, 20/60, 20/80, etc.). To read normal size print, most children need to have only 20/50 or 20/60 vision. Remember, children have a very good ability to focus close up even when their distance vision is poor. To see a blackboard in school, vision of 20/60 or 20/80 may be sufficient, as most teachers' writing is quite large, particularly in the elementary years. However, if the vision is worse, special visual aids may be necessary. These are beyond the scope of this chapter, and it is suggested that the educator who is faced with a visually challenged child consult a local ophthalmologist, optometrist, or school for the visually impaired for advice on management in the mainstream classroom.

Children with marked visual impairment, even total blindness, often function remarkably well in a normal classroom setting with the help of visual aids, which might range from Braille materials to small handheld telescopes and large-print books. Teachers who work with children with visual impairments can subscribe to the newsletters published by the following agencies to learn more about methods of intervention, as well as the trials and tribulations of parenting a visually impaired child: the National Association for Parents of the Visually Impaired (NAPVI, Inc., P.O. Box 317, Watertown, MA 02272-0317) and the Institute for Families of Blind Children (Mail Stop 111, P.O. Box 54700, Los Angeles, CA 90054-0700). In Canada, the Canadian National Institute for the Blind (67 King Street, Brantford, Ontario N3T 3C8) can provide information.

# DYSLEXIA

*Dyslexia* is a collective term that refers to a number of learning problems, including problems with tracking, copying, letter reversal, word substitution, writing on line, and other tasks of learning. There also are many nondyslexic causes of learning disability, including emotional immaturity, subnormal intellect, psychosocial problems, and attention-deficit disorder (see Chapter 15). Even in the absence of these latter problems, true dyslexia, a disorder that more commonly affects boys than girls, can be a source of great difficulty in the classroom. Although the original understanding of dyslexia several decades ago referred to the eyes as the major cause, it is presently known that the eyeballs themselves are rarely an issue. Rather, dyslexia, and all of the learning disabilities that it encompasses, is a disorder of processing of visual information. In other words, the eyeballs present to the brain a perfectly coordinated 20/20 image, then the brain has difficulty in making sense of this image and using it appropriately. Researchers have come to understand that this processing also involves the speech and hearing centers of the brain. To illustrate this point, notice as you are reading these words that you hear the words spoken in your brain. In fact, it is impossible to read "in silence." You cannot turn off this verbal and auditory part of visual processing. Studies now show that it is the integration of these various brain functions that is abnormal in dyslexia. Therefore, interventions that attempt to train the eyeball are not helpful because the eyeballs are normal.

Unfortunately, a large and lucrative market has been created for the use of visual training in the correction of dyslexia and other learning problems. Such visual training is not offered at any medical children's hospital or medical eye hospital in all of North America. Yet, in nonphysician settings, this training continues to be offered, often at great cost. Visual training may involve exercises in hand–eye coordination, balance boards, video games, eye exercises, the use of color overlays to treat "scotopic sensitivity syndrome," or prisms in glasses ("yoked prisms"). All of these treatments have not stood the trial of rigorous scientific testing. Nevertheless, unscientific anecdotal and personal reports continue to emerge, claiming benefits from these unproven treatments, which cost parents thousands of dollars as they search desperately for a solution to their child's learning problem.

This conflict resulted in a statement issued jointly by the American Academy of Pediatrics Committee on Children with Disabilities, the American Association for Pediatric Ophthalmology and Strabismus, and the American Academy of Ophthalmology (1988). An excerpt follows:

> Eye defects, subtle or severe, do not cause reversal of letters, words, or numbers. No scientific evidence supports claims that the academic abilities of dyslexic or learning-disabled children can be improved with treatment based on (a) visual training, including muscle exercises, ocular pursuit, tracking exercises, or "training" glasses (with or without bifocals or prisms); (b) neurologic organizational training (laterality training, crawling, balance board, perceptual training); or (c) tinted or colored lenses. Some controversial methods of treatment result in a false sense of security that may delay or even prevent proper instruction or remediation. The expense of these methods is unwarranted, and they cannot be substituted for appropriate remedial educational measures. Claims of improved reading and learning after visual training, neurological organization training or use of tinted or colored lenses are typically based on poorly controlled studies that rely on anecdotal information or testimony. (p. 1217)

Perhaps all children who show learning difficulties should have a complete ophthalmic examination. Once this examination shows that vision is normal, further evaluation and treatment should rest within the educational system rather then in the hands of "visual trainers."

# SYMPTOMS AND SIGNS
# OF POSSIBLE VISUAL DISORDERS

Educators often ask for guidelines to help in assessing children with learning difficulties for early recognition of potential visual disorders. Some signs have been discussed previously in this chapter. The following sections discuss several symptoms and signs that are often ascribed to the visual system, some correctly and others incorrectly.

## Headaches

Headaches are only infrequently due to problems in the visual system. In fact, only children with very specific uncorrected refractive errors develop this symptom. Most headaches are related to tension and stress or other disorders (see Chapter 13). It is more prudent to refer a child with headaches to the family physician or pediatrician than to an eye doctor, as the latter referral rarely results in the identification of a cause. Headaches that are prolonged, debilitating, associated with nausea or vomiting, and accompanied by visual symptoms, such as an aversion to bright lights (photophobia), or unusual visual phenomena, such as flashing lights or changes in the colors or shapes of objects, may suggest a migraine with an ocular component. Once again, although an eye examination might be part of the overall evaluation, it is suggested that this symptom first be evaluated by the primary medical caretaker.

## Eye Pain

A child who complains of a foreign body sensation ("it feels like there is something in my eye") rarely has a visual disorder. Typically, the sensation indicates some disruption of the eyeball surface, such as a small scratch on the surface of the eye or a foreign particle resting somewhere on the eyeball or under the eyelids. Careful inspection by the school nurse or a medical caretaker may result in identification of the problem.

## Dryness of the Eyes

Dry eyes is a symptom that affects adults much more than children. If a child has problems with dryness (or "stickiness"), the child should be referred for an eye examination.

## Red Eye

Most red eyes are caused by local irritation and are noncontagious infections. However, some red eyes (pink eye) are due to viral conjunctivitis, which can spread rapidly throughout a classroom. If a child develops a red eye, particularly a red eye that spreads from one eye to the other, it is prudent to have this child evaluated by a pediatrician or family doctor to see if further referral to an ophthalmologist is indicated. If viral conjunctivitis is suspected, a child may need to be out of the classroom for as long as 21 days (or until the eye is no longer red) to prevent infection of others. A particularly ominous sign for contagious conjunctivitis is a recent history of multiple family members or classmates simultaneously affected. Not every red eye represents a contagious problem, yet the potential for spread must be ruled out in each case when there is no clear cause for the redness, such as trauma or exposure to a noxious substance.

Herpes, one form of viral infection, can be devastating and result in vision loss if not treated promptly. Most children have recurrent episodes and therefore recognize an occurrence. If the parents have had the foresight to notify the teacher, then at every episode of red eye, especially if it is painful and recognized by the child as a recurrence, the teacher should notify the family so that appropriate medications can be started.

If there is a known exposure to a noxious substance (e.g., a chemistry experiment), then it is of great importance to irrigate the eyes *before medical consultation*. Any type of water can be used, including water from the nearest sink, to irrigate the eyeballs copiously. Even if this requires having the child lie down and pouring water onto the eye's surface, it is essential to perform this treatment to eliminate, as early as possible, any ongoing contact with the offending agent. School nurses should be well versed in this technique.

# OTHER EYE DISORDERS

It is beyond the scope of this chapter to address the multitude of possible eye disorders. Rather, a few brief comments will be made regarding those disorders that might be seen more commonly in the classroom.

## Ptosis

*Ptosis* is a droopy eyelid that may be present at birth or may be acquired later in childhood, particularly after trauma. As long as the droopy lid does not cross the center of vision (center of the pupil), the child may experience no visual deficit. Once again, as with all the ocular disorders discussed in this chapter, if the other eye is entirely normal, then the child will function normally. Ptosis can be repaired by surgery.

## Nystagmus

The term *nystagmus* refers to "shaky eyes." The eyes seem to jiggle in place. This problem is usually congenital and is found either in isolation or in combination with other eye problems. Children with nystagmus do not see a shaky image. The brain is capable, like a computer, of taking microsecond samples of information to provide the child with a still image. However, the nystagmus does cause visual blurring and may even cause legal blindness. Many children with nystagmus hold their heads in an awkward position while looking straight ahead (e.g., turn their face to the left to put their eyes in right gaze). This position unconsciously is found to create the least amount of shaking. Children should be allowed to turn their faces into these seemingly awkward positions, as this maneuver will provide them with better visual acuity.

## Cataract

Any opacity in the normally clear lens of the eye, which sits behind the pupil, is called a cataract. Many cataracts are tiny and do not affect the vision. However, when a cataract becomes more significant, the vision is blurred. There is no harm in having a cataract in your eye, other than its effect on vision. In young children, cataracts are particularly dangerous, as they can lead to profound amblyopia. Surgery is necessary to remove the cataract; however, the cataract cannot be extracted without removing the entire lens of the eye. Therefore, postoperatively these children need something to replace the natural focusing mechanism of their eye (the lens). This can be accomplished with glasses, contact lenses, or the insertion of an artificial lens (e.g., implants, intraocular lens). Lens implants are the most common option selected for school-age children. Occasionally, a human donor cornea is used to fashion a contact lens, which is permanently sewn onto the patient's eye (*epikeratophakia*). Provided that there is no significant amblyopia, once the cataract is removed and the patient is rehabilitated using one of these methods, visual function is restored to normal.

Sometimes, however, particularly when the cataract surgery was done in both eyes, reading glasses may be necessary. This is because the patient has lost his or her natural lens, which had the ability to focus automatically at any distance. Contact lenses, glasses, and lens implants have only certain ranges of clear vision. They usually cannot focus up close. Reading glasses allow that to happen. If the cataract surgery was done in only one eye, and the other eye sees normally, then the child can use the nonoperated eye to read without reading glasses. Even with lens implants, some children still need glasses or contact lenses for distance.

## Albinism

Although we often think of albinism as a completely white individual with pink eyes, there are multiple kinds of albinism, many of which do not give such a severe appearance. *Albinism* is a disorder in which the body cannot effectively make pigment. It may affect the skin, hair, and eyes, or just the eyes alone. It causes nystagmus and reduced vision, and is often associated with strabismus or a need for glasses. There is no treatment for albinism. These children may have difficulties with glare and bright lights. Therefore, seating that reduces glare on the blackboard may be helpful. Most children with albinism do well in a normal classroom setting, although they may need visual aids, particularly for distance vision.

## Glaucoma

A microscopic increase in the pressure of the fluid that normally fills the inside of the eyeball can lead to damage to the optic nerve, the nerve that sends the messages of vision between the eye and brain. This small elevation in pressure cannot cause the eye to explode. Usually, glaucoma is entirely without symptoms in the school-age child. Fortunately, glaucoma occurs very rarely in children. Many of these children will require eye drops or oral medications, one dose of which may need to be taken during school. Surgery may also be required.

## Iritis

*Iritis* is actually a family of disorders with many causes, all of which result in inflammation inside the eyeball. Common causes are eye injury and joint problems (e.g., juvenile rheumatoid arthritis). The eye may or may not be painful, the pupil constricted, and the eye red. Once diagnosed by an ophthalmologist, frequent eye drops may be needed, including administration during school hours. Drops that dilate the pupil and make the pupil unreactive may also be required. Except for the inconvenience of frequent dosing, and possible annoyance by bright lights, children can usually proceed with school uninterrupted. The eye doctor may recommend against gym or sports until the inflammation is under control. If drops that cause the pupils to enlarge are being given to both eyes, the child's vision may be blurry for reading. In this case, reading glasses, even if purchased over the counter at a local pharmacy, can be helpful.

# GENETIC EYE DISEASE

The field of ophthalmology has been a leader in the recognition of the role of genetics in human disease. Many eye disorders, including glaucoma, cataracts, and even nearsightedness may be due to genetic influences. As genes are being discovered, doctors may be able to identify children at risk for conditions such as cataracts, thus leading to screening, early recognition, and prompt sight-restoring treatment. Genetic discoveries may some day also lead to new treatments.

If a child has a family history of the same eye disorder, then inheritance may very well play a role. Teenagers may worry whether they can pass their eye disease on to their children some day. Parents may harbor guilt that they passed their eye disease on to a child. It is important for teachers to recognize such anxieties, as they can potentially affect a child's school performance. In addition, when other family members are affected, they may be helpful in educating the teacher about the disorder, its effect on learning, and potential interventions.

# FUNCTIONAL VISION DISORDERS

Children may present with a variety of unusual symptoms with no true medical disease. These symptoms are not truly psychosomatic in the sense that they do not usually represent significant psychiatric disease. Rather, many children, particularly between the ages of 5 and the early teens, will develop recurrent problems, such as blinking, photophobia, intermittent visual loss, or eyelid pulling, that represent a kind of transient habit. Although these children should be evaluated by an ophthalmologist to rule out the presence of true medical disease, most of these symptoms will resolve within 3 months after seeing the eye doctor. If symptoms persist, recur, or are replaced by other unusual symptoms (substitution), further consultation with the child's pediatrician or family physician is indicated.

# EYE CARE PROFESSIONALS:
# A GLOSSARY

Although the roles and responsibilities of the various professionals involved in eye care may differ from place to place, the following definitions are offered here as a guide:

**Oculist.** Makes prosthetic eye shells. Is not a doctor. Does not do eye examinations or treat eye disease.

**Optician.** Makes and sells glasses but usually cannot examine eyes or prescribe glasses.

**Optometrist.** Is not a physician. Is graduate of a specific training program in diagnosis of eye disorders. Can prescribe and dispense contact lenses or glasses. Often has expertise in low vision assistance. In some jurisdictions, may be able to prescribe some level of eye medication. Cannot perform eye surgery.

**Ophthalmologist.** Is a medical doctor who has graduated from medical school. Is trained in the diagnosis and treatment of all diseases of the body. Can treat all eye disorders and perform eye surgery, having graduated from a minimum of 3 to 4 years of ophthalmology residency (a pediatric ophthalmologist undergoes an additional minimum of 1 year of specialty training).

## SUGGESTED READING

Crawford, J. S., & Morin, J. D. (Eds). (1983). *The eye in childhood.* Toronto, Ontario, Canada: Grune & Stratton.

Frey, T. (1991). Dyslexia and learning disabilities. *Binocular Vision Quarterly, 6*(1), 25–30.

Nelson, L. B. (Ed.). (1998). *Harley's pediatric ophthalmology* (4th ed.). Philadelphia: Saunders.

Vaughan, D., Asbury, T., & Riordan-Eva, P. (1999). *General ophthalmology* (15th ed.). Stamford, CT: Appleton & Lange.

Vellutino, F. R. (1987). Dyslexia. *Scientific American, 256*(3), 34–41.

Vrabec, T. R., Levin, A. V., & Nelson, L. B. (1989). Functional blinking in childhood. *Pediatrics, 83*(6), 967–970.

## REFERENCE

American Academy of Pediatrics Committee on Children with Disabilities, American Association for Pediatric Ophthalmology and Strabismus, & American Academy of Ophthalmology. (1988). Learning disabilities, dyslexia, and vision: A subject review. *Pediatrics, 102*(5), 1217–1219.

# CHAPTER 9

# Hearing Disorders in the Classroom

Vicky Papaioannou

For many years, children who are deaf and hard of hearing have made up the largest group of students requiring special services in schools (Flexer, Wray, & Ireland, 1989). In addition, most of these students have been mainstreamed into general education classrooms in regular schools. In the last 10 years, universal newborn hearing screening programs have become more common across North America. It is the ultimate intent of these programs to identify children with hearing loss early (usually before 6 months of age) and to allow these children access to the services that will enable them to enter the school system with the same level of communication as their peers with normal hearing. Should these goals be realized, it is likely that even more children will be educated in the mainstream. For these children to succeed in this environment, teachers need to have a basic understanding of hearing, hearing loss and its consequences, amplification and assistive listening devices, and educational and classroom management strategies. For individuals interested in more on this topic, a Suggested Reading list is included at the end of this chapter.

## STRUCTURE AND FUNCTION

In describing the structure and function of the auditory system, it is useful to consider four portions:

1. The *outer ear* includes the ear itself (auricle or pinna) and the ear canal (external auditory canal).

2. The *middle ear* includes the eardrum (tympanic membrane), the three middle ear bones (ossicles) with their associated muscles and tendons, and the eustachian tube.

3. The *inner ear* contains both the organs of balance and hearing. Only part of the inner ear, the cochlea, belongs to the auditory system.

4. The *central auditory nervous system* includes all the auditory interconnections between and including the auditory nerve and the auditory cortex.

## Outer Ear

The outer ear consists of the external skin flap (the pinna) and the external auditory canal channel, which direct sound to the eardrum. There is great variation in terms of pinna shape and size from individual to individual. Functionally, the pinna is important for sound localization.

The external auditory canal is an oval tube, approximately 1 in. (2.5 cm) in length, that ends at the eardrum. The path of the canal is not straight and varies across individuals. In the canal, there are hair follicles and glands that secrete cerumen, commonly referred to as earwax. The wax helps moisten the skin of the canal and also serves a protective function. The outer ear structures are illustrated in Figure 9.1.

## Middle Ear

The middle ear is a small air-filled cavity within the skull. The eardrum is the thin, oval-shaped, semitransparent membrane that lies at the end of the external auditory canal and separates the outer ear from the middle ear.

The middle ear contains the three bones of hearing, the malleus, the incus, and the stapes (more commonly known as the hammer, anvil, and stirrup), that transmit sound from the eardrum to the inner ear. The largest of these bones, the malleus, is attached to the eardrum. The incus is the middle bone, which transfers sound vibrations from the malleus to the stapes. The footplate of the smallest bone (in fact, the smallest bone in the body), the stapes, is implanted in an area leading to the inner ear known as the oval window. Movements of the stapes and the oval window transmit sound vibrations to the fluid-filled cochlea. A second "window" into the

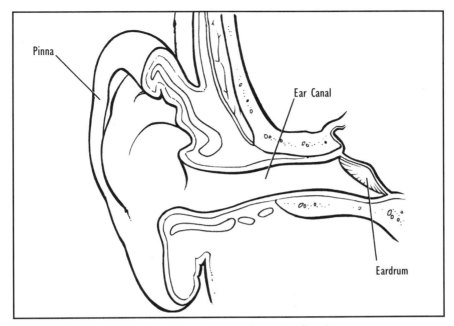

**FIGURE 9.1.** The outer ear and tympanic membrane (eardrum).

cochlea, the round window, is covered by a thin membrane and allows fluids within the cochlea to move and stimulate the sensory cells of hearing.

Two small muscles are found in the middle ear. The tensor tympani is attached to the malleus and functions to tense the eardrum by pulling on the malleus medially. The stapedius muscle is attached to the stapes and serves to prevent excessive movements of this bone by pulling the stapes posteriorly. Together, these muscles provide the ear some protection from very loud sounds.

The eustachian tube connects the middle ear and the nasopharynx (back of the nose). It functions to equalize pressure on both sides of the eardrum and for drainage of fluid from the middle ear space. Figure 9.2 illustrates the middle ear structures.

## Inner Ear

The fluid-filled cochlea, or inner ear, resembles a snail's shell. The cochlea itself is divided into three compartments: the scala vestibuli, scala tympani,

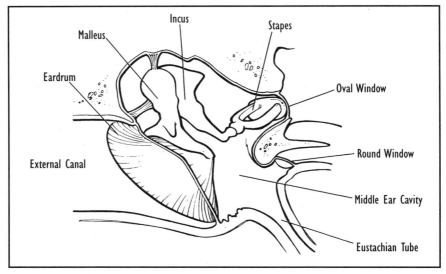

**FIGURE 9.2.** The external auditory canal and the middle ear structures.

and scala media or cochlear duct. The scala vestibuli and scala tympani contain a fluid called perilymph. The scala media is found between the two compartments and contains a different fluid called endolymph. These fluids act to transmit vibrations from the stapes footplate in the oval window to the sensory receptors.

The basilar membrane separates the scala media from the scala tympani. Attached to the basilar membrane is the organ of Corti, formed by a group of sensory cells and related supporting structures. This is the actual receptor organ for hearing. The sensory or receptor cells themselves are called hair cells. The structures of the inner ear are shown in Figure 9.3.

## Central Auditory Nervous System

The sensory hair cells in the inner ear connect to nerve fibers that transmit sound information in the form of neural impulses to the central auditory nervous system. The nerve fibers make up the auditory nerve. Sound information is processed at various levels within the auditory pathway. A person's awareness of sound and recognition of speech are the result of processes at the highest cortical levels. A view of the auditory system up to and including the auditory nerve is illustrated in Figure 9.4.

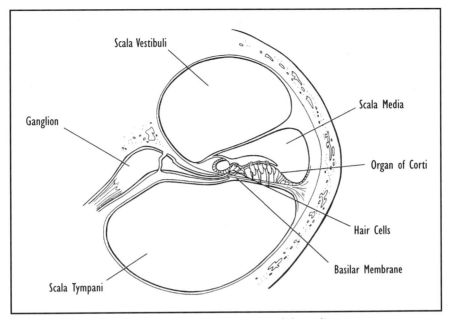

**FIGURE 9.3.** The cochlear portion of the inner ear and the auditory nerve.

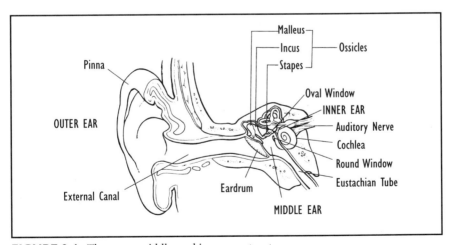

**FIGURE 9.4.** The outer, middle, and inner ear structures.

# TYPES OF HEARING LOSS

As described, the auditory system can be divided into different portions. A problem can occur in any one of these areas or in more than one area. The locations of the problem in different types of hearing loss are described in the following sections.

## Conductive

In a conductive hearing loss, an abnormality exists in the outer or middle ear and causes sound to be attenuated before it reaches the inner ear, which functions normally. This type of loss can often be treated with either medication or surgery. The most common conductive hearing loss in children is caused by otitis media (ear infections causing accumulation of fluid in the middle ear). Other causes include extreme wax buildup, eardrum perforation, small or absent ear canals or pinnas, and ossicular abnormalities.

## Sensorineural

In sensorineural hearing loss, the problem lies in the inner ear or in the transmission of impulses along the auditory nerve. Within the cochlea, the site of damage is usually the sensory hair cells. As a result of the hearing loss, not only does the individual notice decreased sensitivity to sound, but there is often a decrease in the clarity of sound as well. Sound may reach the inner ear, but because of damage to the cochlea or auditory nerve, it is not received clearly by the brain, even if it is made sufficiently loud through the use of amplification. There is usually no medical treatment for this type of hearing loss and it is, therefore, generally permanent. Potential causes include heredity, anatomical abnormalities, noise exposure, certain drugs, head injuries, prolonged high fevers, meningitis, mumps, and measles. In many cases, especially when the child is born with the hearing loss, the cause remains unknown.

## Mixed

A mixed hearing loss is a combination of both a conductive and a sensorineural hearing loss. Usually, the conductive component can be treated with medication or surgery, but no medical treatment is available for the sensorineural component.

## Central or Cortical

A central or cortical hearing loss refers to the inability of the brain to interpret sound information even though peripheral hearing sensitivity is essentially normal. Varying degrees of auditory comprehension result.

## Unilateral or Bilateral

Hearing loss is also referred to as either unilateral or bilateral, depending on whether one or both ears are affected. In a unilateral hearing loss, there is a hearing loss in one ear and normal hearing in the other. Unlike children with bilateral hearing loss, these children typically respond to normal conversation and environmental sounds and demonstrate normal speech and language development. Because of this, the average age at which a child with a unilateral hearing loss is identified is generally later than that of a child with a bilateral hearing loss. Thus, many of these children are not identified until they are in school. Individuals with unilateral hearing loss find sound localization extremely difficult. That is, they have problems determining from where a sound originates. These children also have difficulty hearing in background noise. These are important considerations in terms of the classroom management of these children. Many of the educational implications for children with bilateral hearing loss hold for a child with a unilateral hearing loss as well.

## Auditory Neuropathy

Over the last two decades, another disorder has appeared to surface that is often confusing to both parents and professionals. Auditory neuropathy is not a new disorder, but one that has become better defined and recognized. Typically, children with auditory neuropathy present with hearing loss, absent or severely abnormal auditory brainstem responses (ABR), and normal otoacoustic emissions. These individuals present as somewhat of a challenge because they have some common indicators of normal hearing (normal otoacoustic emissions) but some indicators of hearing loss (absent ABR).

Auditory neuropathy can occur in isolation or with various other symptoms and conditions, which can make management even more difficult. In addition, individuals with this disorder often present very differently. For example, there is significant variation in terms of the audiometric thresholds found in individuals with auditory neuropathy, which vary from the normal hearing range to the profound hearing loss range. One relatively consistent finding among these individuals is their difficulty hearing in noisy environments.

The large variability in how these children present makes it difficult for doctors to counsel parents and other professionals, including educators, in terms of management options and prognosis. The treatment plan must definitely be individualized for each child and must remain flexible. Considerations include whether hearing aids will help given that the child has normal otoacoustic emissions, and whether the child should communicate using speech, language, and listening; sign language; or both. There may seem to be more questions than answers, but hopefully research into this disorder will fill in these knowledge gaps before too long.

## Classifications of Hearing Loss

Individuals have a wide range of hearing abilities, from those deemed to have normal hearing to those who are deaf. The term *deaf* is usually reserved for those individuals who do not use speech as their mode of communication, but rather use American Sign Language and are part of the deaf culture. For those children who use their residual hearing to learn speech and language and who use spoken language at least some of the time, the term *hard of hearing* is generally used.

## Hearing Assessment

The sounds that we hear can be measured by pitch (frequency) and loudness (intensity). Humans have the ability to hear sounds as low in frequency as 20 hertz (Hz) and as high in frequency as 20,000 Hz. The current practice in audiology is to measure hearing in the range of 250 Hz to 8000 Hz, as most speech sounds are found in this range. Intensity is measured in decibels (dB), which are expressed in reference to normal hearing level (dB HL). Sounds can be presented at very quiet levels (0 dB HL) or at very loud levels (120 dB HL). Conversational speech occurs at approximately 50 dB HL.

The audiogram is a graph illustrating the faintest sound that an individual can hear (his or her threshold) at various frequencies. It shows frequency along the horizontal axis and intensity along the vertical axis. Figure 9.5 illustrates an audiogram of an individual with normal hearing. Information below the threshold line is audible, whereas sounds above the line cannot be heard. Because the decibel scale is logarithmic, hearing loss *cannot* be expressed in terms of a percentage. Instead, hearing loss is described in terms of severity, as listed in Table 9.1.

Hearing thresholds are first measured under headphones, in a test called air conduction audiometry. This assesses the performance of the auditory system from the external ear right through to the neural pathways. Puretone stimuli are presented to the child at the various frequencies, and the intensity of the tone that is just heard (the threshold) is noted for each frequency tested. Details of methods used to test hearing sensitivity are discussed later in this chapter.

Bone conduction audiometry may also be performed. In this test, puretone thresholds are obtained using a bone conduction oscillator that is placed on the mastoid bone behind the ear or on the forehead and directly vibrates the skull, thus stimulating the cochlea and neural pathways. In this case, the sound signal bypasses the middle ear system and, therefore, assesses the function of the cochlea and neural pathways directly. If an individual has a conductive hearing loss, bone conduction thresholds will be within normal limits, while air conduction thresholds will show a hearing loss (see Figure 9.6).

Testing is also performed using speech stimuli. The speech reception threshold is the quietest level at which an individual can repeat back 50% of the two-syllable words presented. This test serves to verify puretone thresholds. Word recognition testing assesses the individual's ability to understand speech at a comfortable loudness level under optimal listening conditions. This information may be of assistance in determining hearing aid candidacy. If the child has poor speech, and thus cannot take part in the test verbally, a picture-pointing task may be used.

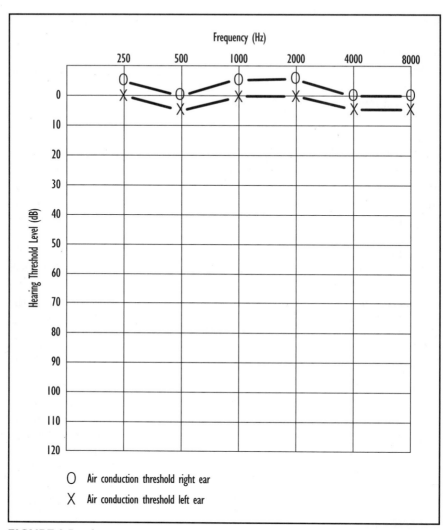

**FIGURE 9.5.** Characteristic puretone audiogram of an individual with normal hearing.

**TABLE 9.1**

The Classification and Implications of Hearing Loss

| Average Hearing Threshold (in dB HL)[a] | Classification | Implications |
|---|---|---|
| −10 to 15 | Normal hearing | The child is able to detect speech even at very soft levels. |
| 16 to 25 | Slight hearing loss | Some children will experience difficulty with quiet or distant speech, especially if the classroom is noisy. |
| 26 to 40 | Mild hearing loss | The child will miss some of the speech signal. Difficulty increases with distance from the teacher and background noise levels. Speech and language development may be afffected. Hearing aid(s) will likely be of benefit to the child. |
| 41 to 55 | Moderate hearing loss | The child is able to hear and understand speech only at very close range without amplification. Speech and language will likely be affected. The child requires hearing aid(s). |
| 56 to 70 | Moderately severe hearing loss | The child is only able to detect speech without hearing aids. Speech and language development will likely be delayed. The child requires hearing aid(s). |
| 71 to 90 | Severe hearing loss | The child is able to detect loud environmental sounds. The child requires hearing aid(s) for speech and language development. |
| 91+ | Profound hearing loss | The child is likely aware of vibrations more than sounds. The child may or may not receive benefit from traditional hearing aids. Hearing aids or a cochlear implant would be necessary if speech and language development is desired. |

[a] The average puretone air conduction threshold of 500 Hz, 1000 Hz, and 2000 Hz.

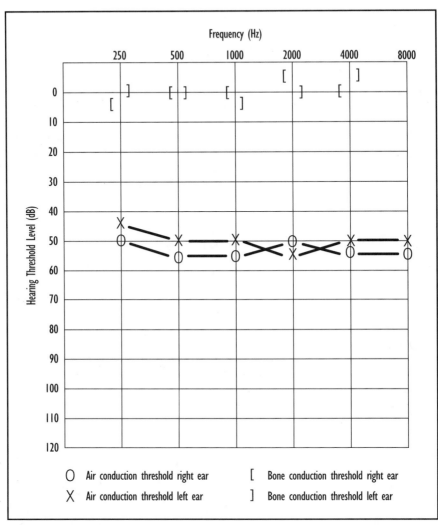

**FIGURE 9.6.** Audiogram illustrating a conductive hearing loss.

# TEST METHODOLOGY

An audiologist administers a variety of tests in a sound-treated booth. No child is too young to have hearing tested; however, assessment methods vary depending on the child's age or developmental ability. Assessment techniques generally fall into one of two categories: objective and behavioral.

## Objective Test Methods

Objective tests neither require a behavioral response by the child nor require the child to actively participate in the test session. Three types of objective tests are described in the following sections.

### Auditory Brainstem Response Testing or Brainstem Evoked Response Audiometry

In auditory brainstem response testing or brainstem evoked response audiometry, recording electrodes are attached to the child's scalp in order to measure changes in brainstem activity occurring with the presentation of sound to each ear using headphones. Infants may be tested using this procedure during natural sleep or while resting quietly. If testing is not possible under these conditions, a mild sedative or even a general anesthetic may be required. This test is generally used with infants or with children who cannot be accurately tested using other test procedures. Information regarding the hearing status in each ear is obtained.

### Otoacoustic Emissions Testing

Otoacoustic emissions testing is very common in universal newborn hearing screening programs and is often used clinically as well. It is basically a screening test of cochlear function and is based on the discovery that there are sounds, measurable within the ear canal, that are generated by the cochlea in response to sound stimulation. Otoacoustic emissions are measured by placing a probe in the ear canal that both produces a test signal and measures for very soft sounds that may be present in the ear canal. The presence of an otoacoustic emission suggests that the outer hair cells within the cochlea respond normally to sound. The absence of an oto-acoustic emission when there are no middle ear problems suggests that the outer hair cells within the cochlea are not responding normally and further testing is required to determine the degree of hearing loss.

## Impedance/Immittance Audiometry

Impedance/immittance audiometry is not a hearing test; rather, this procedure assesses the status of the middle ear system (see Figure 9.2). It allows the audiologist access to information regarding middle ear pressure, eardrum and ossicular mobility, ear canal volume, and eustachian tube function. A probe is inserted into the child's ear canal and sound is presented. The air pressure within the ear canal is varied, and the amount of sound reflected back from the eardrum is measured. Information is recorded on a graph called a tympanogram. Certain combinations of results are associated with specific middle ear problems (e.g., ear infection, eardrum perforation).

## Behavioral Test Methods

Behavioral test methods generally require some type of observable behavioral response by the child. They are described based on appropriateness for a child's developmental age, starting from youngest to oldest. Test methods change as the child develops and is able to be a more active participant in the test procedures. Developmental delays affect the choice of method at any given age.

### Behavior Observation Audiometry

Behavior observation audiometry is not used very often given the availability of objective tests for young children. If used, it is generally appropriate for children with a developmental age of less than 6 months, who are usually unable to turn in response to a sound. Speech and frequency-specific tones are most often presented to the child through loudspeakers, although different types of headphones can be used. Following signal presentation, the examiner watches for changes in the child's behavior or facial expressions. Examples of responses include a startle to loud sounds, an eye shift or widening of the eyes, searching behavior (infant appears to be looking for the sound source), as well as changes in limb movement, breathing, or sucking activities.

## Visual Reinforcement Audiometry or Conditioned Orientation Reflex Audiometry

Visual reinforcement audiometry or conditioned orientation reflex audiometry is generally used for children who are able to turn in response to the presentation of a sound (usually at least 6 months of age), but who are unable to perform conditioned play audiometry (the method discussed next). Using this procedure, if the child turns to a sound that is presented, the child is reinforced using an animated toy or lights. The toy is housed in a dark Plexiglas enclosure that lights up when the child looks for the sound. If the child will tolerate headphones, visual reinforcement audiometry can be attempted while the child wears headphones.

### Conditioned Play Audiometry

Usually when the child is about 3 years of age, conditioned play audiometry becomes the test method of choice. The child is conditioned to give a certain response each time the auditory signal is presented. The response by the child can be putting pegs in a pegboard, stacking rings, dropping blocks in a bucket, or any similar task that the child finds enjoyable. The stimulus is ideally presented through headphones in order to obtain information about each ear. If the child will not tolerate headphones, loudspeakers are used.

### Conventional Audiometry

With children who are approximately 4 or 5 years of age, audiologists can use essentially the same test methods they use with adults. Children are instructed to respond to the softest sound that they can hear. Depending on the child's age and interest level, several options exist. The child could raise a hand, push a button on a handheld device, say "yes," or clap hands when he or she hears a sound.

# AUDIOLOGICAL (RE)HABILITATION

Once doctors have determined that nothing can be done medically to restore a child's hearing to "normal," the child will likely be fitted with one or two hearing aids depending on whether one or both ears are affected. Hearing aids simply amplify sound at frequencies that the child can hear. A clinical audiologist will usually prescribe the hearing aids and will choose the hearing aids based on the individual's hearing loss, lifestyle, educational environment, and personal preferences.

All hearing aids consist of three main components: a microphone, an amplifier, and a receiver. The microphone receives the sound into the hearing aid, the amplifier makes it louder, and the receiver directs the sound from the hearing aid into the ear via the earmold or earpiece. Other components usually found on the hearing aid are an on/off and T switch and a volume control, although features vary with the type of hearing aid. The T switch activates the hearing aid's telecoil and is often used when the individual uses a telephone or FM system. Hearing aids, of course, need a power source, and different sizes of batteries are found in different types of hearing aids.

Three general categories of hearing aids exist:

1. Custom hearing aids, which include in-the-ear (ITE), in-the-canal (ITC), and completely in-the-canal (CIC) hearing aids

2. Behind-the-ear (BTE) hearing aids

3. Body-worn hearing aids

Figure 9.7 shows examples of several types of hearing aids.

The most commonly prescribed hearing aids for adults in North America are generally the custom hearing aids. These are selected because they are smaller and felt by many to be more cosmetically appealing than other hearing aids. These hearing aids are housed entirely within the individual's ear. In general, ITC hearing aids are prescribed for mild and perhaps moderate hearing losses, whereas ITE and CIC hearing aids are prescribed for mild, moderate, or perhaps moderately severe hearing losses.

Behind-the-ear (BTE) hearing aids can be used for any degree of hearing loss. They actually consist of two parts, the hearing aid itself, which fits snugly over and behind the individual's ear, and the earmold, which allows for sound to reach the eardrum.

BTE hearing aids are often preferred for children for several reasons. The earmold material prescribed for children should be soft so that during the rough-and-tumble activities of childhood, the child is not hurt by a blow to the head or ear. An earmold made of a hard material or a custom hearing aid would cause discomfort to the child in such a situation. Fur-

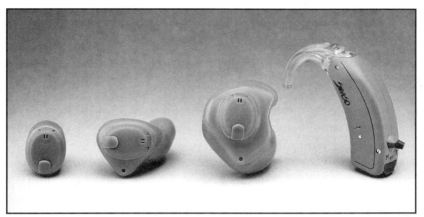

**FIGURE 9.7.** From left to right, completely in-the-canal (CIC), in-the-canal (ITC), in-the-ear (ITE), and behind-the-ear (BTE) hearing aids, provided by Widex, Canada.

thermore, earmolds can be replaced as the child grows, much more quickly and easily and often at less expense, than recasing a custom hearing aid. Growing children may need to have their earmolds replaced as often as every 3 months. A sign that the child needs a new earmold, or a custom hearing aid recased, is a squealing noise (called feedback) coming from the hearing aid when the child is wearing the hearing aid at its usual volume. Another advantage of BTE hearing aids is their compatibility with various assistive listening devices. This compatibility is especially important in an educational environment, and is discussed later in the chapter.

Body-worn hearing aids are rarely used. If this type of hearing aid is used, it is usually for a child with a profound hearing loss. Sometimes children with poor head control make use of body-worn hearing aids to reduce the chance of feedback occurring when their ear is in close proximity to an object (e.g., wheelchair headrest). Body-worn hearing aids, like BTE hearing aids, are coupled to earmolds, which deliver the amplified sound from the hearing aid to the child's ear.

For children with absent pinnas or external auditory canals or children with chronically draining ears due to ear infections, and thus a conductive hearing loss, a different type of hearing aid is used. A bone conduction hearing aid delivers sound to a vibrator, usually placed on the mastoid bone behind the ear and held in place either using a headband or double-sided tape. The sound vibrations are transmitted through the skull and to the inner ear, thus allowing the child to hear.

Some children receive little benefit from traditional amplification due to the severity of their hearing loss. A vibrotactile aid is occasionally used and may help an individual receive sounds by allowing that person to feel the vibrations generated by the sound. In this type of aid, sound is received by a microphone and sent to one or more vibrators, usually worn on the forearm or sternum, which vibrate softly on the person's skin. In devices with more than one vibrator, each vibrator responds to a different frequency region. Thus, users may be better able to discriminate frequency information because this information is coded spatially on different areas of the skin. Loudness changes are represented by the intensity of the vibrations. The device does not help the individual to hear; it may simply help the individual to better interpret incoming sound information.

A cochlear implant is another device that may be used for children who receive little benefit from hearing aids or for whom hearing aids do not allow sufficient access to speech and language. To be considered for an implant, the child must have a bilateral severe to profound sensorineural hearing loss and receive minimal benefit from hearing aids, vibrotactile aids, or personal FM systems.

The cochlear implant does *not* restore normal hearing. In fact, the child "hears" in an entirely different manner. A microphone contained in a device resembling a behind-the-ear hearing aid picks up the speech signal. The signal is sent down a wire to the speech processor, where the signal is coded and sent back up the wire to the transmitting coil. The transmitting coil is attached to the scalp with a magnet. The signal is transmitted across the scalp via a radio signal to the internal receiver/ stimulator, which is implanted in the mastoid bone behind the ear. The receiver/stimulator receives this signal and sends it to the electrode array found within the cochlea. Parts of the cochlear implant are seen in Figure 9.8. A more recent development is the behind-the-ear speech processor, which, in time, may eliminate the need for body-worn speech processors (see Figure 9.9).

## FM Systems

Unfortunately, hearing aids are generally not sufficient for a child with a hearing impairment to hear well in the poor listening conditions found in most classroom environments. Anyone who has worn a hearing aid knows

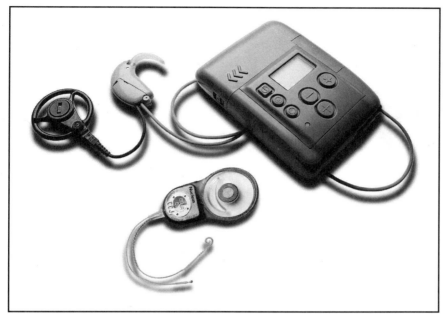

**FIGURE 9.8.** Body-worn processor, including microphone and transmitting coil with internal receiver/stimulator and electrode array, provided by Cochlear Corporation, Englewood, CO.

about the poor performance of many of these instruments in conditions with an abundance of background noise. To deal with the effects of background noise, reverberation or echo, and the listener's distance from the speaker, all common in classrooms, a child may require more than personal hearing aids or preferential seating.

Background noise, reverberation, and distance are all related to what is referred to as the signal-to-noise ratio (S/N). This is the relationship between the sound that the student wants to hear (signal) and all the other sounds present in the environment (noise). A person with difficulty hearing, whether wearing a hearing aid or not, needs a more positive S/N in order to understand speech than does a normal hearing person. For those with normal hearing, speech is easily accessible as long as the speech signal is twice as loud as sounds in the background. For students who have difficulty hearing, speech needs to be almost 10 times as loud as the background sounds to be perceived as intelligible (Flexer et al., 1989). An adequate S/N is often not possible in the classroom without the use of assistive listening devices.

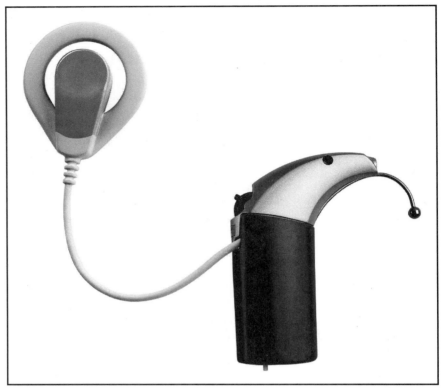

**FIGURE 9.9.** Behind-the-ear speech processor, provided by Cochlear Corporation, Englewood, CO.

An FM system is one type of assistive listening device. It works in a fashion similar to a radio station. The teacher has a microphone worn close to his or her mouth; this serves to prevent the decrease in the signal strength as it travels from the teacher's mouth to the child's ear or hearing aid. The microphone is attached to an FM transmitter via a wire. The teacher's message is transformed to an electrical signal by the microphone. The transmitter, in turn, superimposes this signal onto a radio signal that is then transmitted to the child's FM receiver. Thus, using the radio analogy, the teacher would be similar to the disc jockey at a radio station speaking into the microphone. The student would be the radio listener tuned in to the teacher's radio station. The student and teacher are not connected by wires and have a free range of movement up to approximately 200 feet (Flexer et al., 1989). A personal FM system is illustrated in Figure 9.10.

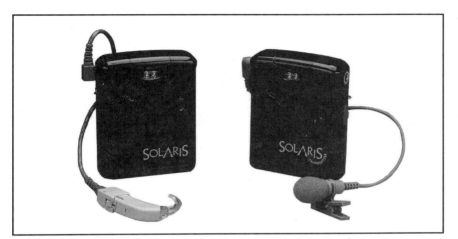

**FIGURE 9.10.** Personal FM system, including FM receiver attached to behind-the-ear hearing aid (left) and FM transmitter with microphone (right), provided by Phonic Ear, Canada.

## Personal FM Equipment

The FM signal can travel from the child's FM receiver to his or her ear in many different ways. These include button receivers with an earmold, direct audio input to the child's hearing aids, a neckloop with the child's hearing aids, a silhouette inductor arrangement, headphones, a behind-the-ear FM system, and an FM receiver audio shoe.

With a basic FM system arrangement, the signal reaches the child's ears via cords attached to button receivers that snap into the child's earmolds. This is often referred to as an auditory trainer. A child may wear this device all the time or only at school, wearing behind-the-ear hearing aids outside of school.

Direct audio input to the child's hearing aids applies mainly to behind-the-ear hearing aids, although it sometimes is used with in-the-ear hearing aids. A cord runs from the student's FM receiver to an audio boot (also known as an audio shoe) that fits over the bottom portion of the hearing aid itself. The sound, therefore, reaches the child's ears through the child's own hearing aids and earmolds.

A neckloop is a special loop of thick wire worn around the student's neck on the shoulders. The electrical signal from the FM receiver is delivered to the loop. The electrical current flowing through this loop creates a small magnetic field. The signal is picked up when the student's hearing aids are switched to the T (telecoil) position. Again, the sound is delivered to the child through the hearing aids and earmolds.

A silhouette inductor arrangement operates similarly to the neckloop. The difference lies in the device that generates the magnetic field. In the silhouette arrangement, the magnetic field is created in a thin structure often resembling the shape of the hearing aid itself. This is worn between the head and the hearing aids, and the student's hearing aids operate in the T position. The sound is delivered to the child through the hearing aids and earmolds.

An FM system also can deliver the signal to the child's ears using headphones. Because this arrangement looks similar to that of a "Walkman," it may be more readily accepted by some children and their peers. Unfortunately, many students find this arrangement uncomfortable when worn for extended periods of time.

The behind-the-ear FM system is a convenient alternative to separate hearing aids and FM receivers as it alleviates the problems of cords, neckloops, silhouette inductors, and headphones. Furthermore, the child is not required to carry a separate FM receiver box. These systems are available in different styles depending on whether the child has a hearing loss. If the child has a hearing loss, the hearing aid and FM receiver functions are combined in a single device. For children with minimal hearing loss, fluctuating hearing loss, unilateral hearing loss, attention-deficit disorder, or central auditory processing disorders who do not wear hearing aids, a miniature behind-the-ear FM receiver exists. This is a nice alternative to the FM systems traditionally worn by these children, which would have included personal FM systems with headphones, soundfield FM systems, or toteable systems.

A relatively recent development has been the miniature FM receiver built into the audio shoe of the hearing instrument. This receiver offers the advantage of being truly wireless and is powered by the battery of the child's hearing aid. It is currently the smallest FM system available (see Figures 9.11 and 9.12) and, again, delivers the sound to the child through the hearing aids and earmolds.

## Soundfield FM Equipment

A freefield or soundfield FM system works on the same premise as the personal FM system. The teacher speaks into a microphone that is worn close to the mouth. This is attached to an FM transmitter that sends the signal to

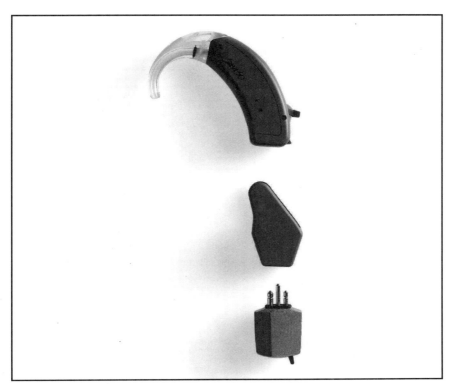

**FIGURE 9.11.** Miniature FM receiver, audio shoe, and hearing aid, provided by Widex, Canada.

two (or more) loudspeakers strategically positioned in the classroom to permit equal loudness levels in all areas (see Figure 9.13). Soundfield FM systems facilitate the reception of the teacher's voice for all students. For example, children with unilateral hearing losses, fluctuating hearing losses, attentional difficulties, learning disabilities, articulation disorders, and developmental delays may all receive benefit from this device, as may children who are learning English as their second language.

## Toteable FM System

The toteable FM system works in the same manner as a freefield or soundfield FM system. Rather than transmitting speech to strategically positioned

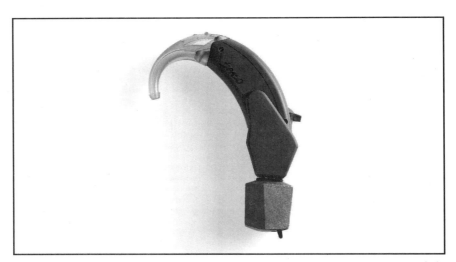

**FIGURE 9.12.** Behind-the-ear hearing aid attached to miniature FM receiver, provided by Widex, Canada.

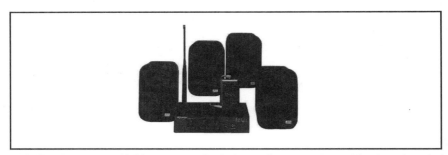

**FIGURE 9.13.** Soundfield FM system (includes teacher transmitter with microphone, amplifier/receiver, and four speakers), provided by Phonic Ear, Canada.

loudspeakers, however, the system transmits sound to a small speaker usually placed on the child's desk or table. In this way, the child can take the system to more than one location, which is not possible with a soundfield system (see Figure 9.14).

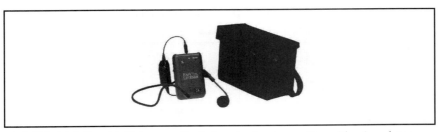

**FIGURE 9.14** Toteable FM system (includes a teacher transmitter with microphone and a receiver in a tote bag with built-in speaker and amplifier), provided by Phonic Ear, Canada.

## IN THE CLASSROOM

Hearing loss is often, but not always, detected before the child reaches school age. For a wide variety of reasons, a child may slip through the cracks and a hearing loss may go unnoticed. A child may have acquired the hearing loss later in life, or a child may come from an environment where management of hearing loss is unavailable. In any case, the symptoms of hearing loss vary greatly from child to child. Factors such as type, degree, and duration of the hearing loss; etiology of the hearing loss; and even the child's intelligence may affect how the child responds to his or her hearing difficulty. A list of behaviors a teacher may notice in a child with a hearing problem is found in Table 9.2. If a student exhibits any signs of hearing loss, it is essential to determine whether a hearing loss does exist. A number of options are available to the teacher and several are listed in Table 9.3.

### Daily Devices Check

Hearing aids and FM systems, like any pieces of electronic equipment, can malfunction. Given that much of a child's school day requires listening, these devices should be checked each morning. At a relatively young age, most children can be responsible for at least some components of the listening check. Table 9.4 lists the components of a daily hearing aid check.

FM systems must be monitored on a daily basis as well. Their benefit is minimized and they may actually hinder the child's performance if they

**TABLE 9.2**

Signs of Hearing Loss That Teachers May Observe in a Child

Demonstrates signs of inattentiveness.

Appears to daydream frequently.

Demonstrates signs of frustration.

Has frequent colds and earaches.

Often fails to respond to his or her name when it is called.

Often requests repetition of what was said.

Appears confused while the teacher is providing instructions.

Engages in inappropriate behaviors, even when given very precise instructions.

Watches what other children do and then imitates their actions.

Responds inappropriately to questions.

Speaks either very quietly or very loudly.

Has articulation errors, especially with high-frequency sounds like s, z, t, k, and f.

Appears fatigued before the day is through.

Watches the speaker's facial expressions and lip movements more than other children do.

Shows an inability to hear in group situations or in noisy environments.

Directs one ear toward the speaker in an attempt to hear better.

Withdraws from the group, often preferring to work or to play alone.

Prefers to interact with younger children, who often accept the child more readily.

**TABLE 9.3**

Strategies Available to Teachers Once a Hearing Loss Is Suspected

Contact the child's parents to discuss your observations.

Examine the student's records for previous evidence of hearing loss, including hearing test results.

Consult with the school nurse, speech–language pathologist, or educational audiologist, discussing your concerns and what to do about them.

Suggest to the child's parents that the student's hearing be checked, recommending an audiological assessment through the child's physician.

If the student is old enough, discuss the suspected hearing difficulties with the student.

**TABLE 9.4**

Components of a Daily Hearing Aid Check

1. Test the hearing aid battery with a battery tester. Replace the battery if it is dead or dying.[a] (Parents should provide extras to keep at school.)

2. Visually check the hearing aid and earmold for cracks, dents, moisture, broken parts, or wax buildup.[a]

3. Attach each hearing aid to a listening stethoscope. While speaking into the microphone, repeat the sounds *oo, ah, ee, sh, s,* and *m.* This is called the Ling six sound test and will give an indication of the clarity of sounds across the entire frequency range of speech.[b] Consider the following:

   Does the hearing aid seem as loud as it usually is?

   Does the hearing aid sound as clear as it usually does?

   Adjust the hearing aid volume louder and softer and listen for static, distortion, or intermittency. Return the hearing aid volume to its original setting.

Send a note home to the parents if any step is eventful. It is even important for parents to know when a hearing aid battery has been replaced because more frequent replacement than usual may indicate a problem with the hearing aid.

[a] Some children may be able to do this.

[b] The teacher should do this.

are not working properly. Different types of FM systems require different test methods. Some ideas for verifying the performance of various systems are presented in Table 9.5.

## Classroom Strategies

Communication can be extremely difficult for students who are deaf and hard of hearing. Whether the student is using an interpreter, has an FM system with or without hearing aids, or uses hearing aids alone, communication is difficult and tedious work, especially in the mainstream classroom. The student must concentrate intently and, because of this, may tire more easily than his or her hearing peers. The classroom teacher needs to arrange the lesson schedule so the student has time to rest and rejuvenate

**TABLE 9.5**

Strategies for a Daily FM System Check

---

1. Different FM systems are powered differently. Check the power source daily and replace or recharge as necessary.

2. Check that both the transmitter and the receiver are on the same frequency if this applies to the FM system being used. This is especially important if more than one FM system is used in a class or if the child travels from class to class with the FM system.

3. Make sure that the FM transmitter microphone is plugged into the correct receptor.

4. Connect the student's FM receiver to the hearing aids and set any FM controls (e.g., volume, on/off, T-switch) appropriately.

5. Engage the child in a listening activity that the child can perform consistently. Move across the room to determine if the signal is transmitting. The child can repeat words, repeat sounds, or raise a hand when he or she hears a sound. If the child cannot do this reliably, the microphone and the transmitter can be left close to a radio or with another person and the teacher can attach the child's hearing aids (already attached to the FM system) to a listening stethoscope and ensure that the FM system is transmitting properly. For soundfield and toteable systems, each speaker should be checked to ensure that it is functioning.

---

during the day. Periods in which the student is not required to focus his or her attention on listening are imperative.

Numerous strategies are available for teachers with students who are deaf and hard of hearing. With time and experience, many strategies will become second nature. Several suggestions are discussed below.

## The Classroom Environment

When deciding on a child's classroom placement, self-contained classrooms are preferred over those that are open concept. A classroom that is free from unnecessary noises and reverberation offers an environment that is conducive to both teaching and learning. It is beneficial for all students in the class and limits vocal strain for the teacher.

The noise or reverberation found in classrooms with an abundance of hard, flat surfaces must be reduced. The fewer hard surfaces in the classroom, the better. This includes the floor. A carpet is a good solution. If a carpet is not an option, felt sliding pads or tennis balls placed on the legs of tables and chairs also reduce noise. Acoustic tile on the ceiling and absorbent material on the walls will reduce reverberation and absorb room noise too. Absorbent material includes the children's artwork displayed on the walls or a corkboard or bulletin board covering the walls. To further reduce reverberant noise, teachers can pull curtains shut to reduce the reflection of sound from the glass of the windows. This also potentially reduces glare, which can have an impact on speechreading. Proper lighting in the classroom is imperative. A shadow on the speaker's face makes speechreading extremely difficult. Light that shines from above and in front of the teacher's face is best to avoid shadows.

Open windows increase noise in the classroom. If this is the only ventilation source, external noise can be limited by landscaping with hedges, trees, and earth mounds or solid fences.

## Seating

Older children may have discovered the seating location that works best for them. If this is the case, the teacher should allow the student to choose a seat. In general, optimal seating for students who are deaf or hard of hearing in a traditional classroom arranged in rows is near the front of the classroom. If the child has a better ear, this ear should be closest to and facing the teacher. It is important that the student is able to view the speaker's face. The view should be unobstructed, so that the child is not constantly fidgeting to get a better view. Students who are deaf and hard of hearing should be permitted to turn around in their seats to view classmates during group discussions. Furthermore, it is often a good idea to allow older students the freedom to change seats if the teacher moves or if the auditory signal comes from a different source.

If the classroom is arranged for learning centers or group discussions, the student who is deaf or hard of hearing will function better if seated at a round table rather than one that is rectangular. At a round table, the student has better visual access to all others seated at the table.

The student should be seated away from high traffic areas, such as hallways, the entrance to the classroom, and the route to the pencil sharpener.

He or she should not be seated near noise sources in the classroom, such as fans, radiators, and aquariums, if at all possible.

## Teaching Strategies

Because the student who is deaf or hard of hearing needs access to the complete auditory and visual signal, the teacher should try to always face the class while speaking. The teacher should avoid speaking while writing on the blackboard or giving instructions while the lights are off during a video or slide presentation.

Another difficult situation for the speechreader is attempting to speech-read a moving target. The teacher should try to avoid walking around the room while speaking. Speechreading an individual who is standing still is difficult enough. It is also important for teachers to keep their hands away from their face while speaking, as this can obstruct the student's view. Chewing gum, drinking, or eating while lecturing will also create difficulties.

When talking to an individual who is deaf or hard of hearing, it is not necessary to use exaggerated lip movements or an overly loud voice. In fact, both make speechreading and comprehension more difficult. It is best to use the same articulation patterns and vocal intensity that one would with anyone else. The student's peers should be made aware of this as well.

A common complaint from teachers is that their students who are deaf or hard of hearing do not pay attention. In an attempt to prevent this, the teacher should obtain the student's attention before beginning a lesson or giving instructions. It is not necessary to call the individual's name to get his or her attention, however. The teacher could gently touch or tap the student or turn the lights quickly on and off. This would help to ensure that this student is not always the one singled out.

In classroom discussions, the teacher should instruct class members to wait until the student who is deaf or hard of hearing has made eye contact before beginning to speak. The teacher can help by identifying by name the student who is about to speak, as well as by pointing out this individual. It would also be beneficial for the teacher to restate or to rephrase what the classmate has said once that person has finished speaking.

Comprehension checks are also important for students who are deaf or hard of hearing, as they allow the teacher to recognize when a student has been unable to follow the lesson. These checks can be overt, such as asking the student to restate a key point, or more subtle, such as making eye contact with the student and the student nodding. Having the student paraphrase information is preferred to asking the student a question demanding a yes or no answer, but more subtle comprehension checks are often important for older students who do not want to stand out from the rest of the class. The teacher and the student can discuss these checks in advance. If the student is having difficulty understanding something, it may be helpful for the teacher to restate the information in a different way rather than simply repeating what was just said.

The use of visual aids and visual information to complement lessons and announcements can greatly enhance student comprehension. Material that is presented auditorily is short-lived and requires immediate processing. Visually presented material lasts longer and can be referred to after the lesson is over. Key words and summaries can be written on the blackboard or on overhead transparencies. Spoken names of people and places, dates, page numbers, and new vocabulary will be especially difficult for students who are deaf and hard of hearing. Diagrams, illustrations, photographs, and charts should be used as much as possible for visual reinforcement of concepts presented auditorily and will benefit all students in the classroom.

Preteaching or pretutoring is a useful technique with students who are deaf and hard of hearing. The day before a planned lesson, the teacher can give new and unusual words and material to the child to investigate as homework. The child also can practice these words at home with family members or in the mirror to become familiar with the lip movements required for each word. The student can then follow the lesson more easily.

Postteaching or posttutoring can serve as a review of important lessons. In this way, the teacher can clarify whether the child has any misunderstandings before it is too late. This task can be something carried out by the teacher, an educational assistant, a resource teacher, a student buddy, or a parent.

A buddy system may help the student who is deaf or hard of hearing. The buddy can have a large or a small role, depending on the buddy's abilities and the partner's needs. The buddy may simply provide the student with brief explanations and clarifications, or he or she may have a bigger role, whereby the buddy writes out homework and assignments or is a notetaker for the student who is deaf or hard of hearing. Notetakers are especially important for older students, due to the greater complexity of material. It is extremely difficult, if not impossible, to take good notes while attempting to speechread. As mentioned above, the buddy may help tutor the student as well. If the buddy is to act as a tutor, he or she should have a good knowledge of the subject area. Different tutors, and therefore buddies, may be required for different subject areas.

The student's peers are often very curious about their classmate who is deaf or hard of hearing. Teachers could use this opportunity to teach the children in the class about hearing and hearing loss. Understanding peers will go a long way in creating a cooperative learning environment for all of the children in the class.

# COMMON MISCONCEPTIONS ABOUT DEAFNESS

- **A hearing aid restores normal hearing.**

  A hearing aid merely amplifies sound. Thus, speech is made louder and *not* clearer. Although hearing aids are fit to compensate for a child's particular hearing loss, they do not give the child "normal" hearing. Because hearing aids amplify sound and because they cannot differentiate between speech and unwanted background noise, in noisy environments *all* sound is amplified. FM systems, directional microphones on hearing aids, and digital hearing aids improve matters, but do not restore normal hearing either.

- **Deaf people are good lipreaders.**

  Lipreading, more accurately referred to as speechreading, involves the interpretation of an utterance through the observation of the speaker's lip and jaw movements, facial expressions, body language, and gestures. It is often assumed that because an individual is deaf or hard of hearing, the individual will be a good speechreader. In fact, it is no easier for these individuals to speechread than it is for hearing individuals. There will be deaf and hearing individuals who are good speechreaders, and deaf and hearing individuals who are poor speechreaders.

  Speechreading is not an easy task. Many sounds look exactly like others on the lips (e.g., *b, p,* and *m; f* and *v*), and many other sounds are not visible on the lips (e.g., *k, g,* and *h*). Because of this, very few people can rely on speechreading alone to understand a speaker's message.

- *Audibility* **is the same as** *intelligibility.*

  This is often a difficult concept to understand. Even though a child may be able to hear a teacher's voice, he or she may not be able to understand what is being said. To demonstrate this point, turn on a radio to a point where it is barely audible. At this point, one is able to detect that sound is being produced, but the message is not intelligible. It is evident, then, that one cannot assume that simply because a child can *hear* the teacher, he or she can *understand* what is being said.

# CURRENT ISSUES IN THE FIELD

One of the biggest issues in the field of deaf education relates to the communication modality used by students who are deaf and hard of hearing. There are basically two camps when it comes to this issue. There are those individuals who believe that children should use their residual hearing and hearing aids in order to communicate using spoken language within a hearing world. These individuals advocate "oralism." Others argue that children who are deaf and hard of hearing should be given language, not necessarily spoken language, and advocate "manualism."

Oralism itself can be broken down further, into various communication methods. The *auditory verbal* method emphasizes the use of whatever residual hearing the child has in order to understand sounds and to develop speech and language. The *aural–oral* method allows the child to use both visual and auditory information. The child watches the face and body of the speaker and uses these speechreading cues to help comprehend spoken language. *Cued speech* uses hand signals on the face along with speech and speechreading cues in order to facilitate the acquisition of spoken language.

Individuals advocating manualism argue that it is unnatural for individuals who are deaf to speak. They state that these individuals should use a language that is more natural to them. They prefer the use of sign language. Although various forms of manually coded English systems exist (e.g., Signing Exact English, Pidgin Sign English, Manual English), use of American Sign Language (ASL) provides individuals who are deaf with entry into the "deaf culture." Supporters of deaf culture argue that individuals who are deaf should belong to a culture that consists of others like themselves, all using a common language. They feel that the deaf community can provide individuals who are deaf with the best environment in which to live and grow. This group shares their own entertainment, social and political activities, athletics, customs, and, most important, language.

*Total Communication* incorporates aspects of both oralism and manualism. It allows the child to communicate in whatever manner is easiest and most effective. Gestures, sign language, fingerspelling, speechreading, listening, and speaking are all used.

## CONCLUSION

The educational needs of students who are deaf and hard of hearing are best served by a team of parents and professionals, all of whom have the individual child's best interests in mind. The classroom teacher is the professional most directly responsible for the child in the school environment. A teacher with a basic understanding of hearing, hearing loss, and the consequences of hearing loss will greatly facilitate the student's educational career. Teachers should feel at ease with students who are deaf and hard of hearing and realize that they, as teachers, perhaps more than any other professional, have a great opportunity to contribute to the overall education and psychosocial adjustment of these students.

## SUGGESTED READING

Culbertson, J. L., & Gilbert, L. E. (1986). Children with unilateral sensorineural hearing loss: Cognitive, academic, and social development. *Ear and Hearing, 7*(1), 38–42.

Estabrooks, W. (1998). *Cochlear implants for kids.* Washington, DC: A. G. Bell Association for the Deaf.

Flexer, C. (1999). *Facilitating hearing and listening in young children* (2nd ed.). San Diego, CA: Singular.

Maxon, A. B., & Brackett, D. (1992). *The hearing impaired child: Infancy through high-school years.* Boston: Andover Medical.

Sacks, O. (1989). *Seeing voices: A journey into the world of the deaf.* Los Angeles: University of California Press.

Sininger, Y., & Starr, A. (Eds.). (2001). *Auditory neuropathy: A new perspective on hearing disorders.* San Diego, CA: Singular.

# REFERENCE

Flexer, C., Wray, D., & Ireland, J. (1989). Preferential seating is not enough: Issues in classroom management of hearing-impaired students. *Language, Speech, and Hearing Services in Schools, 20,* 11–21.

# CHAPTER 10

# Communication Disorders Associated with Medical Problems

Mary Anne Witzel

Speech and language disorders occur in 10% to 15% of school-age children, and many of these problems are associated with an underlying medical illness or condition. Awareness and understanding of the communication disorders associated with medical problems by teachers, special educators, psychologists, speech–language pathologists, and other professionals in the educational system will enhance the curriculum planning and delivery as well as therapy intervention and classroom adaptation for these children. In some cases, previously unidentified medical conditions may be detected first by the communication disorders that they cause.

The purpose of this chapter is to provide teachers and other education professionals with a working knowledge of the types of communication disorders associated with various medical conditions and the role that teachers can play in the identification and management of these problems in the classroom. The medical conditions described were selected to cover the range of communication disorders that the classroom teacher may encounter. The Suggested Reading list and addresses in Appendix 10.A can be useful to individuals who wish to learn more about communication disorders associated with medical problems.

## COMPONENTS OF SPEECH AND LANGUAGE

### Articulation

*Articulation* is defined as a motor skill involving the use of the articulators, including the lips, tongue, teeth, vocal cords, and hard and soft palate, to form the consonant and vowel sounds of speech by shaping the air exhaled from the lungs as it flows through the vocal tract (see Figure 10.1). The articulation of speech sounds may be classified according to either the place in the vocal tract and the specific articulators used to form the sounds or the manner of formation, which is the degree of constriction of the airstream and the direction of the airflow, either oral or nasal (see Table 10.1). For example, /p/ and /b/ are classified as bilabial sounds for place of articulation because they are produced at the lips. They also are classified as stop sounds for manner of formation because the lip closure stops or occludes the airflow through the vocal tract for an instant to allow explosive air pressure to build up. When the lips are opened, the air is expelled with increased pressure, making the sound audible.

The place of production for /s/ and /z/ is lingual alveolar because the tongue (lingua) approximates the alveolar area of the hard palate. The manner of formation of these sounds is classified as fricative because the tongue approximates the alveolar area, narrowing the airstream and causing the turbulence and frication that makes these sounds audible and recognizable. Affricate sounds involve both an occlusion of the airstream and a narrow release of air; the glide and lateral sounds are produced with a relaxed narrowing of the vocal tract and less turbulent noise than the fricative

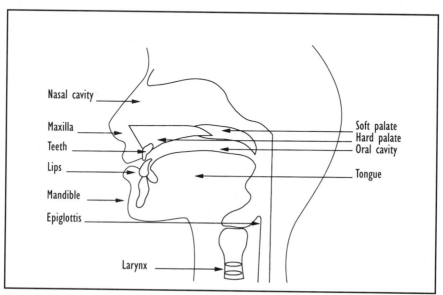

**FIGURE 10.1.** The human vocal tract.

**TABLE 10.1**
Place and Manner of Formation of Consonant Sounds in the Vocal Tract

| Sound | Place | Stop | Fricative | Affricate | Glide | Lateral | Nasal |
|---|---|---|---|---|---|---|---|
| | | | **Manner of Formation** | | | | |
| /p, b, w, m/ | Bilabial | /p, b/ | | | /w/ | | /m/ |
| /f, v/ | Labiodental | | /f, v/ | | | | |
| /th/ | Lingual dental | | /th/ | | | | |
| /t, d, l, n, s, z/ | Lingual alveolar | /t, d/ | /s, z/ | | | /l/ | /n/ |
| /sh, zh, ch, j, y, r/ | Lingual palatal | | /sh, zh/ | /ch, j/ | /y, r/ | | |
| /k, g, ng/ | Lingual velar | /k, g/ | | | | | /ng/ |
| /h/ | Glottal | | /h/ | | | | |

sounds; and the nasal sounds are produced with an occlusion in the oral cavity and the airflow directed through the nose by an open soft palate. Almost all consonant sounds are paired for both place and manner of formation (e.g., /p, b/, /t, d/, /s, z/). Voicing, or vibration from the vocal folds, distinguishes one sound from the other in a pair. For the paired sounds /s/ and /z/, place and manner of formation are identical; however, /s/ does not have vibration from the vocal folds since the larynx is open, whereas /z/ does (see Figure 10.2).

## Voice

*Phonation* is the production of sound by the vibration of the vocal folds of the larynx as they are approximated or adducted (see Figure 10.2B). These sounds are known as voiced sounds. The characteristics of phonation of voice include quality, pitch, and loudness. Vowels are produced with phonation and changes in vocal tract shape by the tongue, lips, and soft palate. Some consonants (e.g., /p/, /t/, and /s/) are produced without phonation or voicing, since the vocal folds of the larynx are open, or abducted, and do not generate vibration during these sounds (see Figure 10.2A). These sounds, known as voiceless sounds, become audible because they have noise caused by hisses, clicks, and small explosions of air.

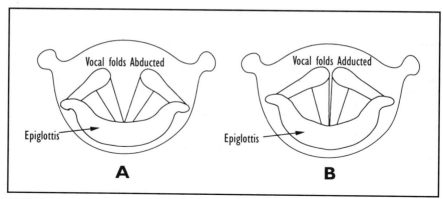

**FIGURE 10.2.** (A) Schematic drawing of vocal folds in open, or abducted, position for the voiceless consonant sound /s/. (B) Schematic drawing of the vocal folds in closed, or adducted, position for the voiced consonant sound /z/.

The noise associated with these consonants is produced when the articulators (tongue and lips) narrow, or occlude, the airstream as it flows through the vocal tract. Other consonants (e.g., /b/, /d/, and /z/) are produced with both phonation and noise. They are referred to as the voiced consonants.

Resonance is defined as the amplification of sound waves generated by vibration of the vocal folds (phonation) and constrictions of the airstream in the vocal tract (noise), which increases the perception of specific vocal tones. Resonance varies according to vocal tract size and shape. The resonance required for the nasal sounds /m/, /n/, and /ng/ is achieved by using the entire vocal tract, including the nasal and oral cavities (see Figure 10.3A); the normal resonance required for the oral sounds—that is, vowels and all other consonants—is achieved by preventing airflow from entering the nasal cavity by closing the soft palate and surrounding musculature (see Figure 10.3B).

## Fluency

Fluency is the flow of speech. Fluent speech is effortless, uninterrupted, and smooth. Fluent speech is free of abnormal pauses, hesitations, prolongations, and repetitions. In fluent speech, the rate or speed does not detract from its intelligibility.

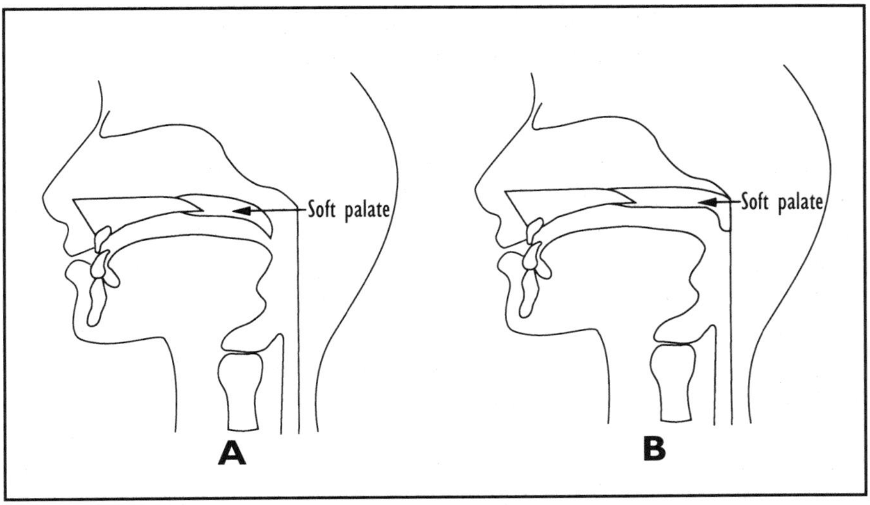

**FIGURE 10.3.** (A) Schematic drawing of the vocal tract with the soft palate open and tongue tip in position for the sound /n/. (B) Schematic drawing of the vocal tract with the soft palate closed and tongue tip in position for the fricative sound /s/.

## Language

*Language* is defined as a communication system involving the use of words or meaningful units combined by a system of rules. It can be divided into two major components: receptive and expressive. Receptive language is the comprehension and understanding of spoken, written, or sign language, whereas expressive language is the verbal, written, or signed expression of an individual's thoughts, ideas, needs, and responses using the symbols and rules of a language. Expressive language consists of three major components: form, content, and use (Bloom & Lahey, 1978). *Form* includes phonology (rules that govern the sequencing and distribution of phonemes, sound units, or sound combinations of a language), syntax (rules that determine the form or structure of a sentence), and morphology (modification of word meanings by use of number, verb tense, possession, extension, etc.). *Content* includes semantics, or that aspect of language concerned with the meaning of words, whereas *use* involves pragmatics, or the social appropriateness and use of language within a communication situation.

# SPEECH PRODUCTION
# AND DEVELOPMENT

Speech production is an integrated, complex process involving neurophysiology and respiration to make airflow from the lungs audible and recognizable by phonation, noise, resonance, and movements of the articulators. Speech development begins with the motor control abilities that emerge in the first year of life. During the first 6 months, the infant coos and babbles, which is followed by unintelligible speech utterances known as jargon. Simple, recognizable words occur around the child's first birthday. Vowel development is usually complete by the time the child is 3, whereas consonant development often continues to age 5. The consistent correct pronunciation of consonants in blends (e.g., *st* as in *stop*) and clusters (e.g., *spr* as in *sprinkle*) may not be achieved in the normal speaking child until age 7 or 8. There is great variability in the normal development of speech in children, and the age of mastery of speech sounds may vary as much as 3 years (Owens, 1994).

## Neurophysiology

Speech production uses the nerves, muscles, cartilage, and bones of the head, neck, and trunk. Speech begins with nerve impulses that are fired from the brain to other areas of the nervous system, causing contraction of certain muscles. The nervous system consists of the central nervous system (CNS), which includes the brain and spinal cord, and the peripheral nervous system (PNS), which includes the cranial nerves and spinal nerves. The CNS and PNS are composed of a network of specialized cells known as neurons. Neurons may be motor or sensory. Motor neurons conduct impulses away from the CNS, usually to muscles in the periphery, and sensory neurons conduct impulses from the periphery toward the CNS. For example, when a person decides to close his or her lips, motor neurons carry the signal or impulse to the lip and jaw muscles, causing them to contract. When the lips contract, this stimulates the sensory receptors near the surface of the skin, and information that the lips have closed is carried along the sensory neurons to the brain (Borden, Harris, & Raphael, 1994).

## Respiration

Respiration involves the spinal and thoracic peripheral nerves; the diaphragm, intercostal, and abdominal muscles; and sensory feedback to the CNS to allow the flow of air into and out of the lungs. Inspiration and expiration of air are necessary not only for breathing but also for speech. In general, the volume of air inspired and exhaled for speech sounds is greater than that needed for quiet breathing. Irregularities and abnormalities in respiratory patterns for breathing are often seen in those patients with speech problems. Inspiration occurs when the air pressure in the lungs is negative compared to atmospheric pressure and air is inhaled into the lungs through the respiratory–vocal tract to equalize the air pressure. Expiration occurs when the muscles of respiration contract, increasing the air pressure within the lungs compared to atmospheric pressure. Air is then exhaled through the tract to again equalize the air pressure with atmospheric pressure. The modulation or shaping of airflow exhaled from the lungs through the vocal tract produces the sounds of speech.

## Phonation

For voiced sounds, nerve impulses from the brain bring the arytenoid cartilages of the larynx together, causing the vocal folds to approximate and putting them in position to vibrate (see Figure 10.2B). As air is exhaled from the lungs and passes between the folds, the increased air pressure causes the vocal folds to vibrate and produce sound. This vibration of the vocal folds is attributed to the pressure of the airstream rather than to nerve impulses. The vocal folds are positioned closer together for vowels than for voiced consonants.

## Noise

For voiceless sounds, the nerve impulses from the brain keep the vocal folds open (see Figure 10.2A). Air then passes freely from the lungs into the oral cavity, where the articulators create noise by briefly stopping or narrowing the airstream to create turbulence.

## Resonance

All objects have a capacity to resonate. The vocal tract (see Figure 10.1) functions as the resonating chamber for speech. It changes in shape and size depending on the position of the articulators and whether the soft palate musculature is open or closed (see Figure 10.3). When the soft palate musculature is open, the resonating chamber of the vocal tract is enlarged, because it includes the nasal cavity. This contributes to the differences in resonance that are perceived between the oral sounds and the nasal sounds (/m/, /n/, /ng/) of speech (see Figure 10.3). When specific vibrations from the vocal folds are similar in frequency to those of the individual vocal tract, these vibrations are enhanced. Those vibrations that are not similar are attenuated. This filtering of the vibrations from the vocal folds through the vocal tract results in the individual's *vocal resonance,* which helps to distinguish one individual's voice from another's.

## Articulation

Articulation of vowels and consonants of speech results from the constriction of the vocal tract by the lips, tongue, jaws, and soft palate to either narrow or briefly stop the airstream. Movement of the articulators, particularly the opening and closing of the soft palate musculature, also directs the airstream through the nose for nasal sounds or through the mouth for oral sounds. Each sound of a language has a specific location in the vocal tract where it is produced, a specific degree of constriction of the vocal tract, and a specific direction of the airflow (see Figure 10.3 and Table 10.1).

# LANGUAGE COMPETENCE

The brain and cortical function, in combination with adequate hearing, speech production, and appropriate social environment, is necessary for the development and use of language. Language is dependent on the individual's ability to learn and integrate the symbols and rule systems. Language development begins in the first months of life and is dramatic and rapid during the preschool years, with particular emphasis on semantics and pragmatics. By the time the child enters school, he or she exhibits the basic aspects of adult language, including a knowledge of the individual sound units and sound-symbol sequences, discrimination between sounds, extensive vocabulary development, and a solid knowledge of rules for combining units of meaning to convey specific ideas. The child is able to understand functional language and express thoughts, ideas, and desires. Growth of the five components of language continues in the school-age years, albeit at a slower rate, and even into adulthood. In the school-age years, refinements in the use of language are developed, particularly in the areas of semantics, syntax, and morphology. Metalinguistic abilities that allow the child to think about and reflect on language occur, and there is an emphasis on written language and reading. School-age children become increasingly able to deal with abstract concepts, attend to and follow complex directions, appreciate jokes, recognize the ambiguities of language, understand metaphors and similes, and narrate stories and thoughts (Landman, 1989).

# TYPES OF
# COMMUNICATION DISORDERS

## Speech

*Articulation disorders* consist of errors in the formation of individual sounds of speech. Errors may be classified as substitutions, omissions, or distortions. These errors are usually related to difficulties in the anatomy or physiology of the motor production system or in the neuromotor control system. For example, speech sound errors may be due to physical abnormalities of the vocal tract, as found in children with cleft palate or neuromotor impairments associated with cerebral palsy. An articulation disorder also may be known as a phonetic disorder.

*Voice disorders* include abnormalities in phonation (e.g., pitch, loudness, quality) and abnormalities in resonance. Abnormalities in pitch include excessively high or low pitch or unusual pitch fluctuations, abnormalities in loudness include excessively high or low volume of voice, and abnormalities in vocal quality include hoarseness (due to irregularities in the contact surface of the vocal folds) and breathiness (incomplete adduction of the vocal folds during phonation). Abnormalities in resonance include hypernasality (excessive resonance for oral sounds due to use of both the oral and nasal cavities as resonating chambers), which may occur in individuals with cleft palate, and hyponasality (decreased resonance of the nasal sounds due to partial or total blockage of the nasal cavity as a resonating chamber for the nasal sounds). This type of resonance also is heard when a head cold or allergies block a speaker's nasal passages. Voice disorders may be due to abnormalities in anatomy or function of the larynx, nasal cavity, or soft palate musculature during speech.

*Stuttering* and other disorders of fluency include abnormal pauses, hesitations, prolongations, interjections, repetitions, blockages, or excessive rates of speech that interrupt the flow of speech. Stuttering may be accompanied by secondary characteristics, such as excessive muscular tension in the vocal tract, eye blinking, and other abnormal body movements during speech. There are many theories about the causation of stuttering, including effects of genetics, neuroses, development, learning, and conditioning (Shames & Ramig, 1994).

## Language

A *phonological disorder* is defined as abnormal organization of the individual's phonological system or a significant deficit in speech production or perception. Phonological disorders involve the cognitive and linguistic components of the speech sound system. Phonological disorders include:

> (a) widespread patterns of errors (e.g., omissions of final consonants in words, production of one group of sounds for another), (b) severe limitations in the range of sounds produced (e.g., the child produces *t* in place of a wide variety of consonants), (c) limitations in syllable structure of words produced (e.g., only the stressed syllables of words are produced), and (d) interactions of sounds and syllable structures (e.g., a child ends all words with *s*) or production of words in which one sound influences the other sounds in the word (e.g., in words with more than one consonant, the two consonants are produced so that they are identical or nearly identical with no direct physical cause). (Schwartz, 1994, p. 256)

*Semantic disorders* include poor vocabulary development, inappropriate use of word meanings, and an inability to comprehend word meanings. *Syntax difficulties* include abnormalities in average length of phrases and sentences and difficulty in interpreting word order and grammar. *Morpho-*

*logical difficulties* include abnormal use of prefixes and suffixes, abnormal structure of words, and abnormalities in use of tenses, plurals, and possessive forms. Finally, *pragmatics problems* involve the inability to comprehend or use language appropriately in context and inappropriate or inadequate use of language in conversation.

# THE EFFECT OF ANATOMICAL ABNORMALITIES ON COMMUNICATION

## Brain

Abnormalities in the structural, metabolic, or electrophysiologic aspects of the brain or CNS may impair receptive and expressive language and speech production, as well as learning, reading, attention, and behavior. Congenital anomalies of the brain documented in various medical conditions include microcephaly (abnormally small brain), macrocephaly (abnormally large brain), holoprosencephaly (impaired midline cleavage of the forebrain), agenesis or absence of the corpus callosum, Arnold Chiari malformation, hydrocephaly, tumors, and encephaloceles. Seizures and increased intracranial pressure also may occur. Acquired conditions, such as traumatic head injury, tumors, infections, and seizures, also will influence communication abilities, often resulting in regression of developed language abilities. Congenital and acquired conditions of the nervous system, such as myasthenia gravis and hypotonia, often affect the coordinated production of speech (Schaefer, Mathy-Lakko, & Bodensteiner, 1992).

## Ear

Abnormalities in the anatomy and function of the components of the ear, including the inner ear, middle ear, eustachian tube, tympanic membrane, and outer ear, may cause varying types and degrees of hearing loss (see Chapter 9). Hearing loss can impede development and production of speech, development and competence of language, and behavior and learning.

## Nose

Resonance of voice may be affected by abnormalities in the size and shape of the nose, because the nasal cavity is an important resonating cavity for speech. Deviation of the septum, enlarged nasal turbinates, or other blockages in the nose will increase nasal resistance in the nose. If this is significant, hyponasal resonance and an audible turbulent sound will occur during production of the nasal sounds.

## Lips

Articulation of sounds such as /p/, /b/, /w/, and /m/, which require lip closure or rounding, or sounds such as /l/ and /v/, which require the lower lip to contact the upper teeth, may be affected if the lips are unable to close or contact the teeth due to abnormal position of the maxilla or mandible, abnormal nerve innervation, or a repaired cleft lip with severe scarring.

## Jaws

If the size and position of the upper jaw (maxilla) or lower jaw (mandible) are in disproportion to each other, the articulation of bilabial, labiodental, lingual alveolar, and lingual palatal sounds may be affected. Speech may sound unusual if the lips and tongue assume abnormal positions for sound production.

## Teeth

### Occlusion

Abnormalities in the occlusion of the teeth are often implicated in articulation problems. When the upper incisor teeth are abnormally protrusive, the child may have difficulty achieving lip closure for the bilabial sounds. When the lower teeth are abnormally protrusive, the labiodental sounds /f/ and /v/ may be produced in reverse, with the lower incisors against the upper lip. When there is a space between the upper and lower incisor teeth during occlusion of the molar teeth (open bite), the lingual dental, lingual alveolar, and lingual palatal sounds may be distorted as the tongue protrudes through this space (see Figure 10.4).

## Interdental Spacing and Missing Teeth

Missing, rotated, or abnormally spaced incisor teeth, resulting in large spaces in the dental arch, often cause abnormal tongue position for the lingual alveolar sounds /s/ and /z/. This may result in a lisp-type distortion of these sounds.

## Tongue

In some craniofacial syndromes, the tongue may be abnormally large (macroglossia) or abnormally small (microglossia) or have abnormal func-

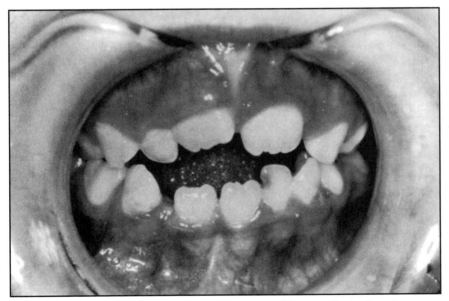

**FIGURE 10.4.** An open bite malocclusion. *Note.* From "Communicative Impairment Associated with Clefting," by M. A. Witzel, 1994, in *Cleft Palate Speech Management: A Multidisciplinary Approach* (p. 154), edited by R. J. Shprintzen and J. Bardach, St. Louis, MO: Mosby. Copyright 1994 by Mosby. Reprinted with permission.

tion due to cranial nerve anomalies. In some cases these abnormalities are true growth anomalies, whereas in others they are relative anomalies due to the size of the oral cavity. For example, in Down syndrome the tongue often appears excessively large and protrusive. Some of these children have a relative macroglossia due to the small size of the oral cavity (see Figure 10.5). These abnormalities of the tongue often affect articulation of the lingual dental, lingual alveolar, lingual palatal, and lingual velar sounds.

## Hard Palate

Sometimes the hard palate has a fistula (hole or opening) due to an unrepaired cleft palate, incomplete surgical closure of the palate, maxillary collapse, or other abnormality. In such cases, the placement of the tongue for palatal sounds, as well as airflow through the oral cavity, is affected (see Figure 10.6).

## Soft Palate and Velopharynx

An inability to close the soft palate and surrounding musculature that allows airflow into the nasal cavity during oral speech sounds results in hypernasal resonance of speech. This condition is known as velopharyngeal inadequacy, or VPI (see Figure 10.7). In addition to hypernasal resonance, the articulation of the oral sounds may be abnormal and sound weak, or there may be unusual substitutions or omission of sounds. This may occur in a child with a repaired cleft palate, submucous cleft palate (bifid uvula and muscle deficiency in the soft palate; see Figure 10.8), or, in rare cases, after adenoidectomy when there is an anatomical disproportion in the size of the structures. VPI also may be due to primary disorders of the central nervous system, which may alter the timing of velopharyngeal closure during speech.

## Tonsils and Adenoids

Abnormally large tonsils often result in excessive tongue protrusion during speech, distorting the anterior tongue sounds. Abnormally large adenoids can impede the flow of air through the nose during speech, resulting in hyponasal resonance.

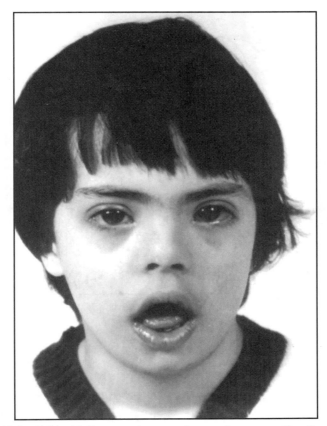

**FIGURE 10.5.** Child with Down syndrome and protrusive tongue. *Note.* From "Speech Problems in Patients with Dentofacial or Craniofacial Deformities," by M. A. Witzel and L. Vallino, 1992, in *Modern Practice of Orthognathic and Reconstructive Surgery* (Vol. 2, p. 1700), edited by W. H. Bell, Philadelphia: W. B. Saunders. Copyright 1992 by W. B. Saunders. Reprinted with permission.

## Larynx

Abnormalities in the anatomy and function of the larynx result in problems with the pitch, loudness, and quality of phonation of voice. A common voice problem in school-age children is hoarseness due to use of the vocal folds with excessive energy. This results in edema or swelling of the folds or, in more severe cases, vocal nodules or calluses on the vocal folds.

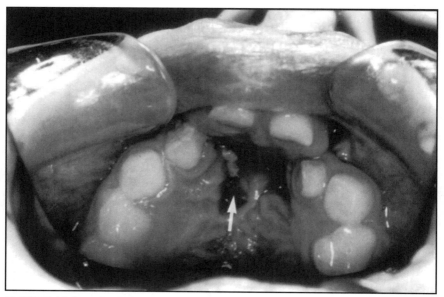

**FIGURE 10.6.** A fistula (see arrow) remaining in the hard palate of a child with repaired bilateral cleft lip and palate.

# MEDICAL CONDITIONS AT RISK FOR COMMUNICATION DISORDERS

Medical conditions are either congenital (present at birth) or acquired after birth. The causes, or etiology, of medical conditions are various. Congenital conditions usually are classified as chromosomal, single-gene, polygenic–multifactorial teratogenic, mechanically induced, or of unknown causation (Jones, 1988; Jung, 1989).

- **Chromosomal**

    Human somatic cells normally contain 46 chromosomes (23 pairs). Chromosomal conditions occur due to abnormalities in the number or structure of one or more of these chromosomes. They are not usually inherited (see Chapter 7).

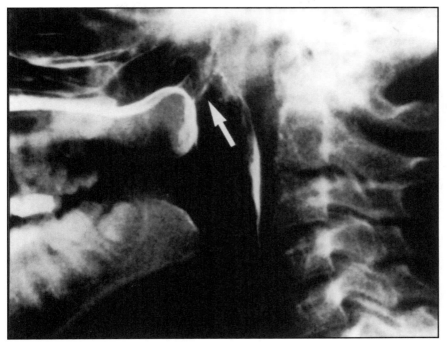

**FIGURE 10.7.** Child with velopharyngeal insufficiency. The soft palate fails to contact the pharynx during speech (see arrow). *Note.* From "Speech Problems in Patients with Dentofacial or Craniofacial Deformities," by M. A. Witzel and L. Vallino, 1992, in *Modern Practice of Orthognathic and Reconstructive Surgery* (Vol. 2, p. 1704), edited by W. H. Bell, Philadelphia: W. B. Saunders. Copyright 1992 by W. B. Saunders. Reprinted with permission.

## • Single-Gene

A single-gene disease or condition is transmitted from one or both parents according to Mendelian laws of inheritance. These conditions are classified as autosomal dominant (individual has a single dose of an abnormal gene received from one parent, where one chromosome of a pair is affected) or autosomal recessive (individual has received the abnormal gene from each parent—thus a double dose).

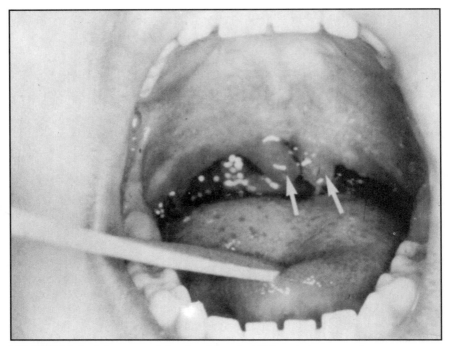

**FIGURE 10.8.** Submucous cleft palate. Note the bifid uvula (see arrows).

- **Polygenic–Multifactorial**

  A polygenic–multifactorial disease or condition is one whose likely cause is a combination of the environment and the effects of more than one gene.

- **Teratogenic**

  Various teratogenic factors, such as exposure to drugs, infection, or environmental agents such as radiation during pregnancy, may cause abnormal development of an embryo or fetus.

- **Mechanically Induced**

  An external factor such as an amniotic band impinges on the developing embryo or fetus, causing an abnormal shape or disruption to the developing body parts.

- **Unknown Causation**

 Some conditions have no apparent cause. These cannot be categorized in any of the previous types of congenital conditions.

# CONGENITAL MEDICAL CONDITIONS

All medical conditions have an associated *phenotypic spectrum,* or a series of abnormal observable features. Some individuals with a particular medical condition have all of the features of the condition, whereas others have only a portion of the features. Some features occur more frequently than others, and the severity of phenotypic features is often variable from patient to patient. This is known as *variable expression.* The *natural history* of the condition refers to the progress of the condition as the individual develops and ages. *Prognosis* indicates the expected outcome or effect of the condition on the individual and the expected response to treatment.

 The following is a partial list of congenital medical conditions due to abnormal chromosomes, single or multiple genes, or teratogenic causes. This list includes a brief description of the general phenotypic spectrum and a more detailed description of the spectrum of communication difficulties that these children may have or are at risk to have. Also included is information on the natural history of the condition and prognosis for improvement of communication skills with intervention. Prognosis is described as *excellent* (reasonable expectation of normal or near-normal speech and language), *fair* (reasonable expectation of functional communication skills), *guarded* (little improvement to be expected due to limiting factors of condition), or *poor* (no improvement expected due to limiting factors of the condition).

## Chromosomal Disorders

### Down Syndrome

**ETIOLOGY:** Chromosome disorder

## PHENOTYPIC SPECTRUM

**GENERAL:** Typical facies (see Figure 10.5), protruding tongue, cardiac malformations, gastrointestinal malformations, developmental delay, small ears, hearing loss, cleft palate

### COMMUNICATION

**Articulation**—substitutions, omissions, distortions, delayed onset

**Voice phonation**—breathy, husky, low pitch, increased loudness

**Voice resonance**—hypernasal

**Fluency**—stuttering, rapid rate of speech

**Phonology**—delayed onset

**Semantics**—delayed

**Syntax**—delayed

**Morphology**—delayed

**Pragmatics**—delayed, difficulty communicating abstract concepts

**NATURAL HISTORY:** Delayed motor, speech, and language development; cognitive deficits; frequent upper respiratory infections; increased risk for early Alzheimer's disease and psychological disorders. Protrusive tongue may influence eating and speech.

**PROGNOSIS FOR COMMUNICATION SKILLS:** Prognosis is excellent to guarded for communication skills. Infant stimulation programs are beneficial in helping the child reach his or her developmental potential. Speech and language therapy in the preschool and school-age years is beneficial in improving speech intelligibility, articulation, voice, fluency, and all aspects of language. Tongue reduction surgery may improve appearance and eating, but it has not been found to improve overall speech intelligibility (Klaiman, Witzel, Margar-Bacal, & Munro, 1988; Margar-Bacal, Witzel, & Munro, 1987).

## Fragile X

**ETIOLOGY:** Chromosome disorder, X-linked

## PHENOTYPIC SPECTRUM

**GENERAL:** Typical facies (see Figure 10.9), including prominent lower jaw and large ears; mental retardation; testicular enlargement;

speech and language disorders; emotional instability; autistic-like behaviors such as severe hand-biting. Occurs primarily in males (Jung, 1989).

### COMMUNICATION

**Articulation**—substitutions, omissions, distortions, delayed onset

**Voice phonation**—difficulty monitoring loudness

**Voice resonance**—normal

**Fluency**—perseverations, cluttering

**Phonology**—delayed onset

**Semantics**—delayed

**Syntax**—delayed

**Morphology**—delayed

**Pragmatics**—delayed; difficulty communicating abstract concepts; use of jargon, echolalia, self-talk

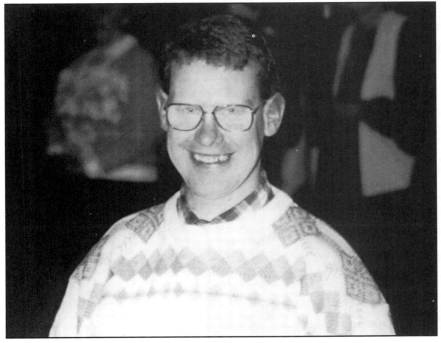

**FIGURE 10.9.** Adolescent with fragile X syndrome. (Photo courtesy of Dr. D. Chitayat.)

**NATURAL HISTORY:** Life span is normal. Cognitive abilities affect development of speech, language, behavior, and social interaction. Some individuals will have normal intelligence; however, most have significant mental retardation. The symptoms of the condition are usually less severe in carrier females than in affected males. Speech problems are variable; most have a generalized language disability (Howard-Peebles, Stoddard, & Mims, 1979; Jung, 1989).

**PROGNOSIS FOR COMMUNICATION SKILLS:** Prognosis for speech and language abilities is primarily dependent on cognitive abilities and ranges from excellent to poor. Speech and language therapy is recommended to improve intelligibility of speech and functional use of language.

## Single-Gene Disorders

## Crouzon Syndrome

**ETIOLOGY:** Autosomal dominant, variable expression

**PHENOTYPIC SPECTRUM**

**GENERAL:** Craniosynostosis, shallow orbits with exophthalmos (prominent eyes), hypertelorism, hearing loss, maxillary hypoplasia (underdevelopment) with significant malocclusion (see Figure 10.10), and attention problems. Some children require tracheostomy in the preschool years due to respiratory difficulties. Cleft palate or submucous cleft palate may occur, but this is not a frequent finding.

**COMMUNICATION**

**Articulation**—substitutions, omissions, distortions, delayed onset

**Voice phonation**—normal

**Voice resonance**—hyponasal, hypernasal

**Fluency**—normal

**Phonology**—normal to delayed onset

**Semantics**—normal to delayed

**Syntax**—normal to delayed

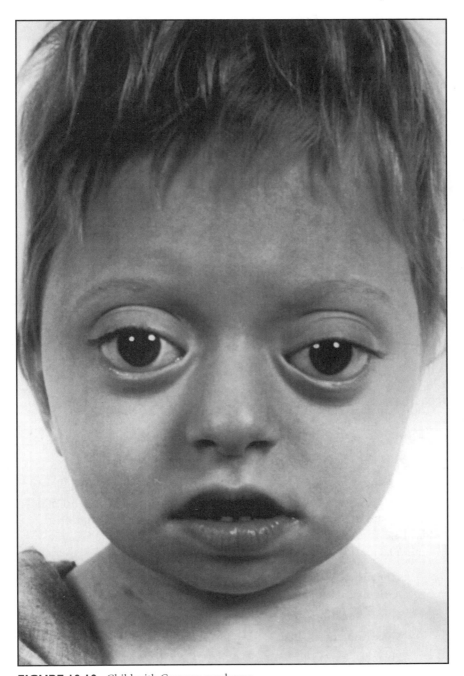

**FIGURE 10.10.** Child with Crouzon syndrome.

Morphology—normal to delayed

Pragmatics—normal to delayed

**NATURAL HISTORY:** Although some children with Crouzon syndrome have delayed cognitive skills, many have normal development and cognitive function, particularly if craniosynostosis and hearing are surgically treated in infancy or in the preschool years. Poor development of the maxilla results in a significant malocclusion and forward positioning of the tongue, contributing to articulation difficulties. The nasal airway is reduced due to the abnormal anatomy of the nasal and pharyngeal cavity. This results in a hyponasal resonance quality. Hypernasal resonance will occur in those with velopharyngeal incompetency. Language abilities are variable and should be monitored. Speech and language therapy in the preschool and school-age years is recommended to optimize the child's potential (Witzel, 1983; Witzel & Vallino, 1992).

**PROGNOSIS FOR COMMUNICATION SKILLS:** The severity of expression of the syndrome will affect speech, language, and cognitive function. The prognosis for communication ranges from excellent to fair. Surgical and orthodontic treatment will improve the oral cavity for articulation.

## Treacher Collins Syndrome

**ETIOLOGY:** Autosomal dominant, variable expression

**PHENOTYPIC SPECTRUM**

**GENERAL:** Malar hypoplasia with down-slanting palpebral fissures; defect of the lower eyelid; mandibular hypoplasia and malocclusion; malformations of the external ear, auditory canal, and middle and inner ear structures; hearing loss; cleft palate (see Figure 10.11).

**COMMUNICATION**

Articulation—substitutions, omissions, distortions, delayed onset

Voice phonation—normal

Voice resonance—hypernasal, muffled

Fluency—normal

Phonology—normal to delayed onset

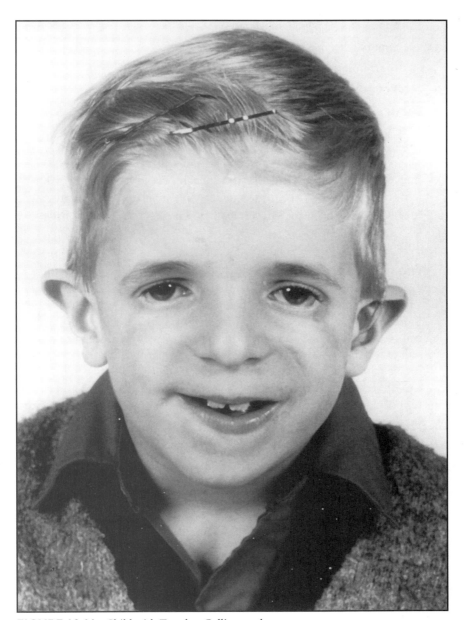

**FIGURE 10.11.** Child with Treacher Collins syndrome.

**Semantics**—normal to delayed

**Syntax**—normal to delayed

**Morphology**—normal to delayed

**Pragmatics**—normal to delayed

**NATURAL HISTORY:** Life span is normal. Tracheostomy may be required in very severe cases in the preschool years due to small airway. Intelligence and cognitive function are usually normal, especially when hearing problems are managed early. Developmental delays may occur due to hearing loss and speech problems. Hearing problems are managed with surgery or hearing aids; speech and language problems are managed with therapy or surgery. Surgical closure of cleft palate, craniofacial surgery, and orthodontics improve appearance and oral function (Witzel & Vallino, 1992).

**PROGNOSIS FOR COMMUNICATION SKILLS:** Prognosis ranges from excellent to fair and is related to the severity of the condition and the timing of management of the facial, occlusal, and hearing problems. Early amplification is stressed. Surgery and orthodontic treatment improve appearance and function, articulation, and resonance. Cleft palate repair may also improve resonance, although muffled resonance may persist. When speech and language problems occur, they can be successfully managed with therapy in the preschool and early school-age years. Surgery and orthodontic treatment to improve the occlusion and facial form will also benefit speech production.

### Velocardiofacial Syndrome

**ETIOLOGY:** Autosomal dominant, variable expression

**PHENOTYPIC SPECTRUM**

**GENERAL:** Most cases have a deletion on chromosome 22q11.2, learning disabilities, cleft palate and velopharyngeal insufficiency, cardiac malformations, behavior and attention-deficit difficulties, and fluctuating hearing loss due to middle ear disease. More than 30 other phenotypic features have been described (Goldberg, Motzkin, Marion, Scambler, & Shprintzen, 1993). The syndrome is also known as Shprintzen (1997) syndrome or 22q11 deletion syndrome (see Figure 10.12).

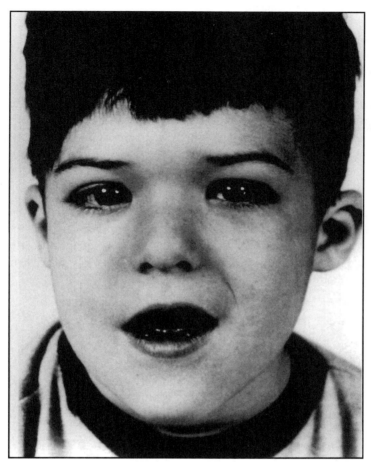

**FIGURE 10.12.** Six-year-old boy with Velocardiofacial syndrome. *Note.* From "Communicative Impairment Associated with Clefting," by M. A. Witzel, 1994, in *Cleft Palate Speech Management: A Multidisciplinary Approach* (p. 151), edited by R. J. Shprintzen and J. Bardach, St. Louis, MO: Mosby. Copyright 1994 by Mosby. Reprinted with permission.

## COMMUNICATION

**Articulation**—substitutions, omissions, distortions, delayed onset

**Voice phonation**—high pitch in preschool and early school years

**Voice resonance**—hypernasal

**Fluency**—normal

**Phonology**—delayed onset

Semantics—delayed

Syntax—delayed

Morphology—delayed

Pragmatics—delayed, difficulty communicating abstract concepts

**NATURAL HISTORY:** Life span is usually normal unless the cardiac condition or mental illness is severe. Attention and behavioral difficulties may present management problems for parents and educational professionals, particularly for children in the preschool and school-age years. Some young adults develop schizophrenia or other forms of mental illness.

**PROGNOSIS FOR COMMUNICATION SKILLS:** Prognosis is excellent to fair for speech and language. Speech problems respond well to therapy and surgical or prosthetic management. Language and attention difficulties are improved with therapy, particularly when a structured approach to therapy is emphasized.

## Polygenic–Multifactorial Syndromes

### Cleft Lip and Palate, Cleft Palate, Submucous Cleft Palate

**ETIOLOGY:** Multifactorial, variable expression

**PHENOTYPIC SPECTRUM**

**GENERAL:** May occur as an isolated defect or as a phenotypic feature of a syndrome; cleft lip may be unilateral or bilateral; cleft palate and submucous cleft palate may occur with cleft lip or as an isolated defect; feeding problems at birth; fluctuating hearing loss due to middle ear disease; maxillary hypoplasia, malocclusion, velopharyngeal insufficiency, and reading and learning disabilities in some cases (see Figures 10.8 and 10.13).

**COMMUNICATION**

Articulation—at risk for substitutions, omissions, distortions, delayed onset

Voice phonation—possible hoarseness

Voice resonance—hypernasal

Fluency—normal

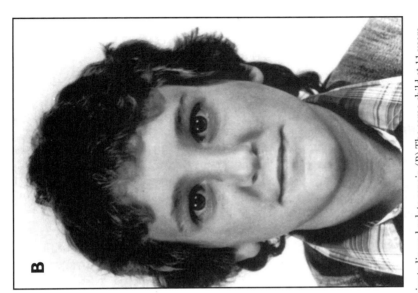

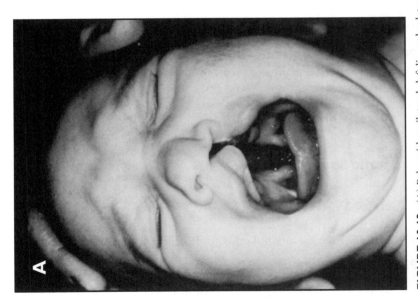

**FIGURE 10.13.** (A) Baby with unilateral cleft lip and palate prior to lip and palate repair. (B) The same child at 11 years of age. (Photos courtesy of Dr. W. K. Lindsay.)

Phonology—delayed onset

Semantics—normal, at risk

Syntax—normal, at risk

Morphology—normal, at risk

Pragmatics—normal, at risk

**NATURAL HISTORY:** Life span is normal, and intellect follows the distribution of the population in general. Surgical repair of the lip and palate in the first year of life improves feeding problems and assists speech and language development. Early management of middle ear disease is necessary for speech and language competence. Secondary surgical treatment of velopharyngeal function in the school-age years is required in 10% to 25% of cases. Definitive treatment of facial growth problems and malocclusion usually does not occur until teenage years. Secondary surgical treatment for the appearance of the lip and nose is usually undertaken in the school-age years. Early therapy intervention for speech and language problems is recommended; this also may be required in the primary grades (McWilliams & Witzel, 1994).

**PROGNOSIS FOR COMMUNICATION SKILLS:** Prognosis is excellent. Speech problems usually are resolved with surgical, orthodontic, and therapy interventions. Some cases require prosthodontic interventions. Language problems respond to therapy.

## Teratogenic Syndromes

### Fetal Alcohol Syndrome

**ETIOLOGY:** Maternal alcohol consumption during pregnancy

**PHENOTYPIC SPECTRUM**

**GENERAL:** Growth deficiency, typical facies, microcephaly, cardiac defects, cleft palate, cognitive deficiency, learning and attention disabilities related to the severity of the cognitive deficit (see Figure 10.14). In those cases with cleft palate or velopharyngeal insufficiency, surgical treatment may improve resonance and articulation (see Chapter 2).

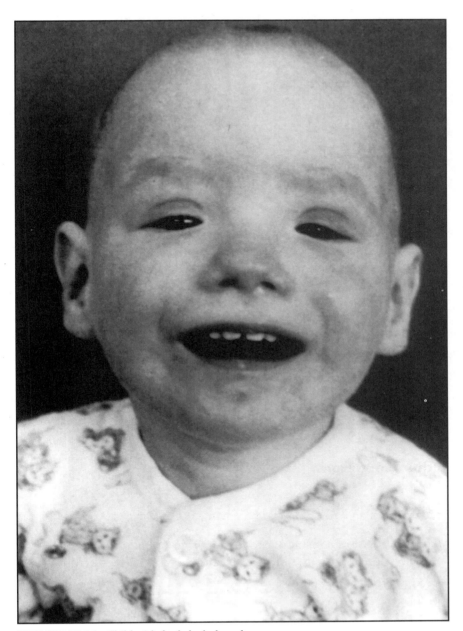

**FIGURE 10.14.** Child with fetal alcohol syndrome.

**COMMUNICATION**

**Articulation**—substitutions, omissions, distortions, delayed onset

**Voice phonation**—abnormal, may have hoarseness

**Voice resonance**—hypernasal

**Fluency**—stuttering

**Phonology**—delayed onset

**Semantics**—delayed

**Syntax**—delayed

**Morphology**—delayed

**Pragmatics**—abnormal

**NATURAL HISTORY:** Growth is deficient. Hyperactivity, behavior difficulties, and learning problems are common and related to cognitive function. Most children have speech and language problems, and individualized intervention in the preschool and school-age years is beneficial. For individuals who have velopharyngeal incompetency, surgical treatment is recommended to improve resonance and articulation.

**PROGNOSIS FOR COMMUNICATION SKILLS:** Prognosis is excellent to fair. Speech, language, and learning abilities and outcomes of therapy are influenced by the severity of the cognitive deficit and the psychosocial environment (Jung, 1989).

## Other Conditions

### Cerebral Palsy

**ETIOLOGY:** Brain insult due to hemorrhage and oxygen deprivation before, during, or after birth. The cause in most cases is unknown.

**PHENOTYPIC SPECTRUM**

**GENERAL:** Neuromotor dysfunction, including flaccidity, hypertonia, hypotonia, hyperkinesia, hypokinesia, ataxia, respiratory system dysfunction, cognitive delay or deficiency; feeding and speech problems attributed to neuromotor abnormalities and cognitive deficiencies; language problems attributed to difficulties in speech production and cognitive deficits. There also is a high incidence of associated seizures (see Chapter 14).

### COMMUNICATION

**Articulation**—dysarthria (slurred speech), substitutions, omissions, distortions, delayed onset

**Voice phonation**—breathy; strained; inconsistent pitch, loudness, and syllable duration

**Voice resonance**—hypernasal

**Fluency**—normal

**Phonology**—delayed onset

**Semantics**—delayed

**Syntax**—delayed

**Morphology**—delayed

**Pragmatics**—delayed

**NATURAL HISTORY:** Hypotonia present in some newborns often develops into spasticity or dyskinesia. Speech and language development are often delayed due to a combination of cognitive deficits, the neuromotor disorder, and difficulty in coordinating the respiratory and speech musculature. Early intervention to develop functional communication strategies is beneficial.

**PROGNOSIS FOR COMMUNICATION SKILLS:** Prognosis is excellent to guarded. The severity of the communication problem is related to the severity of the neuromuscular and cognitive problems. Some children have little difficulty in verbal communication, whereas others achieve functional oral communication with therapy. Some are unable to achieve intelligible oral speech; they communicate with the assistance of alternative or augmentative devices, such as picture symbols, electronic scanning systems, and digitized or synthesized speech. The very severe cases have limited communication abilities (Hardy, 1994).

## Autism

**ETIOLOGY:** Unknown; neuroanatomical abnormalities suspected

## PHENOTYPIC SPECTRUM

**GENERAL:** Significant social deficits, inability to relate to other persons, failure to develop appropriate verbal and nonverbal communication skills, under- or overreaction to sensory stimuli, deficient play skills, repetitive or ritualistic behaviors, poor eye contact. Expression of the impairments is variable (see Chapter 18).

### COMMUNICATION

**Articulation**—substitutions, omissions, distortions, delayed onset

**Voice phonation**—monotone, grunting sounds, may be mute

**Voice resonance**—normal

**Fluency**—stuttering, unusual rhythm

**Phonology**—delayed onset

**Semantics**—delayed, severe echolalia

**Syntax**—delayed, pronoun confusions

**Morphology**—delayed

**Pragmatics**—abnormal, unable to initiate or maintain conversation

**NATURAL HISTORY:** Deviant social development, delayed or unusual language, ritualistic and repetitive behaviors. Some or all of these behaviors can be detected before the age of 3 years. Early intervention is beneficial in improving communication and reducing destructive behaviors.

**PROGNOSIS FOR COMMUNICATION SKILLS:** Prognosis ranges from excellent to poor, depending on the severity of the condition.

## Acquired Brain Injury

**ETIOLOGY:** Cerebral vascular accident, hematoma, encephalitis, trauma, infection

### PHENOTYPIC SPECTRUM

**GENERAL:** Motor abnormalities; cognitive difficulties; difficulty with attention, perception, and memory; impulsivity; difficulty with abstraction, problem solving, judgment, decision making; and inappropriate social behavior.

**COMMUNICATION**

**Articulation**—dysarthria, substitutions, omissions, distortions

**Voice phonation**—abnormal pitch with fluctuations

**Voice resonance**—hypernasal

**Fluency**—normal

**Phonology**—may be affected

**Semantics**—may be affected

**Syntax**—may be affected

**Morphology**—may be affected

**Pragmatics**—may be affected

**NATURAL HISTORY:** Acquired brain injury may involve brain lesions, hemorrhage within the brain, or swelling of the brain. Damage may be localized or pervasive, and there may be loss of consciousness or coma. Recovery is variable and may continue over a period of months or years. Motor, sensory, and cognitive functions may be impaired. Improvement in function from the time of the initial trauma often occurs both spontaneously and with interventions.

**PROGNOSIS FOR COMMUNICATION SKILLS:** Prognosis ranges from excellent to poor, depending on location and extent of head injury, rehabilitation program, family support, previous abilities, and individual motivation. Speech and language therapy is an important part of the rehabilitation program.

# ASSESSMENT AND MANAGEMENT OF MEDICALLY BASED COMMUNICATION DISORDERS

## Interdisciplinary Care

When a congenital or acquired medical condition affects one or more body systems and several health care and education professionals are involved in the habilitation or rehabilitation of the child, interdisciplinary team assessment and treatment is beneficial in planning and delivering the most effective and efficient care. Interdisciplinary team care implies coordinated interaction among the professionals and with the child and family to improve the function and development of the child. This type of coordinated care is common for assessment and management of many medical conditions. Interdisciplinary teams are usually hospital based but also may be based in children's treatment or rehabilitation centers. More recently, interdisciplinary teams have been used in educational settings as an alternative model for service delivery. Teams involving classroom teachers, special education teachers, speech–language pathologists, psychologists, and parents facilitate the identification of children's language and speech problems and as a team are more likely to create a program that is relevant to the child in the classroom setting.

One of the most common interdisciplinary teams for medical conditions is the cleft lip and palate team. Hospital-based interdisciplinary team care for individuals with cleft lip or palate was developed in the 1940s, and this type of care is now the standard throughout the developed world for both cleft lip and palate and other craniofacial anomalies (Witzel, 1993). These teams provide assessment, diagnosis, intervention, referral, and follow-up. Children with cleft lip and palate usually are evaluated yearly or every other year by an interdisciplinary team until their late teens or early 20s. Surgical, orthodontic, and speech interventions occur at various stages and often are determined by the child's growth and development. Surgical and some medical interventions are conducted by the appropriate members of the hospital-based team; however, orthodontic and speech–language pathology interventions usually are conducted in the child's community. Therapy intervention for school-age children with cleft lip and palate who exhibit speech and language difficulties is often best undertaken in the school setting, as this reduces the time away from school, improves the frequency of attendance, and reduces the child's feeling of being different. For these cases, an open line of communication must be maintained between the team speech–language pathologist and his or her counterpart in the education system to assure agreement and understanding about the goals of management and the intervention techniques. Although professionals in education are not usually primary members of these teams, they are important secondary members, and timely and pertinent communication between the health care and education professionals is important for effective and efficient management of the child's communication problems.

## Assessment

The assessment of speech and language problems related to a medical condition is conducted primarily by the speech–language pathologist on the interdisciplinary team. However, input from parents and professionals in audiology, medicine, dentistry, psychology, and education is often necessary to determine the complete nature of the problem, the most effective intervention, the timing of the intervention, and the prognosis. Any assessment of a speech or language disorder must involve a detailed case history, screening of hearing abilities, and an examination of the child's mouth to determine the presence of structural anomalies that might explain the speech patterns.

Assessment of the components of speech involves perceptual ratings of articulation, phonation, resonance, and fluency using rating scales and analysis of speech samples; signal processing techniques to analyze the acoustic signals of speech using electronic instrumentation; and vocal tract imaging using X-ray or fiber optics to examine the anatomy and function of the vocal tract during speech. Although perceptual testing of speech can readily be accomplished in the school setting, the use of signal processing techniques and vocal tract imaging is usually done in a hospital or medical setting, as the technique and interpretation often involve an interdisciplinary approach.

Assessment of the components of language involves analyses of the child's phonology, semantics, syntax, morphology, and pragmatics in comparison to the expected performance for his or her age. This is accomplished through the administration of standardized norm-referenced tests and analyses of spontaneous conversational language samples. Most school boards provide complete assessment of language abilities. To complete the assessment, determine the diagnosis, and recommend appropriate intervention, the school, with the parent's approval, may refer the child for one or more of the following: neuropsychological testing, neurology examination, brain imaging, and genetic testing.

# MANAGEMENT OF SPEECH AND LANGUAGE PROBLEMS

The goals of management of speech and language problems include early identification and elimination of the communication problem (secondary prevention) or reduction of the severity of the disorder to enhance or establish functional communication abilities (tertiary prevention; Witzel, 1990). The goals are selected for each child based on the medical condition, its severity of expression, and the limiting factors such as neuromotor status and cognitive deficits. Management of articulation, specific voice problems, and stuttering includes direct individual or group therapy, often with an ongoing home program. Reconstructive craniofacial or orthognathic surgery is used to correct or improve anatomical or functional problems in the vocal tract, such as abnormalities of the larynx, cleft palate, velopharyngeal insufficiency, and severe jaw growth problems with malocclusion. Orthodontic treatment with or without surgery improves speech problems caused by malocclusion. A prosthetic speech obturator may be used to improve hypernasality due to velopharyngeal insufficiency in selected cases where surgical intervention is not possible.

Language problems in school-age children often are related to learning abilities. Management of language problems recently has involved a more holistic approach that emphasizes the interaction of language, cognition, and social context (Wiig & Secord, 1994). This type of approach involves the following:

- collaborative consultation in which the speech–language pathologist, special educator, classroom teacher, and school psychologist plan and implement intervention as teams;

- contextual–pragmatic intervention in which language and communication training are provided in the contexts in which they are to be used;

- curriculum-related intervention in which language and communication training is related directly to the content and demands of the curriculum (e.g., stories, texts, poems, social studies, verbal math);

- strategy-based intervention in which training involves active problem solving and decision making and focuses on teaching and learning effective approaches and strategies for using effective language in different contexts and for different purposes;

- whole language approaches in which reading, writing, listening and speaking are integrated in whole situations, and the focus is on meaning and not on language itself in authentic speech and literacy events. (Wiig & Secord, 1994, p. 240)

# THE TEACHER'S ROLE

Teachers have an important role in the management of children with communication problems, particularly in schools where interdisciplinary teamwork is used for service delivery. Children who have speech and language disorders often benefit from coordinated programming by speech–language pathologists, teachers, and psychologists. In some cases, the teacher may discover previously undetected communication problems and assist the child and parents in referral to a speech–language pathologist or appropriate hospital-based interdisciplinary team. In other cases, the educator may assist the speech–language pathologist in the carryover aspects of therapy that can be conducted in the classroom. The teacher is often the ideal person to assist the family and speech–language pathologist in monitoring the outcome of therapy interventions and determining the need for continued therapy by observing the child's communication abilities in the educational setting and against the social demands of his or her peers.

For children with significant communication problems or observable medical conditions, such as cleft lip and palate, craniofacial anomalies, or cerebral palsy, the teacher can help to ease the social impact and isolation for the child and reduce teasing by educating other children in the classroom and school about the condition. For example, the AboutFace program (see contact information in Appendix 10.A) is a package that can be used by teachers to explain facial differences to children. Ability OnLine (see Appendix 10.A) is a support network that provides a public forum where children, teens, and young adults with and without disabilities can share ideas, opinions, and knowledge electronically using a computer bulletin board system. Everybody looks and sounds the same on-line, and this computer network helps children with disabilities, including motor disorders, facial deformities, and communication problems, to feel less isolated from other children by promoting communication.

# SUMMARY

A child's speech and language problems may be associated with an underlying medical condition, which will affect the diagnosis, treatment, and predicted outcome of the communication disorder. Teachers may play a significant role in the identification and referral of children who would benefit from detailed assessment of their communication skills, coordinated interdisciplinary programming, and development of strategies within the classroom to enhance and improve communication and behavior. Intervention outcome in both communication disorders and education is improved by an understanding of the underlying pathology, its limitations, and its prognosis. The interaction among the family, teacher, other professionals in education, and health-care professionals is often critical to the improvement of the child's communication difficulties and his or her emotional health.

# APPENDIX 10.A

# Professional Associations and Consumer Groups

The following is a partial list of professional associations and consumer groups that provide information about speech, language, and hearing problems and some of the medical conditions described in this chapter. For a more complete listing, contact the American Speech-Language-Hearing Association and the Council for Exceptional Children (see addresses below).

Ability OnLine
1120 Finch Avenue West
Toronto, ON M3J 3H7
Canada
Phone 416/650-6207
Fax 416/650-5073
http://www.abilityonline.org

AboutFace International
*(For individuals with a facial difference and their families.)*
International Office
123 Edward Street, Suite 1003
Toronto, ON M5G 1E2
Canada
Phone 800/665-FACE
Fax 416/944-2488
http://www.aboutfaceinternational.org

AboutFace USA
P.O. Box 458
Crystal Lake, IL 60014
Phone 888/486-1209
Fax 630/665-8945
http://www.aboutfaceusa.org

American Cleft Palate–Craniofacial
   Association and Cleft Palate
   Foundation
104 South Estes Drive, Suite 204
Chapel Hill, NC 27514
Phone 800/24C-LEFT
Fax 919/933-9604
http://www.cleft.org

American Speech-Language-Hearing
   Association
10801 Rockville Pike
Rockville, MD 20852
Phone 800/638-8255
Fax 301/571-0457
http://www.asha.org

Canadian Association of Speech-
   Language Pathologists and
   Audiologists
401-200 Elgin Street
Ottawa, ON K2P 1L5
Canada
Phone 800/259-8519
Fax 613/567-2859
http://www.caslpa.ca

Canadian Hearing Society
271 Spadina Road
Toronto, ON M5R 2V3
Canada
Phone 416/964-9595
Fax 416/964-2066
http://www.chs.ca

Council for Exceptional Children
1110 North Glebe Road, Suite 300
Arlington, VA 22201-5704
Phone 703/620-3660
Fax 703/264-9494
http://www.cec.sped.org

Velo-Cardio-Facial Syndrome
  Educational Foundation
Jacobsen Hall, Room 708
Upstate Medical University, University
  Hospital
750 East Adams Street
Syracuse, NY 13210
Phone 315/464-6590
Fax 315/464-6593
http://www.vcfsef.org

# SUGGESTED READING

Gorlin, R. J., Cohen, M. M., & Levin, R. S. (1990). *Syndromes of the head and neck* (3rd ed.). New York: Oxford University Press.

Paasche, C. L., Gorrill, L., & Strom, B. (1990). *Children with special needs in early childhood settings: Identification, intervention, mainstreaming.* Menlo Park, CA: Addison-Wesley.

Shames, G., Wiig, E., & Secord, W. (1994). *Human communication disorders: An introduction.* New York: Merrill.

# VIDEOTAPE

Pollock, H., Ferketic, M., Shprintzen, R. J., & Witzel, M. A. (1993). *Delineation and diagnosis of craniofacial syndromes: Effect on case management.* Rockville Pike, MD: American Speech-Language-Hearing Association.

# REFERENCES

Bloom, L., & Lahey, M. (1978). *Language development and language disorders.* New York: Wiley.

Borden, G. J., Harris, K. S., & Raphael, L. J. (1994). *Speech science primer.* Baltimore: Williams & Wilkins.

Goldberg, R., Motzkin, B., Marion, R., Scambler, P. J., & Shprintzen, R. J. (1993). Velocardiofacial syndrome: A review of 120 patients. *American Journal of Medical Genetics, 45,* 313.

Hardy, J. C. (1994). Cerebral palsy. In G. H. Shames, E. H. Wiig, & W. A. Secord (Eds.), *Human communication disorders: An introduction.* New York: Merrill.

Howard-Peebles, P., Stoddard, G., & Mims, M. (1979). Familial linked mental retardation, verbal disability and marker X chromosomes. *American Journal of Human Genetics, 31,* 214.

Jones, K. L. (1988). *Smith's recognizable patterns of human malformation.* Philadelphia: Saunders.

Jung, J. H. (1989). *Genetic syndromes in communication disorders.* Boston: College-Hill.

Klaiman, P. G., Witzel, M A., Margar-Bacal, F. M., & Munro, I. R. (1988). Changes in aesthetic appearance and intelligibility of speech after partial glossectomy in patients with Down syndrome. *Plastic and Reconstructive Surgery, 82,* 403.

Landman, G. B. (1989). Language development from six to twelve. *Pediatric Annals, 18,* 373–379.

Margar-Bacal, F. M., Witzel, M. A., & Munro, I. R. (1987). Speech intelligibility after partial glossectomy in children with Down syndrome. *Plastic and Reconstructive Surgery, 79,* 44.

McWilliams, B. J., & Witzel, M. A. (1994). Cleft palate. In G. H. Shames, E. H. Wiig, & W. A. Secord (Eds.), *Human communication disorders: An introduction.* New York: Merrill.

Owens, B. R., Jr. (1994). Development of communication, language and speech. In G. H. Shames, E. H. Wiig, & W. A. Secord (Eds.), *Human communication disorders: An introduction.* New York: Merrill.

Schaefer, G. B., Mathy-Lakko, P., & Bodensteiner, J. B. (1992). Neurogenetic aspects of communication disorders. *Clinics in Communication Disorders, 2,* 9.

Schwartz, R. G. (1994). Phonological disorders. In G. H. Shames, E. H. Wiig, & W. A. Secord (Eds.), *Human communication disorders: An introduction.* New York: Merrill.

Shames, G. H., & Ramig, P. R. (1994). Stuttering and other disorders of fluency. In G. H. Shames, E. H. Wiig, & W. A. Secord (Eds.), *Human communication disorders: An introduction.* New York: Merrill.

Shprintzen, R. J. (1997). *Genetics, syndromes, and communication disorders.* San Diego, CA: Singular.

Wiig, E. H., & Secord, W. A. (1994). Language disabilities in children and youth. In G. H. Shames, E. H. Wiig, & W. A. Secord (Eds.), *Human communication disorders: An introduction.* New York: Merrill.

Witzel, M. A. (1983). Speech problems in craniofacial anomalies. *Communication Disorders, 8, 45.*

Witzel, M. A. (1990). Craniofacial anomalies. *Seminars in Speech and Language, 11,* 145.

Witzel, M. A. (1993). Cleft lip and palate and craniofacial treatment. *Magazine of the American Speech-Language-Hearing Association, 35,* 42.

Witzel, M. A. (1994). Communicative impairment associated with clefting. In R. J. Shprintzen & J. Bardach (Eds.), *Cleft palate speech management: A multidisciplinary approach.* St. Louis, MO: Mosby.

Witzel, M. A., & Vallino, L. (1992). Speech problems in patients with dentofacial or craniofacial deformities. In W. H. Bell (Ed.), *Modern practice in orthognathic and reconstructive surgery* (Vol. 2). Philadelphia: Saunders.

# CHAPTER 11

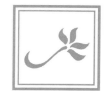

# Childhood Dental Disorders

Douglas H. Johnston
and David J. Kenny

O ver the past 25 years, there has been a dramatic increase in the science of dentistry that has led to improvements in both dental care for children and dental education. As a consequence, dental caries on average have decreased for the total pediatric and adolescent population because of dietary fluoride, and a number of advances have improved preventive and restorative dentistry. Nevertheless, dental caries are still rampant in some children, congenital anomalies of the head and neck affect the way jaws and teeth grow, children continue to have accidents, and those with certain chronic illnesses and disabilities have special dental needs. The purpose of this chapter is to describe acquired dental problems and those congenital anomalies and medical conditions that affect the oral cavity.

## DENTAL CARIES AND DENTAL CARE

### Primary Dentition

Teachers of 3- to 6-year-olds are well aware of the ravages of early decay of the primary dentition in some children. Often the damage was produced during the preschool years and the effects of multiple extractions are still apparent. Factors involved in rampant decay of the primary teeth include the effects of extended bottle feeding, demand breast-feeding during sleep

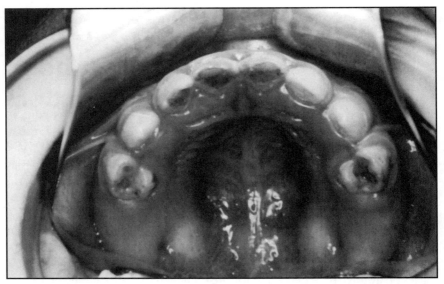

**FIGURE 11.1.** Upper teeth of an 18-month-old child with a history of extended nursing bottle use that included nap time. Nursing habit must be changed immediately and the teeth restored as quickly as possible.

time with the absence of adequate oral hygiene, oral liquid medications containing sugar, and the habit of storing liquid for extended periods in the mouth (see Figure 11.1).

The prolonged use of a bottle with a nipple or a juice cup with a spout to drink liquids, especially those that contain fermentable carbohydrates (sugars), can cause dental caries. The problem is further exacerbated if the child takes the bottle to bed. Some of the mystery of why one child in a family can go to bed with a bottle and have minimal or no caries yet another can have severe damage is explained by an investigation that demonstrates that some children sip and hold liquid in their mouths for prolonged periods while asleep (Schwartz, Rosivack, & Michelotti, 1993). Sleeping with a juice or milk bottle bathes the teeth in sugar (fructose and lactose), the raw material for increased acid production and caries. The issue is complicated by the fact that saliva and oral hygiene, as well as the makeup of the teeth, vary between individuals, even in the same family.

Members of the La Leche League International (LLLI; 1994) contend that a small percentage of breast-fed children develop dental caries in spite of breastfeeding, not because of it. The LLLI and dentists agree that breast-feeding should be encouraged but must be accompanied by a careful parental brushing regime that is started early after the eruption of the first tooth (about 6 months of age).

Another group of children who are at risk for early dental caries are those who have to take multiple doses of oral liquid sugar–based medications for a prolonged period of time. Repeated middle ear infections, epilepsy, or congenital heart disease all require prolonged use of sugar-based drugs for their management. Almost all childhood medications contain 10% to 50% sucrose, to add bulk, thickness, and flavor, and contribute to significant dental decay in these children (Kenny & Somaya, 1988). Even the smallest amount of sugar is sufficient to provide the substrate for plaque bacteria to produce acid, which in turn can dissolve the soft enamel of newly erupted teeth. Teachers regularly see children who have obvious dental decay of the primary teeth or who have had extensive restorative treatment or extractions due exclusively to early dental caries.

Dental caries and abscesses of the primary dentition can produce halitosis from food lodged in the teeth or the presence of pus in the mouth. Once the dentition has been restored, the halitosis may continue but be caused by nondental factors, such as mouth breathing, infected tonsils, nasopharyngeal secretions, or regurgitation.

Some children become involved in early phases of orthodontic treatment, called interceptive orthodontics or guidance of the occlusion. At its simplest, this consists of space maintainers, brackets and arch wires, or removable appliances. Thumb sucking usually extinguishes naturally by 4 years of age, but parents often ask dentists to help with control of the habit before that time, usually for social reasons. Although children can radically alter the shape of their primary dentition by early thumb, finger, or soother sucking, dentists do not usually intervene unless the child has collapsed the upper arch so that one or both sides fit inside rather than outside of the lower arch (cross bite) (see Figure 11.2). If thumb sucking continues after eruption of the permanent incisors, then habit control and comprehensive orthodontic treatment will most likely be required.

## Permanent Dentition

The remarkable control of caries in the young permanent dentition that has occurred in North America has been evident for only slightly more than two decades. With the exception of certain pockets of high-risk children, most school-age children have fewer than three decayed teeth. Early control of

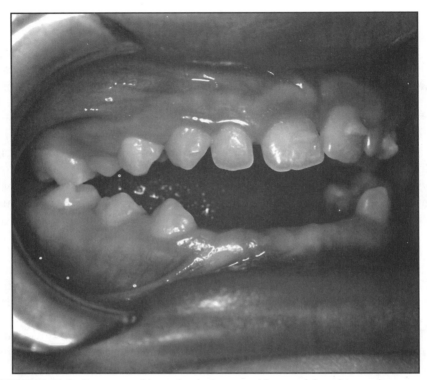

**FIGURE 11.2.**  Severe open bite malocclusion caused by mouth breathing and tongue thrust. Therapy involves correction of the tongue thrust and orthodontics. In severe long-standing cases, craniofacial surgery may be necessary.

decay in primary teeth means that the first permanent molars erupt into a caries-free mouth with a controlled bacterial flora. The vigilance of dentists leads to early detection of biting surface (occlusal) fissures that form in the first permanent molars of almost 40% of children. These fissures are opened and the tooth restored, or they are sealed with a plastic (pit and fissure sealant) material that prevents rapid early damage. As children get beyond 7 or 8 years without decay, their manual dexterity improves and education plus societal concerns for total health seem to further assist the decline of dental caries. The current generation of North American children can expect to keep almost all of their teeth for their lifetime; this fact has changed the cost–benefit ratio in favor of orthodontic treatment for children with tooth and jaw irregularities in order to establish a good occlusion for life.

By age 6 most children in a classroom will be changing their front teeth for permanent incisors, and by age 10 most will be changing their primary side teeth for permanent canines and premolars. Once the side teeth begin to be replaced, classrooms blossom with children "wired" for orthodontics. Aesthetics and improved mastication through the establishment of a proper occlusion are the primary drivers for orthodontic treatment.

## Fluoride and Fluorosis

With the understanding of the caries-inhibiting properties of fluoride and with the introduction of systemic fluoride in water systems, as well as topical fluoride application by dentists and through the medium of toothpastes, there has been a tremendous reduction in caries over the past 35 years. Interestingly enough, however, the decline in caries seems to have reached a plateau in the 1990s. It is also interesting that the greatest benefit from fluoride occurs for children 5 to 11 years of age, who are 75% caries free. In general, water fluoridation affords the greatest protection to the primary dentition of children from the lowest socioeconomic groups. Fluoride as a caries preventative agent works in three ways:

1. It inhibits bacterial metabolism.
2. It slows down demineralization during an acid attack.
3. It promotes remineralization of damaged tooth structure.

Generally, after eating food containing fermentable carbohydrates, the pH of the mouth declines from a neutral 7 to an acidic 4.5 within 5 minutes. If the mouth is permitted to rest with normal salivary flow, the pH returns to normal within 25 minutes. Saliva is important in the prevention and reversal of early caries, as it contains phosphate, calcium, and proteins. With the presence of small amounts of fluoride at 0.04 parts per million in saliva, remineralization is enhanced.

In recent years, there has been a noticeable increase in fluorosis, which is the result of the ingestion of too much fluoride over an extended period of time. Some teeth may have had too much of a good thing. Fluorosis ranges from white areas on teeth in its mild version to actual mottling with surface imperfections in more severe cases, and this can occur in primary and permanent teeth (see Figure 11.3). Most dental fluorosis is so mild, it is barely perceptible. Part of the increase in fluorosis may be due to increased reporting, rather than an increased incidence. Most

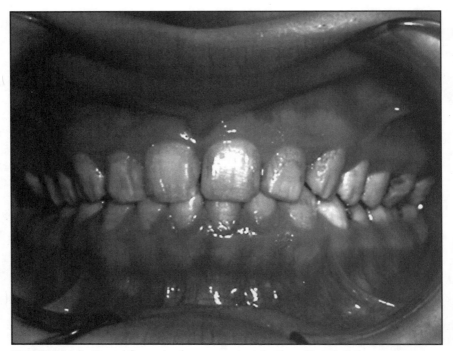

**FIGURE 11.3.** Dental fluorosis of a severe nature that has affected all the permanent teeth, causing brown staining and mottling.

communities have elected to reduce the amount of fluoride in drinking water, and community dentists recommend supplemental fluoride only if there is no water fluoridation or for those who are at high risk of caries or those who have medical problems that make dental restorative procedures risky.

# DENTAL TRAUMA

## Primary Dentition

The major cause of injuries to primary teeth is falls. Toddlers and early school-age children most commonly knock their upper incisors inward, backward, or forward. They also knock these teeth right out of the mouth (avulsion). If the tooth is not visible in the mouth and cannot be physically located or visualized by a dental radiograph, then the child should have a chest auscultation by a physician and perhaps a chest radiograph to rule out aspiration. If a tooth is aspirated into a lung, it can produce a lung abscess, which is a serious medical situation. Primary incisors that have been avulsed are not replanted, as, unlike permanent teeth, there is inadequate scientific literature to support this practice. Primary teeth with root fractures are usually extracted. Teeth that have been bumped may bleed internally within the dental pulp space. With time, the released blood products will be incorporated into the tooth itself and a brown or gray incisor will be the result. If the child is healthy and the tooth has not caused discomfort or signs of an abscess, then these teeth are not routinely treated. However, they need to be examined radiographically every 6 months to rule out abscess formation. In some cases, a root canal treatment can be performed in the primary tooth to improve its appearance and prevent an abscess. Root canal treatment for primary teeth is much simpler than for permanent teeth as the primary tooth will later be shed. Removal of the blood vessels and nerve of a primary tooth (root canal treatment) does not affect the pulp of the permanent tooth that will replace it, as it is a separate tooth.

Primary incisors that have small chips taken out of them can be polished with a fine dental abrasive wheel. Larger chips may involve the pulpal tissue, and a root canal may be necessary prior to restoration of the tooth. Generally, because of development and natural loss of root structure of the primary incisors, root canals in these teeth are not indicated after age 4½ unless the child's dentition is very delayed or there is no permanent tooth successor. Upper front permanent incisors generally begin eruption about age 6.

## Permanent Dentition

Once the permanent incisors have erupted, they too are at risk of injury due to falls, direct hits, or collisions. These mishaps may be caused by falls due to untied shoelaces, schoolyard violence, pick-up sports activities, or vehicular accidents. (For a comprehensive review, see Andreasen & Andreasen, 1994.)

Between the ages of approximately 6 and 14 years, the supporting bone of the maxilla is still easily deformed. During this time, blunt trauma to the region of the upper jaw is apt to cause one or more incisor teeth to be knocked right out of the jaw (avulsed). Very few experienced teachers have not seen the results of such accidents. Clinical investigations have shown that the most important factor for success of replantation of an avulsed permanent tooth is the immediate replacement of the tooth into the socket (if the child will cooperate). If the tooth is dirty, it should be immediately placed in cold milk (which is gentler to the cells of the tooth root than water, which can cause additional damage) and transported with the student to a dentist or hospital that is experienced in management of such injuries. It would be wise to know in advance where to take such children because time is critical. In almost every case of avulsion, the replanted tooth requires root canal treatment. The long-term success of retaining such teeth is much lower than popular perception. Much scientific research is actively under way to examine success of various storage media for avulsed teeth during transit, as well as materials that are painted on the root structure to promote successful reattachment. The success of osseointegrated (titanium) implants to replace missing teeth, should the replantation not be successful, is very high.

Fractures of the tooth crown can be repaired with new adhesive composite resin materials, and conventional root canal treatment can be performed if necessary following the restoration of the fractured area. When teeth have to be removed due to extensive trauma, children who are accident prone or active in sports may be better off with removable appliances during their high-risk years. More lasting dental reconstruction, such as implants and bridgework, can be delayed until growth is completed and the individuals no longer participate in activities that might lead to repeated trauma.

## Prevention

Organized contact sports now require the use of either mouth guards or facial protection in conjunction with a helmet. The use of both a mouth guard and a helmet affords the ultimate in protection, and has virtually eliminated oral trauma while engaged in sports. Facial protection without a mouth guard leaves the teeth vulnerable for blows to the lower jaw that result in rapid contact of the teeth, leading to fracture. Many sports such as basketball and soccer do not require oral protection, and traumatic injuries are still common. The most vulnerable sport is the pickup game of any variety where there is no protection at all. By far the most severe oral traumatic injuries treated at The Hospital for Sick Children are those resulting from nonorganized sport activities. Parents and teachers should encourage young athletes to wear oral protection while engaged in any type of sport.

Many parents ask whether the inexpensive "boilable" mouth guard is as good as a dentist's fabricated guard. In general, the answer is no, but if this is the only kind a family can afford, it is far better than nothing. Because the fit is commonly not as good, wearing compliance is diminished and the guard often ends up in the child's pocket.

# CONGENITAL ANOMALIES

A number of birth defects or congenital anomalies are described in Chapter 7. These inherited conditions are present in the school population, and their associated dental problems may be evident along with other outward signs.

## Cleft Lip and Palate

The child who was born with a cleft lip with or without cleft palate usually undergoes two separate operations before school begins. In the first operation the lip is repaired, and the second operation closes the palate. As a consequence of the cleft palate, two or more upper incisor teeth may be absent, and as a consequence of the palatal closure, the upper dental arch may be contracted, adversely affecting speech production. The end result is that children with cleft lip and palate anomalies spend a significant amount of time with the dentist for routine care, orthodontics, and eventually prosthetic treatment. The bulk of the time away from school stretches from around Grade 5 into high school. In addition, plastic surgery and oral surgery procedures may be needed to adjust jaw dimensions and correct nasal function and aesthetics once growth is complete.

## Ectodermal Dysplasia

Children with ectodermal dysplasia fail to develop many tooth buds and, as a consequence, have very few teeth. Those teeth that do form erupt late and the front teeth have a characteristic conical appearance (see Figure 11.4). The children usually have these teeth reshaped to a more normal anatomy and wear removable dentures. Dental care for children with this

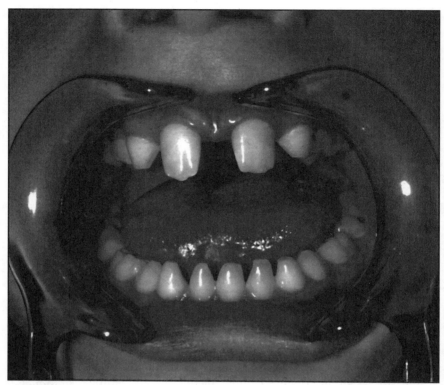

**FIGURE 11.4.** Ectodermal dysplasia with associated conically shaped teeth and congenitally missing teeth. Orthodontics, surgery, and prosthetics are required to correct the dentition.

condition stretches throughout the entire school period. The absence of molar teeth means that the jawbones are not built up with the alveolar bone that normally surrounds and holds the teeth, and the jaws are characteristically overclosed, which may give the appearance of an adult without dentures. In addition, children with this condition may have sparse hair, a pronounced ridge above the eyes, and the inability to sweat. The child may require removable replacement teeth or overdentures as school begins to avoid teasing and to improve masticatory function. Orthodontic, prosthodontic, and oral and maxillofacial care is typically required at various stages during development. Early use of implants is now under scientific investigation to improve function and aesthetics earlier in life for these individuals.

## Amelogenesis Imperfecta

Amelogenesis imperfecta and the next condition discussed, dentinogenesis imperfecta, may produce discolored primary and permanent teeth. By the time the child is of school age, this inherited condition may have been diagnosed. In the case of amelogenesis imperfecta, the enamel is improperly formed and treatment is by plastic or porcelain restorations in the front of the mouth and stainless steel crowns or later gold alloy crowns in the back. Children with this condition will spend much time with the dentist, but the long-term prognosis for maintenance of the teeth is quite good as long as there are sufficient funds for the complicated dental treatment that is required.

## Dentinogenesis Imperfecta

Dentinogenesis imperfecta usually produces darkened brown or gray primary and permanent teeth. The inner dentin is improperly formed, resulting in enamel that literally falls off the teeth. As a consequence, the restoration of the appearance and function of the teeth by plastic or porcelain restorations, stainless steel crowns, or later gold alloy crowns has a more guarded outcome. Some of these teeth unpredictably become infected and form cysts and have to be extracted. Although expensive, the use of osseointegrated implants to anchor prostheses (dentures) offers the first major advance in the care of patients with conditions like ectodermal dysplasia or defects of enamel or dentin. The use of such implants in children is still relatively new, but the history of success in adults is encouraging.

## Severe Malocclusion

Sometimes the combination of face shape and tooth size is so disparate that improvement of dental function and facial aesthetics requires a combined orthodontic and surgical approach (see Figure 11.5). In the case of severe malocclusion, it is possible to assess the bony structure of the face and prepare the patient for surgical orthodontics so that once growth has stopped (late teens for girls and late teens to early 20s for boys), one or both jaws can be moved forward or back and the chin or cheekbones surgically augmented.

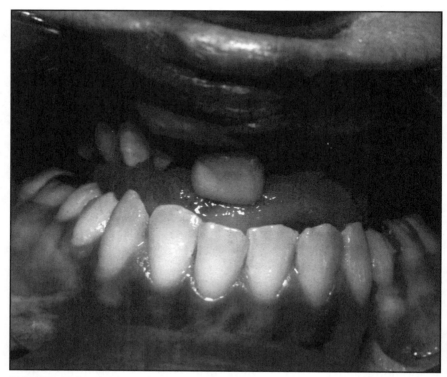

**FIGURE 11.5.** Cleft lip and palate with severe malocclusion. Upper dentition is completely contained within the lower dentition because of postsurgical contraction.

Once again, the increased popularity of such operations is based on the success in controlling dental caries and the realistic expectation that the majority of teeth will last the lifetime of the patient.

## Tongue Thrust

Tongue thrust is the subject of a variety of treatments even though it often is simply the adaptation of the tongue to deal with swallowing as a result of the loss of primary front teeth. When the permanent incisors erupt into normal occlusion, the "tongue thrust" resolves. In other situations, the forward movement of the tongue is eliminated by conventional orthodontic treatment. Unfortunately, in a few cases, there is such a strong neural drive that the tongue causes any orthodontic treatment to relapse. In these rare cases, the only way to protect the patient from relapse is by various means of ongoing retention appliances or cemented devices.

## Webs and Frena

Some children are born with their tongues bound to the bottom of their mouths by a web of tissue (lingual frena). These children cannot extend their tongues to their top lip and may use their fingers to place or manipulate their food. The inability of the tongue to manipulate the food bolus can be dangerous and lead to choking. The natural process of removing food trapped in the cheek folds by a mobile tongue cannot occur, leading to bad breath and caries. This condition, called *ankyloglossia,* is easily re-solved by a variety of surgical techniques.

A thick web of intraoral tissue in the midline from below the nose to between the upper incisors or in the lower jaw from the chin area to the lower incisors can pull on the gum tissue or hold the central incisors apart. These labial frena do not always have to be removed and are managed by a simple operation. Many of the upper frena are torn in childhood falls. Although they may bleed profusely, bleeding is readily controlled by firm finger pressure on the upper lip for 5 minutes.

# ORAL MANIFESTATIONS OF SYSTEMIC DISEASES

## Congenital Heart Disease

Children with congenital heart disease usually have had multiple hospitalizations and much liquid medication during their early years. Often parents and caregivers of children with life-threatening medical problems have indulged them with sweets and have been understandably very lenient in their child rearing. These children may already have had extensive dentistry either in the dental office, in the hospital clinic, or under general anesthesia. Children whose hearts produce blood turbulence or who have prosthetic valves need to be protected by antibiotic coverage in advance of any dental surgery that invades the oral mucosa to prevent the complication of bacterial endocarditis. Occasionally, congenital heart disease may produce a V-shaped upper dental arch. There are no contraindications to orthodontic treatment as long as antibiotic coverage is used during appointments that are apt to cause bleeding (e.g., molar banding).

## Blood Dyscrasias

Children with hemophilia, leukemia, and inherited bleeding disorders usually receive their dental treatment in hospital clinics, because their medical conditions require an interdisciplinary approach and they benefit from the proximity of services within a hospital. Their dental problems are not typically extraordinary, but treatment can be complicated by their medical diagnoses. Preventive dentistry becomes the critical focus, and medical management is required if dental surgery is needed.

## Juvenile Arthritis

In the past, children with juvenile arthritis took large quantities of aspirin, which produced an acid attack to their teeth and increased decay. More recently, the use of nonsteroidal anti-inflammatory drugs (NSAIDs) has reduced this problem. The effects of arthritis on their jaw joints (temporomandibular joints) can produce limited movement that affects chewing, and the effects of steroids used for treatment of some cases can affect the growth centers of the jaws. Dental problems now are mainly orthodontic related and more common during adolescence.

## Immunosuppression

The population of children with suppressed immune systems is rapidly rising and includes those who were intentionally immunosuppressed for organ transplants, as well as those who have childhood cancer or active acquired immunodeficiency syndrome (AIDS). The dental management of these patients is closely linked to their medical management. Their problems are usually related to intraoral infections that affect their tongues, gums, and palate and cheek mucosa. They get periodic intraoral overgrowth of bacteria or fungal microorganisms. They may be more prone to dental decay, which is usually related to diet alterations or the medications that accompany their disabilities. Some medications used to produce immunosuppression can cause increased growth of gum tissue.

# ORAL MANIFESTATIONS OF NEUROLOGICAL DISORDERS

## Cerebral Palsy

Children with cerebral palsy are more prone to dental malocclusion than those who are neurologically normal. This may be the result of sensory loss; muscle imbalance between the tongue, cheeks, and lips; mouth breathing; or even their face shape. Most of these children have normal teeth and, in North America, no more dental caries than other children. However, the protective jaw and lip reflexes and the uncontrolled movement that may be part of their condition complicate dental hygiene. Although uncomplicated restorative dental treatment can often be accomplished in the dental chair, uncontrolled movements and extensive treatment may require that procedures be accomplished under general anesthesia to assure safety, speed, and precision of dental restorations.

## Epilepsy

Young children with epilepsy often take oral liquid medication to control their seizures. They may have additional conditions that demand the use of other medications as well. These medications can negatively affect their dental condition. Once they are old enough to take their medication in pill form, their dental condition approaches that of the general population. Children who have seizures are often more comfortable having their treatment performed by pediatric dentists who can treat them in a hospital; the appeal is the clinician's familiarity with seizures and their management. In the past, many children with epilepsy used a drug, phenytoin (e.g., Dilantin), that produced overgrowth of the gums as a side effect.

Although it is still used for some children, and the growth of gum tissue is dose related, physicians may prescribe newer drugs such as carbamazepine (e.g., Tegretol) that has significantly reduced their dental problems. When gum tissue has overgrown to such an extent that it affects the ability to chew or poses a risk for food stagnation and dental caries, the gum tissue is removed surgically. If phenytoin therapy is continued, the gum tissue will begin again to hypertrophy. Meticulous oral hygiene will reduce the rate at which the gum tissue regrows.

## Autism

Children with autism (see Chapter 18) are usually upset by the invasion of an intraoral examination and are unable to cooperate for dental treatment. Physical restraint to perform treatment is discouraged due to the intense perception of intraoral dental manipulations these children experience. Because children with autism often have restricted sugar intake and are orally active and hypertonic, they tend to have a low dental caries attack rate. If dental problems are visible, radiographic examination, diagnosis, and treatment are usually performed under general anesthesia.

## Developmental Delay (Including Down Syndrome)

A large population of children with trainable and educable developmental delays have their routine dental care accomplished by conventional means. This may include treatment in a private office or an institution clinic. They are cared for by their parents or live in group homes and are as good or better with their personal hygiene than the less managed general population of children and adolescents. Their diets are generally controlled by their caregivers, and their dental problems are minimal but in some cases characteristic of their condition. For example, children with Down syndrome often have a retracted upper jaw that produces crowding when the permanent incisors erupt. Intentional timed extraction of selected primary teeth may prevent overlapping of the crowded permanent teeth. The crowding later may resolve itself as some of the permanent side teeth are characteristically smaller than usual, whereas others can be congenitally absent.

# THE TEACHER'S ROLE

Although dental caries have been on the decline for more than two decades, caries are still prevalent in the pediatric population. Teachers and school nurses are in a position to detect dental defects early and can make recommendations to parents and caregivers to seek early treatment before the child develops pain or infection, or requires hospitalization. Early referral and care are frequently much less expensive and traumatic to the child.

Early detection of fluorosis in the primary dentition by the teacher could alert the parent that the child is receiving too much dietary fluoride. Upon consultation with a dental professional, damage to the permanent dentition could be averted.

Dental trauma can occur in the school yard and during sporting events. Immediate replantation of an avulsed permanent tooth can mean the difference between success and failure caused by delay. Early referrals of other traumatic injuries can also make the difference between a success and long-term failure. Failure to treat simple trauma early can lead to expensive rehabilitation later, including bridgework and implants.

Teachers are in a unique and very important position when it comes to a child's dental health. They can potentially spend more time with a child during the day than the parents do, and may be in a position to make a significant contribution to the child's well-being through good oral health.

# SUMMARY

Every classroom includes a number of children with dental conditions that affect speech, chewing, and possibly facial appearance. These conditions may be congenital or may have been acquired through trauma, such as a motor vehicle accident. In the primary dentition, the leading causes of loss of upper incisors are nursing decay and trauma, usually due to falls. Children with permanent teeth may have missing teeth due to congenital anomalies described elsewhere in this text or to accidents. Some of the congenital conditions, such as cleft lip and palate, enamel and dentin defects, and multiple missing teeth, require extensive dental reconstruction. Teachers should feel comfortable to discuss ways to limit loss of class time with both dentists and families. In this way, the necessary compromises can be made to blend both the academic and health needs of the child.

# REFERENCES

Andreasen, J. O., & Andreasen, F. M. (Eds.). (1994). *Textbook and color atlas of traumatic injuries to the teeth* (3rd ed.). Boston: Mosby.

Kenny, D. J., & Somaya, P. (1988). Sugar load of liquid medications in chronically ill children. *Journal of the Canadian Dental Association, 55,* 43–46.

La Leche League International. (1994). *Breastfeeding and dental caries* (LLLI Statement). Schaumburg, IL: Author.

Schwartz, S. S., Rosivack, R. G., & Michelotti, P. (1993). A child's sleeping habit as a cause of nursing caries. *Journal of Dentistry for Children, 60,* 22–25.

# CHAPTER 12

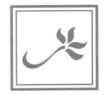

# Orthopedic Problems and Sports Injuries in Children

James Harder

The term *orthopedic* literally means "straight child." The field of orthopedics, therefore, deals primarily with deformity and disease of the locomotor system. This includes muscle, bone, and joint problems, as well as problems with the neurological system as it influences the development and control of locomotion. For example, when a child walks with an obvious limp, possible causes are wide ranging. The limp may be painful or pain free. The limp may be secondary to an injury, faulty biomechanical alignment, or an underlying metabolic disorder such as rickets. Therefore, when recognizing a symptom or clinical sign that suggests an abnormality of the locomotor system, it is important to realize that the specific cause may result from a host of factors.

This chapter reviews some of the orthopedic problems and sports injuries common to the school-age child. Through better understanding, the teacher may assist in the recognition, identification, and early management of many orthopedic conditions. Early diagnosis will result in improved outcomes, and an understanding of the disease process will assist the teaching staff in maintaining the child's education while the child is recovering from an illness or injury. Lists of suggested reading materials and other resources are included at the end of the chapter for individuals wishing to read more on the topics covered in this chapter.

## DISORDERS OF THE SPINE

### Scoliosis

Scoliosis is a curvature of the spine in a helical formation. The abnormal curvature may be congenital or present at birth, or it may develop later in childhood or adolescence. If it develops after birth, it is referred to as acquired scoliosis. The most common types of acquired scoliosis are the idiopathic variety and the neurogenic variety. The word *idiopathic* means "without known cause." Examples of *neurogenic* scoliosis are curves caused by spina bifida, cerebral palsy, or poliomyelitis. The helical curve, in addition to having a side-to-side or lateral component of curvature, also has a rotatory component. This rotation results in the chest's turning to either the right or the left as the lateral curvature takes place. On forward bending, therefore, if one were to observe the shoulder blades, the rotational component would cause one shoulder blade to be at a different level than the other or more prominent than the other. This phenomenon, known as a rib hump, is associated with a significant degree of scoliosis. The forward-bending test is commonly performed by physicians, health nurses, or trained laypeople, to identify children with scoliosis (see Figure 12.1). The forward-bending test is a very sensitive test in that it will show a rib hump or a bump in the lower back region even with the smallest curves. Another common sign of scoliosis is an asymmetry of the waistline. This may be caused by scoliosis or by one leg being shorter than the other.

The most common type of acquired scoliosis is of the idiopathic variety. Females are more frequently affected than males (ratio of 9:1), and it is commonly observed from ages 10 to 16 years. There is usually no complaint of pain or illness associated with scoliosis. The curve is detected incidentally on physical examination by the family physician or by the parents or teacher noticing an asymmetry in posture of the shoulder blades or waistline. The curve may progress or worsen with growth.

The treatment of idiopathic scoliosis depends on the severity of the curve as measured by X-ray at the time of detection. As a general rule, curves between 0 and 20 degrees are simply observed and treated conservatively. School screening programs have found that 70% of curves less than 20 degrees have a tendency to wax and wane, do not progress or cause any serious difficulties, and require no significant treatment in the long term. The child is examined at regular intervals and advised to be fully active with no restrictions. The muscles of the abdomen and spine of an individual this age should be in excellent physical condition, and if there is any question of inactivity, an exercise program is prescribed.

The second category of idiopathic curve measures between 20 and 40 degrees. This degree of scoliosis demands active treatment. If the child is young and has considerable growth remaining, the potential for the curve to progress is significant. Curves in this range are treated with braces that are worn in an attempt to hold the curve stationary. *The brace never corrects the*

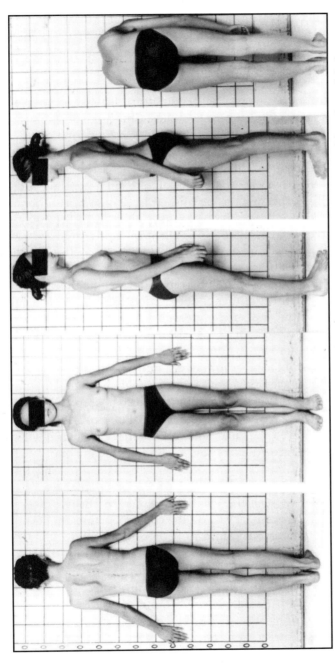

**FIGURE 12.1.** Multiple views of an adolescent with idiopathic scoliosis. In particular, note the curvature of the spine and the hump deformity of the ribs on the right when the child is bending forward.

*curve.* Successful brace treatment will allow the curve to be held between 20 and 40 degrees while the child completes growth. The child is then gradually weaned from the brace and continues into adulthood brace-free, while the curve typically remains stable between 20 and 40 degrees. A small minority of curves, however, continue to slowly progress beyond the 40-degree range and require further treatment. These children are therefore examined at regular intervals until growth has been completed, and annually thereafter to ensure that the scoliosis does not continue to increase after maturity.

Braces for scoliosis are of many varieties, but all have one thing in common. They form a rigid cage around the pelvis, abdomen, and chest. The rigid outer body jacket holds the spine in alignment or, through pad placement, allows the spine to be pushed into alignment. There are two common varieties of brace. The Milwaukee brace has a firm plastic pelvic girdle and three metal uprights, one in the front and two in the back. They meet under the jaw at a neck ring (see Figure 12.2). With the addition of supportive pads, the brace acts as a firm cage in which the position of the spine can be controlled. The second type of brace, the thoracolumbar orthosis, fits more tightly to the skin. It is an underarm brace, which is much more cosmetic and is measured especially for the patient. Pads are placed inside the shell to correct the posture of the spine within the jacket.

These braces are worn approximately 14 to 16 out of 24 hours, with about 8 hours out of the brace for exercise and daily hygiene. This allows the child to wear the brace from about 5 P.M. through the night and then take it off in the morning. Physical activity is encouraged to keep the spinal muscles strong and to maintain a normal range of spinal motion. As the child grows, the spine is monitored at regular intervals and the brace may be altered. The brace is worn until growth is complete (about age 14 in girls).

The "surface" electrical stimulator device and the internally implanted muscle stimulator were used in place of the brace in the early to mid-1980s. They are no longer in use in North America. The electrical stimulators caused a muscle contraction on the convex portion of the curve. The surface stimulator was not found to be effective in controlling scoliosis. The implanted stimulator was found to be as effective as the brace but is no longer produced for the North American market.

The third category of idiopathic curve measures over 40 degrees. It may be associated with a significant asymmetry on forward bending, and the child may be off balance. Depending on a variety of factors, this curve may be considered for surgical intervention. Surgical intervention consists of straightening the curve almost completely by the use of instruments that hook to the spine, and then providing a bone fusion in the area of the

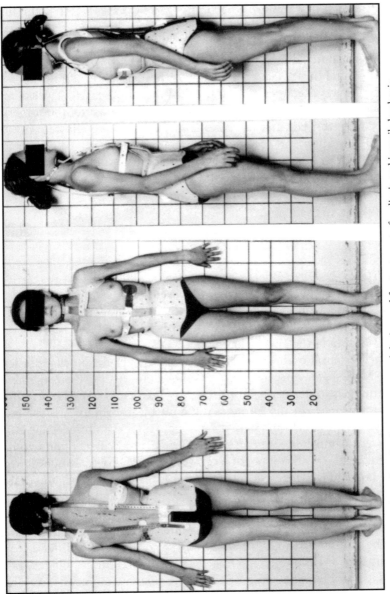

**FIGURE 12.2.**    The Milwaukee brace, an external device used for treatment of scoliosis and juvenile kyphosis.

curvature such that the spine becomes rigid in that area. After the fusion has healed, the spine is stable in the area of the fusion and an increasing curvature is no longer possible. The common name for such an operation is spinal instrumentation and fusion (see Figure 12.3). The child is admitted to the hospital on the day of the surgery, and stays for about 5 to 7 days after the surgery. Recuperation time at home is another 2 to 3 weeks before the child returns to school. Sometimes a brace is worn after the surgery for about 3 months. Normal activities of daily living are allowed; however, physical education and sports are not allowed for about 1 full year while the fusion heals into place. Excessive movement of the vertebral bodies in the fusion mass is detrimental to the healing process.

## Spondylolysis and Spondylolisthesis

*Spondylolysis* refers to a defect of the spine. *Spondylolisthesis* is a term that indicates a spondylolysis defect of the spine that has further resulted in displacement of one vertebra over another. The most common site for spondylolisthesis is where the lowermost lumbar vertebra meets the first sacral vertebra in the low back region.

The vertebral bodies are normally stacked up like blocks in a tower. These blocks are separated and cushioned by a disc that resembles a doughnut. The outer sturdy fibrous ring of the disc holds gelatinous material in the center. The disc protects the spine by absorbing various physical forces during exercise and activity. The spinal cord and nerves lie behind the vertebral body, surrounded by a protective bony canal. Spondylolisthesis occurs in the posterior portion of two vertebral bodies, which allows the upper body to slip forward on the lower one. The cause of the defect is often unknown. The child develops low backache with activity. The pain will sometimes radiate into the legs. The child may walk with an unusual posture, and complain of low backache after participating in sports activities. The hamstring muscles may be tight and the child will have trouble bending forward and touching fingers to the floor. Rest usually relieves the pain. This problem may become clinically apparent as early as 6 or 7 years of age, and is therefore a diagnostic consideration in children with back pain from elementary school onward.

Once the diagnosis of a spondylolytic defect is made by X-ray, it is important to monitor the lower spine by X-ray in case of slippage, which may occur during times of rapid growth. Treatment consists of allowing the child

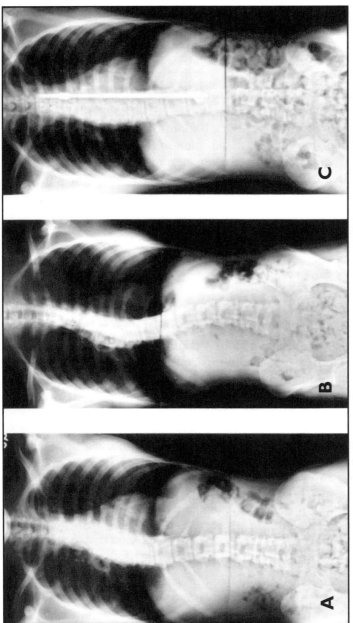

**FIGURE 12.3.** Radiographs (X-rays) of a 16-year-old female with idiopathic scoliosis (A) lying supine showing curvature of the vertebrae, (B) standing erect, and (C) following surgery and the insertion of a steel rod for stabilization.

full activity within the limits of his or her pain tolerance. If the child is obese, nutrition counseling may be of assistance as weight loss may decrease the displacement of the vertebrae. A lower back support may be of help for short periods, and a specific exercise program is initiated to improve muscle tone and support. If the child shows persistent pain or rapid displacement by X-ray, it may be necessary to surgically stabilize the slipping segments by means of a spinal fusion. Spinal fusion is a major surgical procedure, which is generally successful in relieving back discomfort and preventing further slippage. Following surgical stabilization of the vertebrae, the child may be required to wear a brace and be completely restricted from sports, but otherwise may attend school and take part in usual activities. The restrictions will apply until complete spinal fusion has taken place between the two affected vertebral bodies, which may take as long as 10 to 12 months.

## Torticollis

Torticollis, or wryneck, is a condition characterized by a peculiar tilting and turning of the head to one side. The child may be unable to hold the head completely upright and look straight forward. Torticollis may be congenital or acquired. Congenital torticollis presents shortly after birth with a firm swelling in the sternomastoid (strap) muscle on one side of the neck. The swelling ultimately results in shortening of the muscle, which exerts an uneven force on the head, causing it to tilt and turn. Treatment consists of stretching the shortened muscle and is usually successful in correcting the posture and allowing normal function if therapy is initiated at an early stage. If the condition remains untreated, it may result in permanent wryneck and facial asymmetry because of the constant stretch upon the head and neck muscles. If physical therapy is unsuccessful, surgical intervention may be necessary to lengthen the muscle. Surgery is followed by stretching exercises to maintain muscle length and allow normal neck movement and facial growth.

The Klippel-Feil syndrome, a form of torticollis, results from a congenital deformity of the bones and muscles of the neck (see Figure 12.4). The neck appears short, and range of movement in all directions is usually reduced. The diagnosis is confirmed by X-ray. Depending on the severity of the condition, sporting activities may be curtailed, especially if contact is likely. Contact sports such as football, gymnastics, rugby, and wrestling are particularly high risk for a neck injury.

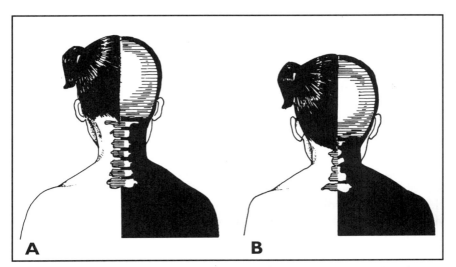

**FIGURE 12.4.** (A) A normal individual. (B) An individual with Klippel-Feil syndrome. Note the patient's shortened neck with malformed vertebrae.

Acquired torticollis may result from a host of causes. For example, tonsillitis resulting in inflamed lymph nodes in the neck may irritate one side of the neck and cause a child to tilt the head. A child who has hearing or visual problems may tilt the head consistently in order to enhance hearing or vision. If the child has had an injury to the neck during play or sport, the protective muscle spasm and inflammation may result in torticollis. Treatment of acquired torticollis is simply treatment of the specific cause. Traumatic torticollis or torticollis secondary to injury may sometimes require a short period of traction in the hospital, combined with anti-inflammatory medication and possibly a collar to support the neck for a short period. Hearing and visual problems should be investigated and corrected.

## Kyphosis

Kyphosis of the spine is an abnormal forward bending or round back deformity that is generally most evident in the shoulder blade area. It may involve a large segment of the spine which is characterized by a long gradual curve, or it may be confined to a localized segment which, on bending forward, appears as a hump. The etiology of kyphosis in children and adolescents covers a wide spectrum of conditions. Congenital abnormalities, which alter the shape or size of the vertebral bodies, may result in abnormal growth and forward bending of the spine.

A much more common cause of a rounded back is Scheuermann's kyphosis, which generally appears in the adolescent age group. The student complains of backache in the shoulder blade area, particularly after sitting for long periods or after activities that involve forward stooping. Inspection of the spine shows a rounded appearance. Lying on a flat surface to straighten the spine generally relaxes the muscle spasm in the area and relieves pain. The etiology of Scheuermann's kyphosis is unknown. The condition is associated with an inflammatory response in the anterior or front portion of the spinal column in the area of the rib cage, and a forward wedging of consecutive vertebral bodies. The disease is self-limiting, and eventually resolves during the late teens. Treatment consists of a regular exercise program to strengthen the back muscles and improve posture. Occasionally, a mild anti-inflammatory drug may be added to relieve pain. The degree of kyphosis is then followed along with growth, and if a significant increase in forward bending is noted, a brace may be necessary (see Figure 12.5). The brace holds the spine in the corrected position and prevents further forward bending while the inflammatory process resolves. The brace is worn in the daytime while the individual is erect, and is removed while recumbent. If bracing is unsuccessful, or if the kyphosis is localized and quite severe, a surgical procedure may be indicated to straighten the spine. This surgery consists of the implantation of corrective hooks and rods to the affected area of the spine, and a spinal fusion in the area of the curvature. The child may return to school following recovery from the operation, but participation in sporting activities is completely restricted for approximately 1 year.

## Disc Protrusion

Disc protrusion (herniated disc) is generally a condition of early and later adulthood; it can also, though rarely, affect the growing child. As stated earlier, the disc is an anatomical unit or spacer between each vertebral body. It is shaped like a doughnut, with an outer ring of strong fibrous material and an inner portion filled with a viscous substance. If a defect were to occur in the firm fibrous outer ring, mechanical forces would allow the

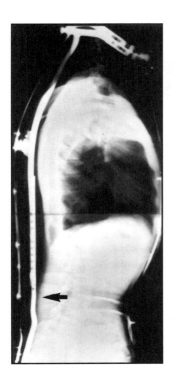

**FIGURE 12.5.** Roundback deformity (juvenile kyphosis). An X-ray shows a hump formation (arrow) in the region of the waist. A Milwaukee brace is in place as a part of the treatment.

gelatinous central portion to extrude through the disrupted ring area. Mechanical defects in the fibrous ring generally occur posteriorly or at the back of the ring where the stress is greatest. This is also the area where the spinal cord and nerves are situated. When the gelatinous disc material is extruded, it may impinge upon the spinal nerve or cord, causing back and leg pain or weakness in a lower extremity (see Figure 12.6). The back pain is enhanced by exercise, coughing, or sneezing. The patient will not be able to touch toes on forward bending and, on trying to do so, may complain of increased back and leg pain.

Following investigation to confirm the diagnosis, a period of complete bed rest is instituted for as long as 4 weeks. The inflammation and swelling may then subside, and the pain and weakness disappear. A computerized tomography (CT) scan or a magnetic resonance imaging (MRI) scan will be helpful in showing the damaged disc and any fragments of the disc that may be pushing on the nerves or spinal cord. In the event that bed rest is unsuccessful in reducing the symptoms, surgical intervention with removal of the offending portion of the extruding disc material may be necessary. This

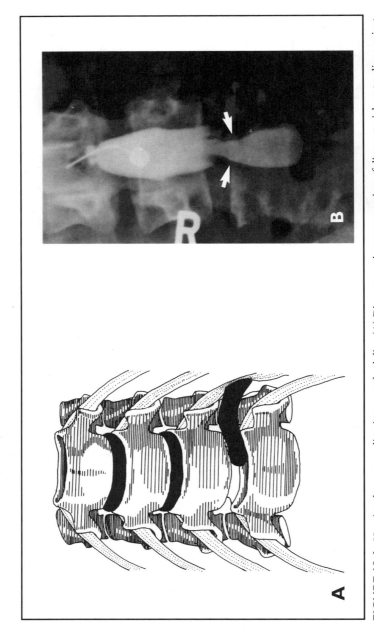

**FIGURE 12.6.** Herniated or protruding intervertebral disc. (A) Diagrammatic representation of disc material protruding against a nerve root. (B) A myelogram (insertion of dye that outlines the space surrounding the spinal cord) showing a defect indicating a disc protrusion. The arrows point to the compression of the spinal column (white mass) by the disc.

operation can be done with microsurgical techniques, which minimize time in hospital and speed recovery. Following the operation, a back brace may be worn and sporting activities are curtailed for 3 to 4 months. In selected cases, particularly when the disc protrusion is not too extensive, a protein-digesting substance called chymopapain can be injected into the disc area. The surgeon injects chymopapain derived from the papaya tree directly into the disc material, which serves to dissolve or shrink the abnormal disc. Through this procedure, an operation may be averted and the patient may return to normal activities in a very short period of time.

## Sprengel's Deformity

Sprengel's deformity is a congenital problem in which one shoulder blade is abnormally higher than the other. The affected shoulder blade does not allow full movement of the arm (see Figure 12.7). The diagnosis can be made by observing that one shoulder is higher than the other and that movement to the affected arm and shoulder is restricted. Generally, the treatment is surgical and the operation is performed between 3 to 6 years of age. The operative procedure usually improves the appearance of the shoulder and may enhance the motor function of the arm.

## Cerebral Palsy

Cerebral palsy is a complex disorder resulting from damage to the brain (see Chapter 14). The cause of the brain damage is, in many instances, not clear. Some of these children are born with brain defects due to abnormalities of formation, and other children have brain injuries due to exposure to toxic substances, lack of oxygen, or direct trauma. The areas of the brain that are affected vary, and effects range from loss of gross and fine motor muscle control to dysfunction of speech, cognitive functions, vision, hearing, and behavior. Involvement may be minimal or severe. Although people often think that someone with cerebral palsy is severely handicapped, this is not true. Sometimes a mild gait or movement abnormality is the only sign when damage to the brain has been minimal.

There are two common types of cerebral palsy, spastic and athetoid. The spastic variety is characterized by tight muscles with increased tone. Initiation of movement and control over movement are both difficult.

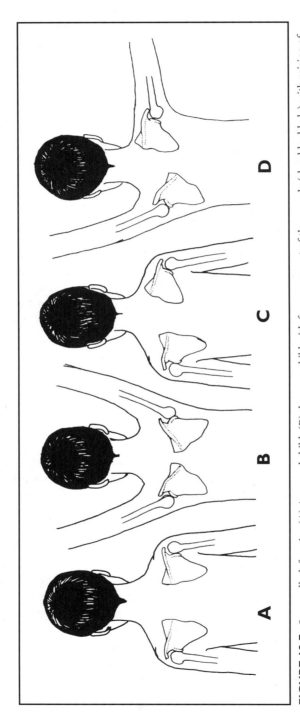

**FIGURE 12.7.** Sprengel's deformity. (A) A normal child; (B) the same child with free movement of the scapula (shoulder blade) with raising of the arms; (C) decreased size and abnormal elevation of the right scapula in an affected patient; (D) limitation of shoulder movement because of the deformity.

Severity is variable and the disorder may affect only one limb or may involve all four limbs, as well as the head, neck, and spine. The athetoid variety of cerebral palsy is characterized by involuntary movements of the body. The movements are spontaneous and made worse when the person is excited. Purposeful activity can be accomplished within the maze of constant involuntary movement, but requires a considerable amount of patience from the patient and the caregiver.

During their growing years, children with spastic cerebral palsy may undergo numerous surgical procedures directed toward improving the level of motor function. A rhizotomy is a surgical procedure on the spinal cord which reduces spasticity. Other common procedures include tendon lengthening or transfer and operations to prevent the hip from dislocating. Hospitalization may be brief; however, the child is usually required to wear a cast for some weeks after the procedure. Attendance at school should be encouraged as soon as possible after the surgery.

Scoliosis may develop secondary to unbalanced spastic spinal muscles. Not all children with cerebral palsy will have scoliosis. It is most common in those children who are confined to a wheelchair. The spinal curvature will present as early as age 5 or 6 years, and will gradually progress with growth. Bracing the scoliosis is not effective. If the curve shows relentless progression, surgical intervention is indicated. Scoliosis secondary to cerebral palsy can be difficult to stabilize, due to the constant pull of the spastic muscles. Instrumentation and fusion of the spine are sometimes necessary from the front of the spine as well as the back in order to build a durable fusion mass to hold the spine straight. This extensive surgery allows the continued balanced sitting necessary for hands-free function. Improved spinal instrumentation systems now allow sitting without a supportive jacket, immediately after the surgery. Hospitalization time for spinal surgery is usually 10 to 14 days, and recuperation time at home may be another 2 to 3 weeks before school attendance is again possible.

# DISORDERS OF THE HIP JOINT

## Congenital Dislocation of the Hip

As the name implies, congenital dislocation of the hip is present at the time of birth. The hip joint consists of a ball and a socket. The relationship of the ball at the top end of the thigh bone (femur) and the cup (acetabulum) in which it usually resides, has been disrupted. The ball is no longer associated with the cup; the joint is dislocated. The dislocatible hip allows the femoral head, or ball part of the socket, to be easily brought in and out of the cup. The muscles in and around the hip joint are of normal length, and the femoral head has been normally related to the cup or at least in the vicinity of the cup for the majority of the 40 weeks of gestation. The hip joint is found to be dislocatible after the child is born. There may be abnormalities or deficiencies in the cup portion of the hip joint in addition to the generalized ligamentous laxity associated with the birth process. This combination of bone and cartilage abnormality as well as ligamentous laxity readily allows the ball to slip out of the cup.

Early detection is critical in this condition. In the newborn period, while the hip is still dislocatible, it is simple in the majority of cases to relocate the hip in the acetabulum or cup and hold it there until soft tissue structures around the hip joint tighten up; this then allows the ball to be held in the abnormal acetabulum. If treatment were discontinued at this stage, the cup might not completely normalize and early adult arthritis of the hip joint might be the end result. Treatment, therefore, must be continued with braces to position the leg and promote normal growth and development of the acetabulum. The earlier the treatment begins, the better the result. This can be illustrated by a comparison of two children. One child's dislocatible hip was discovered by routine examination in the newborn nursery. The child was treated using a special harness to position the lower limbs and then followed on a regular basis as the hip joint gradually normalized over a 12-week period. The other child, an 18-month-old, had a waddling gait pattern or limp because of an undetected congenitally dislocated hip. Relocation and normalization of this hip required an extended hospital stay, traction, operative procedures, and body casting, and was fraught with numerous complications. Fortunately, over the past two decades, great emphasis has been placed on early detection and treatment of infants with a congenitally dislocated hip, and all health professionals who come into contact with a newborn are alerted to the characteristic clinical signs. The number of children with this condition who are detected late is gradually decreasing.

It is important, however, to briefly outline how a school-age child might appear if one or both hips were dislocated. Because the ball is no longer in the socket, there is a pistoning movement in the area of the hip joint. The thigh is not held firmly against the pelvis and pistons up and down with walking. This results in a waddling gait. The child swings his or her upper torso over the dislocated hip while stepping down. If the right hip were dislocated, the child would swing to the right while bearing weight on the right leg. The child would not complain of pain and would be fully active. The right thigh would be short and thick and the skin creases asymmetrical compared to the opposite thigh. The child would have great difficulty participating in any activity that required the legs to be spread wide apart.

The child whose hip dislocation is detected late will require continuing treatment as he or she progresses through school. The treatment may involve physiotherapy, traction in the hospital, or surgical procedures involving the soft tissues or bone around the hip. In general, surgical procedures of the hip involving muscle and tendon require hospitalization ranging from 2 to 3 days and rehabilitative periods with restriction of activity that could last as long as 2 to 3 months. In contrast, bony surgical procedures require a slightly longer stay in a hospital. Postoperatively, crutches may be used to keep weight off the affected limb or the child may be placed in a spica or body cast to completely immobilize the hip joint. Because it is difficult for a child to ambulate successfully in a body cast, a reclining wheelchair may be necessary in the home and at school. A home teaching program is sometimes necessary to enable the child to continue with schooling. Following the removal of the body cast, a rehabilitation program is instituted and the child gradually returns to normal activity over the next 4 to 6 months.

## Legg-Calvé-Perthes Disease

Legg-Calvé-Perthes disease is a condition of unknown etiology that results in partial or complete destruction of the ball portion of the hip joint. In the newborn, the ball consists completely of cartilage. As the child grows, the cartilaginous ball begins to change into bone. By adulthood, the head of the femur has completed its bony growth, with only the outer surface as cartilage to serve as a slippery interface between the cup and the ball. For reasons that are unclear, in children with Legg-Calvé-Perthes disease, the tiny center of growing bone in the middle of the cartilage ball loses its blood supply and degenerates. Boys are affected more commonly than girls, with a ratio of 5:1, and the problem occurs between 4 to 8 years of age. Interruption of the blood supply to the ball is commonly known as *avascular necrosis*. The body recognizes the avascular portion of bone, and sets about to replace it with new bone. The process of bony regeneration in a 5-year-old boy may take

6 to 8 months, and in an 8-year-old may persist as long as 2 years. During regeneration, the hip undergoes two important phases. The first stage, known as the irritable phase, is characterized by complaints of pain in and around the knee or the hip. The pain may be present in the morning and is often associated with stiffness following awakening, or the pain may become more obvious after physical activity and cause the child to limp. The diagnosis of Legg-Calvé-Perthes disease is confirmed by X-ray.

Treatment consists of resting the hip and regaining full range of motion. With the help of anti-inflammatory medications, crutches to help take the weight off the hip, and regular physiotherapy, the hip is gradually mobilized. The child may be admitted to the hospital for a short period as physiotherapists gradually mobilize the hip. Once full range of hip motion is established, it is necessary to protect the ball during the critical regenerative phase. The ball loses some of its strength while the destroyed bone is being removed and the new bone is laid down. To protect the new bone from injury (an indentation as sometimes seen in a ping-pong ball), it is necessary for the ball to be protected and covered by the cup, or acetabulum, during the healing process. In a young child age 5 or younger, the acetabulum will generally supply enough coverage for the soft ball. In the older child, in whom healing takes longer, it is sometimes necessary to use a brace to help cover the soft femoral head. The brace will hold the legs wide apart, thereby turning the ball into the cup as much as possible. Weight bearing in this position is safe. The brace must be worn whenever the child is weight bearing, and until there is substantial evidence of healing. The child under the age of 5 years is seldom braced. Studies have shown that, due to the rapid healing time, the majority of children under age 5 do well as long as range of motion is maintained and the children are closely observed. The child who is wearing a brace may participate in sporting events provided the brace is worn. For swimming, however, the brace can be safely removed as long as the water is chest deep. The student with Legg-Calvé-Perthes disease who does not require a brace may participate in all activities except those involving jumps from heights.

The surgical management of Legg-Calvé-Perthes disease consists of two phases. First, if the hip cannot be readily mobilized due to muscle tightness and shortening, it may be necessary to surgically lengthen the affected muscles to allow full range of motion to the hip joint. This minor soft tissue procedure usually takes place during the initial phase of hospitalization and is followed by bracing as described above. Second, the hip joint is reconfigured such that coverage of the ball is provided by the acetabulum or cup when the child is in the normal standing position. Following surgery, the patient may be treated with a body cast or crutches that may allow partial weight bearing. About 2 months later, the hip joint is mobilized and strengthened. After muscle strength and range of motion have been restored, full activity without restriction is permitted. The coverage provided the ball by the surgical procedure acts like a built-in brace and allows the ball to be protected while it heals.

## Slipped Capital Femoral Epiphysis

Slipped capital femoral epiphysis is a condition of the hip joint in which the ball slides off the shaft of the femur. This occurs much the same way as a scoop of ice cream would melt and slide from a cone. The etiology of slipped capital femoral epiphysis is obscure. The growth plate between the bony shaft and the ball of the femur may be weakened in certain children. Various hormonal conditions and body builds have been implicated as responsible for weakening the growth plate. The obese male child between 10 and 14 years of age is at greatest risk for developing slipped capital femoral epiphysis. The other body type, which is much more rare, is the very tall and slender child. Males are affected much more frequently than females. During the early stages of the disease, the hip will become irritable. Often the child's only complaint will be knee pain when really the problem lies in the hip. As the slip continues, the child's gait becomes abnormal and a limp develops. Instead of walking with the feet facing forward, the child with a slipped capital femoral epiphysis will walk with the affected leg externally rotated or turned outward. The child will not be able to hold the knees together and bring them to the chest when lying on the back. The knee on the affected side will move outward as it is brought toward the chest.

It is important for slipped capital femoral epiphysis to be diagnosed early. If the slip is mild to moderate, the ball portion of the hip joint is surgically pinned in place. If the slip is severe, traction may be necessary prior to surgical stabilization in an attempt to improve the relationship of the ball to the femur. The pinning procedure requires a 2-day hospital stay. The patient then can ambulate with crutches. Contact sports will likely not be allowed until there is good evidence of healing, which may take as long as 12 to 18 months. The most serious complication of slipped capital femoral epiphysis is injury to the blood supply to the ball. If this happens, the body must reconstitute the blood supply and replace all the dead bone with new bone, much the same as in Legg-Calvé-Perthes disease. Unfortunately, the healing process in the adolescent is prolonged and the hip joint may never return to normal due to irreversible arthritic changes.

## Toxic Synovitis of the Hip Joint

Toxic synovitis is the most common cause of a painful hip in a child under 10 years of age. It is an acute, nonspecific inflammatory condition, the cause of which is unknown. Trauma (injury), infection (a virus), and allergy have all been implicated. The child walks with a limp and complains of pain localized to the groin or knee, similar to slipped capital femoral epiphysis. A fever may be evident and there is often a history of an upper respiratory tract infection within the previous 2 weeks. On examination, the child protects the hip but allows a reasonable amount of movement, although not to the fullest extent. Following appropriate blood tests, and an X-ray of the leg to rule out a fracture, the child is treated with bed rest and perhaps anti-inflammatory medication. After 2 or 3 days, the child is allowed to be up and around with gradually increasing activity. Mild anti-inflammatory medications may be continued to decrease pain and muscle spasm and improve the range of motion. The prognosis for complete recovery is excellent. Approximately 1% of these children will go on to develop Legg-Calvé-Perthes disease.

## Pyogenic Arthritis of the Hip

The most feared, destructive, and permanently disabling condition of the hip is an infection within the hip joint. For whatever reason, a transient bacteremia or bacteria in the blood stream, which occasionally occurs in everybody, results in lodging of the *Staphylococcus aureus* bacteria near the growth plate between the neck and the head of the femur. The blood circulation normally slows quite considerably near the growth plate, and if the bacteria becomes established in this area, body defenses cannot be mobilized as quickly as elsewhere, and a rapidly enlarging abscess may result. Because the growth area in the head of the femur is included as part of the hip joint, rupture of the abscess outside the bone results in contamination of the hip joint. The child will appear ill with a high fever and lethargy. The affected hip joint will be very painful and the child will refuse to allow movement of the leg. Following appropriate laboratory tests and confirmation of the diagnosis, the pus within the hip joint must be surgically drained and the joint rinsed out. Intravenous antibiotics will be instituted until all signs of systemic infection have disappeared. Thereafter, oral antibiotics will be continued for approximately 1 to 3 months. The hip will be at rest during the acute phase. Mobilization of the hip will begin after the infection is gone and inflammation is settling. The child will likely use crutches for weight bearing and return to normal activity over a period of 8 to 12 weeks. It is imperative to make the diagnosis early, as undue delay can result in permanent damage to the hip joint. Initially, it is often difficult to differentiate benign toxic synovitis from the much more serious pyogenic arthritis of the hip. The physician must use clinical judgment and selected laboratory tests to establish the correct diagnosis.

# AMPUTATIONS

Limb deficiencies can be present at birth (congenital) or be acquired after trauma, malignant tumor (cancer), or infection. A classification describing limb loss has been adopted by the Association of Children's Prosthetic and Orthotic Clinics (ACPOC) of North America (Kay et al., 1975). A deficiency is described as one of two types, transverse or longitudinal, and thereafter one simply describes what is missing (e.g., a transverse partial radius and ulna, proximal one third, would leave a residual limb below the elbow, somewhere in the first one third of the forearm). More information on limb deficiency and the locations for advice and treatment can be obtained on the ACPOC Web site (http://www.ACPOC.org).

## Congenital Limb Deficiency

Congenital limb deficiency is present at the time of birth. The family with a limb-deficient child is devastated at the time of the birth and feels a distinct sense of loss. Adaptation to this loss follows the typical grief response described by Kubler-Ross (1993): initial anger, followed by bargaining, depression, and, finally, resignation. It is important for professionals to recognize this grieving process and to support the family during this time, should they have problems. The child will be aware of the deficiency but will readily accept it at this early age. When the parents have accepted the deficiency, the child will gain in self-esteem and move forward with confidence. Should the family fail to accept the deficiency and tend to hide the limb from others, it will soon be apparent to the child that there is something wrong with him or her that is upsetting the parents. This will lead to feelings of insecurity and confusion.

Most clinics emphasize early intervention with a family who has a limb-deficient child. A member of the hospital's amputee clinic will meet with the family soon after birth, on the obstetrical unit, and begin the process of education, which will lead to reconciling the limb deficiency. Attending parent groups provides an excellent opportunity for the family to become acquainted with others who have a similar problem. Through a process of education and listening, and given time, acceptance will grow.

The introduction of the child into the school system is made much easier by educating the class with respect to the limb deficiency. This is done by inviting a parent, physical therapist, or occupational therapist to show the class a prosthesis, demonstrate how it works, and introduce a person with a limb deficiency. The class members thereby understand the deficiency and adopt a helpful attitude toward the child with the limb deficiency. Teasing is reduced. If the family has not gained acceptance of the limb deficiency, however, the child may experience problems with self-esteem, which will lead to insecurity and either aggression or withdrawal. Peers will sense these behaviors immediately and, due to lack of understanding, not accept the student.

Should this situation be recognized, much work needs to be done by the school counselor or psychologist to help the child begin the grieving process. The process begins with the recognition that the deficiency is causing a significant disability in activities of daily living, in sports, and in accepted appearance. Family and peer support is required during this time. In North America, the ACPOC is an excellent resource, and in Canada, the Child Amputee Program, a branch of the War Amputations of Canada, is helpful in providing support and information. Special computer aids in the classroom for children with more than one limb affected have made a significant difference in their ability to keep up with their peers. Special adaptations have made it possible to participate in sports like cycling, hockey, golf, swimming, and calf roping, to mention a few.

# KNEE JOINT

## Chondromalacia of the Knee

Chondromalacia of the knee is a diffuse inflammatory condition of the kneecap or patella that results in pain with activity. The condition is prevalent in young adolescents and is more common in girls than boys. It usually begins during activities that require an excessive amount of strenuous running. Cycling, running, climbing, and skiing are some of the common examples that often incite chondromalacia. The etiology of chondromalacia is varied. The most common cause is an imbalance in the quadriceps mechanism of muscles. These muscles are responsible for straightening or extending the lower leg. These muscles are responsible for pulling the patella up and down. As the patella glides in a groove, any improper tracking of the patella as it moves back and forth with flexion and extension of the knee results in pain and swelling about the knee. Another cause of painful knee is a marked knock-knee deformity. This angulation at the knee causes abnormal tracking of the patella, making it strike against the outer portion of the groove in which it travels. The abnormal motion of the joint causes wear and tear, allowing microscopic pieces of cartilage to be distributed around the kneecap area. The end result is cartilaginous damage and inflammation of the lining of the knee joint (see Figure 12.8). In addition to knock-knees, partial or total absence of a portion of the quadriceps muscle, atypical insertion of the muscle just below the knee, abnormal formation of the groove in which the patella glides, or asymmetry of the patella may also result in chondromalacia.

Temporary chondromalacia may result from an injury to the patella or occur as a result of rapid growth. During growth, the bones grow very quickly, and the muscle growth occurs secondarily as the muscle stretches to the new bone length. The muscle is therefore thinner, and particularly the four thigh muscles that control the patella may be out of balance. Abnormal patellar tracking occurs in response to the muscle imbalance, and chondromalacia may develop. Warming up and stretching the muscles out to length before sports is therefore very important to the growing child because doing so improves muscle balance and function. If the muscle has been warmed up and stretched out, injuries are prevented. Once the growth spurt has been accomplished, the muscle strength and coordination improve, the

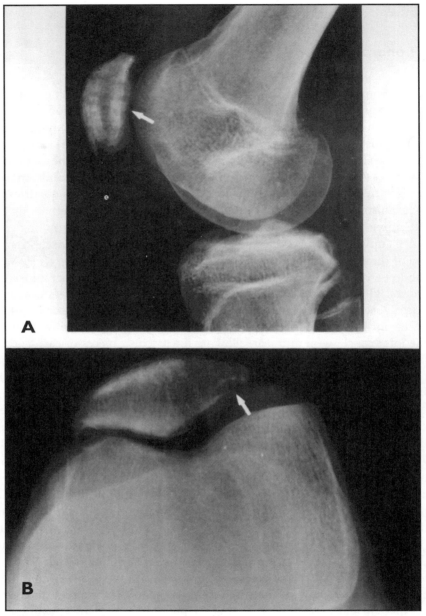

**FIGURE 12.8.** A 12-year-old girl with chondromalacia patella who had a 6-month history of pain and swelling of the right knee. (A) A lateral view of the knee joint shows a ragged appearance (arrow) of the underside of the patella (kneecap). (B) A special X-ray view to show the undersurface of the affected patella.

quadriceps mechanism regains its balance, and the chondromalacia gradually improves and disappears.

Treatment of chondromalacia depends on symptoms. Children continue to participate in all forms of sporting activities to the limit of their discomfort. Warming up and stretching out the muscles is important, as mentioned above. Ice applied to the knee as well as anti-inflammatory agents will help to overcome acute episodes of knee pain. Numerous types of knee braces are available, which help to guide the patella along its course during running activities. The wearing of a knee brace may alleviate pain during sporting activities and increase the participant's endurance. Physiotherapy directed toward vastus medialis muscle strengthening, in conjunction with patellar taping, will improve pain and allow for strengthening. An antipronation running shoe or an orthotic in the shoe will sometimes improve the alignment of the foot and leg. The role of surgery in chondromalacia patella is minor. Although numerous operations have been designed to improve patellar tracking, these have not been very successful unless there is an obvious biomechanical deformity that can be corrected.

## Dislocated Patella

Occasionally, abnormal biomechanics influencing the movement of the patella may cause complete dislocation of the kneecap. Dislocation usually occurs during participation in running sports and is extremely painful. The dislocated patella is observed as a large lump on the outside of the knee. Emergency treatment consists of reducing or replacing the patella into its original position and obtaining an X-ray to rule out a chip fracture of the surrounding bone. Definitive treatment is directed to the surgical reconstruction of the quadriceps mechanism if dislocation is a recurrent problem.

## Osteochondritis Dissecans

Osteochondritis dissecans is a condition of bone and articular cartilage that manifests itself by pain or aching symptoms about a joint. The knee and the ankle are the most commonly affected areas, but the hip, elbow, and shoulder can also be affected. The joint surface is covered by a layer of shiny, bluish-colored cartilage that serves as a slippery surface. It is nourished by the joint fluid. Beneath the covering layer of cartilage lies the supporting bone. In this disease, a small portion of supporting bone, from 1 to 3 centimeters in size, loses its blood supply and degenerates (see Figure 12.9). The destroyed bone is surrounded by normal bone except on the articular surface. The body recognizes the abnormal bone and begins replacing it with new living bone. During the process of replacement, the damaged bone must be removed, new bone laid down, and finally the entire area remodeled to withstand the stress experienced by the joint. As remodeling of the bone proceeds, the surrounding area softens and a piece of the bone and cartilage may swing down into the joint space like a gate on its hinges. The displaced portion of the bone then interferes with the joint mechanics, causing swelling, pain, and locking of the joint. Prior to the piece of bone and cartilage becoming loose, the patient complains of pain in the joint with exercise but has no obvious swelling or redness. If the child is between 6 and 12 years of age, healing takes place fairly quickly, the cartilage usually does not break, and the ultimate result is excellent. In the adolescent, healing is not quite as rapid, and as a consequence the cartilage may finally wear and break along the portion of bone and cartilage and may be displaced into the joint. The absent portion of cartilage (i.e., a hole left in the surface of the joint) has then decreased the weight-bearing surface on the joint, causing increased stresses and inflammation in this area. The loose fragment within the joint generally results in locking and continued inflammation until it is surgically removed. If a diagnosis is made prior to the fragment's loosening in the joint, various operative procedures, including pinning or bone grafting, can be attempted to promote healing of the loose fragment. Degenerative osteoarthritis of the joint may be the end result of osteochondritis dissecans in the adolescent, particularly if diagnosis and treatment are delayed.

## Osgood-Schlatter's Disease

Osgood-Schlatter's disease is a traction apophysitis or chronic inflammation in the proximal tibial area just below the knee joint in the region where the patellar tendon inserts (see Figure 12.10). The child will complain of pain below the knee, and swelling and tenderness will be evident when the area is palpated or pressure is applied. The etiology of Osgood-Schlatter's disease is most often associated with the rapid growth phase in preadolescence, unless there is a history of trauma. When the signal is

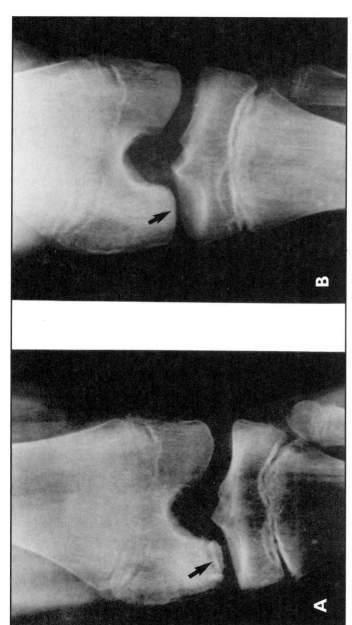

**FIGURE 12.9.** A 10-year-old boy with a history of locking and swelling of the left knee; the diagnosis is osteochondritis dissecans. (A) Defect on weight-bearing surface of femoral condyle (arrow). The fragment may break off and float within the joint. (B) Healing of the defect 16 weeks following surgical drilling through the abnormal cartilage.

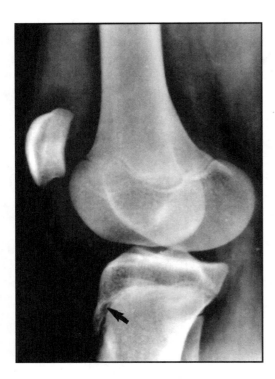

**FIGURE 12.10.** A 13-year-old boy with Osgood-Schlatter's disease with fragmentation of the tibial tubercle (arrow).

received for growth, the bone responds and increases in length; however, the muscle grows in response to stretch and therefore lags behind bone growth. When the muscle is relatively shorter than it should be to accommodate full range of joint motion, undue tension will result within the musculotendinous unit, and this force will be transmitted to the spot where the muscle and tendon insert into the bone (apophysis). Repeated tension at the apophysis, which occurs during vigorous sports, will cause an apophysitis or inflammation in the area due to the repeated excessive traction forces. It is important when establishing the diagnosis of Osgood-Schlatter's disease to be certain that there is no underlying bone pathology that could cause weakness of the bone or tendon in the area. This can be ruled out very simply by an X-ray of the knee joint. After the diagnosis is made, the treatment concentrates on quadriceps stretching to decrease tension at the apophysis. There is no restriction of activity except to participate within the limits of pain tolerance. As pain is the guiding factor, it would be rare for activity to reach such a level that the patellar tendon would be pulled from its bony insertion.

In previous times, Osgood-Schlatter's disease was treated with a straight leg cast. The cast resulted in knee stiffness and severe muscle wasting. Presently, instead of being casted, the patient is treated with anti-inflammatory agents as well as ice to overcome an acute episode, and then taught muscle strengthening and stretching exercises and allowed to participate in sports as long as pain is not severe. A special donut-type brace is available that protects the painful tibial tubercle area from injury. Generally, Osgood-Schlatter's disease runs a course of approximately 12 to 18 months, and then symptoms gradually disappear. A permanent bump in the area of the tibial tubercle may be the only sequela of the condition. Surgical intervention is reserved for the rare instance when total fusion of the area does not occur and a bony spur is associated with continued chronic irritation.

## Bow Legs and Knock-Knees

Genu varum (bow legs) is a deformity or malalignment of the lower leg. If a line is drawn from the upper portion of the hip to a space between the first and second toe, the knee joint in a patient with genu varum would lie to the outside of the imaginary line. Genu valgum (knock-knees) is the opposite of genu varum, in that the knee joint lies inside the imaginary line.

To understand the significance of these deformities, it is important to realize the normal physiological development of the lower extremity. From birth to age 2 years, the majority of normal children have a mild genu varum deformity. It is probable that the mild physiological deformity is developmental. As the child approaches 2 years of age, the genu varum gradually diminishes, and is replaced from age 2 to 7 years by a mild genu valgum deformity. From age 7 years to adulthood, the genu valgum slowly resolves and normal alignment is the rule. However, a group of children seems to fall outside of these parameters and have persistent genu varum or genu valgum. When evaluating children with what seems to be persistent genu varum or genu valgum, it is of utmost importance to determine whether they fit into this exaggerated physiological category or manifest one of the more serious causes of genu varum and genu valgum, such as rickets, rare inherited hormonal diseases, injury to the growth plate, various types of dwarfism, and inherited growth plate abnormalities. A thorough history, physical examination, and X-ray study usually serve to establish the diagnosis. A number of characteristic findings also might make one suspicious of serious problems. These include pain, a unilateral deformity, a rapidly increasing deformity, or associated short stature.

The treatment of exaggerated physiological genu varum or genu valgum is based on the severity of the deformity. If there is persistence of significant genu varum or genu valgum and no apparent resolution with growth, following a period of adequate observation, bracing is instituted. Bracing is usually most successful in the younger child. Surgery plays a minor role in physiological bow legs or knock-knees. Just prior to the completion of bony growth, it is possible to surgically arrest or slow growth on one side of the knee, allowing the opposite side to continue growth, thus straightening the deformity. The operation is known as "stapling the epiphysis." Following a short period of rehabilitation, normal activity is resumed. The staples will be removed after correction is obtained.

# DISORDERS OF THE FEET

## Flat Feet

Pes planovalgus, or flat feet, can be divided into two categories based on the mobility of the hind foot. The flexible flat foot is apparent when walking. The arch is not visible and the ankle seems to be angled inward. This angulation results in the shoe being deformed on the inside. Mild flexible planovalgus is common from age 2 to the mid-teenage years and will resolve as growth is completed. Pain is a rare complaint unless the deformity is moderate to severe and the child is involved in strenuous physical exercise. Following the activity, there may be some discomfort in the arch of the foot or in the calf muscle. On examination, there is flexibility of the hind-, mid-, and forefoot areas, and the deformity corrects nicely when the patient is not weight bearing or is walking on tiptoes. Planovalgus may also be associated with a mild knock-knee deformity. Treatment of the flexible flat foot is based on supporting the foot and may vary from a simple arch support, to a fully molded polypropylene arch support that inserts into the shoe. The type of foot support prescribed is based on the severity of the flat foot, and the ease with which it can be held in the corrected position during weight bearing. Some form of foot support is usually provided until adulthood, when the muscles and tendons may have sufficiently strengthened to maintain the normal contour of the foot. If there is a familial tendency toward flat feet, there may be no improvement in adulthood and the orthotic will continue to be necessary to improve position and decrease aching in the feet.

The second type of pes planovalgus is the rigid flat foot. This foot, as the description implies, remains in the flat foot position whether the child is walking or resting. There is no correction with toe walking. There is sometimes pain in the arch of the foot that may radiate to the calf muscle. The most common cause of the rigid flat foot in the pediatric age group is chronic inflammation of the joints of the hind foot secondary to rheumatoid or related forms of arthritis. As the inflammation resolves, the rigid foot gradually improves. Another cause for a rigid flat foot is a congenital abnormality in which the bones of the hind foot are locked together by bony bridges. In early life, these bony bridges consist of cartilage and are quite flexible and cause no foot discomfort. In the adolescent age group, the cartilage bar becomes more rigid as it turns into bone and the foot hurts in the region of the arch and the top of the foot after activity. The treatment of this type of rigid flat foot is usually surgical, and consists of either removal of the bony bar or fusion of the abnormal joints in the hind foot to completely prevent the painful motion and correct the flat foot deformity at the same time.

## Pes Cavus (High Arched Foot)

Pes cavus is a foot deformity in which the arch of the foot is abnormally high and exaggerated. In most cases, pes cavus is a relatively benign inherited condition, but there are some diseases that are characterized by a high arched foot due to disturbances of the nervous system or muscles. These include Friedreich's ataxia and Charcot-Marie-Tooth disease. The patient usually complains of weakness, loss of balance, leg aches, and repeated ankle sprains due to the abnormal configuration of the foot. Due to the position of the foot, the lateral ligaments of the ankle are easily strained, and walking on uneven ground is particularly liable to result in ankle sprain. The cavus foot is not inherently a painful condition. Management of the high-arched foot begins with modified shoe wear and orthotics. Soft tissue surgical procedures or bony operations can also be of help in rebalancing the foot, depending on the severity of the deformity and the age of the patient.

## Toe Walking

Tiptoe walking is uncommon in normal children beyond 2 years of age. The persistence of toe walking beyond the age of 2 years may be due to a neurological abnormality. Some normal school-age children tend to walk on their tiptoes unless attention is directed to the abnormal gait. With concentration, the child is able to walk with a normal gait pattern, only to resume tiptoe walking a few minutes later. The condition is not painful. Although involvement of both feet is most common, it can be unilateral. The etiology or cause of toe walking includes cerebral palsy, muscular dystrophies, spinal cord tumor, hemiplegia, conditions producing a short leg, and an idiopathic group (cause unknown). If the physical examination is normal and there are no indicators of neurological disease in a child under age 3, the parents and child are reassured and counseled to disregard the toe walking. Sometimes in the very young child, toe walking spontaneously disappears.

If toe walking persists beyond the first 2 years of walking, the child should be taken to the family doctor. This doctor will begin investigations into the cause of the persistent toe walking. Treatment is started with a home program of heel cord stretching exercises, supervised by the physical therapist. The stretching may be augmented by intermittent periods of casting or use of splints. If all has failed and the child continues to toe walk at age 5 or 6 years, then a surgical correction by lengthening the achilles tendon may be indicated. The procedure is not a major one, but does require below-the-knee cast immobilization for 5 to 6 weeks. The casts are then removed, and a period of strengthening is undertaken. It is important to allow controlled exercises and strengthening, but not to permit high-velocity or contact sports until the student can run without limping.

## Toeing In (Pigeon Toe) and Toeing Out

Toeing-in and toeing-out are common problems among children from age 6 months to adolescence. Toeing-in is the more prevalent of the two and is characterized by a gait in which the feet are turned inward. In evaluating this problem, it is important to determine whether the pigeon toe deformity originates in the foot, lower leg, or upper thigh, or from an abnormality of the entire lower extremity. In the preschool child, the most common causes of toeing-in are metatarsus varus (the sole of the foot is turned inward and the child walks on the outer border of the foot) and physiological internal tibial torsion. Fortunately, these two conditions usually spontaneously resolve with growth and the "straightening" forces applied by walking, running, and growing. Pigeon toe in the school-age child is more commonly the result of an abnormality of the femur or thigh, which causes inward rotation of the leg. This condition, known as femoral anteversion, results from an abnormal configuration and relationship between the head and neck of the femur and the shaft of the femur. These children do not complain of hip or knee pain and are quite capable of walking in a normal fashion, if reminded. Many students with femoral anteversion have a propensity to sit in the "W" or tailor position. The neurological and muscle examination is usually completely normal. Studies have shown that surgical treatment to realign the femur is not necessary and that the majority of the children gradually resolve the rotational deformity spontaneously, particularly if they are dissuaded from sitting in the tailor position. The children are encouraged to take part in all types of sports, including skiing, skating, ballet, and gymnastics. There is no need for special shoes or for turning the lower part of the foot outward with braces when the condition ultimately lies in the upper thigh. Persistence of significant inward tibial rotation or metatarsus varus (banana-shaped foot) should be seen and evaluated by the family doctor.

# BONE TUMORS

Bone tumors in children may be benign (noncancerous) or malignant (cancerous). Simple cysts and abnormalities of blood vessels within the bone are examples of common benign bone tumors in the child and young adolescent. The two most common cancerous bone tumors in the child and adolescent are Ewing's sarcoma and osteogenic sarcoma. These bone tumors are highly malignant and commonly affect the thigh or the pelvis. Treatment of Ewing's sarcoma is primarily radiation and chemotherapy, sometimes followed by surgical removal of the tumor. Management of osteogenic sarcoma begins with chemotherapy, then a surgical excision of the tumor, followed by additional chemotherapy. Depending on the location and the extent of the tumor, the surgery may allow limb sparing. Amputation of the limb above the tumor is still sometimes necessary. The 5-year survival for both of these tumors has improved significantly in recent years, and continues to improve through the development of more effective chemotherapeutic agents.

# SPORTS INJURIES

## Sport and Body Build

Participation in sports activities has always played an important role in the school curriculum. In addition to the physiologically beneficial effects of exercise, participation in sports also teaches leadership, team cooperation, winning, and losing, all so important for success in the working world. However, students may respond to sporting activities in varying ways. Some seem to be made for sports. Their coordination is excellent, strength and symmetry of movement are well balanced, and they seem to succeed with ease in all activities. In contrast, other students have body builds that do not allow the same degree of success in sports. The short, obese pupil often moves with great effort and frequently needs to be stimulated to perform; he or she struggles to participate in most activities to a satisfactory level. The child who is very tall and slender may not be balanced by adequate muscle control; this child seems clumsy and awkward. These children are at increased risk of injury when participating in high-velocity or contact sports. In summary, the student's body build tends to predict success and aptitude in various sporting activities. As a result, it is relatively easy to determine which children will require a significant amount of encouragement and patience from teaching staff in order to nurture a positive attitude to exercise.

Physical education in the school is, by necessity, a classroom activity, and does not differentiate aptitudes toward sports. All children are expected to participate in each sport. It is therefore the responsibility of the educator to recognize both the athletic skills and the limitations of the children in the classroom. By using good judgment and careful observation, many injuries can be prevented. Allowing the child to participate to his or her level of ability without shaming will help to ingrain the goal of exercise as a necessity to maintaining good health.

# COMMON ATHLETIC INJURIES

## The Lower Extremity

### Ankle Sprains

A sprained ankle is a common injury brought on by excessive, forceful twisting of the joint. Swelling may occur rather quickly, and the child will walk with a significant, painful limp. The treatment is dictated by the severity of the injury. If significant damage has been done to the ligaments, immobilization is generally required for a period of 7 to 10 days, at which time ice may be applied to reduce the swelling. Controlled range of motion is then instituted, followed by muscle strengthening. An ankle support and a supportive running shoe should then be worn to reduce the likelihood of reinjury.

### Ligament Injuries to the Knee

Injury to the knee is much the same as to the ankle, with one important exception. In the younger child, significant injury about the knee will result in a fracture or separation of the growth area at the end of the tibia or femur instead of tearing of the ligaments around the knee. This type of fracture must be assessed carefully, and X-rays obtained to assure adequate reduction and alignment of the fracture site. Immobilization is accomplished with a cast, and healing takes approximately 3 weeks before protected weight bearing and active range of motion can begin. Rehabilitation may require 4 to 8 weeks, and the child is not allowed to participate in contact sports until the limp has completely disappeared. Permanent injury to the growth area is possible following this growth plate injury, but fortunately is quite rare.

### Fracture of the Femur

The femur, or thigh bone, is the largest bone in the body. This bone is broken after significant force is applied to the bone by a twist or a direct blow to the leg. There will be immediate bleeding into the surrounding soft tissues and deformation of the thigh. Emergency treatment consists of keeping the child warm, preventing further injury to the leg, and calling for help.

The younger child can be treated by realigning the leg under general anesthesia and applying a body cast. The child will be absent from school for about 3 weeks, and then can attend school in a reclining wheelchair. The cast remains in place until the fracture is healed. The time is usually about 1 week for every year of age.

The older child with a fractured femur is managed by inserting temporary rods into the center of the femur to hold it in place. The child may also be casted, depending on the strength of the rods used and the stability of the fracture after fixation with the rods. The child will be discharged from the hospital using a wheelchair and should remain home until all acute pain has subsided and the need for pain medication is minimal. The child can then be trained to walk with crutches and should be able to attend school. If a body cast is used, it is still usually possible for the child to walk with crutches, but sitting may be more difficult. After the bone is healed, the rods are generally removed and the leg rehabilitated. High-velocity or contact sports are not allowed until the child can run without limping, possibly 8 weeks after the fracture is healed.

### Fracture of the Tibia and Fibula

A fracture of the tibia or fibula, the two bones below the knee, is a common injury of childhood and is due to a direct blow, a rotational type of injury, or a combination of both. After alignment of the leg is regained, an above-the-knee cast is applied. The length of immobilization in a cast is related to the child's age and could range from 4 weeks in a 5-year-old to 12 weeks in a 16-year-old. Rehabilitation after cast removal may require 6 to 12 weeks, and high-velocity or contact sports are prohibited as long as a limp is evident.

## The Upper Extremity

Sprained fingers are a common injury in individual and contact sports. These injuries must be assessed on an individual basis to determine whether the injury is limited to the ligaments or also involves a fracture through the bone or growth area. The assessment should be performed by a physician, and X-rays may be necessary to rule out a fracture. Splinting or cast immobilization is then instituted until soft tissue and bony healing is well under way. Immobilization may be necessary for approximately 14 days, then range-of-motion exercises are instituted, but the splint is maintained for protection for at least an additional week.

A hyperextension injury to the elbow with dislocation of the head of the radius (the pulled elbow) is common in school-age children. The injury results in significant pain localized to the outside of the elbow joint. The child is unable to flex the elbow, and a bump may appear on the outer side of the elbow joint. Following examination and X-ray of the elbow joint to eliminate the possibility of a fracture of the radius, the physician reduces the radial head dislocation and applies a splint and a sling for comfort. The splint is worn for approximately 10 days until soft tissue healing has commenced; thereafter, active range-of-motion exercises to the elbow are instituted. Forceful extension of the elbow should be avoided until muscle strength and control are regained.

## Dislocated Shoulder

Some children have lax ligaments and are prone to dislocating their shoulders. The physical activity most frequently associated with shoulder dislocation is one in which the arm is brought up and back, a common position while playing volleyball, racquet sports, or swimming. The child will complain of severe pain around the shoulder joint and a mass will be visible at the front of the shoulder, obliterating the normal roundness of the shoulder. A dislocated shoulder is not often associated with a fracture, but can be combined with an injury to the nerves about the shoulder. It is therefore extremely important for a physician to examine the child before relocation of the shoulder takes place. Once the dislocation has been reduced, the arm must be immobilized for a period of 6 weeks. The shoulder joint must be immobilized except for slow controlled pendulum movements, as excessive early movement of the shoulder joint during the healing phase increases the incidence of recurrent dislocation. The child will not be allowed to participate in any sporting activities during the reparative phase. Once the splint has been removed, the usual rehabilitative process takes place and may require 8 weeks while range of motion is regained and the muscles are strengthened.

## The Fractured Clavicle

A fractured clavicle occurs when the child falls and lands on the point of the shoulder and develops severe pain over the collar bone. There may be immediate swelling in the area. Generally there is no damage to the function of the hand, arm, or underlying nerves and blood vessels. The fracture usually occurs in the middle third of the collar bone, and treatment consists of X-ray followed by appropriate application of a sling or some means of gentle immobilization of the shoulder. Ice packs are applied to the area of swelling, and a pain-relieving medication is prescribed. In approximately 7 to 10 days, the pain tends to disappear and shoulder motion is slowly regained. The shoulder, which was significantly lower than the normal side after the injury, is now symmetrical to the normal side. Healing results in a lump over the area of the break, which in the young child will disappear in a period of 6 to 8 months. In a teenager, the bony lump may persist for as long as 2 or 3 years before remodeling occurs. In the adult, the bump over the fracture site is usually permanent, as the remodeling potential of the bone is limited.

## Fracture of the Radius and Ulna

Fracture of the two forearm bones below the elbow is a common childhood injury. Treatment consists of realigning the fractured bones under general anesthesia and with the assistance of X-ray. Open operation is sometimes necessary, especially if the bone has come out of the skin during the injury. Once satisfactory alignment is obtained, the fracture site is immobilized by a cast that may extend above the elbow. Healing time is generally related to the child's age. Rehabilitation following removal of the cast may take place for another 6 to 8 weeks to redevelop normal range of motion and muscle strength. Swimming is an excellent rehabilitative activity because it helps to regain a full range of motion and improvement in muscle tone without risk of injury. Contact sports should not be permitted until muscle strength has returned.

## Fracture of the Humerus

A supracondylar fracture of the humerus, just above the elbow joint, is a common fracture in childhood. It is usually caused by a fall on the outstretched arm. Treatment is difficult because of its close proximity to the elbow and the risk of accompanying nerve and blood vessel damage. The fracture is managed by realignment under general anesthesia and sometimes the use of pin fixation to hold the fracture fragments in place. After the fracture is healed, the pins are removed and rehabilitation begins. If there has been damage to the nerves around the elbow, rehabilitation is prolonged and may involve additional splinting.

If the joint space is involved by the fracture, a surgical operation is necessary to repair the bone and joint. Treatment of these fractures is difficult, and the prognosis is variable depending on the severity of the injury, the extent of the associated soft tissue injury, and the degree of injury to the growing area of bone.

Fractures to the midsection or upper end of the humerus near the shoulder are common. These injuries occur with a fall or direct blow to the tip of the shoulder. If the fracture is significantly displaced, realignment is necessary. Healing time varies according to the child's age, and rehabilitation of the shoulder and surrounding muscles will take an additional 6 to 8 weeks.

## Neck Injuries

If a child falls or sustains a direct blow to the head and complains of severe pain in the neck region, the child must not be moved until trained personnel are available. Tight clothing around the neck can be carefully loosened to enhance breathing, and the child should be made as comfortable as possible and kept warm. Trained personnel will use spinal precautions to protect the spinal cord from injury during the trip to the emergency room.

# OVERUSE SYNDROMES
# OF THE LOWER EXTREMITIES

Children may develop pain in the extremities following excessive or repetitive exercise over prolonged periods of time. The most common overuse syndromes in children involve the areas around joints where large muscle groups attach to the bone. These attachment areas are regions where growth takes place and cannot sustain prolonged forces.

Sometimes the child may experience pain directly over the heel after repeatedly landing on the tip of the heel during gymnastic dismounts. Injury in this case is usually to the soft tissues surrounding the heel, which may require 6 to 12 weeks to recover. An X-ray should be obtained to rule out an undisplaced stress fracture of the heel bone or a cyst that might have predisposed the heel to injury. Treatment is conservative and normally consists of rest and analgesics.

Pain in and around the ankle that radiates into the front portion of the leg with running suggests shin splints. In this condition, the muscles in the front of the leg that are responsible for lifting the ankle during the swing-through part of gait become very painful. It is generally believed that muscles that develop shin splints lack appropriate blood supply. The lack of blood supply is due to the muscles being squeezed or held too tightly by the fibrous envelope in which they are enclosed. Shin splints of mild to moderate severity can be managed by limiting activity, or modifying shoe wear and running patterns. Taping the ankle at 90 degrees of dorsiflexion is sometimes of help as it prevents excessive stretch of the anterior compartment muscles. Shin splints that are not relieved by rest occasionally require surgical treatment. If the cycle is not broken by relieving the pressure surgically, the muscle will degenerate and function will be lost. Thus, shin splints that do not respond to conservative measures require assessment and treatment. X-rays must be taken to rule out a stress fracture. Stress fractures of the tibia or fibula are commonly due to excessive running on hard surfaces. Most can be visualized with an X-ray, but sometimes a bone scan is necessary to see the stress fracture line. The X-ray also rules out other causes of weakness to the bone, such as osteoporosis or cysts within the bone.

The "march fracture" presents with foot pain after prolonged marching or hiking. It is a stress fracture of the second metatarsal bone near the second toe. Diagnosis is made by history and X-ray or a bone scan. This type of fracture is managed by wearing a sturdy, hard-soled shoe to relieve pain on walking.

Participants in sports that require significant tiptoe weight bearing, such as dancing and gymnastics, may develop pain in the area of the inside of the arch of the foot. This is caused by excessive strain to the navicular bone where the posterior tibial tendon attaches.

# OVERUSE SYNDROMES
# OF THE UPPER EXTREMITIES

Overuse syndromes of the upper extremities, particularly tennis elbow, are relatively common. Tennis elbow is characterized by pain over the outside of the elbow following excessive rotational activity of the forearm. The repetitive activity results in inflammation over the lateral or outside portion of the elbow, with some swelling and excessive pain. Acutely, tennis elbow is treated by resting, applying ice, and using a mild analgesic. Sporting activity should be discontinued until all signs of swelling and tenderness have disappeared. Generally, modifying the arm swing or movement and wearing an elastic support will be sufficient to prevent recurrence of tennis elbow. Occasionally, tennis elbow becomes a chronic problem. The solution is not universally accepted, and treatment is not always successful. For the most part, cortisone injections into the elbow joint in the adolescent are not indicated, and surgical treatment is a last resort. The chronic problem usually is managed by an elastic support, modification of the inciting activity, and participation to the limit of pain tolerance.

# SUMMARY

The medical specialty of orthopedics is directed to the diagnosis and management of disorders of the musculoskeletal system. Orthopedic problems may be congenital and lifelong or results of accidents or injuries. If abnormalities of the muscles, joints, and bones are neglected or untreated in children, a crippling deformity or severe loss of function may result. On the other hand, aggressive therapy of congenital malformations or accidents involving the skeleton can result in an impressive recovery of function. Treatment may require prolonged therapy using surgical procedures, physical therapy, casting, and bracing. This chapter reviewed some orthopedic conditions and sports injuries that are common in school-age children. The teacher is in an unequaled position to detect early symptoms and signs of a child's orthopedic disorder and to initiate timely referral prior to the development of an irreversible disability. Finally, an appreciation by the educator of certain pediatric and adolescent musculoskeletal conditions will serve to support and enhance the affected student's rehabilitation period.

## RESOURCES

Association of Children's Prosthetic & Orthotic Clinics of North America
6300 North River Road, Suite 727
Rosemont, IL 60018-4226
http://www.aaos.org

The War Amputations of Canada
Child Amputee Program
2827 Riverside Drive
Ottawa, ON K1V 0C4
Canada
http://www.waramps.ca

## SUGGESTED READING

Crenshaw, A. H. (1992). *Campell's operative orthopaedics* (8th ed.). St. Louis, MO: Mosby.
Lovell, W. W., & Winter, R. B. (1990). *Pediatric orthopedics* (3rd ed.). Philadelphia: Lippincott.
Tachdjian, M. O. (1990). *Pediatric orthopedics* (2nd ed.). Philadelphia: Saunders.
Weinstein, S. L. (1994). *The pediatric spine*. New York: Raven Press.

## REFERENCES

Kay, H. W., Day, H. J., Henkel, H. L., Kruger, L. M., Lamb, D. W., Marquardt, E., Mitchell, R., Swanson, A. B., & Willert, H. G. (1975). The proposed international terminology for the classification of congenital limb deficiencies. *Developmental and Medical Child Neurology Supplement, 34,* 1–12.
Kubler-Ross, E. (1993). *On death and dying*. New York: Macmillan.

# CHAPTER 13

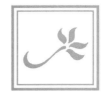

# Common Neurological Disorders in Children

### Robert H. A. Haslam

**T**he intent of this chapter is to outline four neurological disorders prevalent in children that may be encountered by the teacher: headaches, epilepsy, head injuries, and Tourette syndrome. The presenting symptoms are stressed to familiarize the educator with the clinical composition of these common conditions. In particular, certain neurological features are emphasized to illustrate the interaction among the child, the school, and the learning process.

This brief account of common neurological conditions in children should serve to alert the teacher to the inherent complexities associated with disorders of the child's central nervous system. Cooperation on the part of the educator and the physician in sharing knowledge and concerns about these sorts of problems will accomplish a mutual understanding for the ultimate benefit of the child.

## HEADACHE

Headache is a common condition in children and young adults. One study suggested that 48% of children experience headaches, albeit infrequently (Billie, 1962). Another found an incidence of approximately 15% in young adolescents (Hughes & Cooper, 1956). Oster (1972) suggested a prevalence of 20% in children of school age. The effect of headaches on a child's academic performance, personality, memory, and interpersonal relationships, as well as school attendance, depends on their frequency, intensity, and etiology. Thus, if headaches are frequent and incapacitating, they may interfere with intellectual fulfillment and occasionally may represent a life-threatening symptom. For that reason, frequent headaches deserve careful medical scrutiny.

There are many reasons for headaches in the school-age child, but their delineation is often difficult. Contrary to popular belief, refractive errors of vision, strabismus, sinusitis, and malocclusion of the teeth are not common causes. Any child who develops a high fever, for whatever cause, or has a systemic illness (e.g., pneumonia) may develop a headache that tends to parallel the severity of the illness. This headache always disappears with recovery from the primary sickness.

In this section, three major types of headache are discussed: migraines, tension (or muscle contraction) headaches, and headaches caused by increased intracranial pressure. For a comprehensive discussion of other possible sources of headache in children, the reader is referred to other texts (e.g., Barlow, 1984; Friedman & Harms, 1967; Gupta & Rothner, 2001; Shinnar & D'Souza, 1982; Stafstrom, Rostasy, & Minster, 2002).

## Migraines

*Migraine* is defined as a recurrent headache accompanied by symptom-free intervals and at least three of the following symptoms or associated findings: abdominal pain, nausea or vomiting, throbbing headache, unilateral location, associated aura (visual, sensory, motor), relief following sleep, and a positive family history (Prensky & Sommer, 1979). Migraines are relatively common in children. Because these headaches are rarely severe, medical advice is not always sought. The youngest child known to develop migraine was approximately 1 year old (Vahlquist, 1955). Migraine accounts for about 25% of all cases of headache in children. In an extensive, well-organized study in Uppsala, Sweden, Billie (1962) noted a 4% incidence of migraine in school children between the ages of 7 and 15. Prior to adolescence, the gender distribution is equivalent; however, later in life, girls are more frequently affected by migraine.

### Precipitating Factors

In children, migraine headaches tend to have many characteristics that set them apart from migraines in adults. Migraine attacks are precipitated by a multitude of factors: tension; bright, flashing lights such as those from a movie or television screen; excessive physical exertion; mild head trauma; excessive noise, hunger, or alcohol consumption; and oral contraceptive use by the adolescent. One interesting finding is that some children develop migraine headaches following a stressful event, such as undergoing an examination, presenting a speech, participating in an athletic event, or performing in a school play. In contrast to tension headaches, migraine headaches frequently occur on weekend days. Migraine develops in children from all social strata and appears to be more common in compulsive, highly competitive children. Contrary to many reports, migraines can be found in the child with a disability as well as the very bright and intelligent student without a disability.

## Prodome (Aura)

One possible reason for the difficulty in diagnosing migraine headaches in children is that children do not appear to have warning signs (*prodrome* or *aura*) as frequently as do adults. An alternative explanation may be that the child misinterprets these symptoms or gives little significance to them. *Prodromal* (precursory) symptoms are brief and most commonly visual, such as bright, flashing, and often colored lights in the form of stars, zigzag lines, or circles, as well as various crude visual shapes and distortion of body images. A graphic description of visual misinterpretation was depicted by Lewis Carroll, a migraine sufferer, in his *Alice's Adventures in Wonderland* (Carroll, 1865/1984, p. 58). As Alice explains to Caterpillar, "I can't remember things as I used—and I don't keep the same size for ten minutes together!" Other precursory symptoms may include numbness and tingling sensations in the extremities, dizziness, and aphasia.

## Headache Symptoms

The prodromal symptoms are soon followed by the onset of the headache, which may begin in the posterior region of the skull but almost immediately tends to radiate to the forehead, often over an eye or the temple. The headache is described as pounding, pulselike, or throbbing. The headache is frequently not as severe in children as in adults and is usually of shorter duration. During this stage, the child may be extremely confused and belligerent and may prefer to lie down in a quiet, darkened room. Characteristic features that usually accompany the headache are nausea and vomiting, which often are more intense in children. Use of oral medication to alleviate the headache, therefore, is of little benefit to children with these symptoms. Vomiting may be associated with abdominal pain and fever; thus, other conditions such as appendicitis and infection may be incorrectly diagnosed.

The entire migraine attack usually lasts less than 6 hours and is almost always much shorter than what is commonly found in older patients. Afterward, the child awakens from a rather deep sleep in an alert state, asking to be fed and ready to resume normal activities as if nothing had transpired. If migraine attacks are frequent, significant absenteeism from school may result. This can produce anxiety in the child, particularly if school performance diminishes.

## Classification

The Headache Classification Committee of the International Headache Society (1988) recognizes two major types of migraines: without and with aura. Other less common types include migraine variants and complicated migraine.

**COMMON MIGRAINE.** The common migraine is the type that occurs most often in children and is not associated with an aura. A family history, particularly in the mother or her family, exists in approximately 90% of children with common migraine.

**CLASSIC MIGRAINE.** In the classic migraine, an aura precedes headache onset. This aura may consist of blurred vision, depressed vision within the visual field, flashes of light, brilliant white zigzag lines, or irregular distortion of objects. Sensory aura includes numbness of the lips, hands, and feet.

**VARIANTS.** Some individuals experience cyclic vomiting or acute confusional states with migraine. *Cyclic vomiting* consists of periods of intense vomiting on a regular basis, beginning during infancy or the toddler stage. The vomiting may become protracted and lead to dehydration and electrolyte abnormalities, requiring hospitalization and intravenous fluids. Many children with cyclic vomiting have a positive family history of migraine and, as they grow older and become verbal, they describe a typical migraine headache in association with the vomiting. Thus, cyclic vomiting may be the initial manifestation of migraine headache in the preverbal child. *Acute confusional states* may occur during a migraine headache. The child may develop bizarre behavior characterized by confusion, memory disturbances, unresponsiveness, and lethargy, which may persist for several hours.

**COMPLICATED MIGRAINE.** There are three types of complicated migraine. *Basilar migraine* results when the blood vessels that supply the brain stem and cerebellum undergo vasoconstriction. Symptoms include vertigo, double vision, blurred vision, and unsteady gait. Some patients develop alterations in consciousness, such as comatose state, associated with a seizure. *Ophthalmoplegic migraine* is a rare complication in children. It is characterized by a dilated pupil and drooping eyelid on the same side as the headache. *Hemiplegic migraine* is associated with paralysis or weakness on one side of the body. Fortunately, these episodes are rare in children and do not tend to recur.

## Treatment

Treatment for children with migraine headaches can be a challenge for the pediatrician. Before prescribing medication, the doctor must rule out other significant causes of headache. For example, because some symptoms of migraine are similar to epilepsy, an electroencephalogram (EEG) may be considered. Occasionally, the patient may require more specialized studies to rule out abnormalities in the blood vessels (arteriovenous malformation). Thus, a thorough history and physical examination are mandatory. Unfortunately, no laboratory tests ensure a diagnosis of migraine: Results from skull X-rays, computerized tomography (CT) scans, magnetic resonance imaging (MRI), EEG, and blood tests are normal in the child with migraines, in contrast to a patient with epilepsy, arteriovenous malformations, or a brain tumor. Although a thorough psychological examination may demonstrate a compulsive, deliberate, and perhaps insecure student, these findings obviously are not conclusively diagnostic of migraine because they also may be found in many headache-free children.

The initial steps in a treatment regimen should be (a) reassurance of the child and family that the headache is not due to a brain tumor or serious condition, and (b) an attempt to alter or diminish any significant positive causative events. These simple steps significantly reduce the frequency and severity of headaches in most cases. If watching television or movies clearly enhances or provokes migraine headaches, other pleasurable activities should be substituted. Sometimes prolonged parental counseling is necessary to relieve pressures at home or ensure that parents' expectations for the child are realistic. Occasionally, the child with a migraine is in a classroom that is too highly competitive for him or her, necessitating a re-assessment of school placement. Ideally, a conference involving the physician, teacher, and parents will ensure a satisfactory arrangement in most cases. Obviously, the physician and teacher must be cognizant of the pupil who uses headaches as an excuse for not partaking in physical education or other activities that he or she dislikes.

Most migraine headaches in children may be treated simply by the judicious use of acetaminophen or nonsteroidal anti-inflammatory drugs (NSAIDs), particularly if the headaches are relatively mild, infrequent, and of short duration; however, more severe, disabling headaches pose a therapeutic challenge. Ergotamine preparations, which include Cafergot, must be considered for older children and adolescents with severe, classic migraine headaches. These medicines are most efficacious during the early stages of the migraine attack and, for that reason, are of less benefit in children than in adults because children are often unaware of the previously mentioned preliminary symptoms or fail to communicate them to their parents. In addition, as mentioned before, the severe nausea and vomiting so often observed in children preclude the use of orally administered medication.

A major breakthrough in the management of migraine during the past decade has been the discovery that a group of drugs that act as agonists for a vascular 5-hydroxytryptamine receptor subtype (e.g., sumatriptan [Imitrex]) are effective in controlling the headache in acute migraine in adults. Sumatriptan may be given subcutaneously, orally, or by nasal spray. Although this class of drugs has not been formally approved for use in adolescents, recent studies have shown sumatriptan to be an effective drug for the management of acute migraine in adolescents with few undesirable side effects (Winner et al., 2000). Some children with frequent and incapacitating migraine episodes respond favorably to drugs such as propranolol, amitriptyline, phenobarbital, phenytoin (Dilantin), or the calcium-blocking agents; however, they must be administered daily and often produce side effects. Unfortunately, most of these drugs have not been subjected to scientifically well-designed studies of children with migraine. Needless to say, the physician should reevaluate periodically any child on continuous medication for possible harmful drug reactions (including drug dependence and abuse) and, just as important, for the possibility of discontinuing use of the drug. Communication with school personnel may be helpful in this decision.

The teacher may assist the pupil during an acute migraine attack by providing a secluded area in which to rest. In addition, reappraisal of the child's curriculum may demonstrate that undue pressures are being placed on the child. If absenteeism is frequent for a child with migraine, steps should be initiated for medical reevaluation of the student.

Pain management using relaxation techniques and behavior management is an effective treatment for some children and adolescents with migraine. Biofeedback and self-hypnosis programs can be mastered by most children over 8 years of age and have shown positive results in many clinical trials (Olness, MacDonald, & Uden, 1987).

## Tension Headaches

Tension (muscle-contraction) headaches are a relatively common type of headache in children, as in adults. For most children, a tension headache is a rare occurrence and is so clearly related to a stressful, but short-term, situation that treatment is unnecessary. However, for some children these headaches may be frequent and prolonged.

## Symptoms

Tension headaches appear most frequently during school hours, particularly during a test or similar anxiety-provoking circumstance. They rarely occur on weekends and usually have abated by the evening, but may persist for weeks. Some children with tension headaches are found to have parents whose expectations for them—academically or athletically—are far too high. The most common cause of tension headaches in children appears to be unrealistic scholastic goals developed by the parents, teachers, or children themselves. If these headaches occur more often during a vacation period or other time when the child is in greater contact with the parents, parental marital discord or related phenomena may cause the child's anxiety. The student with severe tension headaches frequently has a parent who suffers from similar headaches.

Tension headaches are poorly described by children. They are usually located in the temples, over the forehead, or even in the base of the skull and neck muscles. The headache is usually a steady, dull, aching pain, and is sometimes described as a pressure band constricting the skull. The student may complain of scalp tenderness, particularly during hair combing. These headaches probably are the result of prolonged, unconscious contraction of the muscles of the neck or temples that so often accompanies states of anxiety or tension. Unlike migraine, tension headaches are not associated with nausea or vomiting.

## Diagnosis

The diagnosis of tension headache is made only after excluding other possible causes through use of a careful history and thorough physical and neurological examination. A skull X-ray, EEG, or CT scan is not necessary in most cases because the history and physical examination usually suffice. The physician must then search for possible stressful situations. The teacher may be of great assistance during this phase of the evaluation. Most children have considerable insight into the origin of their emotional problems and, if given the opportunity to speak in confidence with a teacher or pediatrician, will share their concerns. Poor self-image, fear of school failure, and lack of confidence are oft-repeated apprehensions. Occasionally, a child who is depressed will complain of severe headaches (Ling, Oftedal, & Weinberg, 1970). Further questioning may uncover mood changes, lack of energy or excessive fatigue, poor appetite and weight loss, crying spells, and withdrawal from social activities. The term *psychogenic headache* is used to describe headaches caused by severe psychiatric disturbances; children who have this kind are in need of immediate psychiatric evaluation.

## Treatment

The physician's and educator's major responsibility in treatment of tension headaches is to explain to the child that stressful events may culminate in a headache by unconsciously producing isometric contraction of the underlying forehead and temporal muscles. Steps should be taken to alter obvious anxiety-provoking situations. The teacher should be aware of his or her role in this regard. By careful interaction with the child, the teacher can help circumvent certain stressful situations in order to minimize tension-producing episodes. The child and family must be reassured that these headaches are not serious and that a healthy, normal life is to be expected. Acetaminophen, ibuprofen, or other mild analgesics may help in treating tension headaches, but tranquilizers and sedatives are rarely indicated. The physician may choose to hospitalize the child with severe and recurrent tension headaches for observation, particularly if depression is suspected. Biofeedback techniques have proved useful for some children when the previously described measures have been unsuccessful (Baumann, 2002; Diamond, 1979).

## Headaches Due to Increased Intracranial Pressure

Headache may be the earliest symptom of increased pressure within the skull. The causes of increased intracranial pressure in children include brain tumor, chronic lead poisoning, brain abscess, or an abnormal collection of blood clots (subdural hematoma) over the surface of the cortex. In addition, elevation of intracranial pressure may result from hydrocephalus, infection of the central nervous system (meningitis), vitamin A poisoning, water intoxication (the result of water retention and sodium depletion), or, in rare instances, a complication of drug therapy (e.g., tetracycline, an antibiotic, in young children and oral contraceptive agents in female adolescents). The characteristics of the pressure headache vary somewhat, depending on the individual's age and the underlying pathological condition. Sooner or later, other symptoms or neurological signs appear, implying a progressive, destructive process.

The increased pressure headache is the result of abnormal tension or stretching of the cerebral blood vessels and dura, the thick membranous covering of the brain. This kind of headache tends to occur in the early morning hours or shortly after rising. Most children have difficulty describing its location, but it tends to be a diffuse, generalized, often throbbing pain that may be more prominent over the forehead or the occipital region of the skull. Its onset is usually insidious, and in the beginning of the disease process, there may be days or even weeks when the child has no pain. The headache is often made worse by any activity that normally raises the intracranial pressure, such as coughing, sneezing, exercise, or straining during a bowel movement. Certain positions tend to influence the headache: Lying down may enhance the pain, and sitting up or standing may relieve it. Later, the headache becomes more frequent and intense. With increasing intracranial pressure, the child becomes lethargic, uncooperative, and, finally, comatose.

Vomiting may also occur. The child may awaken with a headache and vomit shortly thereafter. He or she usually will not complain of nausea, may eat a normal breakfast immediately following the episode of vomiting, and may remain symptom-free for the duration of the day. Unfortunately, some children who complain of morning vomiting and who appear normal in every other respect are accused of malingering or are thought to display a school phobia. These children require careful medical attention.

## Diagnosis and Treatment

The treatment of intracranial pressure headaches depends on the cause. Every child suspected of increased intracranial pressure must have a thorough examination, including a history, blood pressure determination, and neurological evaluation that includes inspection of the eyegrounds (by using an ophthalmoscope and looking through the pupil to examine the retina) to determine whether the optic nerve is swollen. In addition, certain tests are mandatory. A skull X-ray may show an abnormality suggestive of elevated intracranial pressure (see Figure 13.1).

More specific neuroradiological procedures may clearly outline a specific lesion (see Figures 13.2 and 13.3). The decision as to whether to proceed with further investigation, such as special dye tests or arterial contrast studies (cerebral angiography), is dependent on the outcome of these

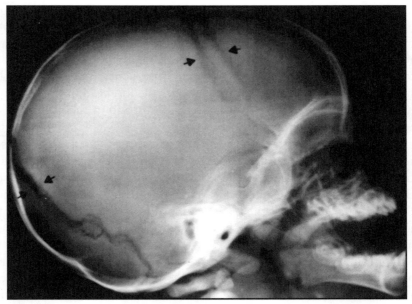

**FIGURE 13.1.** Skull radiograph of an 8-month-old demonstrating separation (arrows) of the sutures (the line of junction of adjacent cranial bones), a reliable sign of increased intracranial pressure.

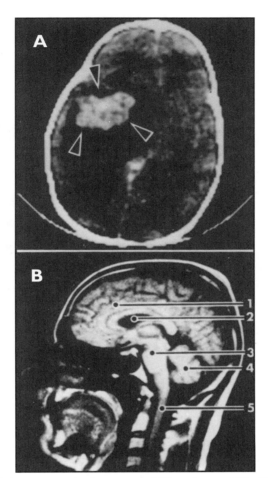

**FIGURE 13.2.** (A) A computerized tomogram (CT scan) on a child with headaches suggestive of increased intracranial pressure. The arrows outline a lobulated tumor that is protruding into the enlarged left lateral ventricle. The tumor, which proved to be a benign choroid plexus papilloma, was successfully removed. The CT scan is an extremely useful and noninvasive method of examining the brain structures. (B) Magnetic resonance imaging (MRI) is the most recently developed noninvasive radiological technique to study the brain and other organs. MRI produces lifelike images and, unlike the CT scan, does not expose the patient to radiation. This sagittal view of a normal patient's head clearly identifies the various components of the brain: 1 = cerebral cortex, 2 = lateral ventricle, 3 = pons, 4 = cerebellum, 5 = spinal cord.

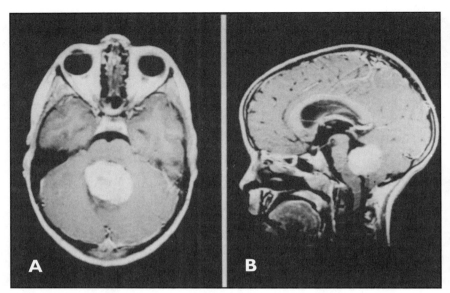

**FIGURE 13.3.** (A) Axial and (B) midsagittal magnetic resonance image (MRI) of a 6-year-old boy with a brain tumor (medulloblastoma) situated in the fourth ventricle. The midsagittal view shows that the tumor is pushing the brain stem forward.

noninvasive studies in conjunction with the patient's neurological findings. If an organic disease process is found, the appropriate medical or surgical therapeutic techniques can be used.

## Symptoms Suggestive of an Organic Cause

Children with recurrent headaches accompanied by other symptoms or signs are more likely to have organic pathology as a cause. A headache that awakens a child during sleep is always of concern. School failure, a change in behavior, or a falloff in linear growth (height) suggest underlying pathology. A seizure in association with a headache, the presence of neurological signs developing during a headache, or visual blurring at the peak of the headache all warrant further investigation by the physician.

# Summary

The investigation and management of headaches in children can be taxing for physicians. A thorough understanding of a child is of considerable importance, particularly if migraine or tension headaches are to be treated successfully. Information from school officials concerning the child's change in personality, decline in school performance, or unusual behavior can be crucial in assisting the physician. The teacher can often initiate a referral to the pediatrician in cooperation with the parents if worrisome symptoms are noted.

Generally speaking, a pattern of recurrent headaches over a prolonged period, with normal behavior and intellectual functioning between episodes, suggests a benign process, such as migraine or tension headaches. The characteristics of the headache—including the inciting factors, location, duration, and associated symptomatology—usually differentiate the two. Many children in this category do not require medical attention because of the sporadic nature and insignificant consequences of their headaches. The educator must be aware of provoking events for the child with more troublesome headaches. Improvement can be expected if the appropriate causative factors can be established and reconciled. Such simple maneuvers as excusing a pupil subject to migraines from observing a movie or participating in functions productive of loud noises (e.g., the school band) may serve to prevent some headaches. Migraine headaches tend to be less severe in adolescence if their onset is prior to 10 years of age (Congdon & Forsythe, 1979). Tension or psychogenic headaches respond favorably to the relief of anxiety-provoking situations and the factors that promote them. Some patients must be taught how to live with their headaches.

Some headaches are worrisome and require prompt medical attention. A sudden, excruciating onset of head pain or an abrupt change in its characteristics suggests an underlying organic disorder, particularly if there is no past history of headache. Any headache that occurs in association with or shortly after head trauma may be extremely serious, no matter how trivial the injury may appear (see the "Head Injuries" section, later in this chapter). All headaches suggestive of increased intracranial pressure justify immediate evaluation. They tend to become more frequent and intense and often are associated with other neurological symptoms in a relatively brief period. The prognosis of headaches due to increased intracranial pressure depends on the underlying abnormality. Early diagnosis and treatment are extremely important as many of these conditions are life-threatening illnesses that can be cured by prompt medical or surgical management.

# EPILEPSY

Epilepsy is a common disorder in school-age children. Most teachers have been confronted by a student with epilepsy; some are fearful of the condition and develop a negative relationship with the child, whereas others become overprotective and solicitous. Even in these modern times, epilepsy is considered by many well-educated but misinformed individuals to represent a host of incredible conditions and aberrations, including mental illness, mental retardation, evil spirits, and perverted thoughts. As a result, the patient with epilepsy may be shunned, shamed, and abused by friends, fellow students, teachers, and even parents.

A *seizure* may be defined as a recurrent involuntary disturbance of brain function that may be manifested as an impairment or loss of consciousness, abnormal motor activity, behavioral abnormality, sensory disturbance, or autonomic dysfunction. It is a symptom of an underlying disorder of the central nervous system. The term *epilepsy* is used to describe a wide variety of disorders due to many different causes and is defined as recurrent seizures unrelated to fever or to an acute cerebral insult. The clinical picture of epilepsy is partially dependent on the age of the child, the etiology of the convulsion, and the area within the brain that is malfunctioning.

Epilepsy occurs in approximately 0.5% of the population, thus affecting about 1 million Americans. The initial presentation commonly occurs during the latter half of the first decade or at the time of adolescence. The causes of convulsions are numerous and include genetic and perinatal factors, complication of a head injury, infections of the central nervous system, congenital malformations, metabolic and degenerative diseases, tumors of the brain, and vascular diseases, as well as poisoning by exogenous substances (Livingston, 1972).

## Classification

It is important for the physician to classify the patient's seizure disorder as precisely as possible. The anticonvulsant medication chosen depends on

## TABLE 13.1
International Classification of Epilepsies and Epilepsy Syndromes

**Localization Related (Focal, Local, Partial) Epilepsies and Epileptic Syndromes**

- *Idiopathic:* Benign childhood epilepsy with centrotemporal spike discharges, childhood epilepsy with occipital paroxysms, primary reading epilepsy

- *Symptomatic:* Temporal lobe, frontal lobe, parietal lobe, and occipital lobe epilepsies; chronic progressive epilepsia partialis continua of childhood

**Generalized Epilepsies and Syndromes**

- *Idiopathic* (with age-related onset): Benign neonatal convulsions, benign neonatal familial convulsions, benign myoclonic epilepsy in infancy, childhood absence epilepsy, juvenile absence epilepsy, juvenile myoclonic epilepsy, epilepsy with grand mal seizures on awakening, epilepsies precipitated by specific modes of activation

- *Cryptogenic or symptomatic:* West syndrome (infantile spasms), Lennox–Gastaut syndrome, epilepsy with myoclonic seizures

- *Symptomatic:* Early myoclonic epilepsy, early infantile encephalopathy, and specific syndromes including disorders in which seizures are a predominant feature

**Epilepsies and Epileptic Syndromes Undetermined Whether Focal or Generalized**

Neonatal seizures, severe myoclonic epilepsy of infancy, acquired epileptic aphasia (Landau–Kleffner syndrome)

**Special Syndromes**

Febrile convulsions, isolated seizures or isolated status epilepticus, seizures occurring only when there is an acute metabolic or toxic event

*Note.* Symptomatic epilepsies have a known etiology, whereas cryptogenic epilepsies do not have a known etiology. Adapted from "Proposal for Revised Classification of Epilepsies and Epileptic Syndromes," by the Commission on Classification and Terminology of the International League Against Epilepsy, 1989, *Epilepsia, 30,* pp. 389–399.

the seizure type. Some conditions may be confused with epilepsy, including breath-holding spells, temper tantrums, rage attacks, sleepwalking, night terrors, fainting, and hysteria (pseudoseizures). These paroxysmal events can only be differentiated from epilepsy by a thorough history, examination, and EEG. The classification of epilepsy, as developed by the Commission on Classification and Terminology of the International League Against Epilepsy (1989), is shown in Table 13.1.

## Partial Seizures

Previously, partial seizures were classified as *psychomotor* or *temporal lobe epilepsy.* Partial seizures are subdivided into simple partial and complex partial seizures.

### Simple Partial Seizures (SPS)

SPS are characterized by clonic or tonic movements that involve the face, neck, or extremities. *Versive seizures,* which consist of the head and eyes turning to one side, are particularly common in SPS. Some children complain of an aura, including chest discomfort or a headache, before the onset of the seizure. The entire seizure persists for 10 to 20 seconds and consciousness is maintained throughout the seizure.

### Complex Partial Seizures (CPS)

CPS may begin as SPS, with or without an aura, and are always followed by a period of altered consciousness. An aura characterized by vague abdominal discomfort or fear is present in approximately one third of children with SPS and CPS. During the period of impaired consciousness, the child may have a blank, "spacey" expression and is unresponsive to verbal commands. During the seizure, approximately 50% to 75% of children with CPS will have *automatisms,* which follow loss of consciousness and consist of lip smacking, chewing, and persistent swallowing movements. Automatisms in older children are characterized by semipurposeful, uncoordinated movements, such as pulling at clothing, buttoning and unbuttoning a garment, repetitive rubbing of objects, or running and clinging to a parent, friend, or object in an uncontrolled and frightened manner. A child with CPS may have a focal or generalized grand mal seizure with spread of the epileptiform discharge (the burst of seizure activity in the brain). With these seizures, the head and eyes may turn to one side, the eyes may blink, and tonic–clonic movements may begin on one side of the body and then become generalized. CPS are associated with EEG abnormalities in the majority of children, especially temporal lobe sharp waves or spikes (see Figure 13.4). CT scanning and especially MRI

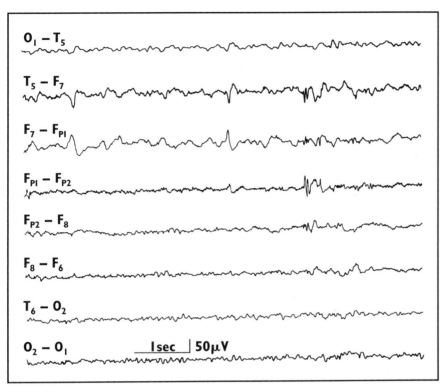

**FIGURE 13.4.** An abnormal electroencephalogram supporting the clinical diagnosis of complex partial epilepsy in a 10-year-old boy. Note the spikes or seizure discharges in $T_5$–$F_7$ and $F_7$–$F_{P1}$.

studies may show a lesion in a temporal lobe in children with CPS, including scar tissue (the result of a head injury, previous prolonged seizure, birth injury, or meningitis), an arteriovenous malformation, or a slow-growing brain tumor.

Students with CPS are at a greater risk for learning disorders than are children without seizures. They may display a shortened attention span or inability to concentrate. A few children tend to display temper tantrums or acting-out behavior, which will require psychiatric consultation. Fortunately, with appropriate medication and counseling, the behavior outbursts and convulsions can usually be controlled.

## Generalized Seizures

### Absence Seizures

Absence (petit mal) seizures commonly have an onset between the ages of 5 and 10 years and are more prevalent in girls. The seizure is manifested by brief episodes of staring, usually less than 30 seconds, and is never associated with an aura. The child momentarily appears to be disinterested and out of contact with reality. There may be lapses of speech and fluttering of the eyelids, but the child does not fall. Automatisms may also occur with absence seizures, confusing the diagnosis with CPS. Absence seizures may occur so frequently that they interfere with a child's concentration and school performance (Freemon, Douglas, & Penry, 1973). Frequent seizures undoubtedly interfere with memory.

The investigation of children with absence epilepsy is often initiated by the teacher. The physician may enhance or demonstrate an episode of this type of epilepsy by asking the child to take deep breaths (hyperventilate) for a period of several minutes. This technique is particularly useful in the EEG laboratory (see Figure 13.5). Unfortunately, absence epilepsy is not

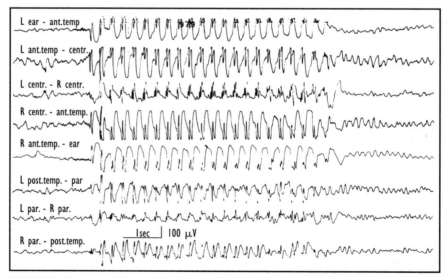

**FIGURE 13.5.** An electroencephalogram showing the typical three-per-second discharges of absence epilepsy. Note the sudden return to normalcy at the termination of the recording.

always diagnosed, and some children with this disorder are disciplined for their general lack of academic interest and enthusiasm. The condition must be differentiated from daydreaming, which is more frequently the result of a boring classroom environment, a tired student, or perhaps a longing anticipation for the events of the upcoming weekend.

## Generalized Tonic–Clonic Seizures

Tonic–clonic (grand mal) convulsions are the most common and, to the uninitiated, the most frightening form of epilepsy. On occasion, the patient can anticipate a seizure minutes or hours prior to its occurrence. A severe headache, tired feeling, or clouding of the sensorium may be warning symptoms.

The convulsion is usually initiated by sudden loss of consciousness. The child may fall, the eyes roll upward, respirations momentarily cease, and the face become slightly dusky. At this point, rhythmic synchronous movements of the extremities and face may develop; these usually persist for a few minutes, but in rare cases for hours. The convulsion may be focal, involving only one side of the body; more frequently, it is generalized. During this phase of the convulsion, the patient's arms and legs are rigid. Within minutes, the child usually becomes relaxed, moans, and may begin to move spontaneously. In most instances, the patient is drowsy following a convulsion and prefers to sleep, although the child can be aroused.

If a patient has persistent or repetitive seizures without regaining consciousness in the interval for a period greater than 30 minutes, a medical emergency exists. The child must be immediately transported to a hospital for treatment of this complication of epilepsy, known as *status epilepticus*. The most important cause of status epilepticus is failure of the patient to take anticonvulsant medication on a regular basis, including sudden unsupervised withdrawal from the drug.

## Myoclonic Seizures

Myoclonic seizures consist of repetitive, brief, symmetric muscular contractions with loss of body tone, which may cause the child to fall, resulting in trauma to the face and mouth. The subtypes of myoclonic epilepsy that most commonly develop during infancy and school-age years are discussed here.

**TYPICAL EARLY CHILDHOOD MYOCLONIC EPILEPSY.** Children with typical myoclonic epilepsy exhibit no symptoms prior to the onset of seizures, which is between 2 and 4 years of age. About 50% of children with this type of epilepsy also have occasional generalized tonic–clonic seizures. At least one third of children with this disorder have a positive family history of epilepsy, which suggests a genetic cause for the disorder. The long-term prognosis is relatively favorable, with at least half of the children becoming seizure-free several years later. Mental retardation develops in a few patients, but learning and language disabilities, as well as behavioral problems, occur in a significant number of these children and require management in a multidisciplinary setting.

**COMPLEX MYOCLONIC EPILEPSY.** Complex myoclonic epilepsy begins with tonic–clonic seizures during the first year of life, followed by the development of myoclonic seizures (see Figure 13.6). Many children with this disorder have developmental delays prior to the onset of seizures. Complex myoclonic seizures are not associated with a positive family history of epilepsy. Unfortunately, these children have a poor prognosis. In spite of anticonvulsant therapy, the seizures persist and are associated with mental retardation and behavioral disabilities in 75% of cases.

**JUVENILE MYOCLONIC EPILEPSY.** Juvenile myoclonic epilepsy typically begins in early adolescence and is characterized by frequent myoclonic jerks, especially on awakening, which makes hair combing and toothbrushing difficult, as the comb or toothbrush is flung from the patient's hand during a seizure. Most of these patients also have generalized tonic–clonic seizures. This form of epilepsy is well controlled with the anticonvulsant valproic acid, and the long-term prognosis is excellent.

**PROGRESSIVE MYOCLONIC EPILEPSY.** Progressive myoclonic epilepsy comprises a heterogeneous group of rare genetic disorders that uniformly have a grave prognosis. Tonic–clonic seizures develop in a previously normal child between 10 and 18 years of age. Within a short period of time, myoclonic seizures become evident. Deterioration of cognitive function and academic performance is apparent within 1 year of the onset of seizures. Neurological abnormalities, including ataxia and poor coordination, are associated with the seizure disorder. The myoclonic seizures are not controlled by anticonvulsants, but the tonic–clonic seizures are prevented by a combination of valproic acid and a benzodiazepine. Progressive myoclonic epilepsy is slowly progressive and often leads to death within 5 to 10 years of the onset of seizures.

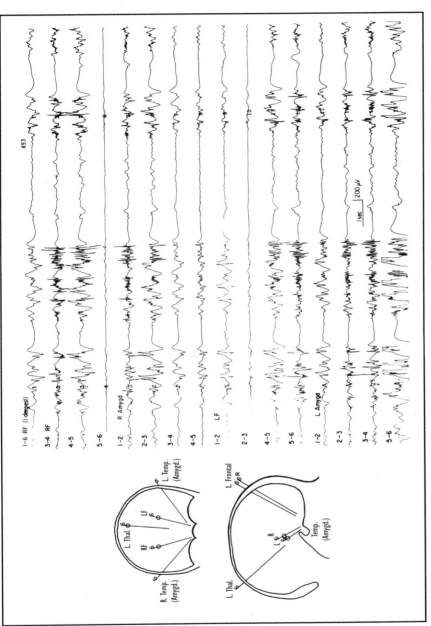

**FIGURE 13.6.**  Intermittent bursts of spikes followed by slowing is a common finding in the electroencephalogram in patients with myoclonic seizures.

## Epilepsy Syndromes

A more recent approach to classifying epilepsy is by syndrome delineation. Many epilepsy syndromes result from a gene mutation, explaining the strong family history of seizures in some patients. Epilepsy syndromes are characterized by a typical age of onset, a specific seizure type, responsiveness to anticonvulsant drugs, and prognosis. The syndromic taxonomy of epilepsy provides a significant advantage compared to previous classifications by providing the physician with guidelines for selecting the most appropriate anticonvulsant, choosing those patients who are most likely to benefit from epilepsy surgery, and counseling patients and families with a reliable prognosis. Examples of epilepsy syndromes include infantile spasms (West syndrome), the Lennox-Gastaut (complex myoclonic epilepsy) syndrome, the Landau-Kleffner syndrome (acquired aphasia), and juvenile myoclonic epilepsy (Janz syndrome). Benign partial epilepsy with centrotemporal spikes (Rolandic epilepsy) is one of the most common epilepsy syndromes in school-age children. The peak onset is between 9 to 10 years of age, with a range from 2 to 14 years. The child's cognitive development and neurological examination are normal. There is often a positive family history of epilepsy. Seizures tend to occur during sleep or upon awakening and typically cause numbness of the tongue and cheek, unilateral tonic contractions of the face and extremities, guttural noises, and excessive salivation. The seizures are usually brief and infrequent and are associated with an excellent prognosis, as most children outgrow them by adolescence. The EEG shows a characteristic spike discharge pattern in the region of the temporal lobe.

## Management

The successful management of a child with epilepsy is dependent on many factors. The patient who has a clear understanding of the disorder is in a better position to cope with frustrations as they occur. The child, physician, parent, and educator must appreciate the many facets of epilepsy to ensure that the child has a normal, happy, and fulfilling existence.

### Emergency First Aid

The only type of epilepsy that warrants emergency assistance is the tonic–clonic variety. The others are often unrecognized and are rarely associated with complications. If a patient is actively convulsing, he or she should be moved from potentially dangerous areas, such as the Bunsen burner in the chemistry laboratory or the kitchen stove in the home economics class. The child should be placed in a horizontal position, preferably lying on the side, and tight or confining garments should be loosened. The patient *must have a free airway:* The mouth and nose should be uncovered and any substances in the oral cavity (including candy, chewing gum, or food) removed, if possible. Blunt objects such as a spoon, stick, or finger should not be forced into a patient's oral cavity during a seizure, as a tooth may be dislodged and aspirated into the lungs. If the convulsive movements are vigorous, the patient can be gently restrained. The majority of major motor convulsions may be managed in this fashion, and complete recovery is anticipated. If the seizure is prolonged (greater than 10 minutes), an ambulance should be summoned and the child given further care by a physician.

## Medical Investigation

The physician initiates a course of management by seeking a cause for the seizure through taking a careful history and performing a physical examination. A complete description of the convulsion by a parent or teacher is an essential component of the investigation, as in most instances the seizure activity has ceased by the time the child reaches the hospital or doctor's office.

After the examination, the pediatrician may perform a variety of blood tests, including a fasting serum glucose and calcium, and perhaps amino acid and lead level analyses. In addition, a CT scan or MRI may be ordered and the cerebrospinal fluid may be examined to determine whether the child has meningitis. These tests are carried out to seek a specific cause for the seizure, enabling the physician to provide a direct approach to its treatment. The interpretation and value of an EEG are misunderstood by many individuals. The physician orders this examination only to confirm the clinical impression. However, the EEG can be quite useful as a diagnostic tool when done in the proper context (see Figure 13.7 for a normal EEG reading).

## Anticonvulsant Therapy

In recent decades, significant advances have been made for the treatment of epilepsy with the discovery of effective anticonvulsant drugs. Examples

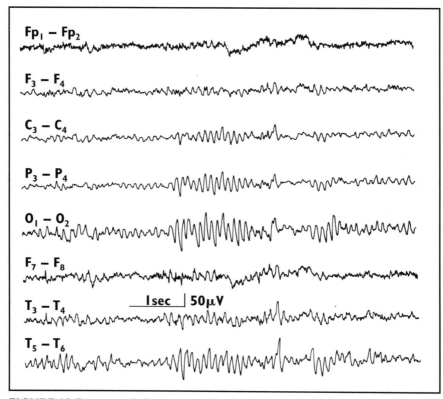

**FIGURE 13.7.** A normal electroencephalogram.

of useful anticonvulsants include valproic acid for the management of absence epilepsy, carbamazepine for partial and generalized epilepsies, and gabapentin for refractory complex partial seizures. The majority of children with complex partial, absence, and tonic–clonic seizures can be expected to become seizure-free through the use of specific anticonvulsant drugs.

The principles of anticonvulsant therapy include the selection of an appropriate drug and the use of one drug (monotherapy), if at all possible, to minimize untoward side effects and prevent drug interaction. It is the physician's responsibility to forewarn the parents and child of potential side effects and to explain the need for routine blood tests to monitor the drug's safety. Table 13.2 summarizes the more commonly used anticonvulsants, the seizure type(s) for which they are most effective, and the unwanted side effects that may be particularly evident in the classroom. A major advance in the management of epilepsy has been the ability to accurately

**TABLE 13.2**
Anticonvulsants: Use and Side Effects

| Generic Drug (Brand) | Seizure Type | Side Effects and Toxicity |
|---|---|---|
| Carbamazepine (Tegretol) | Generalized tonic–clonic, partial | Dizziness, drowsiness, double vision, liver dysfunction, anemia, low white blood cell count |
| Clonazepam (Rivotril, Klonopin) | Absence, myoclonic, partial | Drowsiness, irritability, behavioral abnormalities, depression, salivation |
| Ethosuximide (Zarontin) | Absence | Low white blood count, liver dysfunction |
| Gabapentin (Neurontin) | Complex partial, second-ary generalized | Somnolence, dizziness, ataxia, headache, tremor, vomiting, nystagmus, fatigue |
| Lamotrigine (Lamictal) | Complex partial, absence, myclonic, tonic–clonic | Rash, dizziness, ataxia, headache, nausea, vomiting, somnolence |
| Phenobarbital | Generalized tonic–clonic | Hyperactivity, irritability, short attention span, temper tantrums, altered sleep pattern |
| Phenytoin (Dilantin) | Generalized tonic–clonic, partial | Gum swelling, increased body hair, unsteady gait, skin rash |
| Primidone (Mysoline) | Generalized tonic–clonic, partial | Personality changes, aggressive behavior similar to phenobarbital |
| Topiramate (Topamax) | Complex partial | Fatigue, cognitive depression |
| Valproic acid (Depakene) | Absence, generalized tonic–clonic, myoclonic | Occasional drowsiness, hair loss, weight gain, tremor, liver dysfunction, coma |

measure the quantity of anticonvulsant within the blood. If a child continues to have frequent seizures and the blood level for the specific drug is too low, adjustment of the anticonvulsant may control the convulsions.

Failure to direct therapy to the "whole child" eventually results in lack of cooperation, erratic intake of medication or noncompliance, and gradual reappearance of the seizures. The physician must be in contact with the patient at regular intervals to readjust the anticonvulsant medication, attempt to answer questions, alleviate fears, and assume responsibility for discontinuing the drug when medically feasible.

## Surgery

Surgery should be considered for those children with intractable seizures who are unresponsive to anticonvulsant therapy and who have EEG evidence of a focal onset of seizures. EEG recording with video monitoring for prolonged periods may be necessary to confirm the focal onset of seizures. Children are usually hospitalized for the procedure, and anticonvulsant use is lowered or discontinued in order to record several seizures. The EEG recordings are complemented by neuropsychological studies and neuroimaging tests, including MRI, single photon emission computed tomography (SPECT), or positron emission tomography (PET), to determine if a lesion that coincides with the focal EEG abnormality can be identified. The results of epilepsy surgery are excellent for children with a well-defined focus of epileptogenic activity associated with a structural lesion identified by MRI scanning in the same region of the EEG abnormality (Engel, 1987).

## Long-Term Management

Physicians know that certain events tend to precipitate or enhance seizures. For example, the child with seizures who is experiencing undue emotional stress or who is ill and not sleeping well is at a greater risk for worsening of the convulsive disorder. Some physicians believe that puberty is a particularly vulnerable period in the life of a child with epilepsy.

A concerted effort must be made to allow the child with epilepsy to lead as normal a life as possible. The reasons for long-term anticonvulsant medication should be stressed, and it should be explained that anticonvulsants are not addictive. Most children may be reassured that they will eventually "outgrow" their epilepsy and lead perfectly normal lives. Recent studies suggest that a seizure-free period of 2 years in a neurologically normal child is associated with a good prognosis, so that the physician may elect to taper and eventually discontinue the anticonvulsant at that time (Emerson et al., 1981; Shinnar et al., 1994; Sirven, Sperling, & Wingerchuk, 2001; Thurston, Thurston, Hixon, & Keller, 1982). Children who have seizures that are well controlled should be allowed to engage in activities of all types, with the exception of unsupervised swimming or bathing and participation in contact sports such as football.

## The Teacher's Role

Many parents do not inform school officials of their children's seizure disorders because of the concern that these children may be ostracized. Some schools resist the responsibility of dispensing the child's midday anticonvulsant medication. Thus, the pupil with epilepsy may face the embarrassment of his or her parent personally delivering the medication.

School administrators and educators must take a more positive attitude. Teachers must be aware of the fundamental principles of epilepsy and its management. The educator is in a position to help normalize the life of an epileptic child. The astute educator may use this opportunity to teach the facts of epilepsy to the entire class so that the social stigma of seizures will be lessened and epileptic children allowed to truly function as normal individuals.

Finally, the educator may play an active role in the management of a child with convulsions. The educator's observations of seizure activity in a child with epilepsy will enhance the physician's capability to prescribe accurately the proper quantity of an anticonvulsant drug for the child. Severe seizures may be adequately controlled in the hospital, but with a change in activity at home or at school the seizures may reappear. An educator's observations could be of considerable assistance in such a situation. Is the child excessively drowsy, suggesting too much medication? Has the pupil become hyperactive, combative, or recalcitrant, perhaps indicating an adverse reaction to the drug? Is the child alert, cooperative, and apparently seizure-free? Finally, these children require careful monitoring because learning disabilities are more common in children with epilepsy than in the general population. Most children with epilepsy will have their seizures well controlled by medication, will have normal intelligence, and can be expected to lead normal lives. Cooperation among patient, parent, physician, and educator provides a ready avenue for this goal.

# HEAD INJURIES

Head injury is a common phenomenon in infants and children. It is the rare child who reaches adolescence without experiencing a blow to the head that produces momentary loss of consciousness, a brief period of dazed-ness, or, in some cases, more significant trauma requiring hospitalization. The intent of this section is not to discuss in detail the physiology, pathol-ogy, or acute management of cerebral injury in children, but rather to clas-sify the various types of head trauma and highlight possible complications that may interfere with satisfactory achievement at home and at school.

Approximately 22,000 children and adolescents die of trauma annu-ally in the United States and an additional 600,000 have nonfatal injuries requiring hospitalization, according to the Centers for Disease Control (CDC; 1990a). Statistics compiled by the CDC (1990b) indicate that in 1986 approximately 150,000 children and adolescents younger than age 20 sustained a head injury, leading to 7,000 deaths and 29,000 cases of per-manent disability. Many of the deaths, and a significant number of the long-term sequelae, are preventable by the proper use of seat belts and infant restraints, bicycle helmets, pedestrian pathways, and effective community-based education programs for increasing safety awareness. On a positive note, there has been a substantial reduction of traumatic brain injury–related hospitalizations in the United States since about 1980, particularly for children ages 4 to 14 years. This is likely due to many factors, including injury prevention programs and the ability to make definitive decisions regarding the need for hospitalization for those patients with mild head in-juries following a CT head scan. In spite of these trends, traumatic brain injuries represent a major public health problem which requires more effective methods of injury prevention (Thurman & Guerrero, 1999).

The most common cause of head injury in very young children is a fall from a short distance, which rarely produces neurological problems. Infants and young children subjected to physical abuse, including shaking and striking the head, typically have significant brain injury or die, due to the rotational and deceleration forces that cause shearing of brain sub-stance and acute bleeding. Repeated accidents in children may be reported as falls or clumsiness on the part of the child when, in fact, they are due to abuse on the part of the parent or guardian.

Children are particularly disposed to head injury because of their vari-ous activities, many of which take place in the school yard. Blows to the head from a ball or baseball bat and falls from a swing, bicycle, playground equipment, or tree are all frequent accident causes. Most accidents that pro-duce significant head trauma in children over the age of 3 years are the re-sult of falls, particularly from a bicycle. Children also tend to be injured as pedestrians more commonly than do adults. Boys experience head injury at least twice as frequently as girls. There is strong epidemiological evidence that children with attention-deficit/hyperactivity disorder and learning disabilities are at greater risk for head injury than the general population (Goldstein & Levin, 1987).

The mechanisms of head injury and the resultant brain damage are only partially understood, and it is clear that much is yet to be learned. Various studies have demonstrated that it requires much more force to produce unconsciousness when the head is held in a fixed position than when the skull is freely moving at impact (Denny-Brown & Russell, 1941), explaining the utility of infant restraints and seat belts. The degree of brain trauma is extremely variable and is dependent on the age of the individual, the velocity of the fall or blow, the presence or lack of protective head gear, and whether the injury was a closed or open skull wound. The most immediate response of the brain to significant trauma is the rapid onset of swelling. If the swelling is not recognized and immediately treated, death may ensue.

## Classification

Head injuries may be subdivided into four categories: minor closed head injuries without loss of consciousness, minor closed head injuries with brief loss of consciousness (less than 1 minute), moderate head injury, and severe head injury (American Academy of Pediatrics, 1999). Children with minor head injuries without loss of consciousness have normal mental status and neurological function at the site of the accident. The vast majority experience complete recovery, although a small number experience posttraumatic symptoms, especially vomiting, similar to those children with a mild head injury with loss of consciousness. Moderate and severe head injuries are associated with more extensive injury to the brain; these children are unconscious for greater periods of time than children with minor head injury. Coma, focal neurological signs, and death may ensue.

## Concussion

*Concussion* is the most frequent closed head injury in children and is defined as a traumatically induced alteration in mental status, probably the result of axonal swelling in the brain stem. Contact sports, such as football, boxing, hockey, and martial arts, are the most common causes of concussion. An estimated 250,000 concussions occur annually in the United States (Kelly et al., 1991; see also Durkin, Olsen, Barlow, Virella, & Connolly, 1998).

The duration of amnesia, confusion, and abnormal behavior associated with a concussion may be as brief as a few minutes but frequently persists for several hours. The child is apt to be lethargic, irritable, and pale, and may be confused and disoriented. Vomiting, one of the most common symptoms accompanying a concussion in children, may at times be severe and out of proportion to the apparently mild head trauma. The child also may complain of transient dizziness and headache. The patient prefers to sleep, and, upon awakening a few hours later, he or she usually appears and feels perfectly normal. The child who loses consciousness as a result of a head injury should be transported to a hospital for careful observation. A worsening of the level of consciousness or the evolvement of focal neurological signs (e.g., a dilated pupil, one-sided weakness) suggests the possibility of a more severe injury and warrants further investigation and possible surgical intervention. Any child who is found unconscious without an obvious explanation should be examined and observed by a physician. The Colorado Medical Society (1991) defined the three levels of concussion and steps to be followed when head injury is associated with a sports injury (see Table 13.3).

It is imperative that the child and parents be reassured that the concussion will not produce intellectual deficiency or a physical handicap. The child should be encouraged to return to school and engage in normal activities as soon as feasible.

## Contusion

*Contusion* is a term used to describe an injury to the central nervous system where extensive damage has occurred, including bleeding, bruising, swelling, or laceration of the brain. The lesion may be quite circumscribed but more commonly is widespread; thus, contusion is a more serious injury than concussion.

The clinical findings are dependent on the location or extent of injury, but deep stupor or coma is common. In addition, abnormalities of the pupils, weakness, disturbances of sensation, abnormal body posture, and seizures are frequently encountered signs of brain injury. Needless to say, children displaying these symptoms should be hospitalized immediately for emergency medical and surgical treatment.

**TABLE 13.3**
Colorado Medical Society Guidelines
for the Management of Concussion in Sports

| Concussion Grade | Symptom | Treatment |
|---|---|---|
| 1 | Confusion without amnesia, no loss of consciousness | Remove from contest; examine immediately and every 5 minutes for the development of amnesia or postconcussive symptoms at rest and with exertion; permit return to contest if amnesia does not appear and no symptoms appear for at least 20 minutes. |
| 2 | Confusion with amnesia, no loss of consciousness | Remove from contest and disallow return; examine frequently for signs of evolving intracranial pathology; reexamine the next day; permit return to practice after 1 full week without symptoms. |
| 3 | Loss of consciousness[a] | Transport from field to nearest hospital by ambulance (with cervical spine immobilization if indicated); perform thorough neurologic evaluation immediately; admit to hospital if signs of pathology are detected; if findings are normal, instruct family for overnight observation; permit return to practice only after 2 weeks without symptoms. |

[a] Prolonged unconsciousness, persistent mental status alterations, worsening postconcussion symptoms, or abnormalities on neurologic examination require urgent neurosurgical consultation or transfer to a trauma center.

Note. From *Report of the Sports Medicine Committee: Guidelines for the Management of Concussion in Sports* by Colorado Medical Society, 1991, Denver: Author. Copyright 1991 by Colorado Medical Society. Reprinted with permission.

## Skull Fracture

The presence of a skull fracture following head trauma does not necessarily imply injury to the underlying brain. A child may die following a serious brain injury although the skull may be completely intact. The most common skull fracture is linear (see Figure 13.8). As a rule, this type of fracture does not interfere with the integrity and function of the brain, and the treatment outcome is excellent. If, however, the fracture traverses underlying blood vessels or other important structures, serious complications may result that require immediate medical care. Only an experienced physician, following examination of the child and study of the X-ray, can predict the consequences of a linear skull fracture.

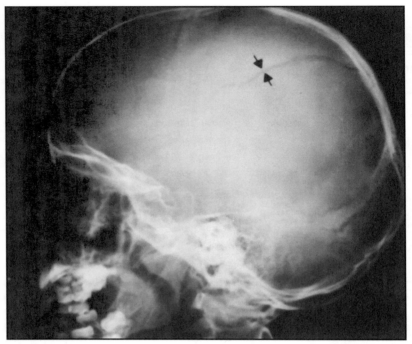

**FIGURE 13.8.** A skull radiograph. Arrows point to a linear skull fracture.

If fractures of the skull are depressed, bony fragments may have penetrated into the substance of the brain. Immediate surgical exploration is necessary to remove any fragments. The base or bottom of the skull may be fractured, which is often the result of a severe injury. Unfortunately, these breaks are difficult to see radiographically. The possibility of a basilar skull fracture becomes a concern when cerebrospinal fluid is dripping from the nostril, blood is observed behind the eardrum, or a bruise develops over the mastoid region. The major concern from a fracture of the base of the skull is the potential for an infection of the central nervous system (meningitis) because of the open entry for bacteria provided by the break.

### Epidural and Subdural Hemorrhage

Because bleeding into the spaces that cover the brain may be fatal, early recognition and therapy are essential. An *epidural hemorrhage* results from disruption of the middle meningeal artery that traverses between the skull and the brain (see Figure 13.9), usually due to a fracture of the overlying bone. The child may very suddenly develop focal neurological signs such as one-sided weakness with rapidly progressive dulling of the sensorium. The outcome is usually favorable if the correct diagnosis and surgical therapy are carried out immediately; if treatment is significantly delayed, the child may die.

A *subdural hematoma* is the consequence of the rupture of fragile veins that drain the cerebral cortex (see Figure 13.10). Large collections of blood interfere with normal cerebral function, may cause herniation (squeezing) of the brain, and can result in death. Although any form of head trauma may produce subdural hematoma, the physically abused child is particularly susceptible to this type of head injury (see Chapter 23).

## Prognosis

The nature and severity of complications and the ultimate prognosis depend on the degree and location of the injured portions of the brain. The Glasgow Coma Scale (Jennett & Teasdale, 1974) can be used as an early predictor of outcome in children with head injuries; an initial score from 3 to 5 is usually associated with a grave prognosis (Grewal & Sutcliffe, 1991) (see Table 13.4). Lieh-Lai et al. (1992) reported that a low Glasgow Coma score does not always accurately predict the outcome in children with a severe traumatic brain injury.

Following head trauma to some children, brief periods of blindness have been observed, often accompanied by restlessness and irritability (Griffith & Dodge, 1968). Fortunately, this phenomenon is reversible. Convulsions are common at the time of the accident, but their presence does not signify long-lasting epilepsy. For the majority of these children, the seizures disappear 1 or 2 days after the accident. However, approximately 5% of children hospitalized for head trauma develop epilepsy. The more severe the injury, the greater the possibility that epilepsy will occur (Caveness, 1976; Englander et al., 2003).

With a severe head injury, a variety of persistent neurological deficits may result, including hemiparesis, disturbances in speech (including aphasia), intellectual deterioration, or behavioral disturbances. As mentioned

(*text continues on p. 386*)

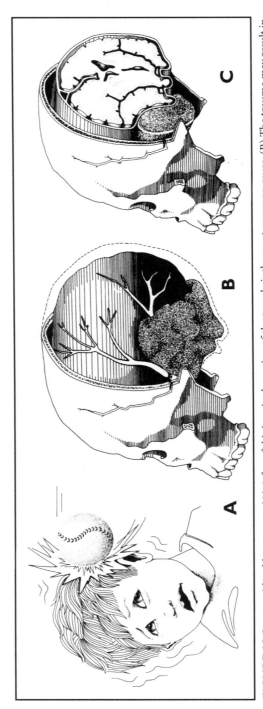

**FIGURE 13.9.** An epidural hematoma. (A) A forceful injury in the region of the temple is the most common cause. (B) The trauma may result in a fractured skull, causing disruption of the middle meningeal artery. Blood collects in the area between the skull and the dura, a tough membrane covering the brain (epidural space). (C) The collection of blood acts as a mass, producing pressure upon vital structures within the brain.

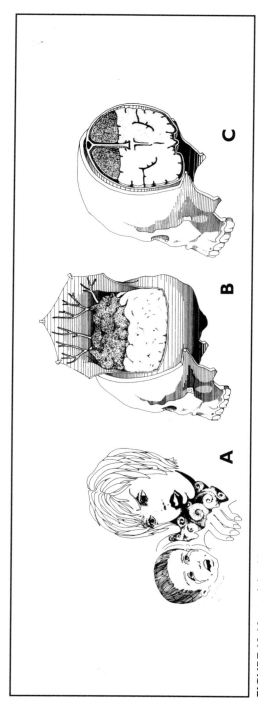

**FIGURE 13.10.** A subdural hematoma. (A) The physically abused child is at risk for a subdural hematoma. (B) The trauma results in rupture of bridging cortical veins due to direct trauma or too vigorous shaking of the child. (C) Venous blood aggregates in a space between the dura and brain (subdural space), often bilaterally. A marked increase in intracranial pressure may result.

**TABLE 13.4**

Scoring of Activities by the Glasgow Coma Scale

| Activity | Best Response | Score |
|---|---|---|
| Eye opening | Spontaneous | 4 |
| | To speech | 3 |
| | To pain | 2 |
| | None | 1 |
| Verbal | Oriented | 5 |
| | Confused | 4 |
| | Inappropriate words | 3 |
| | Nonspecific sounds | 2 |
| | None | 1 |
| Motor | Follows commands | 6 |
| | Localizes pain | 5 |
| | Withdraws to pain | 4 |
| | Abnormal flexion | 3 |
| | Extends | 2 |
| | None | 1 |

previously, many observers have noted that children with personality disorders following serious head injury in fact had unusual behavioral traits prior to their injury that seemed to be enhanced by the accident (Mahoney et al., 1983). Mealey (1968) noted that children who had been culturally and environmentally deprived or emotionally disturbed tended to have more significant posttraumatic personality disturbances than did well-adjusted children.

*Posttraumatic syndrome* may occur in children following relatively minor head trauma (Black, Jeifries, Blumer, Wellner, & Walker, 1969). The essential features of this syndrome include hyperactivity, poor attention span, withdrawal, temper outbursts, and sleep disturbances (Kaufman et al., 2001). Dizziness and headaches occasionally are present as well. Treatment should include a thorough evaluation of the child to eliminate other behavioral causes, followed by reassurance and support, because in most children the condition will improve spontaneously without specific intervention.

The most important determinant of neurological and intellectual recovery in the child with a head injury is the duration of coma. The longer the child is comatose (unresponsive to verbal and physical stimuli), the greater the possibility of neurological, behavioral, or intellectual abnormalities. However, the outcome for these children has improved considerably during the past 10 to 15 years. In Mahoney et al.'s (1983) study of 46 children with severe head trauma and prolonged coma, 38% died. However, upon follow-up examination, one third of the surviving children were found to have recovered fully and an additional one half had returned to school with only mild cognitive or behavioral problems. About 10% had residual motor handicaps but normal intellectual function; the remaining 10% had significant motor and intellectual deficits (Mahoney et al., 1983; see also Scott-Jupp, Marlow, Seddon, & Rosenbloom, 1992).

There are many reasons that the outlook for the child with a severe head injury is better than that for an adult. It is known that the child's brain is more "plastic" than an adult's and generally recovers more completely in a shorter period of time. Important factors in recovery include skilled first aid and stabilization of the patient, including maintenance of the airway, breathing, and circulation at the site of the accident by paramedics and the immediate transport of the child to a hospital trauma center. The treatment of brain swelling with drugs and the close monitoring and treatment of the raised pressure and cerebral circulation within the brain have significantly decreased mortality and long-term sequelae. The ability to perform a CT scan on the child to determine the location, type, and extent of the injury in a quick and noninvasive fashion greatly enhances management of the injury.

Several sophisticated studies of neuropsychological outcomes of children's head injuries have recently been conducted. Children with minor head trauma and brief loss of consciousness have been found to generally function within the normal range (Bijur, Haslum, & Golding, 1990; McKinlay, Dalrymple-Alford, Horwood, & Fergusson, 2002). One study showed that problems with the storage and retrieval of important information and short-term memory were the most common sequelae of significant head injury in children and adolescents (Levin & Eisenberg, 1979). Kionoff, Low, and Clark (1977) followed a cohort of children with head injuries over a 5-year period, using specific neuropsychological tests. They noted a gradual recovery of function that was still evident 5 years following the accident. However, almost one quarter of the children continued to show impairment of cognitive function and related disturbances at the conclusion of the study.

These studies suggest that, although the mortality and morbidity rates for the child with a severe head injury have improved, intellectual and behavioral sequelae are relatively common. Cognitive deficits may not be readily apparent during hospitalization. Neuropsychological evaluation of the child with a severe injury or of the child with a seemingly mild injury who copes poorly in school following the accident is an important method of identifying specific language, memory, or cognitive deficits that may be responsive to special education techniques (Hjern & Nylander, 1962).

## Summary

Most head injuries occurring during childhood are inconsequential. Immediately after an accident, expert medical judgment is necessary to assess the child and to provide medical or surgical care if complications arise (DeVivo & Dodge, 1971; Jennett, 1972).

The use of certain drugs for children may be necessary following a serious head injury. Anticonvulsants may be used for the prevention or treatment of seizures; other specific types of medication may be needed for the management of severe hyperactivity or incapacitating inattentiveness. The educator can assist the parent or physician by relating any apparent benefits or detrimental side effects of these drugs following close observation in the classroom setting. Furthermore, specific rearrangements within the class may be necessary to accommodate the pupil, particularly if a persistent deficit is encountered, such as diminished visual acuity, disturbances of posture, or aberrant speech. The child who has been severely injured may require physical therapy, special language therapy, or remedial instruction. It is extremely important that a child who has sustained a head injury return to school as soon as medically and psychologically feasible. The stimulation of the educational experience and the companionship of colleagues and peers are additional important prescriptions for recovery.

# TOURETTE SYNDROME

Tourette syndrome (TS), a common disorder with a prevalence of approximately 1 in 2,000 children, is inherited as an autosomal dominant trait (Pauls & Leehman, 1986). It occurs more commonly in boys than girls, by a ratio of 3:1. It is characterized by motor and vocal tics. The diagnosis of TS is made when a combination of these tics has been present for longer than 1 year, with an onset prior to 21 years of age. *Motor tics* are brief, jerky, involuntary movements that typically are preceded by a sensation of increasing tension. Fatigue and anxiety exacerbate the motor tics; concentrating on a task usually decreases them. Motor tics tend to be localized to the head and shoulders and include head nodding, eyelid blinking, and shoulder shrugging. *Vocal tics* consist of throat clearing, sniffling and barking, and, rarely, *coprolalia* (the repetitive use of obscene words), *echolalia* (repetition of words addressed to the child), and *palilalia* (repetition of one's own words). Vocal tics tend to develop several months following the onset of motor tics, and the sniffling and throat clearing often are mistakenly ascribed to an allergy. The vocalizations are uncontrollable and may jeopardize the child's social interactions with classmates. The motor tics tend to wax and wane over time; for example, as eyelid blinking or sniffling disappear, a new tic such as head nodding or barking soon follows. The tics become most prominent and vexing during adolescence and on occasion are so severe that they can lead to self-mutilation. Fortunately, these tics become less intense and bothersome in the adult years, and some patients experience prolonged periods of remission.

Obsessive–compulsive behaviors, including uncontrollable touching, licking, repetitive thoughts, and motor actions, occur in approximately 60% of individuals with TS. In addition, attention-deficit/hyperactivity disorder (ADHD) is present in at least 50% of children with TS. In many cases, ADHD precedes the onset of motor and vocal tics by several years. Learning disabilities, particularly problems with mathematics, and behavioral problems are evident in approximately 25% of children with TS. Most children with severe ADHD and TS benefit significantly from stimulant medication. Several reports have implicated stimulant medication (e.g., methylphenidate) as the cause of TS; others have suggested that stimulants may unmask a latent tic disorder. The decision to begin or continue the medication will be determined by the severity of the ADHD and tic disorder (Sverd, Gadow, & Paolicelli, 1988). More recent reports indicate that stimulant drugs rarely enhance the frequency or severity of tics (Gillberg et al., 1997). However, if stimulant drugs are prescribed for a child with TS, it is mandatory that the child be closely followed for worsening of his or her tics and behavior. The cause of TS is unknown, but a genetic etiology is most likely. The symptoms of the condition and the response to specific medications suggest an abnormality in one or more neurotransmitter pathways, particularly the dopamine system.

Motor tics in children are not always due to TS. Transient tics, consisting of eyelid blinking or facial movements, are the most common movement disorder in children. They are most prevalent in boys, and there is often a positive family history. Unlike TS, these tics permanently disappear within 1 year of the onset. Tics may also be observed in children following encephalitis, birth injury, or head trauma, and in rare genetic disorders such as Wilson and Hallevorden-Spatz disease.

Most children with TS do not require treatment with medication because the symptoms are mild and do not interfere with scholastic or social activities. The physician should explain to the child and family that the tics are involuntary and not due to a psychiatric or emotional condition and that punishment of the child or drawing attention to the tics will serve only to heighten the symptoms. The neuroleptic group of drugs, especially haloperidol (a dopamine-blocking agent) and pimozide, are effective in the management of tics in approximately 50% of children with TS. Side effects include cognitive impairment, lethargy, fatigue, and depression, which often preclude their use. Clonidine, an alpha-2-adrenergic agonist that is effective in managing the tics, ADHD, and compulsive behavior, generally has fewer side effects. All children with TS on medication require close medical supervision, especially for untoward side effects (Kurlan, 1989; Shapiro, Shapiro, Young, & Feinberg, 1988).

A teacher is likely to encounter a child with TS sometime during his or her career. A significant number of children display ADHD as the initial manifestation of TS. Ultimately, the characteristic symptoms of TS become evident, including motor and vocal tics. Some children with TS will also have severe learning problems requiring specific remediation. Not surprisingly, behavioral problems are prominent, probably due in part to the reaction of other children and adults to the TS symptoms. Fortunately, in most cases, TS does not significantly interfere with a child's academic achievement or social development; however, if the tics are severe or the ADHD incapacitating, medical management must be considered. As TS is a chronic lifelong disorder, which may be associated with learning, behavioral, and social problems, the educator can play an important role in its multidisciplinary management by serving as an advocate for the child.

# REFERENCES

American Academy of Pediatrics. (1999). The management of closed head injury in children. *Pediatrics, 104,* 1407–1415.

Barlow, C. F. (1984). *Headaches and migraine in childhood.* Philadelphia: Lippincott.

Baumann, R. J. (2002). Behavioral treatment of migraine in children and adolescents. *Pediatric Drugs, 4*(9), 555–561.

Bijur, P. E., Haslum, M., & Golding, J. (1990). Cognitive and behavioral sequelae of mild head injury. *Pediatrics, 86,* 337–343.

Billie, B. (1962). Migraine in school children. *Acta Paediatrica Scandinavia, 51*(Suppl. 136), 1–151.

Black, P., Jeifries, J. J., Blumer, D., Wellner, A., & Walker, A. E. (1969). The post-traumatic syndrome in children. In A. E. Walker, W. F. Caveness, & M. Critchley (Eds.), *The late effects of head injury* (pp. 142–149). Springfield, IL: Thomas.

Carroll, L. (1984). *Alice's adventures in wonderland.* London: Victor Gollancz. (Original work published 1865)

Caveness, W. F. (1976). Epilepsy, a product of trauma in our time. *Epilepsia, 17,* 207–215.

Centers for Disease Control. (1990a). *Childhood injuries in the United States.* Atlanta: U.S. Department of Health and Human Services, Public Health Service.

Centers for Disease Control. (1990b). Childhood injuries in the United States. *American Journal of Diseases of Children, 144,* 627–646.

Colorado Medical Society. (1991). *Report of the Sports Medicine Committee: Guidelines for the management of concussion in sports* (rev.). Denver: Author.

Commission on Classification and Terminology of the International League Against Epilepsy. (1989). Proposal for revised classification of epilepsies and epileptic syndromes. *Epilepsia, 30,* 389–399.

Congdon, P. J., & Forsythe, W. I. (1979). Migraine in childhood: A study of 300 children. *Developmental Medicine and Child Neurology, 21,* 209–216.

Denny-Brown, D., & Russell, W. R. (1941). Experimental cerebral concussion. *Brain, 64,* 93–164.

DeVivo, D. C., & Dodge, P. R. (1971). The critically ill child: Diagnosis and management of head injury. *Pediatrics, 48,* 129–138.

Diamond, S. (1979). Biofeedback and headache. *Headache, 19,* 180–184.

Durkin, M. S., Olsen, S., Barlow, B., Virella, A., & Connolly, E. S., Jr. (1998). The epidemiology of urban pediatric neurological trauma: Evaluation of and implications for injury prevention programs. *Neurosurgery, 42*(2), 300–310.

Emerson, R., D'Souza, B. J., Vining, E. P., Holden, K. R., Mellits, E. D., & Freeman, J. M. (1981). Stopping medication in children with epilepsy: Predictors of outcome. *New England Journal of Medicine, 304,* 1125–1129.

Engel, J. E., Jr. (1987). *Surgical treatment of the epilepsies.* New York: Raven.

Englander, J., Bushnik, T., Duong, T. T., Cifu, D. X., Zafonte, R., & Wright, J. (2003). Analyzing risk factors for late posttraumatic seizures: A prospective, multicenter investigation. *Archives of Physical Medical Rehabilitation, 84*(3), 365–373.

Freemon, F. R., Douglas, E. F. O., & Penry, J. K. (1973). Environmental interaction and memory during petit mal (absence) seizures. *Pediatrics, 51,* 911–918.

Friedman, A. P., & Harms, E. (1967). *Headaches in children.* Springfield, IL: Thomas.

Gillberg, C., Melander, H., von Knorring, A. L., Janols, L. O., Thernlund, G., Hagglof, B., Eidevall-Wallin, L., Gustafsson, P., & Kopp, S. (1997). Long term central stimulant treatment of children with attention-deficit hyperactivity disorder symptoms: A randomized double-blind placebo-controlled trial. *Archives of General Psychiatry, 54,* 857–864.

Goldstein, F. C., & Levin, H. S. (1987). Epidemiology of pediatric closed head injury: Incidence, clinical characteristics, and risk factors. *Learning Disabilities, 20,* 518–525.

Grewal, M., & Sutcliffe, A. J. (1991). Early prediction of outcome following head injury in children: An assessment of the value of Glasgow Coma Score trend and abnormal plantar and pupillary light reflexes. *Journal of Pediatric Surgery, 26,* 1161–1163.

Griffith, J. F., & Dodge, P. R. (1968). Transient blindness following head injury in children. *New England Journal of Medicine, 278,* 648–651.

Gupta, A., & Rothner, A. D. (2001). Treatment of childhood headaches. *Current Neurological & Neuroscience Reprints, 1*(2), 144–154.

Headache Classification Committee of the International Headache Society. (1988). Classification and diagnostic criteria for headache disorders, cranial neuralgia, and facial pain. *Cephalgia, 8*(Suppl. 7), 19–28.

Hjern, B., & Nylander, I. (1962). Late prognosis of severe head injuries in childhood. *Archives of Disease in Childhood, 37,* 113–116.

Hughes, E. L., & Cooper, C. E. (1956). Some observations on headache and eye pain in a group of schoolchildren. *British Medical Journal, 1,* 1138–1141.

Jennett, B. (1972). Head injuries in children. *Developmental Medicine and Child Neurology, 14,* 137–147.

Jennett, B., & Teasdale, G. (1974). Assessment of coma and impaired consciousness: A practical scale. *Lancet, 2,* 81–84.

Kaufman, Y., Tzischinsky, O., Epstein, R., Etzioni, A., Lavie, P., & Pillar, G. (2001). Long-term sleep disturbances in adolescents after minor head injury. *Pediatric Neurology, 24,* 129–134.

Kelly, J. P., Nichols, J. S., Filley, C. M., Lillehei, K. C., Rubinstein, D., & Kleinschmidt-DeMasters, B. K. (1991). Concussion in sports: Guidelines for the prevention of catastrophic outcome. *Journal of the American Medical Association, 266,* 2867–2869.

Kionoff, H., Low, M. D., & Clark, C. (1977). Head injuries in children: A prospective five-year follow-up. *Journal of Neurology, Neurosurgery, and Psychiatry, 40,* 1211–1219.

Kurlan, R. (1989). Tourette's syndrome: Current concepts. *Neurology, 39,* 1625–1630.

Levin, H. S., & Eisenberg, H. M. (1979). Neuropsychological outcome of head injury in children and adolescents. *Child's Brain, 5,* 281–292.

Lieh-Lai, M. W., Theodorou, A. A., Sarnaik, A. P., Meert, K. L., Moylan, P. M., & Canady, A. J. (1992). Limitation of the Glasgow Coma Scale in predicting outcome in children with traumatic brain injury. *Journal of Pediatrics, 120,* 195–199.

Ling, W., Oftedal, G., & Weinberg, W. (1970). Depressive illness in childhood presenting as severe headache. *American Journal of Diseases of Children, 120,* 122–124.

Livingston, S. (1972). *Comprehensive management of epilepsy in infancy, childhood and adolescence.* Springfield, IL: Thomas.

Mahoney, W. J., D'Souza, B. J., Haller, J. A., Rogers, M. C., Epstein, M. H., & Freeman, J. M. (1983). Long-term outcome of children with severe head trauma and prolonged coma. *Pediatrics, 71,* 756–762.

McKinlay, A., Dalrymple-Alford, J. C., Horwood, L. J., & Fergusson, D. M. (2002). Long term psychosocial outcomes after mild head injury in early childhood. *Journal of Neurology, Neurosurgery, and Psychiatry, 73*(3), 281–288.

Mealey, J., Jr. (1968). *Pediatric head injuries.* Springfield, IL: Thomas.

Olness, H., MacDonald, J. T., & Uden, D. L. (1987). Comparison of self-hypnosis and propranolol in the treatment of juvenile classic migraine. *Pediatrics, 79,* 593–597.

Oster, J. (1972). Recurrent abdominal pain, headache, and limb pains in children and adolescents. *Pediatrics, 50,* 429–436.

Pauls, D. L., & Lechman, J. F. (1986). The inheritance of Gilles de la Tourette syndrome and associated behaviors: Evidence for autosomal dominant transmission. *New England Journal of Medicine, 315,* 993–997.

Prensky, A. L., & Sommer, D. (1979). Diagnosis and treatment of migraine in children. *Neurology, 29,* 506–510.

Scott-Jupp, R., Marlow, N., Seddon, N., & Rosenbloom, L. (1992). Rehabilitation and outcome after severe head injury. *Archives of Disease in Childhood, 67,* 222–226.

Shapiro, A. K., Shapiro, E. S., Young, Y. G., & Feinberg, T. E. (1988). *Gilles de la Tourette syndrome* (2nd ed.). New York: Raven.

Shinnar, S., Berg, A. T., Moshe, S. L., Kang, H., O'Dell, C., Alemany, M., Goldensohn, E. S., & Hauser, W. A. (1994). Discontinuing antiepileptic drugs in children: A prospective study. *Annals of Neurology, 35*(5), 509–510.

Shinnar, S., & D'Souza, B. J. (1982). The diagnosis and management of headaches in childhood. *Pediatric Clinics of North America, 29,* 79–94.

Sirven, J. I., Sperling, M., & Wingerchuk, D. M. (2001). Early versus late antiepileptic drug withdrawal for people with epilepsy in remission. *Cochrane Database Systems Review, 3,* CD001902.

Stafstrom, C. E., Rostasy, K., & Minster, A. (2002). The usefulness of children's drawings in the diagnosis of headache. *Pediatrics, 109*(3), 460–472.

Sverd, J., Gadow, K. D., & Paolicelli, L. M. (1988). Methylphenidate treatment of attention-deficit hyperactivity disorder in boys with Tourette's syndrome. *Journal of the American Academy of Child and Adolescent Psychiatry, 28*(4), 574–579.

Thurman, D., & Guerrero, J. (1999). Trends in hospitalization associated with traumatic brain injury. *The Journal of the American Medical Association, 282,* 954–957.

Thurston, J. H., Thurston, D. L., Hixon, B. B., & Keller, A. J. (1982). Prognosis in childhood epilepsy: Additional follow-up of 148 children 15 to 23 years after withdrawal of anticonvulsant therapy. *New England Journal of Medicine, 306,* 831–836.

Vahlquist, B. (1955). Migraine in children. *International Archives of Allergy and Immunology, 7,* 348–355.

Winner, P., Rothner, A.D., Saper, J., Nett, R., Asgharnejad, M., Laurenza, A., Austin, R., & Peykamian, M. (2000). A randomized, double-blind, placebo-controlled study of sumatriptan nasal spray in the treatment of acute migraine in adolescents. *Pediatrics, 106,* 989–997.

# CHAPTER 14

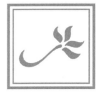

# Cerebral Palsy and Associated Dysfunction

### Peter A. Blasco and Patricia M. Blasco

**P**arents of children with problems related to development typically have vague descriptions of symptoms, such as "He doesn't talk," "He's not sitting (or walking) on time," or "She's too stiff (or floppy)." Sometimes the developmental problems of infants and toddlers are noticed first by early childhood personnel rather than parents. Evaluation of a child with developmental problems may lead to a diagnosis of one or more developmental disabilities (see Table 14.1 for prevalence statistics of various developmental disorders). One of these disabilities, cerebral palsy, is the primary topic of this chapter, although other motor disabilities are also discussed.

## AN APPROACH TO MOTOR DYSFUNCTION

When developmental specialists (developmental pediatricians, pediatric therapists, special educators, etc.) are asked to evaluate children with possible disabilities, the first approach should be to separate the developmental issues (concerns raised by caretakers and findings uncovered on evaluation) into three domains: motor dysfunction, cognitive deficits, and behavioral problems. Although closely interrelated, the three categories are independent. For example, children with severe motor disabilities may be intellectually normal or even gifted. Conversely, the majority of individuals with mental retardation go through normal motor developmental milestones. Individuals with cerebral palsy, despite their physical (motor) limitations and associated medical

**TABLE 14.1**

Developmental Disabilities and Prevalence

| Disability | Percentage of Pediatric Population |
|---|---|
| Learning disabilities and attention-deficit syndromes | 0.5–7.0 |
| Mental retardation | 3.0 |
| Cerebral palsy | 0.2–0.5 |
| Deafness | 0.1 |
| Blindness | 0.05 |
| Autism | 0.04–0.08 |

problems, are active in the classroom and in the workplace. Integration into societal life, as fully as possible, is the ultimate goal, and the classroom is the source of much of the effort in the first two decades of the child's life.

# CEREBRAL PALSY: HISTORICAL PERSPECTIVE

An English orthopedic surgeon, Sir William John Little, initially described the entity of cerebral palsy in 1843 (Little, 1853). He not only presented the first comprehensive clinical description of this motor disorder, but also suggested modalities of therapy such as manipulations, gymnastics, and braces. He emphasized birth trauma and premature delivery as etiologic factors. Subsequently, birth palsies of cerebral origin were referred to as "Little's disease." Sigmund Freud, one of the celebrated founders of psychiatry and psychoanalysis, started his career as a prominent neurologist and neuropathologist and was a pioneer in the cerebral palsy field. In the 1890s, he published his clinical experience of children with Little's disease and described the neuropathology and devised a classification system that was used during the early part of the 20th century and remains the foundation for what is used today. He suggested that there were prenatal causes of cerebral palsy that would be inappropriately attributed to difficulties occurring during delivery:

> Difficult birth and premature birth are not always accidental happenings, but may frequently be the result of a deeper cause or its expressions with-

out being the actual etiological factor. Thus, it may well be possible that the same pathogenic factors that rendered intrauterine development abnormal also extended their influence to parturition; abnormal birth is then the final result of an abnormal pregnancy. (Freud, 1897/1968)

The term *cerebral palsy* was first coined by Sir William Osler in the late 19th century, but it was not commonly used until the 1930s when Winthrop Phelps, an orthopedic surgeon, popularized its use. Over the course of three decades, Phelps oversaw the development of the field of cerebral palsy, demonstrating that these children could be successfully habilitated. He personally trained the lion's share of professionals from many disciplines who specialized in this chronic disorder.

In the late 1950s, Eric Denhoff, a developmental pediatrician, emphasized that cerebral palsy should be viewed as the motor manifestation of an extended spectrum of brain dysfunction. Thus, cerebral palsy was often coupled with cognitive deficits, convulsions, visual or hearing loss, speech difficulty, and behavioral and emotional disturbances (Denhoff & Robinault, 1960). He also made note of the "minimal" end of the spectrum, where the motor and cognitive disabilities are subtle and are frequently accompanied by a particular behavioral disorder, the hallmark of which is inattention. The child with a diagnosis of cerebral palsy needs ongoing surveillance for language development, cognitive abilities, visual motor ability, nutrition and growth, and seizure disorders. These associated deficits need to be delineated in order to provide the child with an educational plan most suitable for his or her needs. In the United States, the Education of the Handicapped Act Amendments of 1986 (Public Law [P.L.] 99-457) provides all children (birth to age 21) with the right to intervention services and educational accommodations to meet their educational, physical, and emotional needs.

Multidisciplinary and interdisciplinary approaches have been adopted in an effort to help identify all the specific problems and orchestrate all the needed services involved with the child and family. The goal of all the players is an educational placement that optimizes learning at a child's cognitive level despite the hurdles of associated deficits.

# DEFINITION

*Cerebral palsy* is defined as a disorder of movement and posture—in other words, a motor disability—resulting from a permanent, nonprogressive insult involving the immature brain (Bax, 1964). Cerebral dysfunction can exist on the basis of a central nervous system (CNS) that has not developed properly from the start, referred to as a developmental malformation or CNS anomaly or, alternatively, can be the consequence of an injury to a previously normally developing nervous system. The insult of cerebral palsy is always *static;* that is, the lesion itself will not get worse. What often does change over time are the manifestations of the motor disorder and the emergence or recognition of associated deficits as the child grows and the nervous system matures. In those instances where the brain insult does get progressively worse over time, we speak in terms of *degenerative* CNS disease.

# PREVALENCE

The epidemiology of cerebral palsy has been confused because of differing assumptions about the population being defined. For example, some studies exclude *all* cases that occur after birth, limiting the population to only prenatal and perinatal etiologies. Without a formal cerebral palsy register in the United States, it is difficult to precisely define its prevalence. In developed countries, rates of cerebral palsy in children are generally quoted in the range of 0.1% to 0.7% of the pediatric population. We favor a rate of 0.5%—that is, about 1 in 200 children have cerebral palsy. We include in our percentage milder cases and a broader age of onset.

There is some disagreement about whether the overall incidence of cerebral palsy is rising or staying stable. A possible rise has been attributed to the increased survival of children born with extremely low birth weights of less than 1,000 g (Hagberg, Hagberg, & Zetterstrom, 1989). Twin gestations also present a much higher risk of cerebral palsy, and multifetal pregnancies have increased significantly in the past two decades (Grether, Nelson, & Cummins, 1993). Regardless of whether cerebral palsy incidence is rising or remaining unchanged, the absolute number of cases is increasing because the overall survival of all high-risk infants has increased over time, resulting in larger numbers of healthy former premies and multiple births, but also increased numbers of children with cerebral palsy.

Risk factors for cerebral palsy identified in a number of studies have included maternal age greater than 35 and less than 20, children born to mothers who have had more than five pregnancies, multiple fetus gestations, intrauterine demise of one fetus in a twin pregnancy, birth weight less than 1,500 g (particularly birth weight less than 1,000 g), and African American racial background (Cummins, Nelson, Grether, & Velie, 1993).

# DIAGNOSIS

On average, cerebral palsy is diagnosed at 12 months of age (Lock, Shapiro, Ross, & Capute, 1986). The diagnosis relies heavily on clinical examination findings. No laboratory or radiographic examination can make or even confirm the clinical diagnosis of cerebral palsy. The following are the criteria used for the clinical diagnosis of cerebral palsy:

- Delayed motor milestones
- Abnormal neurological examination
- Aberrant primitive reflexes and postural reactions
- Positive history for risk or evidence of insult
- No clinical progression based on history or repeat examination
- Age of insult

To make a meaningful statement about a child's motor competence, the examiner should organize data gathered from the history, physical examination, and neurodevelopmental examination according to the following schema (P. A. Blasco, 1992):

1. Motor developmental milestones

2. The classic neurological examination

3. Markers of cerebral neuromotor maturation (the primitive reflexes and postural reactions)

*Motor milestones* are extracted from the developmental history, as well as from observations during the neurodevelopmental examination. A basic reference table of sequential gross and fine motor milestones is needed. Milestone assessment is best summarized as a single motor age (or narrow age range) for the child, allowing one to think of the child in terms of his or her level of motor function. The ratio of the motor age to the chronological age produces the motor quotient (MQ), giving a simple expression of deviation from the norm (P. A. Blasco, 1992). An MQ below 70 is considered abnormal.

Motor milestones do not take into account the quality of a child's movements. The motor portion of the *neurological examination,* including observations of station and gait, take qualitative features into account. Neurological assessments of tone, strength, deep tendon reflexes, and coordination are difficult in the infant because of their subjective nature, compounded by the limited ability for cooperation. Muscle tone (passive resistance) and strength (active resistance) are a challenge to distinguish in the contrary subject. The best clues often come from observation rather than handling of the infant. Spontaneous or prompted motor activities (e.g., weight bearing in sitting or standing) require adequate strength. Weakness may be best appreciated from observing the quality of stationary posture and transition movements. It is important to understand that, although the child's muscle *tone* (passive) may be extremely high, actual *strength* (voluntary) may be quite poor. Clinical experience is essential to gain accurate and useful information. After the child is 2 to 3 years of age, the neurological examination becomes easier and more meaningful, as cooperation improves.

*Station* refers to the posture (body alignment) assumed in sitting or standing and should be viewed from anterior, lateral, and posterior perspectives. *Gait* refers to walking and is examined in progress. Initially, the toddler walks on a wide base, slightly crouched, with the arms abducted and elevated a bit. Forward progression is more staccato than smooth. Movements gradually become more fluid, the base narrows, and an arm swing evolves, leading to an adult pattern of walking by 3 years of age.

The motor *neuromaturational markers* include the *primitive reflexes,* which develop during gestation and generally disappear 3 to 6 months after birth, and the *postural reactions,* which are not present at birth but sequentially develop between 3 and 10 months of age. The Moro, tonic labyrinthine, asymmetric tonic neck, and positive support reflexes are the most clinically useful primitive reflexes. The appearance of postural reactions in sequence beginning after 1 to 2 months of age can provide great insight into the motor potential of young infants. Postural reactions are sought in each of the three major categories of righting, protection, and equilibrium, and they are easy to elicit in the normal infant. (See Baird & Gordon, 1983, and P. A. Blasco, 1992, for more detailed information on individual reflexes.)

Once a motor abnormality has been identified, further assessment as to its exact nature and etiology is essential. This almost always warrants referral to an appropriate subspecialty interdisciplinary team. Categories of motor disability fall into four general areas: static central nervous system disorders, progressive diseases, spinal cord and peripheral nerve injuries, and structural defects.

Motor dysfunction produced by a *static* (i.e., nonprogressive) *brain insult* is the etiology of cerebral palsy. The cerebral insult can happen during early fetal brain development, resulting in a central nervous system anomaly. The anomaly could be the result of improper genetic information (e.g., as in Down syndrome) or a very early biochemical or mechanical insult that permanently alters anatomical development of the brain. Alternatively, a brain developing in a normal fashion can be damaged before, during, or after birth by a variety of insults. Examples are infection (e.g., meningitis, encephalitis), trauma, ischemia (e.g., from dehydration or stroke), poisons (e.g., lead intoxication), metabolic diseases (e.g., phenylketonuria), and so forth. Brain injury resulting in neuron and axon destruction is permanent—little to no true neuronal repair or regrowth takes place. However, intact areas continue to develop during childhood so that some functional improvements may steadily accrue up to a certain point. Maturation of motor areas in the brain has largely reached completion by 7 or 8 years of age. When a motor impairment is due to a brain anomaly or to a nonprogressive insult that took place before midadolescence (others would say before 7 to 8 years of age), the disorder is referred to as cerebral palsy. Specific types of cerebral palsy (spastic, athetoid, etc.) are diagnosed clinically and imply which motor control system in the brain has been primarily damaged. Establishing the type of cerebral palsy has great value in treatment planning and in prognosis. These diagnostic distinctions and the treatment plans based on them are best carried out by a coordinated team of physicians and therapists experienced in the care of children with motor impairments.

*Progressive diseases* of the brain, the nerves, or the muscles produce motor impairment that worsens with time. Although the number of diseases in this category is very large, each individual disease is extremely rare. Therefore, the fraction of all children whose motor impairments are caused by progressive diseases is quite small.

*Spinal cord and peripheral nerve injuries* and anomalies are all static conditions except the rare instance of a growing spine tumor. These conditions differ from cerebral palsy in that future functional loss is much easier to predict and they have different types of associated problems. In this category, the largest single group consists of children with spina bifida, specifically meningomyelocele.

*Structural defects* refer to situations in which some anatomical structure (e.g., a limb) is missing or deformed or in which some support tissue for the nerves and muscles is inadequate (e.g., connective tissue defects, biochemically abnormal bone). Structural defects are usually the most straightforward to understand of all motor-impairing conditions. On the mildest end of the spectrum are a wide variety of fairly common orthopedic deformities that may or may not affect motor development (e.g., club feet, developmental hip dysplasia), whereas other conditions (e.g., osteogenesis imperfecta, many varieties of childhood arthritis) are progressive in nature and may be extremely complex to manage.

Establishing the specific type of progressive disease, the level of spinal cord dysfunction, or the specific structural diagnosis is fundamental to developing a sound treatment program. In addition, the precise diagnosis will carry major implications for genetic counseling.

# CLASSIFICATION

Because different approaches have been employed as the basis for categorizing types of cerebral palsy, classification can be confusing. For example, the site of the cerebral neuropathology, the clinical manifestations, the etiology of the brain injury, and the distribution of extremity involvement (topography) all represent different systems on which cerebral palsy classification can be based. A combined, yet simplified approach is favored by most, based first on the clinical neuromotor manifestations (spastic, extrapyramidal, or mixed) and then on the topographical distribution of involvement:

| Spastic (Pyramidal) | Extrapyramidal | Mixed |
|---|---|---|
| Quadriplegia (tetraplegia) | Rigid | |
| Diplegia | Choreoathetoid | |
| Hemiplegia | Dystonic (dyskinetic) | |
| Triplegia | Ataxic | |
| Monoplegia | Tremor | |
| Paraplegia | Hypotonic | |

*Spastic* (pyramidal) *cerebral palsy,* the most common type, is characterized by an increase in muscle tone that has a "clasp-knife" (spastic) quality, pathologically increased deep tendon reflexes, and a consistent pattern of agonist–antagonist muscle imbalance. For example, in the spastic lower extremity, it is difficult for the child to relax the leg muscles that allow him or her to straighten at the hip and knee and to dorsiflex at the ankle. Therefore, the child always tends to keep the leg postured or move it in a stereotyped pattern of flexion: flexed at the hip, flexed at the knee, and plantar flexed and turned in at the ankle. The term *pyramidal cerebral palsy* is derived from the location of the cerebral insult, which is in the pyramidal system involving the motor cortex in the gray matter of the brain and/or the pyramidal tract fibers leading from the cortex to the spinal cord. These cells usually innervate voluntary muscles (see Figure 14.1). Among spastic types of cerebral palsy, subclassification is based on topographical distribution, that is, which limbs are involved. Spastic quadriplegia involves all four extremities, typically the lower extremities more so than the uppers. In diplegia, all four extremities are again involved, but the lower extremities are dramatically more affected than the uppers. The term *paraplegia* should be reserved for those instances in which the legs are spastic and the arms are normal. Paraplegic cerebral palsy is very rare. *Spastic paraplegia* is primarily associated with spinal cord injury. Hemiplegia is confined to one half of the body, and the arm is usually more affected than the leg. When all four extremities are spastic, with the upper extremities clearly more involved than the lowers, the designation *double hemiplegia* is often used. *Spastic diplegia* and *quadriplegia* may be symmetrical in terms of severity of involvement but as often as not are somewhat asymmetric.

The second main type of cerebral palsy is classified as *extrapyramidal* (or nonspastic). In extrapyramidal cerebral palsy, the involvement is essentially always quadriplegic, so subclassification is determined on the basis of the dominant tone pattern or movement disorder features. *Choreoathetoid, dystonic,* and *rigid* types of cerebral palsy are most commonly seen; *tremor, ataxic,* or *hypotonic* occur less frequently. Sometimes the term *dyskinetic* is used in reference to the choreoathetoid and dystonic subtypes. Extrapyramidal types of cerebral palsy have their origin in the deep gray matter of the brain (the basal ganglia) or in the cerebellum (see Figure 14.2). Extrapyramidal types of cerebral palsy typically affect the upper extremities more than the lower extremities, and the character of increased extremity tone is of a "lead-pipe" (persistently rigid) rather than clasp-knife (i.e., spastic) quality. (Figure 14.3 is a drawing that shows a typical posture of a child with choreoathetosis.) This lead-pipe or putty-like feel will tend to diminish with repetitive active or passive movements. Oral-motor dysfunction is often a prominent feature in children with extrapyramidal cerebral palsy, with

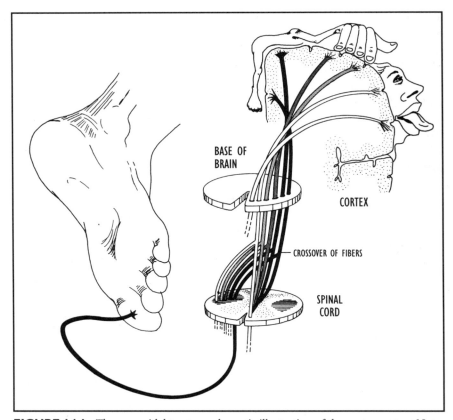

**FIGURE 14.1.** The pyramidal tracts: a schematic illustration of the motor cortex. Note the disproportionate representation of the lower face, tongue, lips, and hand on the motor area of the brain. Injury to the cerebral cortex in the region of the leg (darkest line or tract) will result in spasticity in the opposite extremity.

resultant difficulties in speaking and eating. In children with extrapyramidal cerebral palsy, extra movements and muscle tone become more evident when they become excited or nervous or attempt to perform tasks that require intense effort.

The final major category of cerebral palsy is *mixed,* a combination of both spastic and extrapyramidal patterns of involvement. About 65% of cerebral palsy is spastic, the majority of which is hemiplegic; about 20% is extrapyramidal; and the remaining 15% is mixed. Probably, however, mixed cerebral palsy is underrecognized and misclassified as entirely spastic because the underlying choreoathetosis is unappreciated.

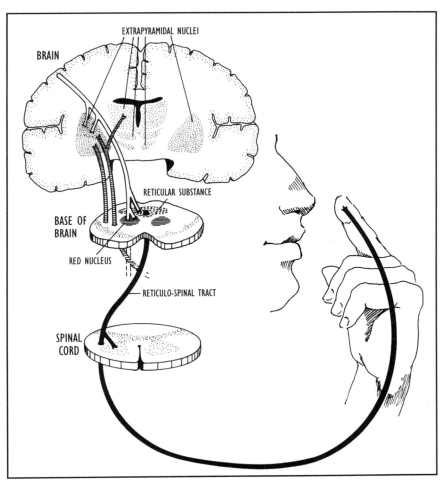

**FIGURE 14.2.** The extrapyramidal tracts. Destruction of the various components of the extrapyramidal nuclei may result in a movement disorder (chorea, athetosis, rigidity, dystonia). The abnormal movements may become pronounced when the child performs certain tasks, such as pointing and writing with a pencil.

It is important to understand the classification of cerebral palsy, both the neuromotor manifestation and the topographic distribution. The type of cerebral palsy often gives insight into the associated perceptual, sensory, and cognitive deficits. For example, children with hemiplegia have a higher incidence of seizures than those with quadriplegia or diplegia. Intelligence tends to be best preserved (generally normal) in spastic diplegia and is a

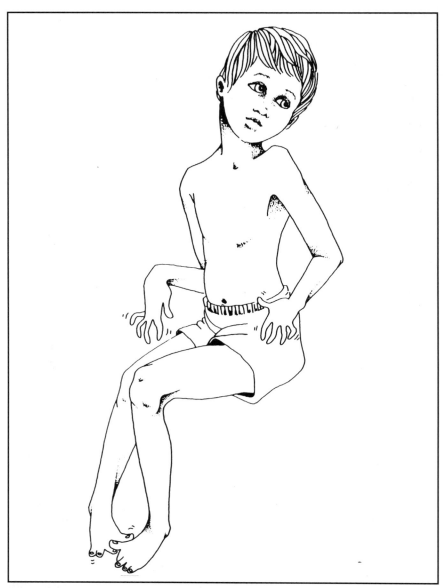

**FIGURE 14.3.** The child with choreoathetosis demonstrates slow writhing movements and assumes abnormal postures.

little lower in hemiplegia (most often in the borderline to mild mental retardation range). Children with spastic quadriplegia virtually always have mental retardation. About 50% of children with hemiplegia have associated sensory impairment of the involved side. This is manifested by the child's inability to recognize an object by touch or feel (*astereognosis*), by diminished awareness of light touch or pain on the affected side, and by neglect of the involved side. This cortical sensory impairment may contribute as much or more to the child's failure to use the limb than does the motor impairment itself (Tizard, Paine, & Crothers, 1954). Additionally, approximately 25% of children with spastic hemiplegia have a loss of vision in a portion of the visual field toward the side of motor weakness (*homonymous hemianopsia*). For children with the choreoathetoid form of cerebral palsy, the motor involvement may be very severe in the face of normal or above normal intelligence (see Nolan, 1987).

As with any disorder, cerebral palsy occurs on a spectrum of severity from very mild to very severe. The most severely involved children may never achieve ambulation or develop intelligible speech. The most mildly involved walk late and, although awkward as children, experience little to no true motor limitation other than in competitive activities. Diagnostically, children at the mildest end of the spectrum may or may not be identified as having cerebral palsy as infants and most often carry either no diagnosis or one of a variety of descriptive designations as school-age children (e.g., minor neuromotor dysfunction, developmental dyspraxia, developmental coordination disorder). Findings in the infant that fulfill the criteria for diagnosing cerebral palsy, albeit mild, often evolve into a more subtle picture in the older child. In that circumstance, clinicians on occasion will use the term "minimal" cerebral palsy but more often choose one of the less pejorative, more descriptive diagnoses noted above.

# ETIOLOGY

Basically, any brain injury to the areas governing motor control can cause cerebral palsy. No single clear etiology of cerebral palsy stands out above the others (see various causes listed in Table 14.2). Certain types of insult tend to result in specific types of motor dysfunction. For example, in the past, choreoathetoid cerebral palsy was most frequently ascribed to bilirubin encephalopathy (kernicterus), but with obstetric advances in the prevention of

**TABLE 14.2**

Causes of Cerebral Palsy

---

**Prenatal (Congenital)**

1. Genetic

   • Chromosomal disorders (e.g., trisomy 18, deletion syndromes)

   • Neurocutaneous syndromes (e.g., tuberous sclerosis)

2. Infectious (e.g., toxoplasmosis, rubella, cytomegalovirus, herpes, syphilis)

3. Toxic/metabolic (e.g., maternal pheylketonuria, maternal iodine deficiency, fetal alcohol syndrome)

4. Other (e.g., unexplained central nervous system [CNS] malformations, prenatal cerebrovascular accidents)

**Acquired**

1. Perinatal (e.g., hypoxic–ischemic insult, prematurity, intraventricular hemorrhage)

2. Postnatal (e.g., head trauma, hypoxia)

   • Infectious (primary CNS infection, such as meningitis or encephalitis, or secondary effects on CNS)

   • Toxic/metabolic (e.g., lead poisoning, inborn errors of metabolism)

   • Neoplastic

   • Other (e.g., cerebrovascular accidents, nutritional deficiency, collagen vascular disease)

---

Rh factor disease, good neonatal surveillance, and improved management of hyperbilirubinemia in the past few decades, choreoathetoid cerebral palsy is now rarely the result of hyperbilirubinemia. More frequently, it is linked to sudden and severe anoxic events in full-term infants. Spastic diplegia results from periventricular leukomalacia as a consequence of hypoxia and altered blood supply to vital portions of the brain in premature infants.

Causes of cerebral palsy are conveniently divided into three categories based on time frame: prenatal, perinatal, and postnatal etiologies. Prenatal causes include central nervous system anomalies, which are structural abnormalities that occur during development of the brain. Prenatal abnormalities of the brain may result from intrauterine infection, such as from cytomegalovirus, toxoplasmosis, rubella, and so on. Additionally, exposure to toxins or drugs can have teratogenic effects on the fetus. Recent concerns relate to the use of cocaine during pregnancy or the existence of a familial predisposition to forming blood clots, either of which may cause strokes *in utero,* resulting in cerebral palsy. Birth asphyxia is a likely contributor to cerebral palsy, but improved obstetric care has reduced the risk of perinatal asphyxia. An infant may experience distress during or following a difficult delivery because of a central nervous system injury or developmental defect that occurred antenatally and that was undetected before birth. Thus, the developmental brain defect and not the delivery is the actual cause of the cerebral palsy (as surmised by Freud so many years ago). Sophisticated brain imaging studies in many cases can pinpoint the nature and the timing of central nervous system lesions and thereby help in the identification of children who had brain pathology existing before delivery. Antenatal screening for specific chemical markers in amniotic fluid and chromosome studies from fetal cells can also help to identify etiologies such as structural anomalies, ischemic injuries, metabolic abnormalities, or specific genetic syndromes prior to birth. These tests are appropriate in pregnancies that are at risk for specific abnormalities because of a positive family history. Metabolic diseases can result in postnatal brain damage that will remain static once the disease is recognized and controlled. The types of cerebral palsy these insults produce are often unusual. They may yield atypical patterns of involvement with unusual progression, or additional insults may be acquired due to episodes when the metabolic disease gets temporarily out of control.

In progressive neurological diseases, the motor disability may be defined as quadriplegia, rigidity, or another term also used to describe types of cerebral palsy, but these disorders should not be lumped together with cerebral palsy because, by the nature of their etiologies, the motor disability will worsen with time. Brain tumors may create a picture of new or progressive motor deterioration, at least as long as the tumor expands. If the tumor is successfully treated, the child may be cured or may be left with a residual motor impairment that is static (i.e., cerebral palsy).

The cause of cerebral palsy cannot be precisely identified in about 15% to 20% of cases. The inability to identify a cause is disconcerting for physicians and frustrating for parents. Knowing the cause may not provide any information useful for treatment but still can be satisfying or relieving for parents who inevitably ask, "Why?" In addition, a particular pattern of disability coupled with radiographic findings may clearly support some causative insult, for example hypoxia, but the exact timing (prenatally, during birth, or shortly afterward) may be unclear.

# ASSOCIATED DEFICITS

It is imperative that the child with cerebral palsy be recognized as being at very high risk for having associated deficits in neurological, cognitive, and perceptual abilities. The motor deficits are generally identified before delays in language or perceptual abilities are evident. Table 14.3 outlines the broad categories of more commonly associated deficits, some of which are discussed in more detail below.

## Orthopedic Deformities

Physical problems associated with cerebral palsy are deformities of the bones and contractures of the tendons and muscles, all of which result from the influence of excessively high or abnormally low muscle tone. Progressive contractures and at times joint dislocations (particularly the hips) are a major problem in spastic forms of cerebral palsy. Scoliosis is also fairly common and warrants careful attention to handling and positioning techniques in an effort to prevent development or progression of spine deformity. As adults, individuals with cerebral palsy complain frequently of musculoskeletal discomfort, especially joint pain associated with osteoarthritis (Andersson & Mattsson, 2001).

## Cognitive Deficits

The insult to the brain that causes cerebral palsy may also result in learning difficulties. Approximately 50% of children with cerebral palsy have varying degrees of mental retardation. Special educators continue to play a primary role in their management, because these children should participate in educational programs appropriate to their level of cognitive functioning. Children with mental retardation, despite the extent of their motor disability, should have as their goals the enhancement of self-help, social, and oral communication skills for living and, if possible, working in the environment that is least restrictive and most suitable to their capabilities. As children with mental retardation and cerebral palsy approach their teenage years, they require vocational training through the school system

### TABLE 14.3
#### Disorders Associated with Cerebral Palsy

| Orthopedic Deformities | Oral-Motor Dysfunction |
|---|---|
| • Muscle and tendon contracture | • Speech deficits (articulation disorders, dysarthria) |
| • Bone deformities and unalignments | • Feeding dysfunction (dysphagia) |
| • Joint dislocation and degeneration | • Swallowing dysfunction (drooling, aspiration) |
| • Scoliosis | • Oral sensory deficits |
| • Osteoporosis and fracture | **Gastroesophageal Reflux** |
| **Cognitive Deficits** | |
| | **Bowel and Bladder Problems** |
| • Mental retardation | |
| • Learning disability | **Seizures** |
| **Poor Growth and Undernutrition** | |
| | **Cervical Neuropathy** |
| **Sensory Deficits** | |
| | **Emotional and Behavioral Disturbances** |
| • Visual impairment | • Organic |
| • Oculomotor disturbance | • Acquired |
| • Hearing loss | |
| • Recurrent otitis | |

and supported or sheltered work environments where they are allowed to practice their vocation while maintaining socialization as well as earning income to enhance self-esteem and assist in their financial support. They will often require planning for long-term supervision or guardianship.

Of the 50% of children with cerebral palsy who do not have mental retardation, a significant but unknown portion have academic challenges due to borderline intelligence scores of 70 to 85 and possibly uneven psychometric profiles indicative of specific learning disabilities, communication disorders, or both. Underlying perceptual and language disorders are common in this subgroup of children, and special teaching methods need to be part of their educational plan. Assistance from speech–language pathologists, occupational therapists, or both should be employed to help with remediation planning and treatment. Because of the motor difficulties caused by cerebral palsy, experienced child psychologists must be available to differentiate abilities that are lacking because of physical limitations from those that are not present because of cognitive limitation.

Physical limitations or other associated deficits that hinder cognitive testing may result in an underestimation of the child's potential. Experienced teachers know better than other professionals the need to allow extra time for the child with cerebral palsy to more fully comprehend and respond to the presented material, and they especially appreciate the great challenge of providing such accommodations in the busy classroom.

## Sensory Deficits

Sensory loss is characteristic of almost every child with a myelomeningo-cele or a spinal cord injury but is generally uncommon among children with cerebral palsy. The exceptions are children with hemiplegia, among whom about 50% have cortical sensory impairments, although not the complete loss of sensation seen in spinal cord dysfunction. Children with extrapyramidal cerebral palsy are suspected of having substantial oral and peri-oral sensory impairment, promoting their tendency to drool. Some children with cerebral palsy seem to have oral sensory irritation (dysesthesia, tactile defensiveness) that further complicates feeding dif-ficulties.

Strabismus (deviation of the eye) occurs in approximately 30% to 35% of individuals with cerebral palsy, and there is a high incidence of refractory errors, which are twice as common in individuals having the spastic type than in those having the extrapyramidal type. Children with athetoid cerebral palsy are more prone to be far-sighted, whereas children with spastic cerebral palsy can be either near- or far-sighted. Visual field defects, as previously noted, occur in approximately 25% of children with hemiplegia. In some children who use their eyes poorly, it is a great challenge to figure out whether visual acuity is the problem or whether visual *attention* is the issue. Again, classroom observations are invaluable.

Children with certain syndromes associated with cerebral palsy due to prematurity or to prenatally or perinatally acquired infections are at high risk for hearing loss. In addition, many children with cerebral palsy, especially those related to genetic syndromes, have great difficulty with recurrent otitis and fluctuating conductive hearing losses. Audiologic screening should be a routine practice for such children.

## Oral-Motor Dysfunction

A continuum of problems related to involvement of the oral-motor and swallowing musculature exists in children with cerebral palsy (see Table 14.3). Mild articulation disorders are common; more severe dysarthria and dysphagia are usually associated with extrapyramidal types of cerebral palsy. There is often a history of poor suckle, difficulty with chewing and swallowing, or gastroesophageal reflux during infancy and the preschool years, the severity of which may preclude adequate nutrition or safe oral feeding. Oral sensory abnormalities, commonly manifested as oral aversion, can greatly aggravate feeding difficulties. Drooling is linked to poor swallowing and can be a major social problem, as well as distracting and even destructive in terms of classroom equipment and educational materials. Early referral to speech–language pathologists is important to establish a program of speech and language intervention, which can be carried out at home as well as in school.

Oral hygiene and dental care are challenges in children with cerebral palsy. Defective tooth enamel, malocclusion, dental caries, and especially periodontal disease are fairly common (see Chapter 11). Children with developmental disabilities are prone to facial and dental trauma as a result of accidental falls, seizures, or self-injurious and self-stimulatory behaviors such as biting and teeth grinding. Acid reflux from the stomach causes dental erosions. Good professional dental care for children with severe disabilities is often extremely difficult for families to access.

## Seizures

Whereas seizure disorders occur in about 0.2% of the general population, they develop in approximately 25% of individuals with cerebral palsy. The frequency of seizures is much greater in individuals with the spastic subtype than in those with the extrapyramidal subtype and is particularly more common in children with hemiplegia. Seizure medications, while invaluable for the suppression of active seizures, may have side effects that interfere with learning. The astute teacher's observations of both seizures and any behavioral changes that might be related to toxic drug effects are invaluable in the balancing act of finding the best medication dose for each child. When a child has a known seizure disorder, it is critical for the classroom teacher to be aware of the type, frequency, and duration of that child's spells so as to manage seizure events properly if needed, and to recognize when events deviate from their usual pattern.

## Emotional and Behavioral Problems

Various behavioral problems are demonstrated by children with cerebral palsy. One subset consists of organically driven abnormalities of activity, emotional lability, attention problems (short attention span, perseveration), low frustration tolerance, impulsivity, and distractibility. These organic behavioral patterns may be observed even in children with cerebral palsy who have normal global intelligence. The behavioral problems may have as significant an impact on the child's family or school environment as do the child's physical limitations. Aggressive environmental modifications, behavioral programming, and medication management may be of great benefit in ameliorating these issues (see Chapter 17).

Another set of behaviors are grounded more in learned responses to situations or people (refusals and opposition, temper tantrums, helplessness, acting out, etc.). Behavioral psychologists can provide considerable assistance by helping caretakers and others devise consistent management plans to modify or eliminate these undesirable behaviors and thus facilitate school performance and peace in the home. Because educators develop over time a working knowledge of the children's primary diagnoses and associated deficits, they can actively participate in the counseling rendered to these families and children.

During adolescence, some individuals with cerebral palsy occasionally appear to lose capabilities in self-help as well as communicative, ambulatory, or social skills. Parents, teachers, and physicians should be concerned as to whether this apparent deterioration is of physical, psychogenic, or organic origin. Physical and psychogenic factors are most likely the underlying cause, because in adolescence there may be a progression of orthopedic deformity or a spurt in bone growth that, when accompanied by insufficient muscular development, may result in the loss of physical skills such as walking. Occasionally, children gain excessive weight, a critical factor in inhibiting physical performance. The child's mental attitude may change, resulting in a pseudo-deterioration after he or she has exerted considerable energy and mental effort for years to learn and perform certain skills and at adolescence begins to seriously question whether the effort was worth it. The exact role of hormones is as yet unknown, but they undoubtedly affect emotional responses at this time. During adolescence, a child with cerebral palsy may experience a greater sense of social isolation as peers begin to date and attend dances, parties, and other events from which the child feels excluded. Perhaps for the first time the child realizes the social effects of having a disability, which can lead to depression, manifested by social and communicative withdrawal, as well as a loss of interest in physical activities. The child with average or superior intelligence who has involuntary movements of all extremities is probably the most prone to developing psychological disturbances during adolescence, with depression being fairly common, although this aspect of cerebral palsy morbidity has been poorly studied.

Mental health counseling should include anticipatory guidance to provide awareness and possibly prevention of emotional problems that may surface during adolescence. Furthermore, some of these youngsters become aware, during childhood, of their physical incapacities and limitations and have developed a poor self-image that may have been compounded by parental overprotection and unwillingness to allow them to participate in many of the social and recreational activities of other children their age. Most children with cerebral palsy need continuous emotional encouragement and sometimes environmental modifications to promote peer interactions in school settings and through extracurricular activities. The hope is for these interactive experiences to generalize socially. The parents and siblings of these children play central roles in rendering emotional support to the family member with a disability, which can lead to a whole spectrum of emotional difficulties for the siblings (Lobato, 1990). It may be possible to eliminate or at least diminish the psychological stress that may confront an adolescent with cerebral palsy by early (i.e., beginning in preschool), periodic mental health counseling for the child and family.

# MANAGEMENT

The treatment of cerebral palsy begins with its identification and initial assessment. Because cerebral palsy is not easily identified in the neonatal period, it is the obligation of pediatricians, family physicians, early childhood specialists, nurse practitioners, and community nurses to do careful surveillance on children at high risk for cerebral palsy. Early neonatal difficulties such as seizures, hypotonia, a history of difficult delivery, and preterm birth should raise suspicion and, therefore, should increase the intensity of sur-veillance. Many centers have been established to closely monitor children at risk, such as neurodevelopmental clinics that provide follow-up evaluations of infants discharged from neonatal intensive care. Infants with very low birth weights are automatically eligible for Supplemental Security Income (SSI) benefits and early intervention evaluation and treatment services in all states.

Treatment interventions can be organized into five broad categories: counseling, hands-on therapy, equipment, medications, and surgery (see Table 14.4). Parents first of all look for guidance and support from their child's physicians, therapists, and teachers, mainly in the form of collabo-rative (sometimes creative) problem solving rather than ultimate decision conferring. Counseling refers to this type of advice, not only for parents, but also for the children themselves and sometimes for siblings. Physicians should have a well thought out approach to "breaking the bad news" coun-seling. Kaminer and Cohen (1988) have offered guidelines for difficult counseling sessions, translating the information and knowledge base into language and concepts that are understandable to parents and that take into account educational, cultural, and ethnic characteristics of the family. The foundation for good communication skills is sensitivity, patience, and especially, good listening skills.

**TABLE 14.4**
Interventions for Children with Cerebral Palsy

| Counseling | Medications |
|---|---|
| **Hands-on Therapy** | • Oral |
| | • Intramuscular |
| • Physical therapy | • Intrathecal |
| • Occupational therapy | **Surgery** |
| • Speech | |
| • Recreational therapy and adapted physical education | • Orthopedics |
| • Special education | • Neurosurgery |
| **Equipment** | • Ophthalmology |
| | • Otolaryngology |
| • Braces | |
| • Adaptive devices | |
| • Electronics | |

Parents frequently ask for literature to clarify a new diagnosis. Such educational material is a desirable and useful adjunct to direct verbal counseling. Because much written literature, as well as information available on the Internet, is inaccurate, misleading, or otherwise unacceptable (P. A. Blasco, Baumgartner, & Mathes, 1983), professionals need to be familiar with the literature generally available and to be prepared to recommend the best resources to families. Among our favorites are *Exceptional Parent* magazine and *Children with Cerebral Palsy: A Parent's Guide* by Geralis (1991).

Physicians and other health care professionals can greatly assist parents to effectively and efficiently meet their children's needs and to address the needs of the *entire* family. A popular term (and important concept) is *empowerment*, that is, providing parents the encouragement and, where needed, the skills to become more effective case managers and advocates. Parents are unable to do this unless they have extensive information regarding the medical, developmental, and psychoeducational interventions their children should be receiving. They are being taught to ask more questions, seek literature, attend professional conferences, and join parent support groups so they can learn as much as possible about disabilities and their management.

The management team for children with cerebral palsy includes a variety of professionals. Physical therapists concentrate on the child's posture and locomotor skills, with particular emphasis on ambulation. They direct and monitor exercise programs to promote strength and endurance and to prevent contractures. They work in conjunction with the orthopedist to determine which orthotic supports are indicated for the child to ambulate to the best of his or her abilities. Braces may be indicated for stability, correction of deformity, or reduction of extraneous movements. Orthotics, canes, walkers, and wheelchairs are often used for mobility assistance.

Occupational therapists focus on upper extremity posture and manipulative skills as a prelude to enhancement of self-help skills and activities of daily living. They focus on such self-help skills as toileting, eating, and dressing. Children with cerebral palsy of the extrapyramidal type commonly have difficulties with oral-motor control and the swallowing mechanism. Occupational therapists, in conjunction with speech and physical therapists, develop seating and positioning systems to reduce tongue thrust and enhance the ability to swallow and to facilitate mobility and the use of adaptive equipment that provides the child with greater independence in activities of daily living and in accessing electronic interfaces.

Speech–language pathologists and assistive technology personnel are also important to the child's management team. In the preschool years, concerns about the child's communication are added to the concerns about his or her motor abilities. Communication depends not only on oral-motor skills, but also on use of the upper extremities. The most efficient and preferred means of communication is verbal; however, children with significant oral-motor dysfunction may be frustrated by unsuccessful efforts to improve their articulation and speech intelligibility. These children may benefit greatly from augmentative means of communication, such as communication boards and electronic devices.

Recreational therapists and adaptive physical educators often get left out in therapy considerations, yet they have a tremendous amount to offer the child with cerebral palsy. Recreational activities, such as hydrotherapy, swimming, and therapeutic horseback riding, not only offer therapy but also boost self-esteem.

The physician managing the child with cerebral palsy may consider the use of medications to reduce muscle tone or involuntary movements. A long list of drugs has been anecdotally reported to be beneficial. For example, diazepam (Valium), trihexyphenidyl (Artane), and baclofen (Lioresal) are helpful to reduce some of the spasticity of pyramidal cerebral palsy or the dystonia of extrapyramidal cerebral palsy. In truth, the majority of children do not benefit substantially from medication. No good data are available, but probably 10% or less of all children with cerebral palsy genuinely benefit from long-term use of oral medications. In the short term, postoperative use of muscle relaxant medications can be extremely helpful following orthopedic surgery. The side effects of medications should not be underestimated because sedation, lethargy, and depression may result, and therefore compromise a child's mental capabilities. The local injection of botulinum toxin into specific muscle groups decreases spasticity but also weakens muscles. An implantable pump device also has been developed to infuse baclofen into the spinal cord (intrathecal baclofen) and greatly diminish spasticity with very low medication doses.

Surgical interventions employed by orthopedists consist most commonly of tendon release or lengthening and bone reconstruction procedures. The intent is to improve function, prevent deformity, or both. On occasion, cosmesis is a factor, but rarely is it the primary indication for orthopedic surgery. Neurosurgeons have also developed techniques, such as selective posterior rhizotomy of the spinal nerve roots, to eliminate spasticity and thereby enhance ambulation in the child with spastic diplegia. In rare instances, stereotactic brain surgery involving the basal ganglia has been used to inhibit severe movement disorders. The neurosurgeon is also involved if the child receives a shunt for the treatment of hydrocephalus. Because of the high prevalence of eye problems and hearing deficits, surgeons in ophthalmology and otolaryngology are often involved in the care of children with cerebral palsy at irregular intervals, mostly early in the child's life.

Thus, the management of the child with cerebral palsy requires the skills and coordinated collaboration of physical and occupational therapists, the recreational therapist or adaptive physical educator, speech–language pathologists, nurses, psychologists, social workers, the orthopedist, the neurosurgeon and other subspecialty surgeons, the orthotist, sometimes the nutritionist, general pediatricians or family physicians, and developmental pediatricians or similar medical subspecialists. The coordination of these professionals, as well as educational and community social and mental health services, is always an enormous challenge.

## PROGNOSIS AND OUTCOME

Most individuals with cerebral palsy are able to live in the community independently or in a somewhat protected environment and to work on their own or in supported or sheltered situations. A smaller subgroup needs total care throughout life. In Sweden, among adults with cerebral palsy but not mental retardation, 75% either lived on their own or with a partner, 54% felt they were not limited in their ability to get around in the community, and 24% reported working full time (Andersson & Mattsson, 2001). With aging, some adults have a hard time with progressive foot deformities and joint pain from osteoarthritis. These changes conspire to cause insecurity in walking, leading to falls and additional injuries (Bottos, Feliciangeli, Sciuto, Gericke, & Vianello, 2001).

The life span of individuals with cerebral palsy is somewhat diminished, but the great majority live well into adulthood. The degree of life shortening is related directly to the severity of motor involvement plus the number and severity of associated deficits (e.g., mental retardation, seizures, nutritional problems). The most profoundly affected individuals have greatly reduced life expectancies and often are predicted to die before or by adolescence. This is an extremely small group, and predictability is rather inaccurate in terms of individual cases, because it is based on chance of survival in a population of similar individuals.

# THE TEACHER'S ROLE

Many children and adults with cerebral palsy used to live out their lives secluded at home or in large institutions. Now, however, children are routinely enrolled in school and in the least restrictive classroom setting. Therefore, the educator is in a unique position to play a vital role in the habilitation of the child and to provide support for the family.

Services, including education, for children with disabilities are now protected in the United States by federal legislation that originated with grassroots efforts in the 1960s. Services then were provided by professionals and dedicated parents in church basements and donated buildings under the auspices of organizations such as the Association for Retarded Citizens and Easter Seals. Subsequently, one of the most important actions by the federal government in support of children with disabilities took place—the passage in 1975 of the Education for All Handicapped Children Act (P.L. 94-142), later amended as P.L. 99-457, then replaced in 1990 by the Individuals with Disabilities Education Act (IDEA; P.L. 101-476). These laws established free, appropriate education for all school-age children with disabilities and early intervention services for preschool-age children (3 years and older) and promised federal incentives for states to establish programs for infants and toddlers (P. M. Blasco, 2001).

During the 1980s, educators realized the significant role of the family, particularly the caretaking parents, as the most influential persons in the child's life. Educators, therapists, and other professionals are transient in the child's life, but families provide ongoing influence. The intervention process that was developed emphasized the importance of family resources, priorities, and concerns, as well as family-directed services. In 1997, Congress reauthorized IDEA and added some changes to the original legislation, the hallmark of which is the Individualized Family Service Plan (IFSP). The following are the key elements of the plan:

- A statement of the child's present developmental status (based on appropriate assessment of the developmental domains listed in eligibility criteria)

- A statement of the family's strengths, resources, concerns, and priorities related to enhancing the development of the child

- A statement of expected outcomes for the child and family (including procedures, criteria for reaching goals, and timelines)

- A list of early intervention services and supports needed, and a plan for service coordination (including frequency, intensity, and method of service delivery)

- A statement of the natural environments in which services will be provided

- The name of the service coordinator who will be responsible for coordinating services and implementing the plan

- A transition plan to support the child and family as they transition to preschool services when appropriate

There are also provisions for ongoing review, evaluation, and revision of the plan.

Today, all children identified through state-required assessment procedures have an Individualized Education Plan (IEP) or IFSP, which is developed with the family and, when appropriate, the child within 30 days of eligibility determination. The child's parents or surrogate parents, other family members, representatives of the local educational agency, the special education teacher and/or general education teacher, and professionals representing other services (e.g., physical therapy, occupational therapy, vision specialists) are invited to participate in the IEP or IFSP meeting. This team works together to develop goals and objectives that are age appropriate for the child in the least restrictive environment. Goals and objectives are based on the student's present level of performance. Family members are included in all decision-making aspects of the IEP process, and they have a right to due process proceedings if they disagree with the rest of the team on placement or educational decisions. Parent advocacy groups, such as PACER (Parent Advocacy Coalition for Education Rights; http://www.pacer.org), are available to help parents locate resources and services. Parents often find additional information on the Internet that they may want to share with the rest of the team.

The provision of services from birth provides a safety net for children diagnosed with cerebral palsy. Many of these children and families are referred for services as they leave the hospital. With early intervention, children with cerebral palsy receive the supports they need to develop to their fullest potential. These supports are best delivered using a coordinated, interagency team-based approach. Teams are most effective when the parents work in partnership to ensure the very best services for their child with cerebral palsy (Bruder, 1996; McGonigel, Woodruff, & Roszmann-Millican, 1994).

The service delivery model varies in each state or province and also at the local educational level. For example, in some states, educational service districts may offer educational services in a resource room with opportunities for inclusion during music, recreation, and meals. The educational service district in the next county may offer full inclusion with supports within the regular general education classroom. Educators need to be informed on what are considered recommended practices in working with children with disabilities. These practices, such as inclusion, are upheld by federal and state or province legislation that sets the standards for educational programs. As this trend continues, educators are assuming an increasingly greater responsibility in the care of the child with cerebral palsy. Their attention to changes in motor performance, intellectual abilities, and behavior plays a critical role in the overall approach to managing the child.

Although children with cerebral palsy may demonstrate normal intellect, as a group they are at significant risk for mental retardation, learning disabilities, or behavioral problems as a result of defects in the cerebral cortex. Thus, children with cerebral palsy have a wide range of intellectual abilities, and the team must also consider all of the associated impairments that may affect the child's learning needs when determining services and placement. Early identification of such learning difficulties and other associated disabilities by a child's teacher may enhance remediation. The IEP should include plans for teaching subject matter and social skills plus recommendations for the use of adaptive equipment and assistive technology in the classroom.

The educator, practicing in an interdisciplinary model with occupational and physical therapists, needs to understand the functional goals and techniques used for classroom positioning and mobility. The teacher may also reinforce the techniques used to work on posture and locomotion skills, with the ultimate goal of motor ability enhancement. Teachers and classroom aides may be called upon to remove and apply orthoses, position children in various mobility or positioning devices, and help operate augmentative communication systems. Teachers also assist by enhancing the activities of daily living or the self-help skills that are so essential for the child to be successful in the home and in the community. The teacher becomes the logical advocate with school authorities to provide modifications within the classroom and the school in order to accommodate the child with cerebral palsy or other special needs. For the child who is taking medication for behavioral difficulties, seizures, or other indications, the teacher plays a vital role in informing parents and physicians whether positive or negative effects of the medications are observed in the academic setting.

Inclusion of children with cerebral palsy can be facilitated by the use of technology. When physical limitations prohibit participation, adaptive devices become a powerful equalizer, providing the means for a child to accomplish classroom assignments and to communicate with peers. Careful assessment of the learner (including positioning, physical ability, visual ability, etc.), the environments, and the tasks expected of the child within each environment will provide a firm basis for selecting possible technology devices to use. Assistive technology includes "any item, piece of equipment, or product system, whether acquired commercially off the shelf, modified, or customized, that is used to increase, maintain, or improve functional capabilities of children with disabilities" (Technology-Related Assistance for Individuals with Disabilities Act of 1988; P.L. 100-407). Technology changes rapidly, and it is the responsibility of the team, including the family, to monitor and evaluate the assistive technology used by the child (Kravik, 2001).

Educators also are encouraged to join organizations that help determine and advocate for recommended practices in the field of special education. The Council for Exceptional Children (CEC) is the largest international professional organization in support of children with disabilities and their families (http://www.canadian.cec.sped.org). CEC provides not only guidelines on professional practices, but also advocacy and ethical standards for professionals working with children. To support some of the unique Canadian needs, the Canadian Council for Exceptional Children was established with its own Board of Directors and its own quarterly publication, *Keeping in Touch.*

# REFERENCES

Andersson, C., & Mattsson, E. (2001). Adults with cerebral palsy: A survey describing problems, needs, and resources, with special emphasis on locomotion. *Developmental Medicine and Child Neurology, 43,* 76–82.

Baird, H. W., & Gordon, E. C. (1983). Neurological evaluation of infants and children. *Clinics in Developmental Medicine* (No. 84/85). Philadelphia: Lippincott.

Bax, M. C. O. (1964). Terminology and classification of cerebral palsy. *Developmental Medicine and Child Neurology, 6,* 295–297.

Blasco, P. A. (1992). Normal and abnormal motor development. *Pediatric Rounds, 1*(2), 1–6.

Blasco, P. A., Baumgartner, M. C., & Mathes, B. C. (1983). Literature for parents of children with cerebral palsy. *Developmental Medicine and Child Neurology, 25,* 642–647.

Blasco, P. M. (2001). *Early intervention services for infants, toddlers, and their families* (pp. 1–8). Boston: Allyn & Bacon.

Bottos, M., Feliciangeli, A., Sciuto, L., Gericke, C., & Vianello, A. (2001). Functional status of adults with cerebral palsy and implications for treatment of children. *Developmental Medicine and Child Neurology, 43,* 516–528.

Bruder, M. B. (1996). Interdisciplinary collaboration in service delivery. In R. A. McWilliam (Ed.), *Rethinking pull-out services in early intervention: A professional resource* (pp. 27–48). Baltimore: Brookes.

Cummins, S. K., Nelson, K. B., Grether, J. K., & Velie, E. M. (1993). Cerebral palsy in four northern California counties, births 1983 through 1985. *Journal of Pediatrics, 123,* 230–237.

Denhoff, E., & Robinault, I. P. (1960). *Cerebral palsy and related disorders.* New York: McGraw-Hill.

Education for All Handicapped Children Act of 1975, 20 U.S.C. § 1400 *et seq.*

Education of the Handicapped Act Amendments of 1986, 20 U.S.C. § 1400 *et seq.*

Freud, S. (1968). *Infantile cerebral paralysis* (L. A. Russin, Trans.). Coral Gables, FL: University of Miami Press. (Original work published 1897)

Geralis, E. (Ed.). (1991). *Children with cerebral palsy: A parent's guide.* Rockville, MD: Woodbine House.

Grether, J. K., Nelson, K. B., & Cummins, S. K. (1993). Twinning and cerebral palsy: Experience in four northern California counties, births 1983–1985. *Pediatrics, 92,* 854–858.

Hagberg, B., Hagberg, G., & Zetterstrom, G. (1989). Decreasing perinatal mortality— Increase in cerebral palsy morbidity? *Acta Paediatrica Scandinavia, 78,* 664–670.

Individuals with Disabilities Education Act of 1990, 20 U.S.C. § 1400 *et seq.*

Individuals with Disabilities Education Act Amendments of 1997, 20 U.S.C. § 1401 (26).

Kaminer, R. K., & Cohen, H. J. (1988). How do you say, "Your child is retarded"? *Contemporary Pediatrics, 5*(5), 36–49.

Kravik, D. J. (2001). Technology and the future. In P. M. Blasco (Ed.), *Early intervention services for infants, toddlers, and their families* (pp. 295–333). Boston: Allyn & Bacon.

Little, W. J. (1853). *On the nature and treatment of the deformities of the human frame: Being a course of lectures delivered at the Royal Orthopedic Hospital in 1843 with numerous notes and additions.* London: Longman, Brown, Greene, and Longmans.

Lobato, D. J. (1990). *Brothers, sisters, and special needs: Information and activities for helping young siblings of children with chronic illnesses and developmental disorders.* Baltimore: Brookes.

Lock, T. H. M., Shapiro, B. K., Ross, A., & Capute, A. J. (1986). Age of presentation of developmental disabilities. *Journal of Developmental and Behavioral Pediatrics, 7,* 340–345.

McGonigel, M. J., Woodruff, G., & Roszmann-Millican, M. (1994). The transdisciplinary team: A model for family-centered early intervention. In L. J. Johnson, R. J. Gallagher, & M. J. LaMontagne (Eds.), *Meeting early intervention challenges: Issues from birth to three* (2nd ed., pp. 95–131). Baltimore: Brookes.

Nolan, C. (1987). *Under the eye of the clock.* New York: St. Martin's Press.

Tizard, J. P., Paine, R. S., & Crothers, B. (1954). Disturbances of sensation in children with hemiplegia. *Journal of the American Medical Association, 155,* 628–632.

# CHAPTER 15

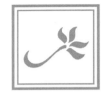

# Attention-Deficit/ Hyperactivity Disorder

Dilip J. Karnik

**A**ttention-deficit/hyperactivity disorder (ADHD) is one of the most common conditions encountered by teachers and physicians who deal with children. ADHD occurs in approximately 3% to 5% of the childhood population. Children affected with ADHD display increased motor activity, impulsiveness, and inattention, with considerable variation in the degree and frequency of these symptoms. When severe, ADHD can affect the ability to learn and can also influence behavior, social skill development, and self-esteem. ADHD can have a significant and lifelong impact on an individual. This chapter covers current concepts in the diagnosis and treatment of ADHD, with particular emphasis on the important role a teacher plays in the management of this condition.

## DIAGNOSTIC CRITERIA

George Still first described the behavioral symptoms of ADHD in 1902 in a series of three lectures to the Royal College of Physicians in England. He presented the case studies of 43 children who displayed problems with attention and behavioral inhibition. Since then, the exponential increase in ADHD research has made this condition one of the most well-studied childhood disorders.

The prevalent features of ADHD, according to the American Psychiatric Association's (2000) *Diagnostic and Statistical Manual of Mental Disorders– Fourth Edition–Text Revision* (DSM–IV–TR), are a persistent pattern of inattention and/or hyperactivity–impulsivity that is more frequent and severe than that observed in individuals of a comparable developmental age. The diagnosis of ADHD is confirmed when six or more of the following symptoms of inattention or hyperactivity–impulsivity have persisted for at least 6 months and are present to a degree that impairs the child's function and development.

### Inattention Group

1. difficulty paying attention to details or makes careless mistakes

2. difficulty sustaining attention

3. difficulty listening when spoken to directly

4. fails to finish schoolwork, chores, and duties, or does not follow instructions

5. difficulty organizing work

6. problems engaging in tasks that require sustained mental effort such as homework

7. frequently loses things such as pencils, books, and assignments

8. forgetful in routine activities

### Hyperactivity–Impulsivity Group

1. fidgety
2. problem remaining seated
3. running about or restless
4. inability to play quietly
5. often "on the go"
6. talks excessively
7. blurts out answers
8. difficulty waiting turn
9. interrupts or intrudes

To be diagnosed with ADHD, a child should have the onset of these symptoms prior to age 7 years, and impairment should be in at least two environments, such as at school and at home.

Based on symptoms, a child can be classified as having one of the following:

• Attention-deficit/hyperactivity disorder, combined type, if the child has both attention and hyperactivity–impulsivity problems

- Attention-deficit/hyperactivity disorder, predominantly inattentive type, if the child has difficulties in attention but not in hyperactivity–impulsivity

- Attention-deficit/hyperactivity disorder, predominantly hyperactivity type, if the child has symptoms in hyperactivity–impulsivity alone

Teachers and parents should be cautious when using the diagnostic label ADHD. Many other conditions may be manifested by similar characteristics and symptoms. When a teacher or parent suspects that a child has ADHD, an evaluation by a qualified professional experienced in the diagnosis and treatment of ADHD should be pursued.

# ASSOCIATED EDUCATIONAL PROBLEMS

Children with ADHD have a greater likelihood of having emotional, cognitive, developmental, and academic problems. These coexisting conditions can significantly affect a child's school performance, social–emotional development, and future vocational success. Not all children with ADHD display all of these problems (summarized in Table 15.1), but many experience at least some of these conditions to a greater extent than do normal children. The symptoms vary in severity.

Children with ADHD may be delayed in intellectual development. Research has shown that children with ADHD score an average of 7 to 15 points below control groups on standardized intelligence tests. However, these children are likely to represent the entire spectrum of intelligence from superior to mild mental retardation (Tripp, Ryan, & Peace, 2002).

**TABLE 15.1**
Learning Problems Associated with ADHD

| | |
|---|---|
| • Mental retardation | • Memory disorder |
| • Learning disability | • Motor coordination disorder |
| • Language disorder | • Dysgraphia |
| • Central auditory processing disorder (CAPD) | |

Learning disabilities can coexist with ADHD. Studies have shown that about 8% to 39% of children with ADHD have a reading disability, 12% to 30% have a mathematical disability, and 12% to 27% have a spelling disorder (Faroane et al., 1993).

Studies also have shown that children with ADHD tend to perform below average on various language evaluations, including tests of simple verbal fluency, complex language fluency, and discourse organization. In addition, children with ADHD appear to produce less speech in response to confrontational questioning and are sometimes less competent at verbal problem-solving tasks. Their story narratives tend to produce less information and are less organized in presentation.

Some children with ADHD demonstrate deficits in the processing of auditory input, despite having no intellectual or hearing impairments. This condition is known as a central auditory processing disorder (CAPD).

Children with ADHD may exhibit deficits in executive functions of the brain, including decreased nonverbal and verbal working memory, impaired planning ability, impaired sense of time, and impairment in behavioral and verbal creativity. These cognitive problems can affect the learning abilities of children with ADHD (Barkley, 1998).

"Soft" neurological signs related to fine motor coordination problems and delayed motor development are found more frequently in children with ADHD than in normal children. Tests of fine motor coordination, including balance tasks, paper–pencil mazes, and tracking activities, reveal that children with ADHD tend to be less coordinated than normal children. As a result, they may have difficulties with handwriting. Their drawing is often sluggish and sloppy. It is frequently characterized by inconsistent letter formation, excessive errors, poor organization on the page, poor fluency of hand movements, odd pencil grasp, and problems with the mechanics of writing, such as spelling, punctuation, and capitalization. All of these characteristics of dysgraphia indicate that children with ADHD experience problems with motor planning, motor control, and motor memory (Mariani & Barkley, 1997).

## ASSOCIATED BEHAVIORAL PROBLEMS

Children with ADHD carry a higher risk for developing other psychiatric disorders, including depression, anxiety disorder, bipolar disorder, conduct disorder, and oppositional defiant disorder. Children with any of these associated behavioral problems will likely have more academic difficulties than children with ADHD alone, as well as problems in their relationships with peers, teachers, and family members. They may be less compliant with parent and teacher requests and be moody or aggressive. The primary identifying symptoms of these conditions include anxiety, defiance, excessive mood swings, aggressive behavior, and depression.

Appropriate evaluation and management is of paramount importance. Children with comorbid psychiatric disorders will require more comprehensive behavioral management strategizing and intervention. Teachers, parents, and professionals should proceed with caution when attempting to diagnose any of these disorders. Sometimes children with ADHD will manifest these symptoms but not warrant a diagnosis of a psychiatric disorder. Conversely, a child who exhibits symptoms of a behavioral disorder in addition to inattention, hyperactivity, or impulsiveness may not necessarily have ADHD. A child with absence seizures manifested by frequent staring episodes may not pay attention in class. A bipolar disorder may initially present with inattention and hyperactivity. Disorders such as pervasive developmental disorder, mild mental retardation, and learning disability can sometimes be mistaken for ADHD. Table 15.2 summarizes some psychiatric disorders or conditions that may be confused with ADHD.

## CAUSES OF ADHD

Despite extensive research in this field, the exact cause of ADHD is not known. Most children with ADHD do not show any evidence of brain in-

**TABLE 15.2**
Associated Psychiatric Disorders or Conditions that May Mimic ADHD

| | |
|---|---|
| • Mood disorder | • Obsessive–compulsive disorder |
| • Anxiety disorder | • Learning disability |
| • Oppositional defiant disorder | • Mental retardation |
| • Bipolar disorder | • Absence (petit mal) seizures |
| • Pervasive developmental disorder | |

jury. Current studies suggest possible genetic, developmental, neurological, neurotransmitter, and molecular genetic factors.

## Genetic Factors

There is an increased incidence of ADHD within family members. The twin of a child with ADHD has a significantly greater chance of developing this condition if he or she is an identical twin rather than a fraternal twin. The younger siblings of children with ADHD are twice as likely to develop ADHD than the siblings of normal children. Children of biological parents who have been diagnosed with ADHD also carry a much greater risk for ADHD than children of adoptive parents. All of these statistical observations suggest a genetic etiology.

## Developmental Factors

Prenatal exposure to toxins such as alcohol and cigarette smoke is associated with an increased risk of hyperactivity, inattention, and disruptive behavior (Bennett, Wolin, & Reiss, 1988; Hartsough & Lambert, 1985; Nichols & Chen, 1981). Fetal distress, toxemia, and low birth weight are also associated with an increased risk of these characteristics. There is some evidence that more children with ADHD are born in September; it appears that prenatal exposure to winter infections may account for this increased incidence (Mick, Biederman, & Faroane, 1996).

## Neurological Factors

Brain injury was initially implicated as a cause of ADHD. Several studies have shown that injury to the frontal lobe often results in symptoms of hyperactivity and inattention (Benton, 1991; Heilman, Voeller, & Nadeau, 1991; Matles, 1980). Neuropsychological tests of frontal lobe function in individuals with ADHD consistently show a disinhibition of behavioral response and impairment of working memory, poor mental planning, decreased verbal fluency, impaired motor sequencing, and other frontal lobe dysfunctions (Barkley, 1997). The injuries can be very subtle and may not be detected by studies such as electroencephalography (EEG) or brain scan. Some of the examples of these factors include head injuries, infections such as meningitis or encephalitis, environmental exposure to toxins, hypoxia, drugs, and structural brain pathologies.

During the last decade, various neurologically based studies using innovative methods have supported the view of a neurodevelopmental origin to the disorder. There is clear evidence of diminished arousal in children with ADHD (Ferguson & Pappas, 1974). Frontal lobe studies have consistently shown an increase in slow waves on quantitative electroencephalogram (QEEG) and evoked response potential (ERP) investigations (Chabot & Serfontein, 1996). These children also have smaller amplitudes on ERP studies in the late positive component that represents the functions of the prefrontal lobe (Klorman et al., 1988).

Numerous studies of individuals with ADHD have shown decreased blood flow to the prefrontal lobe and its pathways (Lou, Henricksen, & Bruhn, 1984, 1990). Studies using positron electron tomography (PET) to measure cerebral glucose metabolism have shown a correlation between the severity of ADHD symptoms in adolescents and diminished metabolic activity in the left anterior frontal region (Zametkin et al., 1993). More recently, studies utilizing techniques such as high-resolution magnetic resonance imaging (MRI) scans (Hynd et al., 1993) and quantitative MRI technology have demonstrated abnormalities in the development of the frontal striatal region (Arnsten, Steere, & Hunt, 1996). Although this latest research is inconclusive, it appears promising in the continued search for answers to the etiology of this disorder.

## • Neurotransmitter Factors

Some research has suggested the existence of a selective deficiency in availability of the brain chemicals dopamine and norepinephrine (Lahoste et al., 1996). However, no indisputable evidence implicates a single brain chemical or neurotransmitter defect. In reality, many brain chemicals may be involved in the etiology of ADHD.

## • Molecular Genetic Factors

Current research has started to unravel the genetic basis for ADHD. Because dopamine is the neurotransmitter linked with attention-related problems, molecular studies have focused on chromosomes that control this chemical. Studies have found that the dopamine D4 receptor gene (DRD4) is located on chromosome 11p15.5. One allele of this gene, the 7-repeat variant, is overrepresented in children with ADHD (Lohoste et al., 1996). This finding could eventually prove to be quite interesting, as this receptor has been reportedly associated with conditions such as Tourette syndrome and high novelty-seeking behavior.

# EVALUATION OF THE CHILD

When a child is identified as having significant symptoms of inattention, impulsiveness, or hyperactivity, a comprehensive evaluation for ADHD is necessary, due to the complex nature of this condition. ADHD can be difficult to diagnose because some children manifest the symptoms in the classroom but not in other environments or situations. Behavioral observations and comments from a teacher may be the only clue that a child has a problem. Frequently, parents, teachers, and physicians struggle to separate a normal behavior from an abnormal one.

If ADHD is suspected, the physician should obtain a detailed history from the student and the parent. A history should also be obtained from the child's teacher through a personal interview or questionnaire. A teacher's candid opinions and good communication with a physician are critical to the evaluation for this disorder. Behavioral questionnaires such as those developed by Conners (1969), Goldstein and Goldstein (1990), and Kendall and Braswell (1985) can be useful in the evaluation for ADHD. An abbreviated Conners's Teacher Questionnaire, as shown in Figure 15.1, can be of help in the evaluation process (see Conners, 1999; Conners, Sitarenios, Parker, & Epstein, 1998).

In addition to obtaining the history, the physician should perform a complete physical and neurological examination. Tests of visual and hearing acuity should also be performed to rule out any sensory disorders affecting vision or hearing.

The diagnosis of an attention-deficit/hyperactivity disorder is essentially a clinical, but subjective diagnosis, as no laboratory tests or neurological scans can identify the disorder with certainty. The physical examination of children with ADHD is generally normal and does not necessarily help in identifying the condition except to rule out other physical or medical conditions that could be causing the symptoms. It is important to ascertain whether the child has any associated conditions. For this reason, the physician should evaluate for motor coordination problems by checking for soft neurological signs. These signs are normally present in very young children

# ABBREVIATED CONNERS'S TEACHER QUESTIONNAIRE

Child's Name _____

Today's Date _____ / _____ / _____
                Month    Day      Year

Parent's Name _____

Teacher's Name _____

**Instructions:** Listed below are items concerning children's behavior or the problems they sometimes have. Read each item carefully and decide how much you think this child has been displaying this behavior at this time. (Check only one box for each row.)

| Observation | Frequency | | | |
|---|---|---|---|---|
| | Not at all | Just a little | Often | Almost always |
| 1. Has difficulty sitting still; is excessively fidgety, restless. | ☐ | ☐ | ☐ | ☐ |
| 2. Has difficulty staying seated; is often on the go. | ☐ | ☐ | ☐ | ☐ |
| 3. Starts things without finishing them; does not complete tasks. | ☐ | ☐ | ☐ | ☐ |
| 4. Does not seem to listen attentively when spoken to. | ☐ | ☐ | ☐ | ☐ |
| 5. Has difficulty following oral directions. | ☐ | ☐ | ☐ | ☐ |
| 6. Is easily distracted; has difficulty concentrating. | ☐ | ☐ | ☐ | ☐ |
| 7. Has difficulty staying with a play activity. | ☐ | ☐ | ☐ | ☐ |
| 8. Acts before thinking. | ☐ | ☐ | ☐ | ☐ |
| 9. Has difficulty organizing work. | ☐ | ☐ | ☐ | ☐ |
| 10. Needs a lot of supervision. | ☐ | ☐ | ☐ | ☐ |
| 11. Interacts poorly with other children. | ☐ | ☐ | ☐ | ☐ |
| 12. Expects demands to be met immediately; is easily frustrated. | ☐ | ☐ | ☐ | ☐ |
| 13. Changes mood quickly; cries; has temper outbursts. | ☐ | ☐ | ☐ | ☐ |

Comments _____
_____
_____

**FIGURE 15.1.** Abbreviated Conners's Teacher Questionnaire. Adapted from "Revision and Restandardization of the Conners' Teacher Rating Scale (CTRS–R): Factor Structure, Reliability, and Criterion Validity," by C. K. Conners, G. Sitarenios, J. D. Parker, and N. Epstein, 1998, *Journal of Abnormal Child Psychology, 26*(4), pp. 279–291.

up to the age of 6 years, but as the brain matures, they generally disappear. Persistence of these signs suggests immaturity of the central nervous system, and they may be present in children with ADHD or motor coordination disorder. If learning disabilities are suspected, the child should be referred for a comprehensive psychometric evaluation that can be accomplished by a school diagnostician or a psychologist.

There are several commercially available standardized tests to identify levels of inattention and impulsivity in children suspected of having ADHD. These tests are not diagnostic by themselves, but can be useful when included as part of a comprehensive diagnostic workup. In addition, such instruments can assist in evaluating a child's response to treatment. These tests are generally referred to as continuous performance tests as they require a child to respond to a target stimulus interspersed among nontarget stimuli and are repetitive in nature. Some of the commonly used instruments include *The Gordon Diagnostic System* (Gordon, 1983), *The Conners Continuous Performance Test* (Conners, 1995), and the *Test of Variables of Attention* (Greenberg & Waldman, 1993). Recently, some advances have been made in the development of laboratory instruments such as Optax to measure activity levels (Teicher, Ito, Glod, & Barber, 1996). However, the use of activity recording devices has thus far not been shown to accurately classify children as having or not having ADHD. These instruments may ultimately prove to be more useful in determining a child's response to treatment.

After careful evaluation, an experienced clinician should be able to make a diagnosis of this condition with some certainty and will be able to rule out many other neuropsychiatric conditions that may resemble ADHD. Neurological investigations such as CAT scan, MRI scans, EEG, brain mapping, allergy testing, or any other scanning is not recommended for ADHD evaluation. These tests are done only if some other physical condition is suspected.

# MANAGEMENT

Research has demonstrated that the use of multiple modalities, including academic support, behavioral counseling, parent training, and pharmacotherapy, is the most successful approach in the treatment of ADHD. Not all children diagnosed with ADHD require medication. Mild cases may respond to educational or behavioral modalities and may not need medication. More severe cases may warrant immediate introduction of drugs. Some physicians may prescribe medications only after a trial of behavioral and educational modalities. Nevertheless, current research suggests that, when compared with the use of nonmedication modalities alone, treatment with psychotropic drugs is statistically more effective in improving ADHD symptoms.

## Counseling

Once ADHD is diagnosed, the physician discusses it with the parents with respect to its nature and treatment options. Every effort is made to give parents a clear picture of this condition and to help them accept the diagnosis and prepare for long-term management. Through counseling, the physician may be able to help remove incorrect ideas and misinformation, guilt, or denial that the parents may have. Ineffective or counterproductive patterns of parenting, if present, are identified and discouraged. Parental overexpectations from the child or the school system are identified and appropriate measures are suggested.

Counseling by a psychologist or a social worker may be warranted, especially if the child has a significant associated condition, such as depression, anxiety, aggression, or antisocial behavior. The counselor may develop a behavioral program that the teacher and parents can follow. Such counseling may consist of individual sessions with the parents to promote more realistic and effective parenting strategies (Barkley, 1990; Wender, 1987). The child may be given specific instruction in the areas of socialization, communication, organization, and better study habits (Furman, 1980).

## Academic Interventions

Managing a child with ADHD can become an overwhelming task for a teacher. Monitoring, recording, and implementing behavioral management strategies can be time consuming and at times impractical. However, appropriate and effective management is critical to the child's success, as well as the teacher's sanity. The following principles and behavioral guidelines are essential to the successful treatment of ADHD in the classroom:

1. Professionals who work with children who have ADHD should understand ADHD as a condition. Educators should become in-

formed by reading books and articles, as well as attending seminars and conferences. Misunderstanding of the disorder can lead to undue stress and adverse relationships.

2. Teachers should be aware that children with ADHD are highly inconsistent in the manifestation of symptoms. A child with ADHD may perform well one day and poorly the next. In addition, the child may seem behaviorally normal in some situations and out of control in others.

3. Professionals should be sensitive to situations in which a child with ADHD might be extremely anxious so as to avoid embarrassing the child, especially in front of peers.

## Teacher's Personality

The extra work and stress incurred in teaching a child with ADHD can cause a teacher to feel overwhelmed. It is important for an educator to consider whether his or her personality is amenable to working with a child with ADHD. Should a teacher feel unable to manage a child with ADHD, he or she should not hesitate to consult with school administrators. School administrators should be supportive in a teacher's efforts to work with children with ADHD but also be open to changes when a teacher is uncomfortable with the addition of a student with ADHD to his or her classroom. Understanding of the following characteristics is important to the successful treatment of children with ADHD and should be considered when assigning a teacher to take on the management of these children.

- **Flexibility**

  Teachers who are open to adjustments will have more success. If the teacher is rigid and inflexible, both the teacher and the child will experience greater difficulty.

- **Creativity**

  Teachers who are creative and innovative in the development and implementation of teaching strategies are more likely to find what works with students who have ADHD.

- **Sensitivity**

  Teachers should understand that many children with ADHD have low self-esteem. Openly commenting on their grades, behavior, or medical condition can certainly exacerbate this problem. In addition, if a child must take medication at school, the teacher should be discreet when assisting with administration of the drug.

## Teaching Style

The following are principles of presentation that teachers may employ with children who have ADHD. Some or all of these approaches may improve a child's classroom behavior and performance.

- An organized presentation benefits all students.

- A vibrant and energetic presentation is much more likely to keep a student's attention than a quiet, monotone delivery.

- A teacher should allow plenty of time for presenting material. A hurried or impatient approach is not effective.

- It is beneficial to emphasize key or important points.

- Eye contact with each student is an important tool in determining whether students are attempting to focus and listen.

- Presentation of material through a variety of teaching aids, such as pictures, hands-on demonstration and manipulation, videos, role-plays, and other audiovisual techniques, can significantly enhance the learning process.

- An interactive presentation is much more likely to sustain students' attention.

- Teachers must establish mutual respect. An authoritarian approach without the respect of students is not effective.

## Management Strategies

Teachers can use a variety of techniques to help the student with ADHD. The following lists include classroom accommodations, child-centered approaches (Barkley, 1985), and teacher-centered approaches. These are followed by a range of suggested classroom behavior management strategies.

## Classroom Accommodations

- Allow the student to sit near the teacher.

- Seat the student near a model student.

- Keep the student away from noisy equipment such as the air conditioner or heating unit.

- Allow the student to sit away from high traffic or distracting areas.

- Keep the student in small groups if at all possible.

- Keep the student away from classroom bullies.

- Keep visual and auditory distractions to a minimum when students are working independently.

- Reduce the disturbance caused by extraneous noise through the use of calming background music or white noise.

- Install an FM system and headphones. Children with ADHD and a central auditory processing disorder may benefit from this method.

- Closely supervise students to be aware of their particular difficulties and challenging subjects. It may be necessary to provide additional time and assistance in instruction of some subjects.

- Some students may require tutoring from an independent source. When possible, pursue tutoring for students who are falling behind in academic development.

- Provide the student with a preview of the material before presenting it to the class. Give the student notes, a copy of the chapter, or books about the subject to read ahead of time. This will help the child become somewhat familiar with the topic and will enhance comprehension and learning.

## Child-Centered Approaches

- Rehearse the instructions. Have the student review and repeat the instructions before starting the task. This can prevent the child from an impulsive and poorly organized start.

- Facilitate planning and organization before the student begins the task. Once the student understands the instructions, help the child plan and organize his or her response by breaking the task down into steps and prioritizing these steps.

- Remember that some students may need to explore other ways of accomplishing the task. Assist the child in choosing the best option for achieving the desired outcome when necessary.

- Teach and demonstrate organizational strategies. Demonstrate how a large and complex assignment can be divided into a series of small assignments that lead to an accurate and timely completion of the task. Also teach students how to use assignment books and time management strategies to help meet deadlines.

- Teach appropriate communication strategies. Teach students to be respectful but assertive when communicating. Encourage students to talk about the effectiveness of various strategies and teaching techniques. This kind of exchange can go a long way in empowering and motivating children with ADHD.

- Monitor behavior. Openly discuss with a student signals that the student thinks can help in correcting inappropriate behavior. Strategies such as standing next to the student, making eye contact, or tapping him or her on the shoulder, might help in redirecting a student and preventing the escalation of inappropriate behavior.

## Teacher-Centered Approaches

- Follow a consistent routine. Children with ADHD tend to do much better in structured programs that follow a regular routine. They do poorly in unorganized, chaotic situations.

- Avoid information overload. Children vary in their ability to attend and concentrate, and in speed of processing. Children with ADHD are particularly vulnerable to problems with the processing of information. Periodically check to see whether a student with ADHD comprehends instructions and information and is not becoming overwhelmed with the amount of material being presented.

- List the primary problems affecting the child with ADHD and concentrate on helping him or her work on these issues. To the extent possible, ignore the problems that do not interfere with learning, such as restlessness, hyperactivity, fidgeting, unusual postures, and noise making or tapping.

- If noise is a problem in the classroom, use a noise meter. Reward the class for keeping noise below a certain level.

## Establishing Consequences

A teacher should identify problem behaviors that need to be extinguished and work on reducing these behaviors by establishing a reward system for appropriate substitute behaviors. Preferred behaviors that might be rewarded include the following:

- Working independently without disturbing others
- Completing assignments
- Remaining seated at desk or workstation
- Taking appropriate notes
- Improving grades

A variety of rewards can be used:

- Homework reduction
- Verbal praise
- Computer access
- Additional recess
- Class job or responsibility (e.g., class monitor)
- Field trip
- Lunch with parent or teacher
- Prize, food, or toy
- Being first in line (leader)
- Show and tell opportunity

Teachers should target the behaviors that are critical to the child's ability to learn and make sure the rewards are meaningful to the child. Parents should be involved in identifying the target behaviors and rewards to the extent possible. It is important to establish positive rewards and avoid negative consequences, such as criticism, insults, or humiliation.

## Point and Token Systems

A variety of methods employ point and token systems (Azvin & Holz, 1966; Duncan, 1997). Teachers may wish to adapt some of these methods or develop their own programs that are tailored to the specific needs of each child.

The primary strategy or goal of these systems is the rewarding of points or tokens for appropriate target behaviors. A system can be set up so that points or tokens are taken away as a consequence for inappropriate behavior, such as talking out of turn, disturbing others, getting out of one's seat, getting off task, and using inappropriate language. A brief explanation should be given as to why a point was taken away. The student should be encouraged to work on the behavior so as to win the point or token back.

The first step in developing a point or token system for behavior modification is to identify the behaviors that most frequently interfere with the child's ability to learn and function appropriately in the classroom. It may be helpful to fill out a behavioral questionnaire such as the Abbreviated Conners's Teacher Questionnaire (in Figure 15.1), and then rank the behaviors based on frequency and severity. Parents also may wish to complete a home situation questionnaire (e.g., Goyette, Conners, & Ulrich, 1978) and provide input during the development of this system. Then the behavior needs to be monitored for improvement. Figure 15.2 is a simple questionnaire that teachers and parents may use to help identify problems and assist them in monitoring progress.

## Extinction Process

Some undesirable behaviors are best ignored when they occur. This technique can be a viable method for weakening and extinguishing behaviors such as whining, pouting, temper tantrums, demanding, complaining, inappropriate noises, foul language, and crying. Generally speaking, ignoring these behaviors and not reacting to them will gradually weaken them over a period of time. The extinction process is not recommended for severe behavior problems such as antisocial acting out or aggressive conduct.

## Proximity Control

The teacher may curtail some undesirable behaviors simply by standing next to the student and assuming a stern body posture and facial expression. Such proximity control techniques can be useful in controlling mild nonaggressive behaviors.

---

## FOLLOW-UP SHEET
## FOR ADHD BEHAVIOR SCORE

Child's Name _____

Parent's Name _____

Teacher's Name _____

Dates: From ____/____/____ To ____/____/____

**Instructions:** Identify the behaviors that need to be extinguished. For each negative behavior, suggest an appropriate or target behavior the child should exhibit instead. Grade the child's behavior by using the following point system. Reward the child if improvement is shown. Counsel the child if no improvement is seen on weekly basis.

| 0—no problem | 2—moderate problem |
|---|---|
| 1—mild problem | 3—severe problem |

| | Points | | | | | Points | | | |
|---|---|---|---|---|---|---|---|---|---|
| **Problem behavior** | 0 | 1 | 2 | 3 | **Suggested behavior** | 0 | 1 | 2 | 3 |
| Gets off task | ☐ | ☐ | ☐ | ☐ | Stays on task | ☐ | ☐ | ☐ | ☐ |
| Interrupts | ☐ | ☐ | ☐ | ☐ | Raises hand/waits turn | ☐ | ☐ | ☐ | ☐ |
| Overactive/fidgety | ☐ | ☐ | ☐ | ☐ | Remains calm | ☐ | ☐ | ☐ | ☐ |
| Forgets assignment | ☐ | ☐ | ☐ | ☐ | Writes down assignment | ☐ | ☐ | ☐ | ☐ |
| Ignores instructions | ☐ | ☐ | ☐ | ☐ | Listens and repeats instructions | ☐ | ☐ | ☐ | ☐ |
| Acts before thinking | ☐ | ☐ | ☐ | ☐ | Thinks before acting | ☐ | ☐ | ☐ | ☐ |
| Talks back | ☐ | ☐ | ☐ | ☐ | Is respectful | ☐ | ☐ | ☐ | ☐ |
| Gets angry | ☐ | ☐ | ☐ | ☐ | Controls anger | ☐ | ☐ | ☐ | ☐ |
| Has difficulty playing | ☐ | ☐ | ☐ | ☐ | Shares/cooperates | ☐ | ☐ | ☐ | ☐ |
| Is not organized | ☐ | ☐ | ☐ | ☐ | Organizes | ☐ | ☐ | ☐ | ☐ |
| Loses things | ☐ | ☐ | ☐ | ☐ | Does not lose things | ☐ | ☐ | ☐ | ☐ |

**Observations:**

Child is making progress at the end of 4 weeks:  ☐ Yes   ☐ No

If yes, progress is:  ☐ Mild   ☐ Moderate   ☐ Significant

**FIGURE 15.2.** Questionnaire for identifying ADHD problems and monitoring progress.

## The Premack Principle

Having the child do unpleasant and difficult work first can help the child complete assignments efficiently. Teachers and parents should consider assigning more difficult tasks at the beginning of the class or homework period. This technique is known as the Premack principle.

## Signal System

Teachers or parents can develop a signal system to reduce undesirable behavior. Examples include using a specific hand signal, calling the child in a different tone of voice, standing near the child's desk, or putting a finger over the lips when the child is talking out of turn.

## Consequences

Action that follows a particular behavior is called a consequence. It can be positive, such as a reward, or negative, such as a punishment. Teachers and parents may use the following rewards:

- Tangible (goods)
- Activities (privileges)
- Social (praise)

The teacher or parent should identify the behavior to be improved and, if the child rectifies the problem, reward the child with positive reinforcement. Rewards are more effective than punishments for improving undesirable behavior.

Negative consequences can be aversive, such as evoking pain or discomfort, or deprivation events, such as taking away a pleasurable object or activity from the child. Research and experience has shown that the aversion method is generally ineffective and there are many short- and long-term undesirable effects.

Children respond best to a behavior modification system if teachers and parents

- are specific about the behavior to improve and suggest the appropriate substitute behavior in language the children understand.

- reward appropriate behavior and punish only the inappropriate ones that cannot be ignored.

- pay minimal attention to minor behavioral problems.

- are consistent with rewards and punishments.

- reward and punish immediately when possible.

- reward with social praise or with privileges that are meaningful to the child.

- avoid the use of physical punishment.

- do not expect big changes in behavior immediately.

## Neuropharmacological Approaches

Some children with ADHD, especially those who have not improved with the use of educational and behavioral modification strategies, may benefit from medication. Research data have clearly demonstrated that appropriate use of medication can significantly benefit children with ADHD.

Response to medication varies across individuals and, although the majority of children will respond to the therapy, some will improve with one form and others need a different medication. Children with difficulties at school but not in other situations may be prescribed medication for school days and may not need the drug over the weekend or the long holidays. Duration of therapy is generally many months to a few years, depending on the child's need. The teacher, parents, and physician should work together to select the most appropriate therapy and monitor the side effects. This collaborative effort is important for the success of managing a child's ADHD.

Given the diverse population with ADHD and the numerous medications available to treat this condition, physicians face a significant challenge in managing the condition. The choice of medications include the following (Kaplan & Sadock, 1997):

- Stimulants
- Antidepressants (tricyclics, bupoprion, venlafaxine)
- Anticonvulsants for aggressive behavior
- Antihypertensives (clonidine, guanefacine)
- Neuroleptics or antipsychotics for aggression

## Stimulants

Stimulants include a variety of medications:

- Methylphenidate group (e.g., Ritalin, Ritalin SR, Concerta, Metadate-ER and CD, Methyline)
- Amphetamine group (e.g., Dexedrine, Adderall, Adderall XR, Dextrostat)
- Newer agents (e.g., dexmethylphenidate (Focalin), Ritalin LA)

The precise mechanism of these medications is unknown. They have been shown to improve selective attention, reduce impulsiveness, increase self-control, and enhance social skills by improving the ability to perceive and integrate social cues (Hunt, Paguin, & Payton, 2001).

Methylphenidate is a short-acting medication with action duration of about 4 hours. Consequently, this drug must be administered two to three times a day. Common side effects include headaches, abdominal pain and discomfort, nausea, loss of appetite, and insomnia. Some children will experience a rebound effect as the drug level tapers off. During this phase, these children become irritable and more impulsive. Use of longer acting preparations may prevent this problem. Stimulants may exacerbate pre-existing tics, and concerns have been raised about growth suppression. Numerous studies have found that about 75% of children with ADHD will improve with the use of stimulants.

Problems with frequent dose administration have recently been solved by the availability of long-acting stimulant medications. Although these newer drugs have the same ingredient, methylphenidate or amphetamine, the structure of the capsule is designed to deliver the medication over a prolonged period of 8 to 12 hours.

Dexedrine is usually the second line of drug choice and used when methylphenidate is found to be ineffective. The side effects are similar to those of methylphenidate.

Pimoline, or Cylert, has been used for many years in the management of ADHD. However, reports of serious liver toxicity in patients treated with this drug have recently surfaced.

## Antidepressants

Various antidepressants have been used to treat ADHD. Although the task performance of children taking these drugs typically improves, antidepressants are generally less effective than stimulants in improving overall behavior. Tricyclic antidepressants, such as imipramine or desipramine, have been used to treat children with ADHD who have depression or insomnia. Cardiovascular side effects necessitate careful monitoring of children who are on these medications.

The use of selective serotonin reuptake inhibitors (SSRIs), such as par-oxitane (Paxil), fluoxetine (Prozac), sertraline (Zoloft), and cetalopram (Celexa), alone are not effective in treating ADHD. However, their concomitant use with stimulants is effective in children with depression, social phobia, or anxiety associated with ADHD. The side effects common to SSRIs include weight gain, diminished libido, blunting of emotions, and sleep difficulties.

Bupropion (Wellbutrin) has been used effectively in patients with ADHD and mood disorder. It is particularly useful in children with substance and tobacco abuse problems. Some of the side effects of this drug include headaches, tremors, malaise, and lower seizure threshold.

Venlafaxine (Effexor) is another relatively new agent useful in patients with ADHD who have associated aggressive or acting out behavior. The medication can reduce oppositional and defiant behavior. Its side effects include sedation.

Mirtazapine (Remeron) is also an antidepressant that can be used to improve behavior in children with ADHD. In low doses at bedtime, it can induce sleep and increase appetite and therefore can be useful in children who experience a loss of appetite and insomnia while on stimulants.

## Other Agents

Drugs such as clonidine and guanfacine have been used in patients with ADHD and tic disorders. These medications decrease the level of activity, tics, and aggressiveness. The common side effects include sedation, a drop in blood pressure, and slowing of heart rate.

Anticonvulsants such as carbamazepine (Tegretol) and valproic acid (Depakote) have been used in special situations, such as in children with ADHD and an associated mood disorder, bipolar disorder, or aggression. Use of the neuroleptic agents such as respiridone, olanzapine, and quentiapine is also restricted to situations when a child with ADHD has other significant psychiatric conditions that are interfering with the student's education or social participation. Use of these drugs is limited due to their significant side effects.

## Unproven Therapies

A number of therapies have been suggested to help children with ADHD without substantial scientific support or appropriate research (Feingold, 1975). These therapies include restricting additives in the diet, avoiding caffeine-containing drinks (Conners, 1980), and megavitamin therapy (Haslam, Dalby, & Rademaker, 1984). Others that do not significantly help include patterning, optometric training, picnogenol, various herbs, brain function–enhancing nutrients or products, and biofeedback. Unproven therapies can be expensive, falsely raise expectations, and delay the appropriate treatment. They should be discouraged.

# THE TEACHER'S ROLE

Attention-deficit/hyperactivity disorder is a common condition that affects a child's education and behavior. If untreated, ADHD may lead to profound and long-term consequences. With proper management, however, most children with ADHD improve and become happier, better adjusted individuals. Although many benefit from medication, the use of medication alone has not been shown to facilitate the best outcome. A multimodality approach, incorporating the use of classroom adaptations, behavior modification strategies, counseling, parent training, tutoring, and therapies, as well as the use of medication when appropriate, is the most effective treatment approach for children with ADHD. Parents, teachers, and physicians all play important roles in assisting these children to achieve good outcomes. However, without a doubt, teachers who work with children with ADHD can make the greatest impact on the ability of these children to learn, achieve, and ultimately feel better about themselves. The classroom teacher has a vital role in both diagnosis and therapy.

# REFERENCES

American Psychiatric Association. (2000). *Diagnostic and statistical manual of mental disorders–fourth edition–text revision.* Washington, DC: Author.

Arnsten, A. F. T., Steere, J. C., & Hunt, R. D. (1996). The contribution of alpa-2-noradrenergic mechanism of prefrontal cortical cognitive function. *Archives of General Psychiatry, 53,* 448–455.

Azvin, H. H., & Holz, W. C. (1966). Punishment in operant behavior. In W. K. Homig (Ed.), *Areas of research and application.* New York: Appleton Century Cross.

Barkley, R. A. (1985). *Defiant children: A clinician's manual for parent training.* New York: Guilford Press.

Barkley, R. A. (1990). *Attention-deficit hyperactivity disorder.* New York: Guilford Press.

Barkley, R. A. (1997). *ADHD and nature of self-control.* New York: Guilford Press.

Barkley, R. A. (1998). *Attention deficit hyperactivity disorder: A handbook for diagnosis and treatment.* New York: Guilford Press.

Bennett, L. A., Wolin, S. J., & Reiss, D. (1988). Cognitive, behavioral and emotional problems among school-aged children of alcoholic parents. *American Journal of Psychiatry, 145,* 185–190.

Benton, A. (1991). Prefrontal injury and behavior in children. *Developmental Neuropsychology, 7,* 275–282.

Chabot, R. J., & Serfontein, G. (1996). Quantitative electroencephalographic profile of children with attention deficit disorder. *Biological Psychiatry, 40,* 952–963.

Conners, C. K. (1969). A teacher rating scale for use in drug studies with children. *American Journal of Psychiatry, 126,* 884–888.

Conners, C. K. (1980). *Food additives and hyperactive children.* New York: Plenum.

Conners, C. K. (1995). *The Conners Continuous Performance Test.* North Tonawanda, NY: MultiHealth Systems.

Conners, C. K. (1999). Clinical use of rating scales in diagnosis and treatment of attention-deficit/hyperactivity disorder. *Pediatric Clinics of North America, 46*(5), 857–870.

Conners, C. K., Sitarenios, G., Parker, J. D., & Epstein, N. (1998). Revision and restandardization of the Conners Teacher Rating Scale (CTRS–R): Factor structure, reliability, and criterion validity. *Journal of Abnormal Child Psychology, 26*(4), 279–291.

Duncan, M. (1997). Practice parameters for assessment and treatment of children, adolescents, and adults with attention-deficit/hyperactivity disorder. *Journal of the American Academy of Child and Adolescent Psychiatry, 36*(Suppl. 10), 85S–121S.

Faraone, S. V., Biederman, J., Lehman, B., Keenan, K. I., Norman, D., Seidman, L. J., Kolodney, R., Kraus, I., Perrin, J., & Chen, W. (1993). Evidence for the independent familial transmission of attention deficit hyperactivity disorder and learning disabilities: Result of a familial genetic study. *American Journal of Psychiatry, 150,* 891–895.

Feingold, B. (1975). *Why your child is hyperactive.* New York: Random House.

Ferguson, H. B., & Pappas, B. A. (1974). Evolution of psychophysiological, neurochemical, and animal moods of hyperactivity. In R. L. Tries (Ed.), *Hyperactivity in children.* Baltimore: University Park Press.

Furman, W. (1980). Promoting social development: Developmental implications for treatment. In B. Lahey & A. Kazden (Eds.), *Advances in clinical child psychology* (pp. 1–40). New York: Plenum.

Goldstein, S., & Goldstein, M. (1990). *Managing attention disorder in children.* New York: Wiley.

Gordon, M. (1983). *The Gordon Diagnostic System.* DeWitt, NY: Gordon System.

Goyette, C. H., Conners, C. K., & Ulrich, R. F. (1978). Normative data on Revised Conners Parent and Teacher Rating Scales. *Journal of Abnormal Child Psychology, 6*(2), 221–236.

Greenberg, L. M., & Waldman, I. D. (1993). Developmental normative data on the Test of Variables of Attention (TOVA). *Journal of Psychology and Psychiatry, 34*(6), 1019–1030.

Hartsough, C. S., & Lambert, N. M. (1985). Medical factors in hyperactivity and normal children: Prenatal development and health history findings. *American Journal of Orthopsychiatry, 55,* 190–210.

Haslam, R. H. A., Dalby, J. T., & Rademaker, A. W. (1984). Effects of megavitamin therapy on children with attention deficit disorders. *Pediatrics, 74*(1), 103–111.

Heilman, K. M., Voeller, K. K. S., & Nadeau, S. E. (1991). A possible pathophysiological substrate of attention deficit hyperactivity disorder. *Journal of Child Neurology, 6,* 74–79.

Hunt, R. D., Paguin, A., & Payton, K. (2001). An update on assessment and treatment of complex attention-deficit hyperactivity disorder. *Pediatric Annals, 30,* 162–172.

Hynd, G. W., Hern, K. L., Novey, E. S., Eliopouous, D., Marshall, R., Gonzalez, J. J., & Voeller, K. K. (1993). Attention deficit hyperactivity disorder and asymmetry of caudate nucleus. *Journal of Child Neurology, 8,* 339–347.

Kaplan, H. I., & Sadock, B. J. (1997). *Attention deficit disorders: Synopsis of psychiatry* (8th ed., pp. 1193–1200). Baltimore: Lippincott Williams and Wilkins.

Kendall, T. C., & Braswell, L. (1985). *Cognitive behavioral therapy for impulsive children.* New York: Guilford Press.

Klorman, R., Brumaghim, J. T., Coons, H. W. I., Peloquin, L., Strauss, J., Lewine, J. D., Borgstedt, A. D., & Goldstein, M. G. (1988). The contribution of event related potential to understand effects of stimulants in information processing in attention deficit disorder. In L. M. Bloomingdale & J. A. Sergeant (Eds.), *Attention deficit disorder, criteria, cognition, intervention* (pp. 198–218). London: Pergamon Press.

Lahoste, G. J., Swanson, J. M., Wigal, S. B., Globe, C., Wigal, T., King, N., & Kennedy, J. L. (1996). Dopamine D4 receptor gene polymorphism is associated with attention deficit hyperactivity disorder. *Molecular Psychiatry, 1,* 121–124.

Lou, H. C., Henricksen, L., & Bruhn, P. (1984). Focal cerebral hyperperfusion in children with dysphasia and/or attention deficit disorder. *Archives of Neurology, 41,* 825–829.

Lou, H. C., Henricksen, L., & Bruhn, P. (1990). Focal cerebral dysfunction in developmental learning disabilities. *Lancet, 335,* 8–11.

Mariani, M., & Barkley, R. A. (1997). Neuropsychological and academic functioning in preschool children with attention deficit disorder. *Developmental Neuropsychology, 13,* 111–129.

Matles, J. A. (1980). The role of frontal lobe dysfunctions in childhood hyperkinesis. *Comprehensive Psychiatry, 21,* 358–369.

Mick, E., Biederman, J., & Faroane, S. V. (1996). Is season of birth a risk factor for attention deficit hyperactivity disorder? *Journal of the American Academy of Child and Adolescent Psychiatry, 35,* 1470–1476.

Nichols, P. L., & Chen, T. C. (1981). *Minimal brain dysfunction: A prospective study.* Hillsdale, NJ: Erlbaum.

Still, G. F. (1902). Some abnormal psychical conditions in children. *Lancet, 1,* 1008–1012, 1077–1082, 1163–1168.

Teicher, M. H., Ito, Y., Glod, C. A., & Barber, N. I. (1996). Objective measurements of hyperactivity and attention problems in ADHD. *Journal of the American Academy of Child and Adolescent Psychiatry, 35,* 334–342.

Tripp, G., Ryan, J., & Peace, K. (2002). Neuropsychological functioning in children with DSM–IV combined type attention deficit hyperactivity disorder. *Australian and New Zealand Journal of Psychiatry, 36*(6), 771–779.

Wender, P. H. (1987). *The hyperactive child, adolescent, and adult—Attention deficit disorder through the lifespan.* New York: Oxford University Press.

Zametkin, A. J., Liebehauve, L. L., Fitzgerald, G. A., King, A. C., Minkumas, D. V., Hersovitch, P., Yamada, F. M., & Cohen, R. M. (1993). Brain metabolism in teenagers with attention deficit hyperactivity disorder. *Archives of General Psychiatry, 50,* 333–340.

# CHAPTER 16

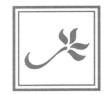

# Mental Retardation

## Pasquale J. Accardo

The understanding of mental retardation has changed dramatically over the past half century. Because the perceptions that many persons have about mental retardation are probably more strongly influenced by impressions left over from a previous generation than by more recent scientific findings taught in university programs, the present chapter focuses on some of the major revisions in thought and practice that now characterize the field of mental retardation. From a medical perspective, most but not all of these changes have been for the better, whereas several offer continuing challenges for the optimal interaction between medicine and the educational profession.

## DEFINITION OF MENTAL RETARDATION

The classic definition of *mental retardation* has three requirements: significantly subaverage intellectual performance, deficits in adaptive functioning, and onset before 18 years of age. The first requirement, significantly subaverage intellectual performance, or "failing" of a general intelligence test, means that the individual performs more than two standard deviations below the mean for that test. Because most recent IQ tests have a

The preparation of this chapter was supported in part by Project #1 T73 MC 00046 04 from the Maternal and Child Health Bureau (Title V, Social Security Act), Health Resources and Services Administration, Department of Health and Human Services.

mean of 100 and a standard deviation of 15, the cutoff for mental retardation would be an IQ below 70 (the mean of 100 less twice the standard deviation of 15). The intelligence test used should measure a wide variety of aspects of cognition. Earlier editions of the *Stanford–Binet Intelligence Scale* were heavily loaded on verbal items and were therefore more likely to misclassify a child with a significant communication disorder as having mental retardation. When using a test with such a bias, it is important to supplement it with tests that tap other facets of intelligence. The *Stanford–Binet Intelligence Scale–Fourth Edition* (Thorndike, Hagen, & Sattler, 1986) and other recent intelligence tests correct this bias by tapping a broader range of cognitive skills.

In addition to the cognitive limitations, the person with mental retardation also needs to exhibit deficits in adaptive functioning; in other words, the intellectual impairment must demonstrate an impact beyond the classroom setting into activities of daily living. This results in excluding children with severe learning disabilities who might do poorly in all academic areas but who can perform more appropriately for age when confronted by the demands of life. In the past, some children with severe learning disabilities might have been misdiagnosed with mental retardation. Such confusion was more likely to occur in an era when professional recognition of and diagnostic testing for learning disabilities was still in an early phase.

The third requirement in the classic definition is onset during the developmental period, or before age 18 years. Most mental retardation is congenital (genetic or related to abnormalities of fetal brain development); it is often present at birth, although it may not be identifiable until years later. Some cases of mental retardation may result from later childhood brain damage due to meningitis, encephalitis, severe head injury, and lead poisoning. Similar severe brain insults may cause significant intellectual impairment in a person over age 18, but this would not be considered mental retardation.

The most recent American Association on Mental Retardation (Luckasson et al., 1992) definition of mental retardation has maintained these basic criteria but notably expanded the concurrent adaptive deficit criterion by requiring that the person exhibit significant deficits in at least 2 out of 10 proposed adaptive skill areas: communication, self-care, home living, social skills, community use, self-direction, health and safety, functional academics, leisure, and work. The difficulty with this expanded definition is that, unlike the IQ score and age of onset requirements, valid instruments to accurately measure all 10 of these areas do not exist. Clarifying the contribution of the adaptive skills criterion is relatively easy with children who are more severely impaired but becomes somewhat more subjective in marginal cases, which tend to be more common than severe cases. The level of needed supports replaces what in the earlier classification was categorized almost exclusively by IQ level. The distinction will be familiar to professionals who participate in the drafting of an Individualized Education Program (IEP): Test scores alone do not define the needed classroom supports. The American Psychiatric Association and the American Psychological Association still use IQ cutoffs to describe levels of severity (American Psychiatric Association, 2000). Although it reflects a very crude approximation, the IQ can describe the rough percentage of the child's chronological age that the child's mental age will achieve. The following are the IQs associated with different levels of severity of mental retardation:

| | |
|---|---|
| Mild mental retardation | 50–55 to approximately 70 |
| Moderate mental retardation | 35–40 to 50–55 |
| Severe mental retardation | 20–25 to 35–40 |
| Profound mental retardation | Below 20–25 |

Using IQ levels to characterize levels of severity allows more consistent association of degrees of brain impairment with various genetic syndromes and other medical etiologies for mental retardation. In other words, regardless of its utility for the classroom setting, to the physician the IQ is a rough neurological marker.

The most important medical statement about mental retardation is that it is not a medical diagnosis. Rather, it is a term that describes a current functional state. The functional state that *mental retardation* describes is, however, most often associated with significant abnormalities of the central nervous system. Although the functional state may or may not change over time, the neurological abnormalities that are the underlying organic substrate for the functional impairment are most often permanent and will continue to exert a negative and limiting impact on cognition and related developmental areas into adulthood. The permanence of the "brain damage" that underlies mental retardation does not, however, mean that a child with mental retardation will remain at a fixed stage in development. All children, even the most severely impaired, continue to make progress—even if, as in severe and profound mental retardation, it is very slow progress. It is the nature of even the most damaged brain to learn and to adapt. Failure to progress and especially regression (the loss of skills) should always be considered indicators for careful medical reevaluation to rule out any complicating, medically treatable conditions. To the physician, mental retardation is a symptom of neurological dysfunction that needs assessment, monitoring, and sometimes further investigation.

It should be mentioned that the United States is the only English-speaking country to continue to use the term *mental retardation*. Great Britain, Canada, and Australia now employ substitute terms such as *global learning difficulties* or *disabilities* and *cognitive impairment*. Although a diagnosis of mental retardation might conceivably be made in a fairly young child, there is an increasing tendency for preschool children to be labeled developmentally delayed instead of mentally retarded. Such terminological substitutions avoid the need to use the emotionally loaded term *mental retardation* with families but have no real impact on the nature and course of the developmental disorder.

# OCCURRENCE RATE
# OF MENTAL RETARDATION

Mental retardation occurs in the general population at a rate of just over 2%. However, this rate varies dramatically in different segments of a population. In the more affluent regions of society, the rate might approximate 1% to 1.5%, whereas in poorer areas, it might rise as high as 15%. The reason for this higher rate in lower socioeconomic groups probably reflects the complex interaction among a number of factors: polygenetic inheritance (a large number of mildly deleterious genes collecting in a population); limited access to prenatal, pediatric well child, and other preventive health care services; and the long-term impact of understimulation and substandard schooling. Except for fluctuations in incidence related to ascertainment and definition, the occurrence of mental retardation seems to have remained relatively constant over the past century. For every condition and etiology related to mental retardation that medical science alleviates, another seems to replace its impact in the overall picture.

An earlier definition of mental retardation included the now-defunct category of borderline mental retardation used to characterize persons with IQs between 70 and 85. With this elevated cutoff, the incidence of mental retardation rose above 15%. Such "slow learners" no longer qualify for the educational and social supports allotted to persons with mental retardation, but they persist in experiencing academic difficulties.

# DIAGNOSIS OF MENTAL RETARDATION

The major presenting concern for a child with mental retardation is developmental delay. The child is not achieving milestones, not doing what he or she should be doing at a given age. The child with mental retardation acts like a much younger aged child in all or most areas of development. Some children with mental retardation will present at first with behavioral problems such as severe tantrums when their developmental delay is not recognized, and they become very frustrated when faced with what are for them impossible (although actually age-appropriate) demands.

Because the motor area is often the least involved in a child with mental retardation, many such children begin to walk on time and do not exhibit serious motor delays. It is not uncommon to encounter parents and even some professionals who are puzzled as to how a child who walked at 12 months of age could possibly be considered "slow." Later, more complex motor planning skills are often impaired.

Language is the most sensitive marker for general cognition, and many children with mental retardation present first with delayed language. It is therefore imperative for infants and young children who present with language delay to have their nonverbal intelligence assessed independently of their language skills in order to differentiate the isolated, and much more common, communication disorder from the less common generalized cognitive impairment. Perhaps one of the most frequent misdiagnoses places a preschool child with communication delay secondary to mental retardation in an intervention program for young children with speech and language problems.

The physical examination of the child with mental retardation includes looking for the presence of nonneurological diseases that might negatively affect development and the presence of dysmorphic features that may be indicators of specific genetic syndromes or nonspecifically of early damage to the developing brain. Higher numbers of dysmorphic features, or "minor malformations," are found in mental retardation, autism, attention-deficit/hyperactivity disorder, learning disabilities, and major psychiatric disorders. The following features are associated with developmental problems:

- Electric hair

- Hairwhorl abnormalities (absent, multiple [cowlicks], poorly defined, counterclockwise, linear, frontal [widow's peak])

- Head circumference (macrocephaly [large head], microcephaly [small head])

- Epicanthic folds

- Hypertelorism (wide space between eyes)

- Pinna (ear) abnormalities (low-set, rotated, rounded, flattened, protuberant, malformed)

- Absent ear lobules (adherent earlobes)

- High-arched or steepled palate

- Geographic tongue

- Clinodactyly (incurving) of the fifth finger

- Brachydactyly (shortness) of the fifth finger

- Palmar crease abnormality (simian, Sydney, hockeystick)

- Sandal gap deformity of (widened space between) first toes

- Syndactyly (decreased space between or partial fusion) of toes two and three

- Long middle toe

Abnormalities on the neurological examination may help to localize brain damage as well as indicate deficits associated with the mental retardation. For example, an abnormal gait associated with unilateral weakness of the extremities may imply injury to the cerebral cortex, or incoordination and "staccato"-like speech may indicate a lesion in the cerebellum.

In the presence of significant delays in any major developmental area, a measure of general intellectual functioning is indicated. If that developmental quotient falls into the mentally retarded range, then a more in-depth multidisciplinary assessment by a team of professionals familiar with the diagnosis of mental retardation should be carried out. Confirmation of the diagnosis should go side by side with attempts to uncover the reason for the presence of the mental retardation. Appropriate parent support, counseling, and educational placement should follow.

With regard to etiology, a detailed medical history should document the presence or absence of a variety of risk factors—with the strong qualification that a *risk factor* is not the same as a *diagnosis*. Most children with risk factors exhibit normal development, and most children with developmental diagnoses do not demonstrate any risk factors. Items to be reviewed include family history, infections or exposure to toxins during pregnancy (with alcohol among the most prominent and preventable of these), severe prematurity, perinatal (the time just preceding and following birth) medical complications, severe illnesses in early childhood, meningitis or encephalitis (brain infections), exposure to high levels of lead, and severe traumatic brain injury. With regard to the last item, the brain injury should be associated with unconsciousness and seizures and is much more severe than the usual falls (with head lacerations or cuts requiring stitches) that are almost routine in early toddlerhood.

There is no routine biomedical assessment (group of medical tests) for children with mental retardation. The selection of tests and procedures to perform is based on a review of the child's developmental history and functional pattern, the physical and neurological findings, and the parents' wishes. (Even some so-called noninvasive tests may require general sedation from which children with mental retardation are at greater risk for complications.) Potential components of a laboratory assessment for mental retardation include thyroid function studies, chromosomal analysis, fragile X testing, deoxyribonucleic acid (DNA) probes for specific syndromes, amino and organic acid levels, electroencephalograms (EEGs), and neuroimaging of the brain (computerized tomography and magnetic resonance imaging scans). Rather than sending blood to the genetics laboratory for chromosomal analysis, it is preferred to send the child with mental retardation for a clinical genetics consultation. The number of DNA probes used to identify specific syndromes associated with mental retardation continues to increase at such a rapid pace that the geneticist should be given the opportunity to evaluate the child for their appropriateness. A "shotgun" approach to evaluations by utilizing every available test is likely to be both expensive and unrewarding.

In a large population of children with mental retardation, 5 out of 6 will be mildly retarded (IQs above 50), whereas only 1 out of the 6 will be moderately to severely retarded (with IQs below 50). Detailed biomedical assessments are likely to uncover a specific etiology in one third of all cases.

That one third, however, is asymmetrically composed of three quarters of those with more severe retardation and only one quarter of those with mild retardation.

It is of concern to note that a number of children with significant mental retardation who have received extensive and repeated multidisciplinary evaluations to determine functional levels may be placed in special education for years without having had any medical assessment other than well-child visits. The professionals competent to perform an appropriate medical evaluation of the child with mental retardation include child neurologists, developmental pediatricians, behavioral pediatricians, and clinical geneticists.

# SYNDROME IDENTIFICATION

A quarter of a century ago, the scientific literature included papers on different aspects of mild and moderate mental retardation. Today, these are almost completely absent. Medical journals instead publish research papers on specific conditions such as Down syndrome, fetal alcohol syndrome (FAS), Prader-Willi syndrome (PWS), fragile X syndrome, and the like. The earlier classification by degrees of severity of intellectual impairment (IQ level) no longer makes sense in the current medical understanding of the neurological substrate of intellectual deficiency. Many syndromes are no longer associated with a specific narrow IQ range, but rather are known to occur with a fairly wide range of IQs. For example, FAS and PWS can occur in the presence of normal intelligence. In these latter examples, although IQ may be in the normal range, the child's learning profile is still affected, so that specific language, learning, behavioral, and attentional problems, often severe, characterize these syndromes.

Today, there is less concern with identifying the IQ range associated with a syndrome than with describing the behavioral and learning profiles (which does include IQ as one of its components) associated with the syndrome (see Table 16.1). This behavioral phenotyping (O'Brien & Yule, 1995) represents one of the frontiers of modern genetics and promises to be of use in the classroom management of children with such syndromes.

**TABLE 16.1**

Behavioral Profiles for Several Mental Retardation Syndromes

| Syndrome | Behavioral Characteristics |
| --- | --- |
| Down syndrome (trisomy 21) | Developmental deceleration, delayed expressive language, sitting down, escape behavior, visual spatial short-term memory (STM) better than auditory STM |
| Williams syndrome (17q11 deletion) | Inflated expressive language ("cocktail party" speech), auditory STM better than visual STM |
| Smith-Magenis syndrome (17p11.2 deletion) | Self-hugging ("spasmodic upper-body squeeze"), onychotillomania (pulling out fingernails and toenails), polyembolokoilamania (insertion of foreign bodies into body orifices) |
| Prader-Willi syndrome (15q11-13 deletion, paternal) | Hyperphagia (overeating, leading to life-threatening obesity if not controlled), obsessive–compulsive traits, skin picking |
| Angelman syndrome (15q11-13 deletion, maternal) | Puppet-like gait, paroxysmal laughter |
| Lesch Nyhan (Xq27-q28 mutation) | Severe self-mutilation |

# MEDICAL MANAGEMENT OF MENTAL RETARDATION

When the human brain is sufficiently impaired to produce global cognitive limitation, there is no traditional medical treatment to "cure" the resulting mental retardation. There are, however, a number of areas in which the physician can contribute to the well-being of the child with mental retardation.

## Primary Medical Care

A half century ago, many children with mental retardation were placed in institutional settings. Their basic medical care was marginal, and their environment fostered the spread of diseases that would ultimately shorten their life span. Today, children with mental retardation live at home and make use of community health and educational resources. The life span of persons with even severe mental retardation more closely approximates the average life span of persons without mental retardation. Providing primary health care to children with mental retardation can be challenging because of limitiations on the child's ability to communicate. With an increasingly improved knowledge of the medical implications of different genetic syndromes, physicians can monitor and anticipate various medical complications as, or even before, they arise (Roizen, 1999; Wilson & Cooley, 2000). Thus, routine thyroid screening is part of the recommended management of children with Down syndrome. The onset of hypothyroidism can explain why a child with Down syndrome becomes more sluggish and apathetic and falls off his or her learning curve; it is also very treatable. The almost normal mild diseases of childhood and sometimes their treatments can have a greater impact on the developmental rate of a child with mental retardation than on a typically developing child.

## Specialty Medical Care

Children with mental retardation syndromes are more likely to exhibit multiple other nondevelopmental medical problems. On the one hand, such children are less likely to complain about or describe these illness patterns; on the other hand, even mild chronic disorders can have a devastating impact on the child's development. A higher percentage of children with mental retardation exhibit seizure disorders. In the treatment of the epilepsy, it is important to avoid exacerbating the cognitive impairment or facilitating problem behaviors with the use of selected anticonvulsants.

## Behavioral Medications

Although some controversy remains about the use of psychotropic medications to manage challenging behaviors in persons with developmental disorders, there is little doubt that the use of such drugs often allows children with mental retardation to function in a less restrictive environment and to make better use of various educational and behavioral interventions. Without discussing particular drugs, two major considerations always need to be kept in mind:

1. If a child is to be maintained long term on a drug, the behavioral improvement should be dramatic and not marginal.

2. The child should experience no side effects from the drug, including sedation and sometimes not so subtle personality changes. *Primum non nocere*—first, do no harm. Medication should facilitate (not force) behavioral improvement in the child.

Over the past several decades, many schools have modified (a) an originally antagonistic attitude toward the use of pharmacotherapeutic agents as not appropriate to an educational program to (b) an almost too eager acceptance of the use of such drugs to minimize the need for intensive behavioral supports in an educational system with increasingly limited fiscal resources. However, the concern should be with each child's needs rather than extreme policy. Again, with behavioral disorders, it is critical to make certain that other medical factors are not contributing to the problem (e.g., when the anticonvulsant phenobarbitol precipitates an out-of-control hyperkinetic and impulsive behavior pattern).

## Prevention

Mental retardation that results from some specific causes can be prevented. For example, a vaccine has virtually eliminated haemophilus influenzae meningitis, a common cause of mental retardation and hearing loss in children (Alexander, 1998). Also, genetic etiologies may pose an identifiable recurrence risk for the family of a child with mental retardation, in which case genetic counseling is important before additional pregnancies. Toxic exposures such as alcohol and lead can also be expected to influence later children in the same family.

So-called medical treatments with a purported neurological basis lack scientific evidence for efficacy in the treatment of mental retardation. These include patterning, masking (intermittent suffocation to induce carbon dioxide rebreathing), nutritional additives (glutamic acid, megavitamins, trace elements, amino acids), elimination diets, music therapy, nootropics (drugs to increase intelligence, such as piracetam), sicca cell therapy, osteopathy (craniosacral therapy or skull massage), hormones (in the absence of documented endocrine deficiencies), antioxidants, and antimold (anti-yeast or anti-Candidiasis) drug treatment.

# THE TEACHER'S ROLE

The teacher is an important participant in the medical management of children with mental retardation. Most important is establishing open communication among the teacher, parents, and medical professionals. The following is a list of ways to benefit children with mental retardation:

- Encourage families to have a primary care pediatrician who is familiar with the child with mental retardation. Sporadic emergency room visits are not an acceptable equivalent for such care.

- Establish open avenues of communication with regard to children with mental retardation who are not experiencing problems in the classroom, in preparation for interaction with physicians when problems do arise.

- Do not specifically recommend the use of medications, but encourage parents of children with mental retardation to make certain that their child's developmental disorder has been adequately medically assessed, with both a careful search for etiologies and an evaluation of possible medical therapies (including medications).

- When children with mental retardation are diagnosed with specific syndromes, ask for information with regard to both the medical and behavioral implications of the diagnosis. The school nurse should be a resource to help the teacher become familiar with these associations.

- When children with mental retardation are placed on specific drugs, ask for information with regard to both the medical and behavioral implications of such drugs. Again, the school nurse can function as a liaison between the teacher and the prescribing physician.

- When responding to physicians or parents with regard to drug effects, include changes noted even if these were not specifically identified as possible effects.

- When a child's behavior or learning deteriorates, consider a medical reassessment even in the absence of obvious signs of physical illness.

Additionally, the following guidelines concern the management of children with mental retardation in the classroom.

- The special education teacher's classroom role is generally carefully spelled out in the child's Individualized Education Program (IEP). When that IEP is negotiated (or reviewed), a reasonable point to address is the identification of any unique needs specific to the child's learning profile and any associated medical condition.

- When the child with mental retardation is mainstreamed into a regular education setting, close communication with the child's special education teacher (and any other specialty service providers) should be maintained.

- Proactive preparatory education to sensitize regular education students for the reception of students with special needs is indicated.

- Significant underachievement with regard to reasonable IEP goals may reflect medically treatable complications to the child's condition and not merely lack of motivation.

# REFERENCES

Alexander, D. (1998). Prevention of mental retardation: Four decades of research. *Mental Retardation and Developmental Disabilities Research Reviews, 4*(1), 50–58.

American Psychiatric Association. (2000). *Diagnostic and statistical manual of mental disorders–fourth edition–text revision.* Washington, DC: Author.

Luckasson, R., Coulter, D. L., Polloway, E. A., Reiss, S., Schalock, R. L., Snell, M. E., Spitalnik, D. M., & Stark, J. A. (1992). *Mental retardation: Definition, classification, and systems of supports* (9th ed.). Washington DC: American Association on Mental Retardation.

O'Brien, G., & Yule, W. (1995). *Behavioural phenotypes* (Clinics in Developmental Medicine No. 138). London: MacKeith Press.

Roizen, N. J. (Ed.). (1999). Down syndrome. *Mental Retardation and Developmental Disabilities Research Reviews, 2*(2), 66–115.

Thorndike, R. L., Hagen, E. D., & Sattler, J. M. (1986). *Stanford–Binet Intelligence Scale–Fourth Edition.* Itasca, IL: Riverside.

Wilson, G. N., & Cooley, W. C. (2000). *Preventive management of children with congenital anomalies and syndromes.* Cambridge, England: Cambridge University Press.

# CHAPTER 17

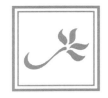

# Emotional and Behavioral Disorders in the Classroom

Jorge E. Gonzalez, Michael H. Epstein, and Ron Nelson

**E**motional disturbance (ED), as defined by the Individuals with Disabilities Education Act of 1990 (IDEA), refers to various disorders in learning, interpersonal relationships, behaviors or feelings, moods, or physical symptoms or fears that persist over long periods of time, are of a marked degree, and adversely affect school performance. In the 1998–99 school year, 463,172 children in the United States were identified as having ED and provided with special education or related services in the public schools (U.S. Department of Education, 2001). Although this number represents approximately 1% of school-age children, epidemiological research suggests that the actual prevalence of ED may be much greater, ranging from 3% to 6% (Kauffman, 2001). Thus, it is not unreasonable to conclude that many children with ED remain underidentified by the schools (Kauffman, 2001). Unfortunately, as the need for services for children with ED grows, the nation continues to fail in developing a cohesive and unified infrastructure to assist these children and their families. Too often, these children and families miss opportunities for early intervention and receive fragmented or low-resource and low-priority services (Department of Health and Human Services, 2000). In this chapter, we clarify who children with ED are; describe the status and scope of this population, a probable path to ED, and major underlying disorders; discuss federal eligibility criteria for inclusion into special education, along with screening procedures, assessment strategies, and sources of data; and conclude with some final thoughts.

# THE POPULATION

Children with ED are overwhelmingly White males who are behaviorally disruptive, noncompliant, verbally abusive, and aggressive. Because their behaviors are so disruptive and irritating, these children often arouse negative feelings in others, thus alienating schoolmates and adults, and ultimately robbing themselves of the benefits of learning opportunities. Moreover, they often experience social rejection or alienation by peers, parents, and teachers (Quinn & Epstein, 1998). When these children do make friends, it does not take them long to alienate them as they do not know how to foster, nurture, and maintain friendships. When they do obtain status among peers, it is usually among deviant groups who reinforce antisocial behavior. Finally, children with ED experience significant educational deficits across numerous academic domains (Kauffman, 2001).

# STATUS AND SCOPE
# OF CHILDREN WITH ED

Data on identification, academic outcomes, graduation rates, absenteeism, employment status, and criminality among children with ED suggest that educating them is a complex, confusing, and often daunting task for educators, related services professionals, and family members (S. W. Smith & Coutinho, 1997). Perhaps the most disturbing finding is that, although a child's problems are noticed at a very early age (usually prior to age 4), it may take about 5 or more years before school personnel formally identify the need for special education services. To make matters worse, virtually no educational, mental health, or related services are provided between the time that problems are first noticed and official identification (Duncan, Forness, & Hartsough, 1995).

Data from the 23rd Annual Report to Congress on the Implementation of IDEA (U.S. Department of Education, 2001) and the National Longitudinal Transition Study (Wagner, Blackorby, Cameto, Hebbeler, & Newman, 1993), along with other research (e.g., Kauffman, 2001; Quinn &

Epstein, 1998), present a rather sobering and challenging picture of the status, scope, and outcomes for children with ED:

- According to the NLTS report, the school dropout rate for youth with ED was 50.3%, a rate 37% higher than the next highest category of special education eligibility.

- When considering students with disabilities, the NLTS found that children with ED demonstrated the highest rate of school failure in both regular (74%) and special education (22.7%) classes.

- According to the 22nd Annual Report, the percentage of Black children with ED receiving special education services (i.e., 26.4%) far exceeded their percentage in the general population percentage (i.e., 12%).

- After graduating from high school, approximately one third of children with ED were either unemployed, not in school, or not receiving any training (Neel, Meadows, Levine, & Edgar, 1988).

# THE PATH TO
# EMOTIONAL DISTURBANCE

ED begins early in life and is evident in some young children by the preschool years (Beare & Lynch, 1986; Campbell, 1990; Patterson, De Baryshe, & Ramsey, 1989). Data from various sources indicate that children diagnosed with ED come from backgrounds in which they are exposed to a myriad of risk factors that over time foster damaging negative experiences with parents, teachers, and peers (Walker & Sprague, 1999; Wehby, Symons, & Hollo, 1997). These risk factors may collectively include long-term residential instability, contact with numerous service agencies, mental illness, poverty, abuse, neglect, harsh and inconsistent parenting, high stress, parental psychopathology, criminality, and drug or alcohol abuse (Quinn & Epstein, 1998). With each negative experience encountered, children become at greater risk of developing chronic social adjustment problems, increasing the probability of special education referral (Walker & Sprague, 1999).

Unfortunately, the prognosis for young children with ED is bleak. Less than half of young children with early signs of maladjusted behavior show remission by the time they reach adolescence (Shaw, Gilliom, & Giovannelli, 2000). Moreover, as adolescents, it becomes increasingly difficult to intervene (Kazdin, 1985; Robbins, 1966). These adolescents often grow up to evince numerous forms of adult maladjustment at a significant cost to society in terms of loss of productivity and continued need for special services.

While debate continues about the dominant causes of ED, the emerging perspective is that individual child characteristics interact with family and environmental factors to place some children at high risk for ED by the time they reach school (Farrington, 1989; Garmezy & Masten, 1994; Kauffman, 2001; Singh, Landrum, Donatelli, Hampton, & Ellis, 1994; Walker & Sprague, 1999). Syntheses of the research have identified major factors that contribute to the development of disruptive behavioral disorders—the most frequently identified disorders among children with ED (Duncan et al., 1995). Among the global factors are family characteristics, child characteristics, and sociological characteristics (Farmer, Quinn, Hussey, & Holahan, 2001; Kauffman, 2001).

## Family Characteristics

Parent–child relationships among children identified as having ED are frequently governed by coercive and reciprocal interaction styles. Using harsh, inconsistent, or erratic discipline practices, parents simultaneously provoke and teach children to escape negative consequences by escalating their problem behaviors (Dishion, French, & Patterson, 1995). In a model outlining the development of disruptive behavior patterns, Walker and Sprague (1999) demonstrated the connecting stepping stones that underlie a clear path from early exposure to risk factors and later development of maladjustment (see Figure 17.1).

As demonstrated in Figure 17.1, the family initially experiences severe stress caused by exposure to one of many risk factors (e.g., poverty, unemployment, family upheaval, neglect, abuse, substance abuse). These stressors subsequently disrupt normal parenting practices, which in turn yield high rates of negative interactions among family members. These negative interactions often develop into coercive processes and aversive control strategies aimed at controlling one another's behavior. This powerful set of circumstances often provides a context for inadvertently teaching antisocial behavior patterns that are virtually impervious to intervention and resistant to change (Walker & Sprague, 1999).

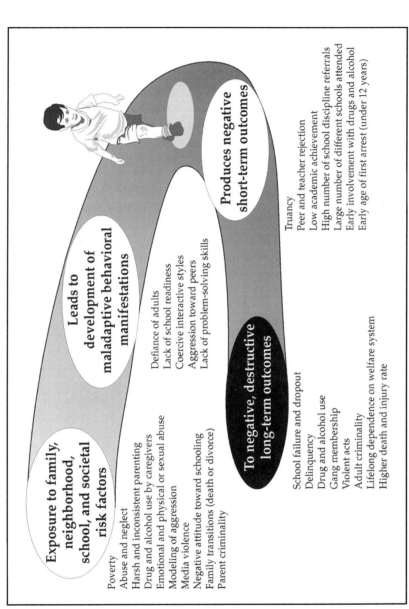

**Exposure to family, neighborhood, school, and societal risk factors**

Poverty
Abuse and neglect
Harsh and inconsistent parenting
Drug and alcohol use by caregivers
Emotional and physical or sexual abuse
Modeling of aggression
Media violence
Negative attitude toward schooling
Family transitions (death or divorce)
Parent criminality

**Leads to development of maladaptive behavioral manifestations**

Defiance of adults
Lack of school readiness
Coercive interactive styles
Aggression toward peers
Lack of problem-solving skills

**Produces negative short-term outcomes**

Truancy
Peer and teacher rejection
Low academic achievement
High number of school discipline referrals
Large number of different schools attended
Early involvement with drugs and alcohol
Early age of first arrest (under 12 years)

**To negative, destructive long-term outcomes**

School failure and dropout
Delinquency
Drug and alcohol use
Gang membership
Violent acts
Adult criminality
Lifelong dependence on welfare system
Higher death and injury rate

**FIGURE 17.1.** The path to emotional disturbance. *Note.* From "The Path to School Failure, Delinquency, and Violence: Causal Factors and Some Potential Solutions," by H. M. Walker and J. R. Sprague, 1999, *Intervention in School and Clinic, 35,* p. 68. Copyright 1999 by PRO-ED, Inc. Reprinted with permission.

## Child Characteristics

### Hyperactivity and Attention

Externalizing behavioral problems are often associated with attention and hyperactivity (Farmer et al., 2001). Evidence reveals that the two most frequently co-occurring psychiatric disorders are attention-deficit/hyperactivity disorder (ADHD) and conduct disorder (CD). In fact, Duncan and colleagues (1995) reported that 59% of the students in their study had CD and ADHD together. The high comorbidity rate for ADHD and CD is problematic given that these children often possess the most deviant features of both disturbances, effectively interfering with appropriate social and academic development (American Psychiatric Association [APA], 2000; Wenar, 1994). When these disorders co-occur, they tend to be a precursor for adult aggression, violence, and criminality (Brier, 1995; Farrington, 1989; Zuckerman, 1999).

### Temperament

In studies examining the relationship between early temperament characteristics and conduct problems, researchers have found that infant and child negative emotionality is modestly related to later oppositional and aggressive behavior through its indirect effect on parenting (Shaw et al., 2000). According to this research, mothers who perceive their infants as high on negativity display less responsiveness to infant and child requests for attention and resort to harsher discipline strategies in response to those requests. Moreover, these researchers found that infants and children who respond with intense, sustained, and prolonged anger to goal attainment frustration, are at a higher risk of developing aggressive behavioral problems. It is important to note, however, that although temperament may play an important role in heightening the risk of developing emotional and behavioral problems, it does so only as it interacts with the child's proximal environment (e.g., parents, caregivers) (Crockenberg & Leekes, 2000; Kauffman, 2001).

### Attachment

Evidence has accumulated that specific infant–primary caregiver relationship patterns determine the quality of the relationship as manifested by the security of the infant's or child's attachment (Crockenberg & Leekes, 2000). Research suggests (e.g., Department of Health and Human Services, 2000) that the relationship between maternal problems (e.g., maternal depression) and family risk factors (e.g., abuse) often predispose children, particularly young children, to form insecure or disorganized attachments. In fact, investigators now believe that the nature and the outcome of the caretaker–child attachment process often predicts later depression and conduct disorders among these infants and children (Department of Health and Human Services, 2000).

## Academic Difficulties

As risk factors, low academic performance and maladaptive behavior patterns are highly related. Although the mechanism of the relationship is unknown, evidence suggests that an association exists between academic and conduct problems that emerges early in a child's development (Brier, 1995; Farrington, 1989). Compared to their classmates, students with ED tend to be academically deficient, often functioning a year or more below expected grade level across most academic areas (Epstein, Kinder, & Bursuck, 1989; Kauffman, 2001). Studies addressing the academic characteristics of youth with ED have found that large numbers of these students meet at least one learning disability definition (Greenbaum et al., 1998). Ruhl and Berlinghoff (1992) suggested that between 33% and 81% of children with behavioral disorders have academic difficulties. As these children grow older, academic problems appear to worsen, as evidenced by the lower than expected graduation rates for youth with ED in comparison to general education students and students with other disabilities (Oswald & Coutinho, 1996).

## Sociological Characteristics

### Peer Relationships

The peer group can be a mechanism that contributes to development of ED in two ways. First, establishing positive and reciprocal peer interactions is critical for normal social development. Children who are unable to foster such positive exchanges are at high risk because the social peer group provides an important link to social learning. Second, socially skilled and adept children can become embedded in undesirable peer groups, which promote maladaptive social response patterns (Kauffman, 2001). Antisocial children who bring this behavior pattern to school are likely to experience peer rejection, to affiliate with deviant peers, and possibly to adopt a delinquent or violent lifestyle (Epstein & Walker, 2001). Their antisocial behavior interferes with the formation of positive peer relations, depriving them of the benefits of peer learning. Rejected by their peers (and teachers), these children become embedded in social networks that reinforce, promote, enhance, and maintain their maladaptive behavior patterns. Over time, antisocial children tend to develop affiliative tendencies toward other youth who value disruptive behavior, thus increasing the likelihood of lifelong antisocial behavior patterns (Farmer et al., 2001; Wehby et al., 1997).

### Economic Disadvantage

Children from families of low socioeconomic status (SES) often demonstrate higher levels of both externalizing and internalizing behavioral problems (Greenberg, Lengua, Coie, & Pinderhughes, 1999). Many of the conditions associated with poverty (e.g., chaotic living conditions, family psychological distress, lack of food, lack of opportunity to learn, violence, school failure), especially extreme poverty, have been linked to the development of ED (Aber, Jones, & Cohen, 2000; Kauffman, 2001) by way of rearing practices. Often these children come from families in which poverty has taken a considerable toll on parents and other caregivers, who are left with little or no energy or skill to foster nurturance or stimulation in their children. These children frequently demonstrate signs of attachment disorders well into middle childhood (Knitzer, 2000).

## MAJOR DISORDERS ASSOCIATED WITH EMOTIONAL DISTURBANCE

Several diagnostic categories are subsumed under the general term *emotional disturbance*. These disorders can be organized into two broad dimensions of disorders: externalizing and internalizing (Achenbach, 1991b). Externalizing disorders refer to a distinct group of behaviors reflecting conflicts with other individuals and their behavioral expectations. In general, these disorders are directed outwardly and viewed as undercontrolled. Internalizing behaviors generally refer to disorders that are directed toward the self (e.g., anxiety, depression, withdrawal from social contact) (Achenbach & Rescorla, 2000). They are generally inner directed such that the core symptoms are often related to the overcontrol of behavior (W. M. Reynolds, 1992b). While a complete description of all the externalizing and internalizing disorders is beyond the scope of this chapter, interested readers may consult the *Diagnostic and Statistical Manual of Mental Disorders–Fourth Edition–Text Revision* (DSM–IV–TR; APA, 2000) for more information.

## Externalizing Disorders

Externalizing disorders are disruptive and outer directed in nature. They represent a domain of disorders characterized by the undercontrol of behavioral impulses (W. M. Reynolds, 1992b). Externalizing problems in the schools are often manifested as conflicted relationships with peers, teachers, and other school-related individuals (House, 1999).

## Conduct Disorder (CD)

According to the DSM–IV–TR, the qualifying feature of CD is "a repetitive and persistent pattern of behavior in which the rights of others or major age-appropriate societal norms or rules are violated" (p. 93). The disorder may manifest itself in aggression toward people or animals, property destruction, theft or deceit, or serious rule violations. These behavioral manifestations often result in difficulties with social, academic, or occupational functioning. Prevalence estimates suggest that rates range from 6% to 16% among males and from 2% to 9% among females. The prognosis for child-onset CD is not encouraging. Children diagnosed with CD often show behavior patterns that meet criteria for later adult antisocial personality disorder (House, 1999). High comorbidity rates are also reported, with the co-occurrence of CD and oppositional disorders, affective disorders, anxiety disorders, and attention-deficit disorders (House, 1999; McConaughy & Skiba, 1994).

## Oppositional Defiant Disorder (ODD)

In ODD, there is an ongoing pattern of uncooperative, defiant, and hostile behavior. These behaviors are directed toward authority figures or others and seriously interfere with a child's daily academic, social, or occupational functioning (APA, 2000). Children with ODD tend to be argumentative with adults, often lose their tempers, appear angry, are prone to spite and vindictiveness, and are easily annoyed by others (APA, 1994; Goldstein, 1995). Prevalence rates of ODD among children range from 2% to 16%. The outcomes for ODD vary. In some children, the disorder evolves into a conduct disorder or other mood disorder. As adults, ODD can develop into passive–aggressive personality disorder or antisocial personality disorder (Goldstein, 1995).

## Attention-Deficit/Hyperactivity Disorder (ADHD)

The diagnostic and treatment questions most frequently asked of school psychologists and other service-related personnel refer to problems of poor impulse control, overactivity, and distractibility (House, 1999). Due to its impact on others, ADHD has been classified, since 1984, as a disruptive behavior disorder (Goldstein, 1995). As discussed in Chapter 15, ADHD involves two classic symptoms: inattention and hyperactivity or impulsivity. Children with ADHD display these characteristics significantly more than their peers do and to a marked degree. Prevalence rates for ADHD among children are 3% to 5%. The course of ADHD appears stable through early adolescence. Prognosis for children with ADHD is not encouraging. Research (APA, 2000) suggests that ADHD in children may be a precursor to adult psychopathology. Follow-up studies have shown that between 25% and 33% of children diagnosed with ADHD develop antisocial and conduct disorders, leading to much higher arrest records in adulthood (Zuckerman, 1999).

## Internalizing Disorders

Internalizing disorders subsume a wide array of inner directed, self-related disorders. Although teachers have no problem spotting children who act out, they often overlook those who may have internalizing disorders (e.g., depression, anxiety) (Kauffman, 2001). The school "problem children" are easily identified because they are unruly, draw attention, and are often scolded for their actions. Teachers, paraprofessionals, and other service-related personnel often devote significant amounts of time to dealing with these students. While teachers and others attend to the externalizing child, the internalizing child who suffers from a potentially serious problem, such as depression or anxiety, may go unnoticed.

## Social Phobia

Children with social phobia (also known as social anxiety disorder) demonstrate extreme anxiety in age-appropriate performance situations where they believe they are being evaluated, because they fear embarrassment, humiliation, and being thought poorly of by peers (House, 1999). These children usually avoid or endure these situations with extreme anxiety. Epidemiological studies have revealed the prevalence of social phobia in the range from 3% to 13%. Although it may diminish during adulthood, the course of social phobia is usually continuous, often being exacerbated or attenuated by stressors (APA, 2000).

## Obsessive–Compulsive Disorder (OCD)

OCD is a debilitating disorder that can have a profoundly negative effect on the individual, family and peer relationships, and academic performance. The obsessive or compulsive behaviors (e.g., hand washing, counting, repeating words silently) are intrusive, recurrent, and time consuming, and they lead to elevated distress or impairment in the child. Because they fear ridicule, children with OCD often perform their compulsive behaviors in secret, resulting in underidentification of this disorder. Recent epidemiological studies suggest that 1 in every 200 children is affected by OCD. Furthermore, the majority of OCD cases are commonly misdiagnosed as depression or anxiety disorder (APA, 1994; House, 1999; Waters, Barrett, & March, 2001). The prognosis for OCD is mixed, with affected children showing periods of elevated disturbance and periods of diminished symptoms (APA, 2000).

## Generalized Anxiety Disorder (GAD)

With children, GAD typically involves excessive and persistent worries about performance in school or social activities. Often, the worries are unrealistic, usually not under their control, and distressing. In response to the distress, children with GAD frequently engage in approval-seeking behaviors, strive for perfectionism, are intolerant of substandard performance, and constantly seek reassurance on their performance. In addition, children with GAD frequently complain of headaches, difficulty sleeping, restlessness, or concentration problems (APA, 1994; UCLA–Neuropsychiatric Institute, 1999). Approximately 17% or more of children diagnosed with some type of anxiety disorder have concurrent diagnoses (e.g., depression) (Goldstein, 1995; Zuckerman, 1999). Estimates put the prevalence of GAD at 3%. GAD tends to be chronic, with the course of GAD waxing and waning as a function of stressors (APA, 2000).

## Posttraumatic Stress Disorder (PTSD)

Perhaps the most controversial of the anxiety disorders is PTSD. The diagnosis of PTSD was developed in an effort to normalize the experiences (e.g., cognitive, emotional, behavioral) observed of individuals following exposure to traumatic events. Part of the controversy can be found in understanding the nature of the stressor in the context of the individual's past. Questions about its validity continue to plague the diagnostic category (Mezey & Robbins, 2001).

Researchers have, however, come to realize that PTSD is far more frequent than previously thought (Goldstein, 1995). A child or adolescent who experiences or is exposed to a catastrophic event may develop PTSD. The traumatic event may involve a situation where someone's life has been threatened (e.g., school shooting, sexual or physical abuse, war), a natural disaster (e.g., tornado), or a severe injury that has occurred or been witnessed (e.g., seeing another person killed, car accident). The probability of developing PTSD relates to the magnitude of the trauma, whether the event is repeated, the child's proximity to the stressor, and his or her affiliation to the victim(s). Often, the stressful event is reexperienced in numerous ways, such as intrusive recollections, flashbacks, dreams, or feelings that the event is recurring. Shortly after the event, children may appear agitated, confused, or disorganized. They may demonstrate extreme fear, helplessness, anger, melancholy, horror, or denial. Some children may even dissociate from the stressful event by demonstrating emotional deadening. Depending on the population sampled, prevalence estimates for PTSD range from 1% to 14%, with some estimates being much higher (e.g., Bosnian refugees exposed to "ethnic cleansing" by Serbians) (Zuckerman, 1999). With treatment, the prognosis for PTSD is good, with most symptoms not persisting beyond 12 months.

## Separation Anxiety Disorder

Children who suffer from separation anxiety disorder often experience intense developmentally inappropriate anxiety when separated from significant attachment figures (usually the mother). These children often avoid any situation that takes them away from home or other familiar surroundings (e.g., going to school). They tend to cling to parents or other attachment figures. When separated, these children often cry uncontrollably, fear being abandoned or not being reunited with parents, or distress over the possibility that some catastrophe will befall loved ones. It is also common for children with separation anxiety disorder to have difficulty sleeping, have nightmares, and complain of physical symptoms (APA, 1994, 2000; House, 1999; Huberty, 1987). The prevalence of separation anxiety disorder among children and adolescents is approximately 4%, with the course of the disorder waxing and waning and decreasing through adolescence (APA, 2000).

## Childhood and Adolescent Depression

Depressive disorders are quite rare in the preschool period, but are more common in middle childhood and adolescence. Moreover, they bear a striking similarity to adulthood manifestations (Kendall, 1991; W. M. Reynolds, 1992a; Wenar, 1994). Depressed children often report feeling down and out about themselves. The most common symptom is dysphoria or a feeling of melancholy. Associated features and symptoms include irritability, tiredness, moodiness, negativism, hostility, anger, aggressive and antisocial behavior, difficulty sleeping, low energy, and appetite disturbances. It is not uncommon for attention, concentration, and memory to be negatively affected as well (Kendall, 1991). Some researchers have posited that academic and behavioral performances can be very sensitive indicators of the sudden onset of depression in children (Goldstein, 1995).

Depending on the age of onset as well as the diagnostic method used, estimates of childhood depression range from a low of 1.9% to a high of 13.9%. Higher prevalence rates are, however, commonly found among special populations such as children referred for diagnostic assessment relating to academic or behavioral problems. Studies show rates as high as 34% to 49% for these populations, with parental psychopathology representing one of the most significant risk factors (Goldstein, 1995; Kendall, 1991). The prognosis for depression among children varies. Large-scale studies have emphasized that all treatments for depression, even psychological ones, do not permanently diminish or reduce the chances of relapsing into depression, but must be maintained at some level to influence the course (Zuckerman, 1999).

## Summary

In sum, given the persistent nature of and negative outcomes associated with ED, educating these children is a complex and overwhelming task. Although the debate continues on the etiology of ED, emerging perspectives suggest that child characteristics interact with family and environmental factors to place some children at higher risk for developing ED. As the previous section outlined, numerous disorders are subsumed under the term *emotional disturbance,* with most disorders falling along externalizing and internalizing dimensions.

# ELIGIBILITY FOR EMOTIONAL DISTURBANCE

Before a student can be declared eligible for special education services, the student must be shown to possess a disability (e.g., ED). The student must also demonstrate an educational or academic problem necessitating the need for special services. Along with federal guidelines, each state has an education code that determines under what conditions a student is considered disabled. Specifically, for children to receive special education services, they must (a) be diagnosed with a disability, (b) possess special learning needs, and (c) require special educational services to promote better educational outcomes (McLoughlin & Lewis, 1994; Salvia & Ysseldyke, 2001). In this section, we discuss (a) the definition of ED, (b) screening for ED, (c) assessment for ED, and (d) sources of assessment data in an ED evaluation.

## Definition

*Emotional disturbance,* as defined in the 1997 reauthorization of IDEA, refers to a condition exhibiting one or more of the following characteristics over a long period of time and to a marked degree that adversely affects a child's educational performance: (a) an inability to learn that cannot be explained by intellectual, sensory, or health factors; (b) an inability to build or maintain satisfactory interpersonal relationships with peers and teachers; (c) inappropriate types of behavior or feelings under normal circumstances; (d) a general pervasive mood of unhappiness or depression; or (e) a tendency to develop physical symptoms or fears associated with personal or school problems. The term includes schizophrenia. The term does not apply to children who are socially maladjusted, unless it is determined that they have an emotional disturbance. [*Federal Register*, 300.7(c)(4), 1997]

As described in the definition, children who possess one or more of the five characteristics of ED must also meet the following three conditions to qualify for special education services: long period of time, marked degree, and adverse educational effects. To meet the long period of time condition, the identified difficulty must have existed much longer than would be expected of reactions to stressful events. Similarly, to meet the marked degree requirement, a child's behavior must be more severe than would be expected for peers of similar age and the same gender. Finally, adverse educational effects require demonstrating low scores on standardized tests or some other overall measure of school functioning (McConaughy, 1993).

The federal definition of children with ED has always been and continues to be problematic because of issues of difficulty in operationalizing the definition, misinterpretation, stigma, and a lack of consensus about the nature of the disorders underlying ED (Forness et al., 2000). Although the qualifier "seriously" was removed in the 1997 reauthorization of IDEA, for several reasons the definition remains neither clear nor comprehensive enough to determine appropriate eligibility as a special education category. First, the five ED criteria are not supported by previous research on various subtypes of children with emotional or behavioral disorders. Second, the notion of adverse educational performance has been literally interpreted to pertain only to "academic" performance, thus effectively excluding "social" and "behavioral" performance as indicators. The final, and arguably the most problematic, feature is the total exclusion of youth with social maladjustment, most notably those with conduct disorders. This exclusion virtually ignores the possibility of comorbidity of mental disorders among youth identified as emotionally disturbed (Cullinan & Epstein, 2001). Indeed, the second emotional disturbance criterion—that is, the inability to build or maintain satisfactory relationships with peers and teachers—practically defines the behavioral repertoire of social maladjustment (Forness, Kavale, & Lopez, 1993).

Despite these definitional concerns, IDEA continues to guide the provision of educational services for children diagnosed with ED (Kaufman, 1997). A clear definition of ED is important because it influences the criteria that students must satisfy to be identified and subsequently receive special education services. Consequently, the definition also influences prevalence estimates for ED. Moreover, the definition influences decisions on such issues as services, research, and funding by policymakers, administrators, and advocacy groups. Intradisciplinary and interdisciplinary communication and discussion about ED are also shaped by the definition used (Epstein & Walker, 2001).

## Screening for Emotional Disorders

Given that many children with ED remain underidentified by the schools (Walker & Sprague, 1999), systematic screening of all children is recommended. The *Systematic Screening for Behavior Disorders* (SSBD; Walker & Severson, 1990) is a multigate system that provides an equal opportunity for all students in a class to be considered and be identified as at risk of having ED. The SSBD provides a solution to the problems of underreferral by providing teachers with uniform behavioral standards for use in identifying candidates for differing levels of intervention. The screening occurs in three stages: (a) general education teachers rank-order all children on their class roster to identify the students who present with the most significant externalizing (e.g., oppositional) or internalizing (e.g., withdrawn) behavior problems; (b) teachers rate the top three ranked externalizers and top three ranked internalizers on three scales that assess each child's behavioral functioning (i.e., critical events, adaptive behaviors, and maladaptive behaviors); and (c) for students who exceed criteria in the second step, teachers conduct direct observation of each student's attention to task and social interaction behaviors in classroom and playground settings. The SSBD has been shown to meet acceptable levels of reliability, validity, cost efficiency, and consumer satisfaction (Phillips, Nelson, & McLaughlin, 1993; Walker & Severson, 1990; Walker et al., 1994).

## Assessment for Emotional Disturbance

School-based assessment typically serves the following purposes: (a) prereferral classroom decisions, (b) entitlement decisions, (c) postentitlement decisions, and (d) accountability and outcome decisions (Salvia & Ysseldyke, 2001). In prereferral classroom decisions, assessment seeks to assist in the provision of special help or enrichment, referral to a teacher assistance team, or provision of intervention assistance. Assessment for entitlement decisions assists in screening, referral, identifying the disability, documenting special learning needs, and determination for special education or related services eligibility. Postentitlement classroom assessment includes testing for instructional planning, determining the best instructional setting, and monitoring progress evaluation. Finally, assessment with regard to accountability and outcomes for individuals assists in program evaluation.

To meet IDEA eligibility criteria for ED, assessment should be guided by a multidimensional (i.e., multimethod, multitrait, multisource, multisetting) approach (McConaughy & Ritter, 1995). The *multimethod* component relies on self-reports, teacher reports, parent reports, behavior rating scales, interviews with the child or adolescent, direct observation, standardized inventories, and projective techniques. The *multitrait* component relies on assessing interpersonal skills, personal coping methods, behavior types and magnitude, affect and mood states, and academic performance. The *multisource* component relies on obtaining information from the child, parents, teachers, other school personnel, health professionals, mental health professionals, and family members. Finally, assessment should be conducted across *multiple settings* to include the home, the school, different classes, different activities in the same room, structured versus unstructured settings, and different teachers in the same and different settings.

Although the process varies from setting to setting, a multidimensional assessment of ED is necessary. Although all assessment techniques make a unique contribution, surveys of school psychologists reveal that not all methods possess utility in guiding intervention practices. In a survey, Cheramie, Griffin, and Morgan (2000) found that interviews (by child, teacher, and parent) were rated highest in terms of guiding classification practices, whereas direct observation was most useful for intervention purposes.

## Sources of Data Collection

### Functional Behavioral Assessment

In recent years, behavioral researchers and practitioners have developed and used functional behavioral assessment procedures in an attempt to improve decision making in the development of treatment plans. The assumption underlying functional behavioral assessment is that treatment effectiveness is enhanced if the treatment matches the function of behavior. The goal of a functional behavioral assessment is to identify relationships between person–environment events and the occurrence and nonoccurrence of a target behavior (Dunlap & Fox, 1996). If performed accurately, this assessment allows an interventionist (e.g., teacher, psychologist) to develop a specific description of the problem behavior, identify the factors that contribute to the occurrence of the behavior, and establish a link between the behavior and a treatment (M. A. Smith, 2001).

Functional behavioral assessment is designed to (a) promote hypotheses-driven treatment, (b) place more emphasis on skill building rather than punishment, (c) increase the prospect of a positive treatment outcome, (d) increase the chance of maintenance and generalization of treatment effects, and (e) contribute to the scientific advancement of treatment efforts (Blakeslee, Sugai, & Grub, 1994). Although researchers use various specific procedures, they tend to use a combination of indirect and direct methods when conducting a functional behavioral assessment. The assumption is that compiling information from a variety of sources can create a more accurate picture of the problem behavior, including its function.

### Standardized Behavior Rating Scales

Rating scales provide an index of various individuals' (e.g., teachers', parents') perceptions of a student's behavior patterns. Respondents are asked to assess the presence or absence of a behavior and to gauge the amount, intensity, or frequency of that behavior (Salvia & Ysseldyke, 2001). Examples of rating scales include the *Child Behavior Checklist* for parents or caregivers, the *Teacher Report Form,* and the *Youth Self-Report* (Achenbach, 1991a, 1991b, 1991c). For preschool children, companion forms are also available (Achenbach & Rescorla, 2000). Another example that also includes teacher, parent and self-report forms is the *Behavior Assessment System for Children* (C. R. Reynolds & Kamphaus, 1992). Because it operationally defines the federal definition of ED, the *Scale for Assessing Emotional Disturbance* (Epstein, Cullinan, & Ryser, 2002) is especially important in helping identify children who qualify for special education services under IDEA's category of ED. In general, rating scales provide a more reliable measure of a child's externalizing and internalizing functioning (McConaughy, 1993).

## Clinical Interview

Parent, child, and teacher interviews should be routinely obtained when conducting an evaluation for ED. These interviews elicit valuable information that is not as readily obtained or is less accessible using other procedures. Most interviews should focus on a child's medical and developmental history, social–emotional functioning, educational and academic progress, and level of community involvement (Salvia & Ysseldyke, 2001). Examples of interview questions are "Have there been any hospitalizations in the past?" "Does your child play well with his or her brother and sisters?" or "Do you have any academic concerns?"

Data derived from interviews is used for clarifying information and in deciding which additional assessment procedures to pursue (McConaughy & Ritter, 1995). In general, several principles for conducting interviews should be used as guidelines (Lentz & Wehmann, 1995) . First, an ecological framework should always underlie the interview. Questions should be directed at the natural and observable constellation of variables surrounding the problem situation, the referring source, and beliefs and perceptions of the interviewee. Second, prior to beginning the interview, explicitly stated outcomes should be clearly articulated. Third, because of time limitations, interviews should always be focused and economical. Fourth, once objectives for the interview are established, questions and responses should be structured for purposes of achieving those objectives. Finally, a plan should be in place for connecting the interview information with decisions about subsequent professional practices (Lentz & Wehmann, 1995).

## Behavioral Observation

When conducting an evaluation for ED, behavioral observation yields the most useful data and, compared with other methods of assessment, represents the most direct and desirable approach to data collection (Goldstein, 1995). In behavioral observations, the observer (a) has a goal of measuring a specific behavior (e.g., counting noncompliant episodes),

(b) has previously defined the behavior of interest, (c) uses procedures for objectively gathering information about the behavior (e.g., frequency count chart), (d) specifically knows when and where the behavior will be observed, and (e) knows how the behaviors will be quantified (e.g., percentage of time noncompliant). Measuring behavior typically relies on four fundamental characteristics: duration (i.e., beginning and end of behavior), latency (i.e., the length of time between a prompt to begin a behavior and actual beginning), frequency (i.e., how often the behavior occurs), and amplitude (i.e., intensity of behavior). In determining which behavior to assess, observers should pick the most salient aspect of the behavior in the most relevant situation (Salvia & Ysseldyke, 2001).

## Personality Assessment

Due to its subjective nature, personality is a complex concept and somewhat difficult to accurately assess. More important, the choice of instruments used to assess personality depends on the theoretical orientation of the assessment personnel. For example, one might expect a psychoanalytic evaluator to focus on an individual's personality traits, whereas a behaviorally oriented evaluator might consider the manner in which someone behaves as a function of situational specificity.

In general, there are three types of personality assessment tools, namely, self-report inventories, projective techniques, and behavioral rating assessments (Ludy, Hopkins, & Nation, 1994). For example, the *Children's Depression Inventory* (Kovacs, 1982) is a self-report, symptom-oriented scale designed for all school-age children and adolescents suspected of depression. Personality assessment also includes strategies that focus on projective techniques. One popular projective test is *Roberts Apperception Test for Children* (McArthur & Roberts, 1994), which is used to subjectively assess and evaluate children's and adolescents' perceptions of common interpersonal situations. Many school psychologists also use projective drawing approaches. One popular instrument is the *Draw A Person: Screening Procedure for Emotional Disturbance* (Naglieri, McNeish, & Bardos, 1991). As the name implies, this instrument is used to screen children who may show signs of ED requiring further evaluation. Finally, many evaluators use behavioral rating scales, such as the *Child Behavior Checklist* (Achenbach, 1991a) or *Scale for Assessing Emotional Disturbance* (Epstein et al., 2002) described earlier.

From a behavioral perspective, projective evaluation techniques represent an ambiguous task at best (Knoff, 1990). Although many tests have objective scoring procedures (e.g., *Draw A Person*), the interpretation of these results relies quite heavily on subjective judgment. Personality assessment procedures that use projective techniques should only be conducted by trained psychologists, never be the primary source of data, and be interpreted with great caution (McConaughy & Ritter, 1995).

## Achievement and Educational Performance

As with all referrals for school-based, diagnostic, comprehensive psychological evaluations, assessment of ED must include information about current levels of academic achievement and performance. Information derived from achievement and performance evaluations is required to assess whether the identified behavioral or emotional difficulty adversely affects educational performance, one of the qualifying conditions for ED as stated in IDEA. Academic assessment generally involves the use of standardized tests, such as the *Woodcock–Johnson III Tests of Achievement* (Woodcock, McGrew, & Mather, 2000), curriculum-based assessment (CBA) (Gickling & Rosenfield, 1995), report cards, and work samples. CBA refers to a group of assessment techniques that serve multiple purposes but are used primarily for instructional planning and progress monitoring in tandem with what is being taught in the classroom. Over time, CBA permits continuous and direct assessment of student progress (Gickling & Rosenfield, 1995).

## Strength-Based Assessment

Up to this point, the focus of all previously discussed models, procedures, instruments, and protocols for the collection of assessment data on children suspected of having, diagnosed with, or identified with ED has been deficit based. Although these data may be necessary for decision-making purposes (e.g., special education placement), they unduly limit the scope and range of information gathered, and in the process stress the negatives at the expense of the positives in a child's functioning (Epstein, 1999). According to Epstein and Sharma (1998),

> strength-based assessment is defined as the measurement of those emotional and behavioral skills, competencies, and characteristics that create a sense of personal accomplishment; contribute to satisfying relationships with family members, peers, and adults; enhances one's ability to

deal with adversity and stress; and promotes one's personal, social, and academic development. (p. 3)

For these reasons, Epstein and Sharma developed the *Behavioral and Emotional Rating Scale: A Strength-Based Approach to Assessment.* Another strength-based assessment instrument is the *Devereux Early Childhood Assessment* (Lebuffe & Naglieri, 1999), which is designed to evaluate within-child protective factors in an effort to generate information about the strengths and areas of need in a child's protective factors (e.g., attachment, self-control, initiative).

# INTERVENTION STRATEGIES FOR CHILDREN WITH ED

Students with ED represent significant challenges to schools. Often these students are the most difficult to teach and manage in the classroom. It is not uncommon for these students to present with a wide range of social and emotional adjustment problems (e.g., conduct disorder, depression, anxiety) that impair their ability to form appropriate relationships and experience academic success. Three-tiered schoolwide prevention models (i.e., primary, secondary, and tertiary prevention programs) have been recommended to assist schools in creating more positive teaching and learning environments for these students (Sugai, Sprague, Horner, & Walker, 2000; Walker et al., 1996; Walker & Sprague, 1999). Three-tiered schoolwide prevention models represent the application of risk factor causal theory (Hawkins, Von Cleve, & Catalano, 1991; Lynam, 1996) in the schools. This theory is rooted in the notion that prolonged and pervasive exposure to one or more key risk factors (e.g., poverty, neglect, abuse) is associated with negative, destructive, and long-term outcomes (Patterson, Reid, & Dishion, 1992). The longer a child is exposed and the greater the number of risks involved, the greater the likelihood the child will develop and sustain a dysfunctional and maladaptive behavioral repertoire (Walker & Sprague, 1999).

Three-tiered schoolwide prevention models are premised on the view that, in any school setting, three types of youth can be seen: (a) typical children not at risk for problems, (b) children at risk (i.e., having one or more risk factors) for developing maladaptive behavior repertoires, and (c) children who show signs of pervasive life-course and persistent maladaptive

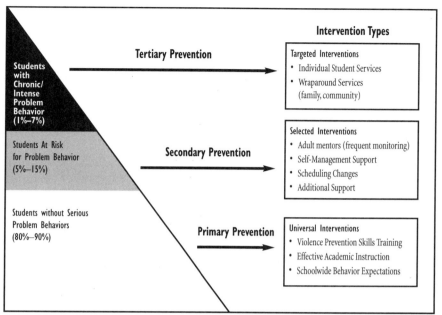

**Intervention Types**

**Tertiary Prevention**

Students with Chronic/ Intense Problem Behavior (1%–7%)

**Targeted Interventions**
• Individual Student Services
• Wraparound Services (family, community)

Students At Risk for Problem Behavior (5%–15%)

**Secondary Prevention**

**Selected Interventions**
• Adult mentors (frequent monitoring)
• Self-Management Support
• Scheduling Changes
• Additional Support

Students without Serious Problem Behaviors (80%–90%)

**Primary Prevention**

**Universal Interventions**
• Violence Prevention Skills Training
• Effective Academic Instruction
• Schoolwide Behavior Expectations

**FIGURE 17.2.** Primary, secondary, and tertiary forms of intervention. *Note.* From "The Path to School Failure, Delinquency, and Violence: Causal Factors and Some Potential Solutions," by H. M. Walker and J. R. Sprague, 1999, *Intervention in School and Clinic, 35,* p. 7. Copyright 1999 by PRO-ED, Inc. Reprinted with permission.

behavioral repertoires (Moffitt, 1993). Children within each category represent candidates for various levels of programs or interventions that provide greater specificity, intensity, comprehensiveness, and costliness (Reid, 1993). Primary, secondary, and tertiary forms of prevention are appropriate for each identified child and adolescent group. School and community approaches that encourage all three of these prevention levels are necessary to maintain the health of children, schools, and communities. Figure 17.2 illustrates primary, secondary, and tertiary forms of prevention, along with estimates of the youth who will likely be recipients of and respond to each type of prevention.

Primary prevention services are aimed at enhancing protective factors (e.g., discipline practices) on a schoolwide basis so that students exposed to this level of intervention do not become at risk for developing problematic and maladaptive behavior patterns. Interventions used for primary prevention are universal in their focus (i.e., all students are exposed to the services). As an example of primary-level prevention strategy, Nelson

(1996) developed one of the few empirically validated schoolwide prevention programs. In systematic fashion, this program addresses (a) adjusting the school's ecological arrangements (e.g., scheduling and use of space in common areas), (b) clearly stated and consistent behavioral expectations, (c) active supervision of students in common areas (e.g., hallways), (d) a consistent classroom disciplinary response connected to a continuum of disciplinary responses, and (e) functional behavioral assessment along with behavioral intervention plans linked to students' curricular and behavioral difficulties. According to the Surgeon General's (U.S. Department of Health and Human Services, 2001) report on violence, other examples of promising primary prevention programs include *Life Skills Training* (Botvin, Miholic, & Grotpeter, 1998) and the *Montreal Longitudinal Study/ Preventative Treatment Program* (Tremblay et al., 1992).

Secondary prevention programs are more intensive and costly. These programs are directed at providing behavioral, social, or academic support and skill development to children who are already demonstrating signs of their at-risk status (Walker & Sprague, 1999). Secondary prevention programs are designed to positively address one or a combination of risk factors before they grow into significant maladaptive behavioral repertoires. *First Step to Success* (Walker et al., 1998) is a secondary-level early intervention program that targets primary-grade children who show clear signs of emerging antisocial behavior patterns (e.g., aggression toward others, oppositional–defiant behavior, tantrums, rule infractions, escalating confrontations with peers and adults). Teachers and/or parents or caregivers participate in the intervention as implementation agents, under the direction and supervision of a school consultant who has primary responsibility for coordinating the intervention. The intervention specifies clear roles and duties for each social agent. *First Step to Success* incorporates many of the strategies, principles, and practices recommended in a comprehensive program. These include continuous assessment and monitoring of progress, provision for the practice of newly learned skills, treatment matched to presenting problems, multicomponent treatment strategies, programming for transfer and maintenance of new skills, commitment to sustaining the intervention, and family involvement (Epstein & Walker, 2001). Other examples of secondary prevention programs include *Functional Family Therapy* (Alexander et al., 1998) and *Second Step* (Beland, 1988).

Tertiary prevention programs are directed to children who evince severe involvement in life-course–persistent maladaptive behavioral repertoires. In general, these youth require services, interventions, and supports that very likely exceed the capacity of the school alone. Successful tertiary-level programs are likely to be intensive, comprehensive, and long term; include involvement of parents, siblings, and peers; and involve interagency collaboration. *Multisystemic therapy* (MST; Henggeler & Borduin, 1990) is a family- and home-based tertiary-level treatment that strives to change how children function in their natural settings—home, school, and neighborhood—in ways that promote positive social behavior while decreasing antisocial behavior. This multisystemic approach characterizes individuals as embedded within a network of interconnected systems that encompass individual, family, and extrafamilial (e.g., peer, school, neighborhood) factors and recognizes that intervention involves a combination of these systems. Most significantly, the conceptual framework of MST fits closely with the known causes of mental health problems, delinquency, and substance abuse. MST addresses these factors in an individualized, comprehensive, and integrated manner.

Based on the belief that the most effective and ethical route to helping children is through helping their families, MST views parents or guardians as valuable resources, even when they have serious and multiple needs of their own. The primary goals of MST are to (a) reduce the frequency and severity of mental health problems, (b) reduce other types of antisocial behavior, and (c) achieve these outcomes at a cost savings by decreasing rates of incarceration and out-of-home placements. MST achieves these goals through adherence to the nine MST treatment principles. Other examples of tertiary programs include *Multidimensional Treatment Foster Care* (Chamberlain & Mihalic, 1998) and *Intensive Protective Supervision Project* (Land, McCall, & Williams, 1992).

In summary, children with ED represent a significant challenge to schools. To create sustained positive teaching and learning environments, three-tiered (i.e., primary, secondary, tertiary) schoolwide prevention models, along with suggested programs, have been outlined. Each of the highlighted programs has the potential to reduce the risk of ED among children and has been identified either as a model or as promising by the Surgeon General's report on youth violence (U.S. Department of Health and Human Services, 2001).

# CONCLUSION

The United States is facing a health crisis in the mental well-being and care of children. Many children in schools have mental health problems that interfere with social and academic development. Evidence by the World Health Organization suggests that by 2020 childhood neuropsychiatric disorders will rise proportionately by over 50%, effectively becoming one of the top five reasons for childhood morbidity, mortality, and disability (U.S. Department of Health and Human Services, 2000). To date, research in the area of ED continues to report a chronic problem of underreferral and underidentification of children, thus creating growing numbers of children at risk of persistent, chronic, and lifelong emotional and behavioral maladjustment. Despite the significant challenges to families, schools, and society that these children present, recent evidence suggests that there is hope. Schoolwide three-tiered prevention programs have shown promise by taking an ecological approach to service delivery that involves multiple systems interacting in synergistic ways to bring about positive outcomes for children at risk for or already diagnosed with ED. Moreover, the Surgeon General, in a report on children's mental health (U.S. Department of Health and Human Services, 2000), has focused attention on evidence-based treatments (i.e., systematically tested treatments). These treatments have been shown to yield positive treatment effects, often comparable to those found in adult outcome research. Unlike untested treatments, these interventions have training manuals, are specific to the identified problems, are durable, and often show maintenance 6 months or more beyond the initial treatment.

# REFERENCES

Aber, J. L., Jones, S., & Cohen, J. (2000). The impact of poverty on the mental health and development of very young children. In C. H. Zeanah (Ed.), *Handbook of infant mental health* (2nd ed., pp. 113–128). New York: Guilford Press.

Achenbach, T. M. (1991a). *Manual for the Child Behavior Checklist.* Burlington: University of Vermont, Department of Psychiatry.

Achenbach, T. M. (1991b). *Manual for the Youth Self Report.* Burlington: University of Vermont, Department of Psychiatry.

Achenbach, T. M. (1991c). *Teacher's Report Form.* Burlington: University of Vermont, Department of Psychiatry.

Achenbach, T. M., & Rescorla, L. A. (2000). *Manual for the ASEBA preschool forms and profiles.* Burlington: University of Vermont, Department of Psychiatry.

Alexander, J., Pugh, C., Parsons, B., Barton, C., Gordon, D., Grotpeter, J., Hansson, K., Harrison, R., Mears, S., Miholic, S., Schulman, S., Waldron, H., & Sexton, J. (1998). Functional family therapy. In D. S. Elliott (Ed.), *Blueprints for violence prevention.* Boulder, CO: Center for the Study and Prevention of Violence.

American Psychiatric Association. (1994). *Diagnostic and statistical manual of mental disorders–fourth edition.* Washington, DC: Author.

American Psychiatric Association. (2000). *Diagnostic and statistical manual of mental disorders* (4th ed., text rev.). Washington, DC: Author.

Beare, P. L., & Lynch, E. C. (1986). Underidentification of preschool children at risk of behavioral disorders. *Behavioral Disorders, 15,* 177–183.

Beland, K. (1988). *Second Step, grades 1–3: Pilot project 1987–1988 summary report.* Seattle, WA: Committee for Children.

Blakeslee, T., Sugai, G., & Grub, J. (1994). A review of functional assessment use in data-based intervention studies. *Journal of Behavioral Education, 4,* 397–413.

Botvin, G. J., Miholic, S. F., & Grotpeter, J. K. (1998). Life skills training. In D. S. Elliott (Ed.), *Blueprints for violence prevention.* Boulder, CO: Center for the Study and Prevention of Violence.

Brier, N. (1995). Predicting antisocial behavior in youngsters displaying poor academic achievement: A review of risk factors. *Developmental and Behavioral Pediatrics, 16,* 271–276.

Campbell, S. B. (1990). *Behavior problems in school children.* Baltimore: Guilford Press.

Chamberlain, P., & Mihalic, S. F. (1998). *Blueprints for violence prevention, book eight: Multidimensional treatment foster care.* Boulder, CO: Center for the Study and Prevention of Violence.

Cheramie, G. M., Griffin, K. M., & Morgan, T. (2000). Usefulness of assessment techniques in assessing classification for emotional disturbance and generating classroom interventions. *Perceptual and Motor Skills, 90,* 250–252.

Crockenberg, S., & Leekes, E. (2000). Infant social and emotional development in family context. In C. H. Zeanah (Ed.), *Handbook of infant mental health.* New York: Guilford Press.

Cullinan, D., & Epstein, M. H. (2001). Comorbidity among students with emotional disturbance. *Behavioral Disorders, 26,* 200–213.

Dishion, T. J., French, D. C., & Patterson, G. R. (1995). The development and ecology of antisocial behavior. In D. Cicchetti & D. J. Cohen (Eds.), *Developmental psychopathology: Risk, disorder, and adaptation* (Vol. 2, pp. 421–471). New York: Wiley.

Duncan, B. B., Forness, S. R., & Hartsough, C. (1995). Students identified as seriously emotionally disturbed in school-based day treatment: Cognitive, psychiatric, and special education characteristics. *Behavioral Disorders, 20,* 238–252.

Dunlap, G., & Fox, L. (1996). Early intervention for serious behavior problems: A comprehensive approach. In L. Koegel & R. L. Koegel (Eds.), *Positive behavior support: Including people with difficult behaviors in the community.* Baltimore: Brookes.

Epstein, M. H. (1999). The development and validation of a scale to assess the emotional and behavioral strengths of children and adolescents. *Remedial & Special Education, 20,* 258–268.

Epstein, M. H., Cullinan, D., & Ryser, G. (2002). Development of a scale to assess emotional disturbance. *Behavioral Disorders, 28,* 5–22.

Epstein, M. H., Kinder, D., & Bursuck, B. (1989). The academic status of adolescents with behavioral disorders. *Behavioral Disorders, 14,* 157–165.

Epstein, M. H., & Sharma, J. M. (1988). *Behavioral and Emotional Rating Scale: A strength-based approach to assessment.* Austin, TX: PRO-ED.

Epstein, M. H., & Walker, H. M. (2001). *Special education: Best practices and* First Step to Success. Unpublished manuscript.

Farmer, T. W., Quinn, M. M., Hussey, W., & Holahan, T. (2001). The development of disruptive behavioral disorders and correlated constraints: Implications for intervention. *Behavioral Disorders, 26,* 117–130.

Farrington, D. P. (1989). Early predictors of adolescent aggression and adult violence. *Violence and Victims, 4,* 79–100.

Forness, S. R., Kavale, K. A., & Lopez, M. (1993). Conduct disorders in school: Special education eligibility and comorbidity. *Journal of Emotional and Behavioral Disorders, 1*(2), 101–108.

Forness, S. R., Serna, L. A., Nielsen, E., Lambros, K., Hale, M. J., & Kavale, K. A. (2000). A model for early detection and primary prevention of emotional and behavioral disorders. *Education and Treatment of Children, 23,* 325–345.

Garmezy, N., & Masten, A. S. (1994). Chronic adversities. In M. Rutter & E. Taylor (Eds.), *Child and adolescent psychiatry* (pp. 191–208). Oxford: Blackwell Scientific.

Gickling, E. E., & Rosenfield, S. (1995). Best practices in curriculum-based assessment. In A. Thomas & J. Grimes (Eds.), *Best practices in school psychology III* (pp. 587–607). Washington, DC: National Association of School Psychologists.

Goldstein, S. (1995). *Understanding and managing children's classroom behavior.* New York: Wiley.

Greenbaum, P. E., Dedrick, R. F., Friedman, R. M., Kutash, K., Brown, E., Lardieri, S. P., & Pugh, A. M. (1998). National Adolescent and Child Treatment Study (NACTS): Outcomes for children with serious emotional and behavioral disturbance. In M. H. Epstein, K. Kutash, & A. Duchnowski (Eds.), *Outcomes for children and youth with behavioral and emotional disorders and their families: Programs and evaluation best practices* (pp. 21–54). Austin, TX: PRO-ED.

Greenberg, M. T., Lengua, L., Coie, J. D., & Pinderhughes, E. E. (1999). Predicting developmental outcomes at school entry using a multiple-risk model: Four American communities. *Developmental Psychology, 35,* 403–417.

Hawkins, J. D., Von Cleve, E., & Catalano, R. F. (1991). Reducing early childhood aggression: Results of a primary prevention program. *Journal of American Academy of Child and Adolescent Psychiatry, 30,* 208–217.

Henggeler, S. W., & Borduin, C. M. (1990). *Family therapy and beyond: A multisystemic approach to treating the behavior problems of children and adolescents.* Pacific Grove, CA: Brooks/Cole.

House, A. E. (1999). *DSM–IV diagnosis in the schools*. New York: Guilford Press.

Huberty, T. J. (1987). Children and anxiety. In A. Thomas & J. Grimes (Eds.), *Children's needs: Psychological perspectives*. Washington, DC: National Association of School Psychologists.

Individuals with Disabilities Education Act of 1990, 20 U.S.C. § 1400 *et seq*.

Individuals with Disabilities Education Act Amendents of 1997, 20 U.S.C. § 1401 (26).

Kauffman, J. M. (1997). *Characteristics of emotional and behavioral disorders* (6th ed.). Columbus, OH: Merrill.

Kauffman, J. M. (2001). *Characteristics of emotional and behavioral disorders of children and youth* (7th ed.). Columbus, OH: Merrill-Prentice Hall.

Kazdin, A. E. (1985). Selection of target behaviors: The relationship of the treatment focus to clinical dysfunction. *Behavioral Assessment, 7*, 33–47.

Kendall, P. C. (1991). *Child and adolescent therapy*. New York: Guilford Press.

Knitzer, J. (2000). *Promoting resilience: Helping young children and parents affected by substance abuse, domestic violence, and depression in the context of welfare reform*. New York: National Center for Children in Poverty.

Knoff, H. (1990). Best practices in personality assessment. In A. Thomas & J. Grimes (Eds.), *Best practices in school psychology II*. Washington, DC: National Association of School Psychologists.

Kovacs, M. (1982). *Children's Depression Inventory*. Washington, DC: Multi-Health Systems.

Land, K. C., McCall, P. L., & Williams, J. R. (1992). Intensive supervision of status offenders: Evidence of continuity of treatment effects for juveniles and a "Hawthorne Effect" for counselors. In J. McCord & R. Tremblay (Eds.), *Preventing antisocial behavior: Interventions from birth through adolescence*. New York: Guilford Press.

Lebuffe, P. A., & Naglieri, J. A. (1999). *Devereux Early Childhood Assessment user's guide*. Lewisville, NC: Kaplan.

Lentz, F. E., & Wehmann, B. A. (1995). Best practices in interviewing. In A. Thomas & J. Grimes (Eds.), *Best practices in school psychology III*. Washington, DC: National Association of School Psychologists.

Ludy, B. T., Hopkins, R., & Nation, J. R. (1994). *Psychology* (3rd ed.). New York: Macmillan.

Lynam, D. R. (1996). Early identification of chronic offenders: Who is a fledgling psychopath? *Psychological Bulletin, 120*, 209–234.

McArthur, D. S., & Roberts, G. E. (1994). *Roberts Apperception Test for Children*. Los Angeles: Western Psychological Services.

McConaughy, S. H. (1993). Evaluating behavioral and emotional disorders with CBCL, TRF, and YSR cross-informant scales. *Journal of Emotional and Behavioral Disorders, 1*, 40–52.

McConaughy, S. H., & Ritter, D. R. (1995). Best practices in multidimensional assessment of emotional or behavioral disorders. In A. Thomas & J. Grimes (Eds.), *Best practices in school psychology III*. Washington, DC: National Association of School Psychologists.

McConaughy, S. H., & Skiba, R. J. (1994). Comorbidity of externalizing and internalizing problems. *School Psychology Review, 22*, 421–436.

McLoughlin, J. A., & Lewis, R. B. (1994). *Assessing special students.* New York: Macmillan College.

Mezey, G., & Robbins, I. (2001). Usefulness and validity of post-traumatic stress disorder as a psychiatric category. *British Medical Journal, 323,* 561–563.

Moffitt, T. E. (1993). Adolescence-limited and life-course–persistant antisocial behavior: A developmental taxonomy. *Psychological Review, 100,* 674–701.

Naglieri, J. A., McNeish, T. J., & Bardos, A. N. (1991). *Draw A Person: Screening procedure for emotional disturbance.* Austin, TX: PRO-ED.

Neel, R. S., Meadows, N., Levine, P., & Edgar, E. B. (1988). What happens after special education: A statewide follow-up study of secondary students who have behavioral disorders. *Behavioral Disorders, 13,* 209–216.

Nelson, J. R. (1996). Designing schools to meet the needs of students who exhibit disruptive behavior. *Journal of Emotional and Behavioral Disorders, 4,* 147–161.

Oswald, D. P., & Coutinho, M. J. (1996). Leaving school: The impact of state economic and demographic factors for students with serious emotional disturbance. *Journal of Emotional and Behavioral Disorders, 4,* 114–125.

Patterson, G., De Baryshe, B. D., & Ramsey, E. (1989). A developmental perspective on antisocial behavior. *American Psychologist, 44,* 329–335.

Patterson, G., Reid, J., & Dishion, T. (1992). *Antisocial boys.* Eugene, OR: Castalia.

Phillips, V., Nelson, C. M., & McLaughlin, J. R. (1993). Systems change and services for students with emotional/behavioral disorders in Kentucky. *Journal of Emotional and Behavioral Disorders, 1,* 155–164.

Quinn, K. P., & Epstein, M. H. (1998). Characteristics of children, youth, and families served by local interagency systems of care. In M. H. Epstein, K. Kutash, & A. Duchnowski (Eds.), *Outcomes for children and youth with emotional and behavioral disorders and their families.* Austin, TX: PRO-ED.

Reid, J. (1993). Prevention of conduct disorder before and after school entry: Relating interventions to developmental findings. *Development and Psychopathology, 5,* 243–262.

Reynolds, C. R., & Kamphaus, R. W. (1992). *Behavior Assessment System for Children.* Circle Pines, MN: American Guidance Service.

Reynolds, W. M. (1992a). Depression in children and adolescents. In W. M. Reynolds (Ed.), *Internalizing disorders in children and adolescents* (pp. 150–253). New York: Wiley.

Reynolds, W. M. (1992b). The study of internalizing disorders in children and adolescents. In W. M. Reynolds (Ed.), *Internalizing disorders in children and adolescents* (pp. 1–18). New York: Wiley.

Robbins, L. N. (1966). *Deviant children grown up.* Baltimore: Williams & Wilkins.

Ruhl, R. L., & Berlinghoff, D. H. (1992). Research on improving behaviorally disordered students' academic performance: A review of the literature. *Behavioral Disorders, 17,* 178–190.

Salvia, J., & Ysseldyke, J. E. (2001). *Assessment* (8th ed.). New York: Houghton Mifflin.

Shaw, D. S., Gilliom, M., & Giovannelli, J. (2000). Aggressive behavior disorders. In C. H. Zeanah Jr. (Ed.), *Handbook of infant mental health* (2nd ed., pp. 397–411). New York: Guilford Press.

Singh, N. N., Landrum, T. J., Donatelli, L. S., Hampton, C., & Ellis, C. R. (1994). Characteristics of children and adolescents with serious emotional disturbance in systems of care: Part I. Partial hospitalization and inpatient psychiatric services. *Journal of Emotional and Behavioral Disorders, 2*(1), 13–20.

Smith, M. A. (2001). Functional assessment of challenging behaviors. In S. Alper, D. L. Ryndak, & C. N. Schloss (Eds.), *Alternative assessment of students with disabilities in inclusive settings* (pp. 256–272). Boston: Allyn & Bacon.

Smith, S. W., & Coutinho, M. J. (1997). Achieving the goals of the national agenda: Progress and prospects. *Journal of Emotional and Behavioral Disorders, 5,* 2–5.

Sugai, G., Sprague, J. R., Horner, R. H., & Walker, H. (2000). Preventing school violence: The use of office discipline referrals to assess and monitor school-wide discipline interventions. *Journal of Emotional and Behavioral Disorders, 8,* 94–101.

Tremblay, R. E., Vitaro, F., Bertrand, L., LeBlanc, M., Benchesne, H., Boileau, H., & David, L. (1992). Parent and child training to prevent early onset of delinquency: The Montreal longitudinal experimental study. In J. McCorea & R. Tremblay (Eds.), *Preventing antisocial behavior: Interventions from birth through adolescence.* New York: Guilford Press.

UCLA–Neuropsychiatric Institute. (1999). *Generalized anxiety disorder in children.* Retrieved November 14, 2001, from http://www.nbi.ucla.edu

U.S. Department of Education. (2001). *Twenty-third annual report to Congress on the implementation of the Individuals with Disabilities Education Act.* Washington, DC: Office of Special Education.

U.S. Department of Health and Human Services. (2000). *Report of the Surgeon General's Conference on Children's Mental Health: A national action agenda.* Washington, DC: Department of Health and Human Services.

U.S. Department of Health and Human Services. (2001). *Youth violence: A report of the surgeon general.* Washington, DC: Office of the Surgeon General.

Wagner, W., Blackorby, J., Cameto, K., Hebbeler, K., & Newman, N. (1993). *The transition experiences of young people with disabilities: A summary of findings from the National Longitudinal Transition Study of Special Education Students.* Menlo Park, CA: SRI International.

Walker, H. M., Horner, R. H., Sugai, G., Bullis, M., Sprague, J. R., Bricker, D., & Kauffman, M. J. (1996). Integrated approaches to preventing anti-social behavior patterns among school-age children and youth. *Journal of Emotional and Behavioral Disorders, 4,* 194–209.

Walker, H. M., Kavanagh, K., Stiller, B., Golly, A., Steverson, H. H., & Feil, E. G. (1998). First Step to Success: An early intervention approach for preventing school antisocial behavior. *Journal of Emotional and Behavioral Disorders, 6,* 66–80.

Walker, H. M., & Severson, H. (1990). *Systematic Screening for Behavior Disorders.* Longmont, CA: Sopris West.

Walker, H. M., Severson, H. H., Nicholson, F., Kehle, T., Jensen, W. R., & Clark, E. (1994). Replication of the Systematic Screening for Behavior Disorders (SSBD) procedure for the identification of at-risk children. *Journal of Emotional and Behavioral Disorders, 2,* 66–77.

Walker, H. M., & Sprague, J. R. (1999). The path to school failure, delinquency, and violence: Causal factors and some potential solutions. *Intervention in School and Clinic, 35,* 67–73.

Waters, T. L., Barrett, P. M., & March, J. S. (2003). Cognitive-behavioral family treatment of childhood obsessive–compulsive disorder: A home-based observation. *American Journal of Psychotherapy, 57,* 80–100.

Wehby, J. H., Symons, F. J., & Hollo, A. (1997). Promote appropriate assessment. *Journal of Emotional and Behavioral Disorders, 5,* 45–54.

Wenar, C. (1994). *Developmental psychopathology* (3rd ed.). New York: McGraw-Hill.

Woodcock, R., McGrew, K., & Mather, N. (2000). *Woodcock–Johnson III Tests of Achievement.* Itasca, IL: Riverside.

Zuckerman, M. (1999). *Vulnerability to psychopathology.* Washington, DC: American Psychological Association.

# CHAPTER 18

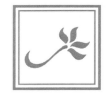

# Autistic Spectrum Disorders
## Autism, Pervasive Developmental Disorder, and Asperger Syndrome

Pasquale J. Accardo

L ong a confusing entity, autism has been identified by the National Institutes of Health of the United States as a major target for research into both its etiology and treatment. It is anticipated that the next decade will see major advances in how this disorder is understood. Already, the prognosis for many autistic children is much improved over what it was a decade or two ago. Autism is a condition with a rapidly changing portrait.

## DESCRIPTION OF AUTISIC SPECTRUM DISORDERS

For several decades after its first description by Leo Kanner in 1943 (thus some older literature refers to Kanner's syndrome), autism was initially considered to be a catastrophic childhood emotional withdrawal precipitated in early infancy by deviant parenting (especially "cold" mothers). Since the 1970s, an increasing body of scientific evidence has completely overturned this interpretation. Autism is now recognized as a neurobehavioral syndrome that is for the most part congenital, caused by genetic factors or other prenatal influences affecting how the baby's brain develops. It is

The preparation of this chapter was supported in part by Project #1 T73 MC 00046 04 from the Maternal and Child Health Bureau (Title V, Social Security Act), Health Resources and Services Administration, Department of Health and Human Services.

**TABLE 18.1**

Diagnostic Features of Autistic Spectrum Disorders

| Qualitative Impairment in Communication | Qualitative Impairment in Social Interaction | Repetitive, Restrictive, Deviant Behaviors |
| --- | --- | --- |
| Language delay | Poor eye contact | Water play |
| Echolalia, immediate and delayed | No joint attention | Perseveration |
| Expressive better than receptive language | No gaze monitoring | Preservation of sameness |
| | Doesn't read faces | Stereotypies |
| Hyperlexia | Treats people like furniture | Rocking |
| Equinus gait | In own little world | Covers ears |
| Refers to self in third person | Laughs for no reason | Spinning/twirling |
| Pronominal reversal | No peer interaction | Likes fans |
| Acts as if deaf | No reciprocity or sharing | Stiff/noncuddly baby |
| Protoimperative but not protodeclarative pointing | | Splinter skills |
| | | Savant behavior |
| Good rote memory | | Inflexible routines and rituals |
| Poor pragmatic language | | Obsessive—compulsive behaviors |
| No imaginative play | | Tone abnormalities |
| | | Blunted affect |
| | | Arching |
| | | Flapping |
| | | Lines up/groups toys |
| | | Preoccupation with parts of objects |
| | | Insensitivity to pain |
| | | Sniffing at things |
| | | Hyperactivity |

important for professionals as well as parents to recognize the magnitude of this reversal in interpretation because many of the popular books that proposed the deviant parenting hypothesis remain on library shelves without any disclaimers.

Autistic spectrum disorders (ASDs) are characterized by the co-occurrence of significant problems in three developmental areas: communication, socialization, and repetitive behaviors. Table 18.1 lists typical diagnostic features of ASD.

The class of ASDs including pervasive developmental disorders includes five relatively distinct entities:

1. *Autism* (previously referred to as early infantile autism) is present when the child exhibits significant impairment in all three domains affected by autism—communication, socialization, and stereotypical behaviors—and does this prior to age 3 years. Autism is often accompanied by a regression in language and socialization between 18 and 24 months of age (*autistic regression*). Autism can occur with varying degrees of mental retardation or with normal to above average intelligence.

2. *Pervasive developmental disorder, not otherwise specified* (PDD-NOS, or atypical autism), is present (a) when impairment is significant in one or two of the three autistic domains but is not severe enough in the third to qualify for a diagnosis of autism, or (b) when the condition has an onset after 3 years of age. Often considered a milder form of autism (since all three areas are not severely affected), it might nevertheless be associated with serious mental retardation. Thus, some children with PDD-NOS are more severely handicapped than some children with autism.

3. *Rett syndrome* is an X-linked (at the site MeCP2) genetic syndrome that occurs in girls who seem to develop relatively normally for at least the first year of life. Sometime during the second year of life, a severe regression in cognitive, language, motor, and socialization skills occurs. Autistic features include stereotypical hand wringing movements and marked gaze avoidance (poor eye contact). One striking physical finding is an acquired microcephaly (i.e., a previously normal-sized head stops growing, and the plateauing head circumference falls farther and farther off its growth curve).

4. *Childhood disintegrative disorder* involves a rapid loss of cognitive and behavioral skills; the child's previously normal developmental curve is reset to a moderately retarded level with the appearance of significant autistic features. Careful investigation will uncover specific degenerative neurological conditions in as many as a third of these cases. It is debated whether children with a specific neurodegenerative disorder should remain in this autism classification or be switched to a purely neurological category.

5. *Asperger syndrome* is characterized by the presence of severe deficits in socialization and stereotypic behaviors; language skills appear normal early in life but later demonstrate significant pragmatic defects (problems with maintaining a conversation or linguistically interacting with another person). Asperger syndrome is probably identical with so-called high-functioning autism in which the IQ (including verbal IQ) is average to high. A major caveat to the diagnosis of Asperger syndrome is that early language should appear normal.

Because the problems presented by the various other autistic spectrum disorders are more severe, they are easier to suspect, diagnose, and approach than the difficulties encountered in Asperger syndrome, which can be quite subtle, almost to the point of being a variant of normal (such as what is sometimes referred to as the "nerdy" child with limited social skills). Thus, it is not uncommon for Asperger syndrome to be diagnosed late, even for autistic spectrum disorders. Because children with Asperger syndrome typically function quite well in formal academics ("little professors"), it is not difficult for their limited social interactions, narrowly restricted interests, and pragmatic language deficits to be downplayed or ignored. Their concrete use of language makes them relatively insensitive to jokes and innuendos. Poor empathy, limited facial expressiveness, motor awkwardness, weak common sense, and no idea of cooperating toward a common goal, all contribute to generating social outcasts. At first insensitive to this exclusion, by the time of adolescence, these children may feel anger and even rage. The extent to which Asperger syndrome differs from autism with high verbal intelligence (so-called high-functioning autism) is a question that is currently the subject of much research, with preliminary data suggesting that the two may be almost identical in their management implications.

A pattern of behavior that is neither part of the diagnosis of autism nor unique to autism but occurs much more commonly in this condition than in any other developmental disability is known as the *savant syndrome*. (The older, derogatory term was *idiot savant*.) In savant syndrome, one or more highly specific cognitive functions are exacerbated and hypertrophied to the point of genius or giftedness. The areas so accelerated can include reading (hyperlexia), but more commonly affect nonverbal or right brain functions such as music (e.g., persons who can reproduce a complex piano piece after hearing it only once and without benefit of any formal lessons), mathematics, and graphic arts. Such savant skills can have significant positive social and vocational advantages, but the extent to which they should be encouraged needs to be decided on an individual basis.

One other syndrome that is often mentioned in connection with autism is acquired epileptic aphasia, or *Landau-Kleffner syndrome*. In this condition, the child develops a seizure disorder, most often with overt and obvious convulsions, and with a localization of the seizure focus over the brain's language areas so that the epilepsy impairs the child's speech and language skills. Because some children develop an active epileptic focus over the language areas of the brain in the absence of obvious seizures, the possibility that some cases diagnosed as autistic regression may be due to an occult seizure disorder needs to be considered. The child who loses language because of Landau-Kleffner syndrome does not exhibit—at least at first—the associated simultaneous emotional withdrawal and loss of social skills that characterize autism not associated with epilepsy. If the Landau-Kleffner syndrome is not identified and effectively treated, however, the prolonged communication impairment can lead to the development of various degrees of emotional withdrawal and loss of social skills so as to effectively imitate an autistic disorder.

# PREVALENCE RATES OF AUTISM

In the past, autism was considered to be quite rare, with a prevalence rate of approximately several children per 10,000. More recently this rate has escalated. In isolated areas, rates as high as 1% (1 in 100 children) have been reported (Bertrand et al., 2001). There are two possible explanations for this dramatic increase: (a) It is a true increase, and there are many more cases of autism than in the past, presumably because of some novel negative environmental influence on fetal brain development, or (b) the increase is artificial and, although there were more cases of autistic spectrum disorders in the past, these were not recognized as such because of decreased professional sensitivity to the diagnosis. In this latter case, many children with autism would probably have been misdiagnosed as mentally retarded. The second option is supported by the fact that the increase in autism has coincided with the following:

- Widespread early intervention and birth-to-age 3 screening and diagnostic activities

- Heightened professional awareness and improved autism education in both preservice training and continuing education programs

- An expanded description of different presentations for autism in the American Psychiatric Association's (2000) *Diagnostic and Statistical Manual of Mental Disorders–Fourth Edition–Text Revision*

As stated previously, children with autism can have many of the same genetic syndromes that produce mental retardation, and the autistic features may be ignored as part of the retardation syndrome. A decade ago, autism was considered rarer in Down syndrome than in the general population; more recently, autism has been considered at least as common in Down syndrome as in the general population. Current research now suggests that autism may be much more common in Down syndrome than in the general population, with an incidence in Down syndrome as high as 7%

(Kent, Evans, Paul, & Sharp, 1999). Thus, a child with Down syndrome who is exhibiting features of autism should be considered for an additional diagnosis that may help to explain unanticipated academic, cognitive, and behavioral underachievement or regression. Recognition of multiple diagnoses is another factor contributing to the explosive increase in the incidence of autism.

# DIAGNOSIS OF AUTISM

Optimally, autism should be diagnosed at 2 to 3 years of age. Unfortunately, autism is more often diagnosed closer to 5 years. The importance of early diagnosis derives from reasonable evidence that an intensive behavioral program (most often referred to as applied behavioral analysis, or ABA) can significantly improve long-term outcome when rigorously employed in the early temporal window of 2 to 5 years (Lovaas, 2000). To miss this window of opportunity is to risk a less than optimal outcome (although ABA is still used to ameliorate autistic behaviors in older children). The three behavioral intervention programs most commonly employed in the treatment of autism are ABA (UCLA Young Autism Project, or the Lovaas method), TEACCH (Treatment and Education of Autistic and Communication Handicapped Children; Schopler, Reichler, & Lansing, 1980), and DIR (Developmental, Individual differences, Relationships model, or the Greenspan approach; Greenspan & Wieder, 1997).

For primary health care providers, close monitoring of children's language at 18 and 24 months of age should allow the earliest recognition of autism (Kanthor, 1999). Children should have 6 to 12 words at 18 months of age (no words at 18 months of age is an automatic indicator for referral) and at least 50 words and several 2-word phrases at 24 months of age. The child with autism usually presents by age 2 years with one of three language patterns:

1. Mute (no expressive language)

2. Less than 50 words and no 2-word phrases (delayed expressive language)

3. At least 50 words and several 2-word phrases (apparently normal expressive language)

In the last case, it is important to determine what if any percentage of the child's vocalizations are echolalic or parrotting (repeated without any communicative intent).

As a marker for autism, social deviance is often suspected much earlier than it is confirmed. Many mothers of children with autism describe their infant as having been "aloof" or not very socially responsive even in the first year of life. That this is a genuine phenomenon has been documented by careful review of family videotapes of such infants.

Three useful markers for the problems with reciprocal social interaction that characterize autism in young children are the absence of

- *pretend play* (e.g., imaginatively encouraging a doll to drink from an empty toy cup filled from a toy kettle)
- *gaze monitoring* (looking in the same direction as someone else)
- *joint attention* (encouraging shared interest)

Children point to indicate they want something by around 1 year of age; beginning at 18 months, they point to name something, such as body parts or pictures in a book. Between 18 and 24 months of age, children begin to point to direct another's attention to something of interest; this *protodeclarative pointing* is a reliable marker for the presence of joint attention.

# MEDICAL ASSESSMENT FOR AUTISM

When asked which biomedical tests and procedures should be employed in a case of autism, the reasonable response is that there are no specific tests for autism. Therefore, the autism itself is not an indication for any test. Rather, indications for any test, based on the history and physical examination, should be separate from the fact of the autism. Thus, the medical assessment for autism is almost the same as that for mental retardation.

*Fragile X syndrome* is sometimes described as an autistic syndrome, and testing for the FMR-1 gene is often considered routine for children with autism. It is, however, more appropriately classified as a mental retardation syndrome in which several to many autistic behaviors are apparent. Autism in a child without mental retardation (or a family history of mental retardation) and without any physical features of fragile X syndrome is very unlikely to yield a positive genetic test for fragile X. Again, autism by itself is not an indication for any specific biomedical test.

That many of the same etiologies are involved in autism and mental retardation should not be surprising since many children with autism are also mentally retarded. No child with Asperger syndrome is mentally retarded, whereas all children with Rett syndrome are severely mentally retarded, and all children with childhood disintegrative disorder are moderately mentally retarded. Children with autism and PDD-NOS can exhibit the full range of IQ levels from profound mental retardation through gifted intelligence.

When describing the cognitive behavioral profile associated with different syndromes, one of the variables used is the presence of a significant verbal–performance discrepancy. Syndromes with a stronger association with autism tend to be those (such as Down syndrome) in which the verbal–performance discrepancy reflects a language weakness.

# TREATMENT FOR AUTISM

As with mental retardation, the medical treatment for children with autism includes the provision of quality primary medical care, the occasional use of psychotropic drugs for the management of challenging behaviors, and genetic counseling for risks to future pregnancies. The use of psychotropic medications for behavior management is much more problematic in children with autism than in children with other developmental and behavioral conditions. Although various drugs are just as likely to improve target behaviors, they seem more likely to precipitate or exacerbate other problem behaviors. The more complicated neurological substrate for autism seems to decrease positive medication responses.

Various so-called medical treatments with a purported neurological basis lack scientific evidence for efficacy in the treatment of autism. These treatments include secretin infusions, megavitamins, facilitated communication, immunoglobulin therapy, music therapy, auditory integration training, treatment for disorders of metal-metabolism/metallothionien, and avoiding antibiotics and infant immunizations.

Because schools routinely require that entering students provide documentation of an up-to-date immunization schedule, some comment about the controversial association of autism with measles–mumps–rubella (MMR) immunization is indicated. Regression is a surprisingly common feature in many cases of autistic spectrum disorder; it is found in all cases of Rett syndrome and disintegrative disorder and in half to two thirds of cases of autism and PDD-NOS, but in no cases of Asperger syndrome. The regression in classic autism typically occurs between 18 and 24 months of age. Almost anything that routinely happens to children between 12 and 18 months of age has been proposed as a possible trigger for if not an actual cause of the onset of autism in the second half of the second year of life. Examples of such culprits include both frequent (almost any number of) episodes of otitis media (ear infections) and the antibiotics used to treat them. Most recently, the combined MMR immunization has been suggested as a cause of autism, and parents have been warned against immunizing their children. Despite much speculation, there is no evidence to support such an association, or rather there is no more evidence than a *post hoc, ergo propter hoc* (after this, therefore because of this) reasoning would assume. Such a fallacy would also indict teething (and any treatment for the teething) as a cause of autism. Whether and when a child received the MMR vaccine was compared to the onset of autistic symptoms, and no association was found; that is, the onset of autism was just as likely to precede as follow the immunization (Halsey, Hyman, & Conference Writing Panel, 2001).

# THE TEACHER'S ROLE

Along with the family and physician, the teacher is an important participant in the management of children with autism. The following are some guidelines for classroom teachers. (For readers who want more information, a Suggested Reading list is provided after these guidelines.)

- With successful behavioral treatment of their specifically autistic symptoms, many children with autistic spectrum disorders will, as they get older, fall into the category of children with mental retardation with an uneven cognitive profile.
- The classroom role of the special education teacher generally is spelled out in detail in the child's Individualized Education Program (IEP); this IEP should itemize both generic interventions and accommodations

for children with autism, as well as more specific recommendations to address the individual's unique behavioral characteristics. Close collaboration between the classroom teacher and the child's speech–language and occupational therapists should help optimize the achievement of defined academic, socialization, and other developmental goals.

- The indications for psychotropic medication are narrower in children with autism, and, as mentioned previously, success is more limited. Nevertheless, medications should be seriously considered whenever disruptive behaviors (hyperactivity, inattention, obsessive–compulsive traits, tantrums, etc.) interfere with classroom progress and threaten the loss of an otherwise appropriate program placement.

- Children with Asperger syndrome (children with some autistic features and with normal to above average intelligence) are the ones most likely to be found in the regular classroom setting. Social skills training, therapy for pragmatic language disorders, and anger management programs are probably best provided by speech–language therapists, psychologists, and counselors. The classroom teacher needs to collaborate closely with these professionals to help positive effects generalize to the larger school social setting.

# SUGGESTED READING

Filipek, P. A., Accardo, P. J., Baranek, G. T., Cooke, E. H., Jr., Dawson, G., Gordon, B., Gravel, J. S., Johnson, C. P., Kallen, R. J., Levy, S. E., Minshew, N. J., Prizant, B. M., Rapin, I., Rogers, S. J., Stone, W. L., Teplin, S., Tuchman, R. F., & Volkmar, F. R. (1999). The screening and diagnosis of autistic spectrum disorders. *Journal of Autism and Developmental Disorders, 29*(6), 439–484.

Filipek, P. A., Accardo, P. J., Ashwal, S., Baranek, G. T., Cook, E. H., Jr., Dawson, G., Gordon, B., Gravel, J. S., Johnson, C. P., Kallen, R. J., Levy, S. E., Minshew, N. J., Ozonoff, S., Johnson, C. P., Prizant, B. M., Rapin, I., Teplin, S., Rogers, S. J., Stone, W. L., Tuchman, R. F., & Volkmar, F. R. (2000). Practice parameter: Screening and diagnosis of autism: Report of the Quality Standards Subcommittee of the American Academy of Neurology and the Child Neurology Society. *Neurology, 54*(4), 468–479.

McIlvane, W. J., Alexander, D., & Bristol, M. (Eds.). (1998). Autism [Special issue]. *Mental Retardation and Developmental Disabilities Research Reviews, 2*(4).

# REFERENCES

American Psychiatric Association. (2000). *Diagnostic and statistical of mental disorders* (4th ed., text rev.). Washington, DC: Author.

Bertrand, J., Mars, A., Boyle, C., Bove, F., Yeargin-Allsopp, M., & Decoufle, P. (2001). Prevalence of autism in a United States population: The Brick Township, New Jersey, investigation. *Pediatrics 108*(5), 1155–1161.

Greenspan, S. I., & Wieder, S. (1997). Developmental patterns and outcomes in infants and children with disorders in relating and communicating: A chart review of 200 cases of children with autistic spectrum disorders. *Journal of Developmental and Learning Disorders, 1,* 87–141.

Halsey, N. A., Hyman, S. L., & the Conference Writing Panel. (2001). Measles–mumps–rubella vaccine and autistic spectrum disorder: Report from the New Challenges in Childhood Immunizations Conference convened in Oak Brook, Illinois, June 12–13, 2000. *Pediatrics, 107*(5), E84.

Kanthor, H. A. (Chair). (1999). *Autism/pervasive developmental disorders: Assessment and intervention for young children (age 0–3 years). Clinical practice guideline: Report of the recommendations* (Publication No. 4215). Albany: New York State Department of Health Early Intervention Program.

Kent, L., Evans, J., Paul, M., & Sharp, M. (1999). Comorbidity of autistic spectrum disorders in children with Down syndrome. *Developmental Medicine and Child Neurology, 41,* 153–158.

Lovaas, I. (2000). Experimental design and cumulative research in early behavioral intervention. In P. J. Accardo, C. Magnusen, & A. J. Capute (Eds.), *Autism: Clinical and research issues* (pp. 133–161). Baltimore: York Press.

Schopler, E., Reichler, R. J., & Lansing, M. (1980). *Individualized assessment and treatment for autistic and developmentally disabled children.* Baltimore: University Park Press.

# CHAPTER 19

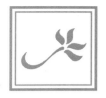

# Adolescent Eating Disorders

### Debra K. Katzman

**E**ating disorders are complex illnesses that are affecting adolescents with increasing frequency. Given this rising incidence, people who work with children and adolescents need to become familiar with these disorders. Schools provide a natural place to teach young people about health issues, including nutrition and exercise. Teachers can play an important role in imparting cultural values and cultivating healthy attitudes toward the body and the self. They thus can have a strong impact on the prevention of eating disorders and the growing preoccupation with weight. They are in an excellent position to soften the impact of the sociocultural factors causing food and weight problems and to help in their early detection and treatment.

This chapter is a summary of current knowledge about eating disorders in the adolescent, with particular attention to the teacher's role. It describes the clinical presentation of anorexia nervosa and bulimia nervosa, medical and developmental issues, and kinds of treatment specific to adolescents. It is my hope that the information presented here will increase the teacher's knowledge about adolescent eating disorders and facilitate prevention, early detection, and referral.

## DIAGNOSIS

*Anorexia nervosa* is characterized by self-imposed starvation. The adolescent refuses to maintain body weight over a minimally normal weight for age and height or fails to make the expected weight gain during a period of growth, leading to a body weight 15% below that expected. In postmenarchal girls, the absence of at least three consecutive menstrual cycles is another sign of this disorder. Patients have an intense drive for thinness or a fear of gaining weight, accompanied by distortions in their perception of body shape, weight, and size. For example, they point to areas they see as too fat when in fact these areas can be described as "skin and bones." They control their weight by restricting both the quantity and type of food and by exercising strenuously to eliminate calories. The criteria from the American Psychiatric Association's (2000) *Diagnostic and Statistical Manual of Mental Disorders–Fourth Edition–Text Revision* (DSM–IV–TR) for anorexia nervosa are presented in Table 19.1.

Commonly, the adolescent begins a weight-reducing diet in response to comments made by friends or family. At first, the patient wants to lose a few pounds and so eliminates sweets and desserts. Gradually, the choice of food becomes more restricted as the patient begins skipping meals and eating only high-protein, low-carbohydrate, no-fat foods that are low in calories. The patient may consume as few as 600 to 800 calories per day (Beaumont, Chambers, Rouse, & Abraham, 1981). Even after significant weight loss, the adolescent is not satisfied and desperately wants a weight buffer so as to be able to indulge in an occasional treat. As weight gets lower and lower, the adolescent develops a sense of accomplishment and begins to feel better. The results of dieting and weight loss often win praise from peers, which encourages the young person to continue the same practices. Individuals with anorexia nervosa often weigh themselves several times a day.

Dieting is accompanied by changing weight goals, social isolation, and increased physical activity. Most of these patients become preoccupied with food and eating. They often entertain magical beliefs about their routines and food, consider many foods forbidden, and eat the same foods at the same time every day. If the caloric allotment is exceeded or a prohibited food eaten, the individual may become overwhelmed with guilt and reduce the caloric intake yet further. The adolescent with anorexia nervosa often likes to cook for family members but refuses to eat the food, and typically avoids meals with other family members by offering numerous excuses: "I've already eaten," "I have the flu," or "I'm going out for dinner." If these young people sit down to a meal with others, they often cut their food into tiny pieces, rearrange it on their plate, or chew food and spit it out.

*Bulimia nervosa* is characterized by recurrent episodes of binge eating and inappropriate compensatory behaviors, such as self-induced vomiting, laxative and diuretic abuse, fasting, and excessive exercise to prevent weight gain. Like individuals with anorexia nervosa, those with bulimia

## TABLE 19.1

DSM–IV–TR Criteria for Anorexia Nervosa and Bulimia Nervosa

**Anorexia Nervosa**

A. Refusal to maintain body weight over a minimally normal weight for age and height (e.g., weight loss leading to to maintenance of body weight 15% below that expected), or failure to make expected weight gain during period of growth, leading to body weight less than 85% of that expected.

B. Intense fear of gaining weight or becoming fat, even though underweight.

C. Disturbance in the way in which one's body weight or shape is experienced, undue influence of body shape and weight on self-evaluation, or denial of the seriousness of current low body weight.

D. In postmenarchal women, amenorrhea (i.e., the absence of at least three consecutive menstrual cycles. A woman is considered to have amenorrhea if her periods occur only following hormone— for example estrogen—administration).

**Restricting type:** During the episode of anorexia nervosa, the person does not regularly engage in binge eating or purging behavior (i.e., self-induced vomiting or the misuse of laxatives or diuretics).

**Binge eating/purging type:** During the episode of anorexia nervosa, the person regularly engages in binge eating or purging behavior (i.e., self-induced vomiting or the misuse of laxatives or diuretics).

**Bulimia Nervosa**

A. Recurrent episodes of binge eating. An episode of binge eating is characterized by both of the following:

   1. eating in a discrete period of time (e.g., within any 2-hour period) an amount of food that is definitely larger than most people would eat in a similar period of time in similar circumstances; and
   2. a sense of lack of control over eating during the episode (e.g., a feeling that one cannot stop eating or control what or how much one is eating).

B. Recurrent inappropriate compensatory behavior in order to prevent weight gain, such as: self-induced vomiting; misuse of laxatives, diuretics, enemas, or other medications; fasting; or excessive exercise.

C. The binge eating and inappropriate compensatory behaviors both occur, on average, at least twice a week for 3 months.

D. Self-evaluation is unduly influenced by body shape and weight.

E. The disturbance does not occur exclusively during episodes of anorexia nervosa.

**Purging type:** The person regularly engages in self-induced vomiting or the misuse of laxatives, diuretics, or enemas.

**Non-purging type:** The person uses other inappropriate compensatory behaviors, such as fasting or excessive exercise, but does not regulary engage in self-induced vomiting or the misuse of laxatives, diuretics, or enemas.

nervosa are overly concerned with their body shape and weight; however, bulimia is more prevalent among those who previously have been obese. Typically, bulimia begins with unwanted weight gain during or following puberty. Research indicates that the onset of bulimic symptoms is often followed by periods of prolonged caloric deprivation (C. L. Johnson, Stuckey, Lewis, & Schwartz, 1982; Pyle, Mitchell, & Eckert, 1981). The DSM–IV–TR criteria for bulimia nervosa are presented in Table 19.1.

Binges occur regularly (at least twice a week for 3 months) and are marked by the rapid and out-of-control consumption of a large amount of high-calorie food in a short period of time. At the start of a binge, the patient typically feels a surge of euphoria, but as the behavior continues, the individual experiences fear, self-disgust, guilt, or anxiety about impending weight gain. The patient may consume as many as 5,000 calories during a binge. A variety of methods are used to induce vomiting; the most common is sticking a finger or toothbrush down the throat. Some patients can vomit spontaneously. Purging produces another episode of euphoria. Several hours after the binge–purge behavior, patients often feel depressed and hopeless. Occasionally, they get desperate enough to hoard or steal food or steal money to buy food. Initially, the binge–purge activity is infrequent, but its frequency may increase to daily or even to many times a day. Both bingeing and purging behaviors are often secretive.

The diagnosis of anorexia nervosa or bulimia nervosa requires ruling out other medical and psychiatric conditions, including malignancy, brain tumors, seizures, inflammatory bowel disease, endocrine and metabolic diseases, infection, and pregnancy. Typically, patients with one of these conditions do not pursue thinness or distort their body image. Weight loss may also occur with psychiatric disorders such as schizophrenia, depression, conversion disorder, and obsessive–compulsive disorder. However, it is important to keep in mind that an eating disorder can occur simultaneously with another medical or psychiatric illness.

# EPIDEMIOLOGY

Since the early 1980s, major changes have occurred in the epidemiology of eating disorders in adolescents. Anorexia nervosa and bulimia nervosa are now considered serious public health problems. As a result, teachers and others who work with teenagers are encountering increasing numbers of adolescents with eating disorders.

The prevalence of anorexia nervosa among girls ages 15 to 19 years is 0.5%, making it the third most common chronic illness among adolescent girls after obesity and asthma (Lucas, Beard, O'Fallon, & Kurland, 1991). The age range of highest risk is thought to be between 12 and 25 years, and the peak ages of onset are 14 and 18 years (Halmi, Casper, Eckert, Goldberg, & Davis, 1979). Girls and women account for 90% to 95% of all reported cases. Approximately 5% to 10% of adolescent and adult patients are boys and men; however, 20% to 30% of children presenting with an eating disorder are male (Bryant-Waugh, 1993).

Bulimia nervosa tends to strike in middle adolescence, either as a result of anorexia nervosa or as an isolated occurrence. The prevalence of bulimia nervosa is 5% of adolescent and young adult women (but fewer than 1% of boys and young men). It is rare in children under 14 years of age (Bryant-Waugh, 1993).

Although some researchers associate anorexia nervosa with middle-class backgrounds (Szmukler, McCance, McCrone, & Hunter, 1986), others maintain that this disorder has been detected in all social classes (Garfinkel & Garner, 1982). One report suggested that children and younger adolescents with the disorder tend to be more often from higher social classes (Bryant-Waugh, 1993). Eating disorders affect individuals from a wide variety of ethnic backgrounds. Those of African and Asian backgrounds, for example, have developed these disorders both in their countries of origin and elsewhere (Bryant-Waugh, 1993).

# RISK FACTORS

Although the exact causes of anorexia nervosa and bulimia nervosa are unknown, biological, psychological, and societal factors all have been implicated. Family studies have suggested a genetic predisposition to the development of an eating disorder. For example, the rate of anorexia nervosa is higher among first- and second-degree relatives of patients with the disorder (Herzog, Keller, Lavori, & Bradburn, 1991; Strober, Lampert, Morrell, Burroughs, & Jacobs, 1990). Also, studies of twins suggest that identical twins have a higher concordance rate for anorexia nervosa than fraternal twins (Holland, Sicotte, & Treasure, 1988). Likewise, the rate of bulimia nervosa is higher among twins of patients with this disorder, and identical twins have a higher concordance rate than fraternal twins (Kendler et al.,

1991). Increased rates of substance abuse, affective disorders, and obesity have been noted in family members of patients with bulimia nervosa (Herzog et al., 1991).

Adolescents with eating disorders have extremely low self-esteem. In one study, those with anorexia nervosa achieved lower scores in areas of body and self-image, social relationships, and sexual attitudes than healthy adolescent controls (Grant & Fodor, 1986). These girls put pressure on themselves to please others and do nothing to please themselves. Patients with eating disorders do not experience pleasure from their bodies. They often believe that they have little control over their world; eating and losing weight become the methods they choose to exert control. During adolescence, young people begin to experience a sense of personal identity. Those who are vulnerable to an eating disorder have difficulty with autonomy and feel ineffectual when they are in situations that place new and different demands on them (Bruch, 1973). They fear the inevitability of maturity and independence.

Cultural trends may contribute to the increased frequency of eating disorders, especially in adolescent girls. Society gives them the message that looking attractive is an important achievement. The media perpetuates this message: Teen role models are usually portrayed as attractive, self-disciplined, in control—and always slender.

Puberty, which usually occurs at the age of 11 years in girls and 13 years in boys, is associated with numerous physical and emotional changes. Pubertal development as a cause of eating disorders is supported by studies showing that dieting and disordered eating increase with both menarche and breast development and appear to be independent of chronological age (Killen et al., 1992). Another report suggested that the early onset of puberty and the tendency to be overweight may predispose a young person to developing an eating disorder (Garfinkel, Garner, & Goldbloom, 1987).

Several studies have reported on family characteristics that may influence the development of an eating disorder. Compared with normal controls, adolescents with anorexia nervosa described their parents as being overly strict; exhibiting increased marital discord; disagreeing more about discipline; being more belittling, critical, rejecting, and neglectful; providing less structure; and having more family secrets (Humphrey, 1988, 1989; Humphrey, Apple, & Kirschenbaum, 1986; Strober, 1981). The families of patients with bulimia nervosa have been characterized as lacking in parental affection; being negative and hostile; and having weaker family interactions, increased parental impulsivity, and more familial obesity

(Strober & Humphrey, 1987). A study of the role of sexual abuse in the origin of eating disorders has led to conflicting conclusions (Connors & Morse, 1993). No studies have examined this issue in relation to adolescents with eating disorders.

Some adolescents have a documented medical illness that places them at a high risk for developing an eating disorder. Studies have suggested relationships between insulin-dependent diabetes mellitus and bulimia (Rodin & Daneman, 1992) and between Turner syndrome and anorexia nervosa. One study found that eating disorders occurred in 20% of females with diabetes (Rodin, Johnson, Garfinkel, Daneman, & Kenshole, 1986), representing a sixfold increase in anorexia nervosa and a twofold increase in bulimia nervosa over the expected prevalences in similar nondiabetic individuals (see Chapter 5).

# CLINICAL CHARACTERISTICS

Patients with anorexia nervosa display distinct clinical characteristics. They often look much younger than their chronological age and are often perceived as active, energetic, and therefore physically well. Patients who are quite ill, on the other hand, may be lethargic and irritable. Their skin is often yellow, they lose scalp or pubic hair and subcutaneous fat, they develop lanugo hair (fine downy hair) on the body, their hands and feet are usually cold and mottled, and they may experience sleep disturbances, cold intolerance, and constipation. Young patients may appear sad, depressed, and socially isolated, and show a decline in school performance. Patients with anorexia nervosa frequently deny their physical and psychological symptoms.

Patients with bulimia nervosa can hide their illness more successfully than can those with anorexia nervosa. They may show signs of weakness, muscle aches, stomach bloating or pain, and a puffy face. In addition, calluses may develop over the back of the hand or knuckles (known as Russell's sign) due to the repeated trauma of the patient's teeth (central incisors) striking the skin of the hand used to stimulate the gag reflex. Other clues to bulimia nervosa include painless swelling of the parotid gland, dental enamel erosion, and tooth decay. These patients may complain of swelling of the hands and feet, chest pain, and fatigue. Patients with both anorexia and bulimia nervosa may exhibit features of both disorders.

# MEDICAL ASPECTS

Although physical complications involving nearly every organ system in the body have been described (Palla & Litt, 1988), many young people with eating disorders are so embarrassed about their illness that they rarely disclose their physical symptoms. Cardiovascular abnormalities are frequent in adolescents with eating disorders and cause significant morbidity and mortality. Electrocardiographic changes occur in up to 75% of hospitalized patients. These include *bradychardia* (slow heart rate) and other abnormalities, and are probably a result of malnutrition or electrolyte depletion. Postural changes in both blood pressure and pulse are common, but these are reversible with hydration and nutritional rehabilitation. Approximately 17% of patients with bulimia induce vomiting with syrup of ipecac, an over-the-counter product used as first aid in cases of accidental poisoning. Ipecac contains a cardiotoxic substance, emetine, which is a muscle poison and can, with repeated use, lead to irreversible *cardiomyopathy* (primary myocardial disease)—with sudden death—or peripheral muscle weakness (Mitchell, Seim, Colon, & Pomeroy, 1987). Changes in cardiac dimensions, including reduction in chamber size, have been described in emaciated patients (Isner, Roberts, Hymsfield, & Yager, 1985). Refeeding of these patients may cause congestive heart failure as a result of an increase in cardiac output, expansion of plasma volume, and increase in metabolic rate. An association between eating disorders and mitral valve prolapse has been reported (G. L. Johnson, Humphries, Shirley, Mazzoleni, & Noonan, 1986).

Abnormalities of fluids and electrolytes can also occur, as the result of starvation, vomiting, laxative or diuretic abuse, and water loading. Low potassium levels, called *hypokalemia,* have been reported to be the most common electrolyte abnormality (Palla & Litt, 1988). Hypokalemia is associated with abnormal cardiac rhythms, muscular weakness, constipation, and cramping. The patient may present with dehydration or abnormal serum levels of sodium, potassium, chloride, carbon dioxide, and blood urea nitrogen. Several renal abnormalities may also be observed. Alterations of kidney function in adolescents with eating disorders have been reported (Palla & Litt, 1988).

Growth retardation and short stature, both known complications of anorexia nervosa, can be very severe when the disorder develops before the growth spurt (Kreipe, 1989; Matthews & Lacey, 1983; Nussbaum, Baird, Sonnenblick, Cowan, & Shenker, 1985; Pfeiffer, Lucas, & Ilstrup, 1986;

Root & Powers, 1983; Russell, 1992; Weiner, 1989). During early adolescence, marked acceleration in weight and modest acceleration in linear growth occur in both girls and boys, averaging 8.8 lb (4 kg) and 2.3 to 2.7 in. (6 to 7 cm) and 13.2 lb (6 kg) and 2.3 to 2.7 in. (6 to 7 cm), respectively (Vaughan & Litt, 1987). Development of an eating disorder during this period can adversely affect adult height (Nussbaum et al., 1985).

Menstrual dysfunction is common with eating disorders. *Amenorrhea* (abnormal absence of menstrual periods) is a characteristic of anorexia nervosa. Reports have indicated that 20% to 50% of females with anorexia nervosa lose their menstrual period even before they lose a significant amount of weight (Kaye, Gwirtsman, & George, 1989). Females with bulimia nervosa may experience irregular menstrual function or absent periods (Newman & Halmi, 1988). Many factors may contribute to the amenorrhea, including loss of body fat, excessive exercising, emotional disturbances, and alterations in the regulation of the hypothalamic–pituitary function (Golden & Shenker, 1992). Moreover, adolescents with anorexia nervosa have delayed sexual maturation. Weight loss not only interferes with the onset of menarche but also inhibits normal pubertal development in the premenarchal girl and causes secondary amenorrhea in the postmenarchal girl. With the onset of an eating disorder during puberty, there is delay of breast and testicular development, depletion of axillary and pubic hair, and loss of growth of pelvic contours in girls.

Osteoporosis is an established complication of anorexia nervosa in adolescent and young adult women. Severe *osteopenia* (reduced bone mass greater than two standard deviations below the normal mean) occurs in 50% to 65% of patients (Bachrach, Guido, Katzman, Litt, & Marcus, 1990; Biller et al., 1989). The reduction in bone mineral may be severe enough to cause painful and disabling pathologic fractures. The extent to which osteopenia in anorexia nervosa is reversible remains uncertain and its management controversial (Ayers, Gidwani, Schmidt, & Gross, 1984; Bachrach et al., 1990; Bachrach, Katzman, Litt, Guido, & Marcus, 1991; Biller et al., 1989; Crosby, Kaplan, Pertschuk, & Mullen, 1985; Joyce, Warren, Humphries, Smith, & Coon, 1990; Newman & Halmi, 1989; Rigotti, Nussbaum, Herzog, & Neer, 1984; Szmukler, Brown, Parson, & Darby, 1985; Treasure, Fogelman, & Russell, 1986; Treasure, Russell, Fogelman, & Murby, 1987). Calcium intake should be 1,200 to 1,500 mg per day, but calcium alone is insufficient to prevent a deficit in bone mineral density (Bachrach et al., 1990; Biller et al., 1989; Rigotti, Neer, Skates, Herzog, & Nussbaum, 1991). Similarly, although exercise has been shown to protect against osteopenia in anorexia nervosa (Rigotti et al., 1991), this finding has not been confirmed

(Bachrach et al., 1990; Biller et al., 1989; Castro, Lazaro, Pons, Halperin, & Toro, 2000). Weight rehabilitation is an effective means of increasing bone mineral density (Bachrach et al., 1991; Charig & Fletcher, 1987). In adolescents with anorexia nervosa, weight gain has been associated with increases in bone mass even before the return of menses. A weight necessary for the resumption of normal menses should be achieved; however, patients with chronic anorexia nervosa may resist weight rehabilitation, with the result that pathological bone fractures remain a clinical risk. High-impact aerobics should be discouraged.

Clinical evidence of mild hypothyroidism is evident in patients with anorexia nervosa. Features include constipation, cold intolerance, bradycardia, dry skin, and relaxation of reflexes. Thyroid function, as determined by the serum levels of thyroxine and thyrotropin, is usually in the low-normal to normal range. Some patients have difficulty concentrating their urine in response to water deprivation, possibly because of defective osmoregulation of the secretion of the hormone vasopressin.

Structural abnormalities in the brain of adolescents with anorexia nervosa are among the earliest and most striking physical consequences. Using magnetic resonance imaging (MRI), one study has demonstrated that acutely ill adolescents with anorexia nervosa have significant deficits in both gray-matter and white-matter volumes (Katzman et al., 1996; Katzman, Zipursky, Lambe, & Mikulis, 1997). In the past, it had been assumed that the brain abnormalities found in patients with anorexia nervosa reverse with weight recovery. However, studies of weight-recovered patients have shown that young people may have persisting deficits in gray-matter volumes (Katzman et al., 1997; Lambe, Katzman, Mikulis, & Zipursky, 1997). Very little is known about the functional significance of these brain abnormalities.

Studies have demonstrated changes in cognitive function in patients with anorexia nervosa, with evidence of impairment in attention and concentration (Fox, 1981; Hamsher, Halmi, & Benton, 1981; Laessle, Krieg, Fichter, & Pirke, 1989), visual associative learning (Witt, Ryan, & Hsu, 1985), visual-spatial abilities, problem solving, and, most notably, attentional–perceptual–motor functions (Szmukler et al., 1992). Subgroups of anorexic patients demonstrated psychomotor slowing (Palazidou, Robinson, & Lishman, 1990) and inflexibility, poor planning, and lack of insight (Szmukler et al., 1992). Although current evidence suggests that there may be some improvement in cognition with weight recovery, it is unclear whether cognitive function recovers fully or equally across all neuropsychological domains. A better understanding of the interactions between structural brain abnormalities and cognition will help promote the development of interventions that improve outcomes for children and adolescents with this disorder. It is essential that teachers be aware of the cognitive deficits associated with the emaciated patient.

Hematologic disturbances in anorexia nervosa include anemia, *leukopenia* (reduction of the number of leukocytes in the blood), and *thrombocytopenia* (reduction of the number of platelets in the blood) (Mant & Faragher, 1972). It does not appear, however, that these patients are more susceptible to infection (Bowers & Eckert, 1978). Gastrointestinal complications occur frequently as a result of starvation, bingeing, vomiting, or purging. Constipation and abdominal pain may result from delayed gastric emptying and slowed intestinal motility. Complaints of bloating after a meal are often reported in this patient group, even after snacks or small meals. Acute dilatation of the stomach (clinically defined as abdominal pain, nausea, distended abdomen, constipation, absence of bowel sounds, and rebound tenderness) is a life-threatening event. Other serious gastrointestinal disorders that have occurred in the course of anorexia nervosa include gastric perforation, *trichobezoar* (a ball of swallowed hair), and acute pancreatitis. As a result of starvation, liver function test results and cholesterol levels are mildly elevated, a condition that seems reversible with refeeding.

Patients with bulimia nervosa expose their teeth to a steady immersion in acid, resulting in enamel erosion and tooth decay. They may also have associated *esophagitis* (inflammation of the esophagus), Mallory-Weiss tears (mucosal tears and bleeding where the esophagus joins the stomach), and even esophageal erosion and rupture. Some patients with bulimia may develop a nonpainful enlargement of the parotid glands.

Patients with anorexia nervosa exhibit abnormal responses to exposure to heat and cold when compared with control subjects (Mecklenberg, Loriaux, Thompson, Anderson, & Lipsett, 1976). Because thermoregulation is located in the hypothalamus, this finding further supports the suggestion that patients with eating disorders suffer from hypothalamic dysfunction.

Young people with eating disorders may develop dermatologic complications as a result of malnutrition, vomiting, or drugs used to lose weight. For example, those with anorexia nervosa may have dry skin, brittle hair and nails, an orange discoloration to the skin, edema, and loss of subcutaneous skin.

# TREATMENT

The successful management of adolescents with eating disorders, as outlined by Comerci (1988), includes four components: early restoration of a normal nutritional and physiologic state, establishment of trust, involvement of the family in the treatment program, and a team approach. Professionals generally accept that a multidisciplinary team approach is most effective in the treatment of adolescent eating disorders (Kreipe & Uphoff, 1992).

Adolescents with eating disorders should be treated at a facility with staff members who understand these problems and have experience in treating young people. Treatment may be carried out on an outpatient, inpatient, or day patient basis. Treatment goals are to diagnose the disorder rapidly and restore the patient's physical and psychological health. Initial goals are medical stabilization and nutritional rehabilitation; these must be achieved before any psychological therapy can be beneficial. Most adolescents with these disorders are admitted to hospitals because of cardiovascular or metabolic instability, profound weight loss, inability to gain weight as an outpatient over an extended period, delayed growth and development, or suicidal behavior. Special consideration should be given to younger adolescents, who lose a higher percentage of body weight sooner and experience delays in growth and sexual development.

Because no single method has been found to be superior in the treatment of adolescent eating disorders, a multidisciplinary approach—including modified behavioral strategies and family, individual, and pharmacotherapy techniques—should be considered. All health care providers must have a clear understanding of adolescent issues: psychosocial, cognitive and physical growth and development, educational achievement, family and peer interaction, substance use, and sexual behaviors.

Inpatients are expected to finish their meals in a specified period of time, and, if unable to do so, may be given a nutritive supplement. The nasogastric tube is used only in rare cases where the patient cannot tolerate oral feeds or is so resistant to progressive weight gain that the situation becomes life threatening. Increasing energy requirements are provided during the course of the hospitalization, supported by a secure and caring milieu.

Outpatient care should focus on monitoring weight, growth and development, menstrual irregularities, bone mineral density, and biochemical indices, and also on providing therapy for the individual, family, or both. Weight gain is slower in this setting. Various types of mental health treatment are available to the adolescent; an approach that combines several techniques offers the greatest hope for success.

Day treatment programs provide an alternative and innovative approach to the management of eating disorders. The patient participates in the therapeutic setting and meals are supervised. Most of these programs function 5 days a week; patients go home for the night and on weekends. Treatment may be provided in groups, on an individual basis, or with the family. This approach encourages autonomy, fosters the ability to test newly acquired skills in regulating eating behavior, and avoids a lengthy separation of the adolescent from the family.

Family therapy is an important part of treatment, because coping with anorexia or bulimia nervosa in one family member affects all other members. One report found that family therapy was the most effective maintenance treatment for younger, less chronically ill patients (Russell, Szmukler, Dare, & Eisler, 1987). Team members, therefore, need to develop an alliance with the family and patient from the outset. The first steps in family therapy are to provide accurate information about the eating disorder and to provide helpful interventions. Later in the course of treatment, issues such as autonomy, expression of individual feelings, and conflict resolution should be explored.

Clinically controlled trials of the efficacy of cognitive behavior therapy in adults with bulimia nervosa have shown it to be effective in 60% to 70% of patients (Mitchell, Raymond, & Specker, 1993). Whether there is an additive effect with pharmacotherapy requires further study. Such trials have not been conducted in adolescent eating disorder patients.

Group therapy often helps both the teenager and the family gain insights and exchange information. Patients also have the opportunity to develop relationships outside the family and to compare their values and feelings with others coping with similar problems. Psychoeducational groups provide both education and support by offering information about physical complications of eating disorders, proper nutrition, parental responsibilities, and eating behaviors. Such knowledge and understanding may help motivate adolescents to change their behavior.

Studies have found pharmacologic treatment using serotonin reuptake inhibitors to be effective in preventing relapse among weight-restored adults, with significant reduction in anxiety, depression, and obsessions and compulsions (Kaye, Gendall, & Strober, 1997). Studies of adults with bulimia nervosa have shown early benefits from use of drug therapy, but these have decreased over time. Only a minority of adults have experienced complete suppression of their symptoms with antidepressant monotherapy (Mitchell et al., 1993). No trials using these medications have been conducted in adolescents with eating disorders.

# THE TEACHER'S ROLE

Although teachers cannot be expected to identify or diagnose psychiatric illness, they should be able to recognize adolescents who are experiencing emotional, psychological, and social difficulties. A teacher is in an advantageous position to make an early identification of a student with an eating disorder and may be the first to observe changes in behavior or appearance. Table 19.2 lists the warning signs of anorexia nervosa and bulimia nervosa. Teachers who suspect that a student has an eating problem should discuss their concerns with other school professionals, such as an educational psychologist, school nurse, or counselor. These discussions may help teachers present their concerns to the student and her or his parents. The teacher's initial approach to the student should take the form of a compassionate and honest conversation rather than a diagnostic interview. School staff need to be respectful and supportive while recognizing the difference between constructive assistance and overinvolvement. The teacher should be informed about the steps in the referral process, and school officials should know about the services available for the diagnosis and treatment of adolescent eating disorders.

For the most part, adolescents with eating disorders do not come to the school's attention because usually their academic performance is high, attendance excellent, and behavior compliant and polite. When the teacher looks more closely, however, it becomes apparent that these adolescents have problems. Their struggles with peer and adult relationships are manifested at school in social withdrawal and isolation. The teacher and school resource staff can assist with issues of self-esteem, social interaction, peer relations, and education about healthy and appropriate nutrition and exercise.

Adolescents with eating disorders often deny their illness or its symptoms and may continue to participate in regular school activities. School staff therefore should be well informed about the medical and psychological complications of these disorders so that they can meet the students' needs. Often the school can adjust a student's schedule, offer a restricted physical education program if weight remains a concern, and help compensate for absence from school because of medical appointments or prolonged hospitalization. The school's involvement and support may help alleviate the patient's anxiety about missing classes.

Students with a serious eating disorder who remain in school should participate in a suitable treatment program and their general medical safety monitored by clinicians. The school can work with the clinician to determine a student's ability to participate in athletic and other extracurricular activities. Students with a serious eating disorder may be advised to take a leave of absence if they are seriously ill.

Teachers and coaches can play a vital role in strengthening these students' self-acceptance and promoting positive attitudes toward body size and shape and the enjoyment of physical activities (Levine, 1987). They should encourage healthy adolescents to participate in physical activity regardless of their body shape, size, or weight, and foster healthy attitudes toward the body and nutrition. Teachers and coaches working with adolescent athletes who are at risk for eating disorders because of participation in certain sports (e.g., gymnastics, ballet, or figure skating for girls; bodybuilding and wrestling for boys) need to be aware of early symptoms of eating disorders. Coaches should be discouraged from performing weekly weigh-ins, announcing body weights, or determining changes in body fat in their students. Even the seemingly benign act of weighing a young person as part of a sports evaluation can be a much more serious psychological experience than one might think.

The school curriculum can be adjusted to help prevent eating disorders by addressing concepts of nutrition, links between food and emotions, appearance values, self-esteem, and the biological, emotional, and psychological changes of adolescence. Prevention should start in health or physical education in the primary grades with the introduction of age-appropriate concepts and continue through the upper grades.

Teachers should be aware of the impact of the mass media on young people. Television, films, videos, magazines, newspapers, and books continue to glamorize thin, beautiful women and sculpted, attractive men, projecting unrealistic images and false symbols of success, self-control, competence, and strength. The role of the school in counteracting these influences is particularly important. In addition, teachers should examine their own views about body size, attitudes about food, and eating behaviors so they can have a positive influence on young people. Their beliefs can unintentionally affect the body images their adolescent students are in the process of forming.

**TABLE 19.2**

Warning Signs of Anorexia Nervosa and Bulimia

**Signs of Either Anorexia Nervosa or Bulimia Nervosa**

**Food and Weight Control**
- Preoccupation with weight, food, calories, and dieting.
- Claims of "feeling fat" when weight is normal or low.
- Guilt and shame about eating.
- Frequent weighing.
- Evidence of binge eating.
- Hoarding food.
- Use of laxatives, diuretics, purgatives, and emetics.
- Use of diet pills.
- Secretive vomiting: leaving for the bathroom immediately after a meal.

**Personality and Emotionality**
- Moodiness and irritability.
- Inflexibility and resistance to changes in routine.
- Low self-esteem.
- Perfectionism and dichotomous thinking ("I'm thin" or "I'm gross").
- Chronic dissatisfaction with grades and with self, regardless of level of performance.
- Social withdrawal and intolerance of others.
- Oversensitivity to criticism.
- Extreme concern about appearances, both physical and behavioral.

**Signs of Anorexia Nervosa**

- Significant weight loss in the absence of related illness.
- Extremely thin appearance.
- Signs of starvation: thinning of hair; hair loss; the appearance of fine, raised white hair (*lanugo*) on the cheeks, neck, forearms, and thighs; repeated gastrointestinal problems; yellowish appearance of the palms or soles of the feet.
- Significant reduction in eating coupled with a denial of hunger.
- Strenuous dieting when not overweight.
- Amenorrhea in women.
- Unusual eating habits: preference for foods of a certain texture or color, compulsively arranging food, unusual mixtures of food.
- Obsessive and prolonged exercising despite weakness, fatigue, or illness.
- Complaints of feeling bloated or nauseated after eating a small or normal amount.

*(continues)*

**TABLE 19.2** *Continued.*

---

**Signs of Bulimia**

---

- Evidence of binge eating: actual observation, verbal reports, large amounts of food missing, stealing money or food.
- Habitual overeating in response to stress.
- Frequent weight fluctuations of 10 lb or more.
- Eating (not sampling) foods such as dough, canned frostings, or maple syrup without preparing them.
- Evidence of purging by vomiting, laxative/diuretic use, emetics (e.g., syrup of ipecac), frequent fasting, excessive exercising.
- Swelling of the glands under the jaw (caused by frequent vomiting), yielding a "chipmunk" appearance.
- Frequent and unusual dental problems.

---

Note. From *How Schools Can Help Combat Student Eating Disorders: Anorexia Nervosa and Bulimia* (pp. 254–255), by M. P. Levine, 1987, Washington, DC: National Education Association of the United States. Copyright 1987 by the National Education Association. Reprinted with permission.

Health care professionals can serve as trainers, coordinators, and professional supports for peer counseling efforts at schools and dormitories (residential schools). School health services and health clinics must be alert to identifying early signs and symptoms of eating disorders.

Finally, teachers, school administrators, school nurses, and guidance counselors need to be prepared for an emergency. Students with eating disorders may demonstrate acute medical symptoms (fainting, vomiting blood, abdominal pain, seizures) as a result of starvation, bingeing, or purging. In some cases, students may be suicidal.

# PROGNOSIS AND OUTCOME

Research studies of the outcome and prognosis of patients with eating disorders have differed so widely in methodology (number of patients studied, populations studied, standardization of diagnostic and recovery criteria, and differences in duration of illness at time of diagnosis) that generalizations are difficult. However, factors that frequently predict a positive outcome in patients with anorexia nervosa include earlier age of onset, good parent–child relationship, and brief duration of illness (Steinhausen, Rauss-Mason, & Seidel, 1991). The literature on prognosis and outcome in patients with bulimia nervosa is inconclusive and contradictory. These patients often have frequent relapses (Herzog & Sacks, 1993). Studies have found that psychiatric symptoms, including alcohol abuse (Lacey, 1983), suicide attempts (Abraham, Mira, & Llewellyn-Jones, 1983), increased depression at follow-up (Swift, Kalin, Wamboltd, Kaslew, & Ritholz, 1985), association of vomiting and other purging behaviors, and association with anorexia nervosa may be predictive of a poor outcome in patients with bulimia nervosa.

The course of anorexia nervosa is typically protracted. Outcome studies show that approximately 50% of patients will have complete resolution of the illness, whereas 30% will have residual features that come and go in severity well into adulthood. The disease will follow a chronic course in 10% of patients and another 10% will die from the disorder (Strober, Freeman, & Morrell, 1997). Although less is known about the long-term prognosis for patients with bulimia nervosa, 50% recover and 20% continue to meet full criteria anywhere from 5 to 10 years after their initial presentation.

# SUMMARY

People who work with children and adolescents should become familiar with eating disorders. Parents, teachers, guidance counselors, and health professionals can help identify and prevent these disorders by understanding the risk factors that are thought to contribute to their development. Early detection of abnormal adolescent eating behaviors may also help reduce morbidity and mortality. Teachers, other school staff members, and parents can help the adolescent deal with issues of self-esteem, self-acceptance, and a healthy lifestyle. Concerned, sensitive, and well-informed school staff are in a position to help make a difference in how adolescents feel and think about themselves.

# REFERENCES

Abraham, S. F., Mira, M., & Llewellyn-Jones, D. (1983). Bulimia: A study of outcome. *International Journal of Eating Disorders, 2,* 175–180.

American Psychiatric Association. (2000). *Diagnostic and statistical manual of mental disorders* (4th ed. text rev.). Washington, DC: Author.

Ayers, J. W. T., Gidwani, G. P., Schmidt, I. M. V., & Gross, M. (1984). Osteopenia in hypestrogenic young women with anorexia nervosa. *Fertility and Sterility, 41,* 224–228.

Bachrach, L. K., Guido, D., Katzman, D. K., Litt, I. F., & Marcus, R. (1990). Decreased bone density in adolescent girls with anorexia nervosa. *Pediatrics, 86,* 440–447.

Bachrach, L., Katzman, D., Litt, I., Guido, D., & Marcus, R. (1991). Recovery from osteopenia in adolescent girls with anorexia nervosa. *Journal of Clinical Endocrinology and Metabolism, 72*(3), 602–606.

Beaumont, P. J., Chambers, T. L., Rouse, L., & Abraham, S. F. (1981). The diet composition and nutritional knowledge of patients with anorexia nervosa. *Journal of Human Nutrition, 35,* 265–273.

Biller, B. M. K., Saxe, V., Herzog, D. B., Rosenthal, D. I., Holzman, S., & Klibanski, A. (1989). Mechanisms of osteoporosis in adult and adolescent women with anorexia nervosa. *Journal of Clinical Endocrinology and Metabolism, 68,* 548–554.

Bowers, T. K., & Eckert, E. (1978). Leukopenia in anorexia nervosa—lack of increased risk of infection. *Archives of Internal Medicine, 138,* 1520–1523.

Bruch, H. (1973). *Eating disorders.* New York: Basic Books.

Bryant-Waugh, R. (1993). Epidemiology. In B. Lask & R. Bryant-Waugh (Eds.), *Childhood onset anorexia nervosa and related eating disorders* (pp. 55–68). East Sussex, England: Erlbaum.

Castro, I., Lazaro, L., Pons, F., Halperin, I., & Toro, J. (2000). Predictors of bone mineral density reduction in adolescents with anorexia nervosa. *Journal of the Academy of Child & Adolescent Psychiatry, 39*(11), 1365–1370.

Charig, M., & Fletcher, E. (1987). Reversible bone loss in anorexia nervosa. *British Medical Journal, 295,* 474–475.

Comerci, G. D. (1988). Eating disorders in adolescents. *Pediatrics in Review, 10*(2), 1–11.

Connors, M. E., & Morse, W. (1993). Sexual abuse and eating disorders: A review. *International Journal of Eating Disorders, 13,* 1–11.

Crosby, L. O., Kaplan, F. S., Pertschuk, M. J., & Mullen, J. L. (1985). The effect of anorexia nervosa on bone morphometry in young women. *Clinical Orthopedics and Related Research, 201,* 271–277.

Fox, C. F. (1981). Neuropsychological correlates of anorexia nervosa. *International Journal of Psychiatry in Medicine, 11,* 285–290.

Garfinkel, P. E., & Garner, D. M. (1982). *Anorexia nervosa: A multidimensional perspective.* New York: Brunner/Mazel.

Garfinkel, P. E., Garner, D. M., & Goldbloom, D. S. (1987). Eating disorders: Implications for the 1990's. *Canadian Journal of Psychiatry, 32,* 624–631.

Golden, N. H., & Shenker, I. R. (1992). Amenorrhea in anorexia nervosa—Etiology and implications. In M. P. Nussbaum & J. T. Dwyer (Eds.), *Adolescent medicine: State of the art reviews: Vol. 3. Adolescent nutrition and eating disorders* (pp. 503–517). Philadelphia: Hanley and Belfus.

Grant, C. L., & Fodor, I. G. (1986). Adolescent attitudes toward body image and anorexic behavior. *Adolescence, 21,* 269–281.

Halmi, K. A., Casper, R. C., Eckert, E. D., Goldberg, S. C., & Davis, J. M. (1979). Unique features associated with the age of onset of anorexia nervosa. *Psychiatric Research, 1,* 209–215.

Hamsher, K. D. S., Halmi, K. A., & Benton, A. L. (1981). Prediction of outcome in anorexia nervosa from neuropsychological status. *Psychiatry Research, 4,* 79–88

Herzog, D. B., Keller, M. B., Lavori, P. W., & Bradburn, I. S. (1991). Bulimia nervosa in adolescence. *Journal of Developmental and Behavioral Pediatrics, 12,* 191–195.

Herzog, D. B., & Sacks, N. R. (1993). Bulimia nervosa—Comparison of treatment responders vs. nonresponders. *Psychopharmacology Bulletin, 29*(1), 121–125.

Holland, A. J., Sicotte, N., & Treasure, J. (1988). Anorexia nervosa—Psychopharmacology evidence for a genetic basis. *Journal of Psychosomatic Research, 32,* 549–554.

Humphrey, L. L. (1988). Relationships within subtypes of anorexic, bulimic and normal families. *Journal of the American Academy of Child and Adolescent Psychiatry, 27,* 544–551.

Humphrey, L. L. (1989). Observed family interactions among subtypes of eating disorders using structural analysis of social behavior. *Journal of Consulting and Clinical Psychology, 57,* 206–214.

Humphrey, L. L., Apple, R. F., & Kirschenbaum, D. S. (1986). Differentiating bulimic-anorexic from normal families using interpersonal and behavioral observation systems. *Journal of Consulting and Clinical Psychiatry, 57,* 190–195.

Isner, J. M., Roberts, W. C., Hymsfield, S. B., & Yager, J. (1985). Anorexia nervosa and sudden death. *Annals of Internal Medicine, 102,* 49–52.

Johnson, C. L., Stuckey, M. K., Lewis, L. D., & Schwartz, D. M. (1982). A descriptive survey of 316 cases. *International Journal of Eating Disorders, 2*(1), 3–16.

Johnson, G. L., Humphries, L. L., Shirley, P. B., Mazzoleni, A., & Noonan, J. A. (1986). Mitral valve prolapse in patients with anorexia nervosa and bulimia. *Archives of Internal Medicine, 146,* 1525–1529.

Joyce, J. M., Warren, D. L., Humphries, L. L., Smith, A. J., & Coon, J. S. (1990). Osteoporosis in women with eating disorders: Comparison of physical parameters, exercise, and menstrual status with SPA and DPA evaluation. *Journal of Nuclear Medicine, 31,* 325–331.

Katzman, D. K., Lambe, E. K., Mikulis, D. J., Ridgley, J. N., Goldbloom, D. S., & Zipursky, R. B. (1996). Cerebral gray matter and white matter volume deficits in adolescent girls with anorexia nervosa. *Journal of Pediatrics, 129,* 794–803.

Katzman, D. K., Zipursky, R. B., Lambe, E. K., & Mikulis, D. J. (1997). A longitudinal magnetic resonance imaging study of brain changes in adolescents with anorexia nervosa. *Archives of Pediatrics and Adolescent Medicine, 151,* 793–797.

Kaye, W., Gendall, K., & Strober, M. (1997). Serotonin neuronal function and selective serotonin reuptake inhibitors in the treatment in anorexia and bulimia nervosa. *Biological Psychiatry, 44,* 825–838.

Kaye, W. H., Gwirtsman, H. E., & George, D. T. (1989). The effect of bingeing and vomiting on hormonal secretion. *Biologic Psychiatry, 25,* 768–780.

Kendler, K. S., MacLean, C., Neale, M., Kessler, R., Heath, A., & Eaves, L. (1991). The genetic epidemiology of bulimia nervosa. *American Journal of Psychiatry, 148,* 1627–1637.

Killen, J. D. S., Hayward, C., Litt, I., Hammer, L. D., Wilson, D. M., Miner, B., Taylor, C. B., Varady, A., & Shisslak, C. (1992). Is puberty a risk factor for eating disorders? *American Journal of Diseases of Children, 146,* 323–325.

Kreipe, R. E. (1989). Short stature in females with anorexia nervosa. *Pediatric Research, 25*, 7A.

Kreipe, R. E., & Uphoff, M. (1992). Treatment and outcome of adolescents with anorexia nervosa: State of the art reviews. *Adolescent Medicine, 3*(3), 519–540.

Lacey, H. (1983). Bulimia nervosa, binge eating, and psychogenic vomiting: A controlled treatment study and long term outcome. *British Medical Journal, 286*, 1609–1613.

Laessle, R. G., Krieg, J. C., Fichter, M. M., & Pirke, K. M. (1989). Cerebral atrophy and vigilance performance in patients with anorexia nervosa and bulimia nervosa. *Neuropsychobiology, 21*, 187–191.

Lambe, E. K., Katzman, D. K., Mikulis, D. J., & Zipursky, R. B. (1997). Cerebral gray matter volume deficits after weight recovery from anorexia nervosa. *Archives of General Psychiatry, 54*, 537–542.

Levine, M. P. (1987). *How schools can help combat student eating disorders: Anorexia nervosa and bulimia.* Washington, DC: National Education Association of the United States.

Lucas, A. R., Beard, C. M., O'Fallon, W. M., & Kurland, L. T. (1991). 50 year trend in the incidence of anorexia nervosa in Rochester, Minn.: A population based study. *American Journal of Psychiatry, 148*, 917–922.

Mant, M. J., & Faragher, B. S. (1972). The haematology of anorexia nervosa. *British Journal of Haematology, 23*, 737–749.

Matthews, B. J., & Lacey, J. H. (1983). Skeletal maturation, growth, and hormonal and nutritional status in anorexia nervosa. *International Journal of Eating Disorders, 2*, 145–150.

Mecklenberg, R. S., Loriaux, D. L., Thompson, R. L., Anderson, A. E., & Lipsett, M. B. (1976). Hypothalamic dysfunction in patients with anorexia nervosa. *Medicine, 53*, 147–157.

Mitchell, J. E., Raymond, M., & Specker, S. (1993). A review of the controlled trials of pharmacotherapy and psychotherapy in the treatment of bulimia nervosa. *International Journal of Eating Disorders, 14*, 229–247.

Mitchell, J. E., Seim, H. C., Colon, E., & Pomeroy, C. (1987). Medical complications and medical management of bulimia. *Annals of Internal Medicine, 107*, 71–77.

Newman, M. M., & Halmi, K. A. (1988). The endocrinology of anorexia nervosa and bulimia nervosa. *Neurologic Clinics, 6*, 195–212.

Newman, M. M., & Halmi, K. A. (1989). Relationship of bone density to estradiol and cortisol in anorexia nervosa and bulimia. *Psychiatry Research, 29*, 105–112.

Nussbaum, M., Baird, D., Sonnenblick, M., Cowan, K., & Shenker, J. R. (1985). Short stature in anorexia nervosa patients. *Journal of Adolescent Health Care, 6*, 453–455.

Palazidou, E., Robinson, P., & Lishman, W. A. (1990). Neuroradiological and neuropsychological assessment in anorexia nervosa. *Psychological Medicine, 20*, 521–527.

Palla, B., & Litt, I. F. (1988). Medical complications of eating disorders in adolescents. *Pediatrics, 81*, 613–623.

Pfeiffer, R. J., Lucas, A. R., & Ilstrup, D. M. (1986). Effects of anorexia nervosa on linear growth. *Clinical Pediatrics, 25*, 7–12.

Pyle, R. L., Mitchell, J. E., & Eckert, E. D. (1981). Bulimia: A report of 34 cases. *Journal of Clinical Psychiatry, 42*(2), 60–64.

Rigotti, N. A., Neer, R. M., Skates, S. J., Herzog, D. B., & Nussbaum, S. R. (1991). The clinical course of osteoporosis in anorexia nervosa: A longitudinal study of cortical bone mass. *Journal of the American Medical Association, 265,* 1133–1138.

Rigotti, N. A., Nussbaum, S. R., Herzog, D. B., & Neer, R. M. (1984). Osteoporosis in women with anorexia nervosa. *New England Journal of Medicine, 311,* 601–606.

Rodin, G. M., & Daneman, D. (1992). Eating disorders and IDDM: A problematic association. *Diabetes Care, 15,* 1402–1412.

Rodin, G. M., Johnson, L. E., Garfinkel, P. E., Daneman, D., & Kenshole, A. B. (1986). Eating disorders in female adolescents with insulin-dependent diabetes mellitus. *International Journal of Psychiatry and Medicine, 16,* 49–57.

Root, A. W., & Powers, P. S. (1983). Anorexia nervosa presenting as growth retardation in adolescents. *Journal of Adolescent Health Care, 4,* 25–30.

Russell, G. F. M. (1992). Anorexia nervosa of early onset and its impact on puberty. In P. F. Cooper & A. Stein (Eds.), *Feeding problems and eating disorders in children and adolescents* (Monographs in Clinical Pediatrics, No. 5, 85–113). Reading, UK: Harwood Academic.

Russell, G. F. M., Szmukler, G. I., Dare, C., & Eisler, I. (1987). An evaluation of family therapy in anorexia nervosa and bulimia nervosa. *Archives of General Psychiatry, 44,* 1047–1056.

Steinhausen, H. C., Rauss-Mason, C., & Seidel, R. (1991). Follow-up studies of anorexia nervosa: A review of four decades of outcome research. *Psychological Medicine, 21,* 447–454.

Strober, M. (1981). The significance of bulimia in juvenile anorexia nervosa: An exploration of possible etiologic factors. *International Journal of Eating Disorders, 1,* 28–43.

Strober, M., Freeman, R., & Morrell, W. (1997). The long-term course of severe anorexia nervosa in adolescents: Survival analysis of recovery, relapse, and outcome predictors over 10–15 years in a prospective study. *International Journal of Eating Disorders, 22,* 339–360.

Strober, M., & Humphrey, L. L. (1987). Familial contributions to the etiology and course of anorexia nervosa and bulimia. *Journal of Consulting and Clinical Psychology, 55,* 654–659.

Strober, M., Lampert, C., Morrell, W., Burroughs, J., & Jacobs, C. (1990). A controlled family study of anorexia nervosa: Evidence of familial aggregation and lack of shared transmission with affective disorders. *International Journal of Eating Disorders, 9,* 239–253.

Swift, W. J., Kalin, N. H., Wamboldt, F. S., Kaslew, N., & Ritholz, M. (1985). Depression in bulimia at 2 to 5 year follow-up. *Psychiatric Research, 16,* 111–122.

Szmukler, G. I., Andrewes, D., Kingston, K., Chen, L., Stargatt, R., & Stanley, R. (1992). Neuropsychological impairment in anorexia nervosa: Before and after refeeding. *Journal of Clinical and Experimental Neuropsychology, 14,* 347–352.

Szmukler, G. I., Brown, S. W., Parson, V., & Darby, A. (1985). Premature loss of bone in chronic anorexia nervosa. *British Medical Journal* (Clinical Research Ed.), *290,* 26–27.

Szmukler, G., McCance, C., McCrone, L., & Hunter, D. (1986). Anorexia nervosa: A psychiatric case register study from Aberdeen. *Psychological Medicine, 16,* 49–58.

Treasure, J. L., Fogelman, I., & Russell, G. F. M. (1986). Osteopenia of the lumbar spine and femoral neck in anorexia nervosa. *Scottish Medical Journal, 31,* 306–307.

Treasure, J. L., Russell, G. F. M., Fogelman, I., & Murby, B. (1987). Reversible bone loss in anorexia nervosa. *British Medical Journal* (Clinical Research Ed.), *295*(6596), 474–475.

Vaughan, V. C., & Litt, I. F. (1987). Growth and development during adolescence. In R. E. Behrman & V. C.Vaughan (Eds.), *Nelson textbook of pediatrics* (13th ed., pp. 20–27). Philadelphia: Saunders.

Weiner, H. (1989). Psycho-endocrinology of anorexia nervosa. *Psychiatry Clinics of North America, 12,* 187–205.

Witt, E. D., Ryan, C., & Hsu, L. K. G. (1985). Learning deficits in adolescents with anorexia nervosa. *Journal of Nervous and Mental Disorders, 173,* 182–184.

# CHAPTER 20

# Teacher Awareness of Drug and Substance Abuse

Margaret Thompson,
Shinya Ito, and Gideon Koren

Substance abuse is a major problem. A number of different government and social service agencies conduct regular surveys of drug use in selected populations. The National Household Survey on Drug Abuse (Substance Abuse and Mental Health Services Administration, 2000) reports that, in 1999, 6.3% of the population admitted to substance use in the previous 30 days, representing approximately 14 million Americans, and 3.1 million individuals used illicit substances. Similarly, the World Drug Report 2000 (United Nations Office for Drug Control and Prevention, 2000) estimates illicit drug use at 4.2% of the worldwide population. For further resources on the scope of the drug problem in youth, see Appendix 20.A.

A pattern of illicit drug use is usually established during youth, in parallel with tobacco use and alcohol drinking, and tends to be carried on into adulthood. In children and adolescents, the use of illicit substances is often associated with educational underachievement, school dropout, serious medical consequences, and various criminal or self-inflicting activities. Also, increased mortality and morbidity (risk of a disease) continue to pose major problems, not only for the users themselves in later life, but also for the society to which they belong. Because substance abuse behavior often begins in childhood, understanding of and education about this problem in the school setting is particularly crucial.

For educators, the first step in the prevention of and intervention in this hazardous behavior is to acknowledge its existence and to address the problem in an honest and knowledgeable fashion. Although there are many different approaches, which are sometimes mutually exclusive (e.g., for and against legalizing marijuana use), nobody can argue against the importance of knowing facts. This chapter is designed to provide educators with basic information on this complicated issue. Historical aspects of substance abuse, recent statistics, and medical issues are discussed. An attempt was made to avoid the use of technical terms, but those that are included are fully explained. Drug and chemical names, as well as commonly used street names, are given in the text. Appendix 20.B provides Web addresses for interesting sites to reference any multitude of other street names and terms. At the conclusion of the chapter, a Suggested Reading list is provided for further information on substance abuse by youth.

# DEFINITIONS

The term *substance abuse* is defined as the self-administration of any substance in a way that oversteps the social norms of a culture. This definition implies that there are medical, social, and cultural contexts to the substance abuse problem. For instance, once a substance is legalized or well accepted, modest use of it may no longer be seen as abuse by society. In contrast, use of currently legal substances may be regarded as abuse in the future. Some children who start substance abuse or use of potentially addictive legal substances develop physical and/or psychological dependence on the substance; however, there is no simple distinction between dependence and nondependent repeated use. In the medical community, diagnosis of *drug dependence* has been based on fulfillment of three or more of the following occurring at any time during the same 12-month period (American Psychiatric Association, 2000):

1.  tolerance, as defined by either of the following:
    a.  a need for markedly increased amounts of the substance to achieve intoxication or desired effect
    b.  markedly diminished effect with continued use of the same amount of the substance
2.  withdrawal, as manifested by either of the following:
    a.  the characteristic withdrawal syndrome for the substance
    b.  the same (or a closely related) substance is taken to relieve or avoid withdrawal symptoms
3.  the substance is often taken in larger amounts or over a longer period than was intended

4. there is a persistent desire or unsuccessful efforts to cut down or control substance use

5. a great deal of time is spent in activities necessary to obtain the substance (e.g., visiting multiple doctors or driving long distances), use the substance (e.g., chain-smoking), or recover from its effects

6. important social, occupational, or recreational activities are given up or reduced because of substance use

7. the substance use is continued despite knowledge of having a persistent or recurrent physical or psychological problem that is likely to have been caused or exacerbated by the substance (e.g., current cocaine use despite recognition of cocaine-induced depression, or continued drinking despite recognition that an ulcer was made worse by alcohol consumption)

*Addiction* implies the severest extreme of physical and/or psychological dependence on the substance and is often associated with damage to the individual and society.

Dependence frequently is associated with *tolerance* to effects caused by the substances; the user needs more and more of the substance to acquire the effects experienced previously. By using more, substance abusers are at a higher risk for the toxic, often fatal effects of the substance.

Sudden discontinuance of drugs after frequent exposure for a sufficiently long period often causes severe symptoms. This condition, collectively called *withdrawal syndrome* or *abstinence symptoms,* is disturbing and sometimes life threatening, especially in the cases of alcohol and sedatives or hypnotics.

# EVOLVEMENT OF SUBSTANCE ABUSE IN AN INDIVIDUAL

"Experimentation" is the most common initial motive for using illicit substances or drugs for nonmedicinal purposes. This is especially true in adolescents, who often lack the ability to exercise mature judgment, and whose peer circle tends to have its own internal standards. Substance-abuse experts recognize that very few abusers correctly predicted that their substance-abusing behavior would result from experimentation. Experimenters believe that they will be in full control of using illicit drugs and that they will be able to stop using them anytime they want to. Unfortunately, some eventually become drug abusers, despite initial confidence in their behavioral immunity against addiction.

In general, children and adolescents who progress to drug addiction experiment with such substances as alcohol and tobacco, which are legal for adults, before initiating use of illicit substances. Among illicit drugs, use of marijuana usually precedes that of cocaine and other substances. This trend is probably due to a combination of availability and magnitude of social acceptance of the behavior. Alcohol, tobacco, and marijuana are viewed as "gateway" substances. Interestingly, of the two age-restricted legal substances preceding marijuana use, male adolescents more commonly use alcohol and smokeless tobacco; regular tobacco smoking is more common in female adolescents (Johnston, O'Malley, & Bachman, 2001). In both genders, marijuana use is often followed by cocaine snorting and, subsequently, by "crack" cocaine smoking. This phenomenon may explain why the majority of drug abusers also use tobacco and drink alcohol.

The age of onset for cigarette smoking and alcohol drinking is also a predictor for subsequent involvement with other abused substances (Kandel & Yamaguchi, 1993). In the study by Kandel and Yamaguchi, adolescents using cocaine reportedly began smoking tobacco, drinking alcohol, or both 2 years earlier than those who did not progress to using cocaine (mean age 11 years vs. 13 years). Similarly, cocaine-using adolescents on average began using marijuana 2 years earlier (13 years of age) than those who did not go on to use cocaine (15 years of age). Although this earlier initiation of the behavior may not be a *cause* of subsequent use of more toxic substances, this is certainly an important marker for identifying children at greater risk of advanced substance abuse.

# RISK FACTORS

Much of the current knowledge about substance abuse has come from studies using animal models. Experimental animals *self-administer* substances of abuse in a similar way to that of humans who abuse drugs. In humans, prevention of initial experimentation and subsequent development of addiction may be the result of many counteracting factors, including social disapproval, family norms against their use, and knowledge about the grave consequences of substance abuse. However, certain family and peer environments may provide children with an atmosphere convenient for experimenting with substances of abuse. Friends, rather than strangers, almost always entice adolescents into substance abuse; hence, family and peer environments that fail to denounce substance abuse undoubtedly are strong risk factors for children.

It is widely accepted that a vulnerability to alcoholism is partly inherited (Cloninger, Dinwiddie, & Reich, 1989), although environmental factors also play an important role, and the mode of inheritance seems extremely complex (Holden, 1991). Genetic predisposition to other substances of abuse is less clear, but there seem to be susceptible personalities, such as those who display rebelliousness, risk-taking, low self-esteem, aggressiveness, and other antisocial characteristics, who are predisposed to drug addiction. Overall rates of substance abuse seem to differ among different ethnic groups; however, when social and environmental conditions are controlled, there are no genetic differences in rates of abuse in different races (Lillie-Blanton, Anthony, & Schuster, 1993).

# PREVENTION AND TREATMENT

There are many drug abuse prevention programs, some of which are incorporated in school systems. Students must be taught the consequences of experimentation and abuse of these substances, although this approach alone is not sufficient. A model program that appears to be successful in school settings provides opportunities for students to become familiar with external and internal pressures leading to substance abuse and to learn how to disregard the prodrug arguments and pressures. If supported by other approaches aimed at parents and the community, this kind of program can be even more effective.

Long-term medical complications and acute overdose require medical treatment, but behavioral and psychological interventions play more crucial roles in sustaining drug-free lifestyles. Medical attention to acute problems of substance abuse should always be followed by the above-mentioned approaches, of which drug rehabilitation programs are important components.

Appendix 20.C lists multiple reliable Web addresses for drug education programs and curricula.

# ABUSED SUBSTANCES

Recreational substances that are abused can usually be categorized in four groups. These include stimulants, sedatives–hypnotics, narcotics, and hallucinogens. Common drugs of abuse are discussed in each category. Special mention is made of "club" or "rave" drugs. The primary focus is on substance abuse by children and adolescents, but children suffering from intrauterine exposure to alcohol, nicotine, marijuana, and cocaine are briefly mentioned because they are relatively common and, ultimately, these children with potential problems will become pupils within the school system. Finally, because of the importance of sports in adolescence, steroid abuse is discussed.

Rather than present, as we did in the third edition of this book, an incomplete and out-of-date table of common street names and slang terms as they relate to substances of abuse, we direct the reader to Appendix 20.B, Web Sites Listing Street Drug Names. We searched all Web addresses listed and found them to be reliable and current sites. Street terms may also be regional; not finding a term on one site may reflect that it is not used in a particular region of the world. Several sites may need to be searched.

For more information on specific substances, Appendix 20.D gives reliable Web sites about the common drugs of abuse that follow.

## Stimulants

### Tobacco

Cigarette smoking and use of smokeless tobacco are closely associated with adolescent alcohol and drug use. About 90% of adults and adolescents who abuse drugs or alcohol also smoke cigarettes (Myers & Brown, 1994). Every day in the United States, 6,000 students start smoking (Jacobs et al., 2001). Findings of the Monitoring the Future survey (Johnston et al., 2001) indicated that approximately 15% of children in Grade 8, 24% in Grade 10, and 31% in Grade 12 admitted to cigarette use in the past 30 days. Daily tobacco use was 5.5%, 12%, and 19%, respectively, for the same grade cohorts. Many of these adolescent smokers carry this habit into adulthood, probably due to a combination of nicotine dependence and a reinforcing environment, unless intervention is implemented. Indeed, 90% of adults who smoke started smoking before the age of 19 (Jacobs et al., 2001).

In experiments (Cox, Goldstein, & Nelson, 1984), animals have been shown to self-administer nicotine repeatedly, indicating the reinforcing actions of the substance (strengthening effects on its own use). In humans, one puff of smoke reaches the brain within 10 seconds of inhalation and stimulates the reward centers of the brain by increasing a brain substance known as dopamine. Nicotine may further facilitate memory and attention, enhance composure, and reduce appetite, leading to decreased weight gain. Another strong reinforcing factor is the positive image of tobacco use endorsed by actors, celebrities, athletes, or other role models for children and adolescents.

The main active component in tobacco is nicotine. During cigarette smoking, nicotine stimulates the body by increasing noradrenaline and adrenaline levels. Mild increases in heart rate, blood pressure, and respiratory rate, comparable to those resulting from mild exercise, occur. Nausea, vomiting, and tremors (typically, fine shaking of hands and fingers) may be seen more frequently in some people, especially first-time smokers or occasional smokers. This same increase in adrenaline levels can lead to the adverse effects of nicotine, including severe blood vessel disruption, causing loss of limbs, gangrene, heart attacks, or blindness.

Tobacco smoke has ill effects distinct from those of nicotine. Various health hazards also result from other combustion substances, such as polycyclic aromatic hydrocarbons (some of which may cause cancer) and carbon monoxide. About 4,000 compounds are estimated to exist in tobacco smoke. Smoke contains substances capable of inducing cancer (i.e., carcinogens). This deadly effect only becomes apparent several decades after the initiation of the smoking habit. Another important clinical implication is that infants and children in a smoker's household, as well as smokers themselves, are at risk for respiratory illness, stunted growth, and learning difficulties due to second-hand smoke.

Cigarette smoking during pregnancy poses risks of growth retardation in the fetus. The fetus is exposed to nicotine, carbon monoxide, and other toxic chemicals when the mother smokes. In fact, the fetus is exposed to nicotine when someone other than the mother exposes the child to second-hand tobacco smoke. Tobacco use should be strongly discouraged in school settings, where the next generations of parents begin forming their social habits.

## Cocaine

Cocaine (street names include coke, crack, C, candy, lady, and line) comes from the leaves of the *Erythroxylon coca* tree. Natives of the South American

Andes have chewed coca leaves for more than 5,000 years to gain feelings of well-being. Medical use of cocaine as a local anesthetic and for various other indications began in the 19th century in Europe, although local anesthesia to the nose for surgical procedures is the sole remaining medical indication for cocaine hydrochloride. Sigmund Freud, the founder of modern psychoanalysis, was one of the first Europeans who studied the clinical uses of cocaine. Interested in brain effects of cocaine, Freud gave the drug to one of his colleagues in an attempt to wean the person from morphine (a potent narcotic). The weaning was successful, but the patient became one of the first-known cocaine addicts. Cocaine was an ingredient in Coca-Cola from 1888 until 1901, when it was removed from the formulation. Cocaine was banned for use in the United States in 1914. Since then, the medicinal use of cocaine is under strict governmental control in most countries.

In the illegal market, cocaine is supplied either as a hydrochloride powder, which is sniffed or injected intravenously after being dissolved into water, or as freebase cocaine ("crack"), which also can be smoked. Because cocaine hydrochloride decomposes under heat from a match or lighter, it cannot be smoked. The name crack stems from the cracking sound generated when clusters of freebase cocaine break upon heat. Crack is sold in small dosage units of "rocks" costing $5 to $10 each. This relatively low price makes crack cocaine within the reach of adolescents.

Data from Monitoring the Future (Johnston et al., 2001) indicated that 5% of high school seniors, 4% of 10th graders, and 2% of 8th graders in the United States had used cocaine hydrochloride in the past year. Approximately 2% of those from all grades surveyed had used crack in the past year. This compares to a high in 1986 of approximately 13%. Whereas 8% of U.S. students in Grade 10 reported having used crack or cocaine hydrochloride in their lifetime (Johnston et al., 2001), 2% of European Grade 10 students reported having done so (Hibell et al., 1999).

Peak blood concentrations of cocaine are achieved 30 minutes to 1 hour after intranasal application, which suggests that absorption is not completed immediately after sniffing. Inhalation of cocaine smoke produces more intense and instantaneous effects, and heavy users may repeat the smoking every 10 to 15 minutes. After intravenous or inhalation application, cocaine is rapidly eliminated from the bloodstream. Although there are substantial variations in cocaine-use behaviors, taking the drug in bouts or binges is common. Binge users may be totally dependent on the drug and out of control in their drug-seeking behavior, even if they do not use it on a daily basis.

Cocaine is also a stimulant. Similar to nicotine, it increases the amount of noradrenaline and adrenaline released. Acute effects of cocaine use include elated mood and increased self-confidence, increased heart rate and blood pressure, dilated pupils, and erratic or aggressive behavior. Headache, seizures, fever, chest pain, irregular heart rhythm, and even heart attack may occur in toxic cases. When the acute effects of cocaine have gone, the user often becomes severely fatigued and mentally depressed.

Symptoms commonly seen in chronic adolescent cocaine users are fatigue, insomnia (sleeplessness), loss of appetite, weight loss, and a chronic cough. Because users of cocaine, especially crack cocaine, are often polysubstance abusers, they may have other health problems attributable to multiple substance exposures.

Cocaine use is associated not only with higher homicide rates but also with increased rates of suicide, which is the second leading cause of death among U.S. adolescents. Among high school students, suicide ideation and attempts are more common in drug users, particularly crack cocaine users (Felts, Chenier, & Barnes, 1992). Moreover, in New York City, cocaine was detected in 64% of "Russian roulette" fatalities and in 35% of those who committed suicide by handgun, suggesting a link between cocaine use and potentially fatal risk-taking behaviors (Marzuk, Tardiff, Smyth, Stajic, & Leon, 1992).

It is not uncommon for newborns to be exposed to cocaine in utero. Many of these children are presently in the school system. Despite tremendous negative publicity, experts now believe that cocaine exposure in utero does not result in birth defects. However, probably because of a combination of poor prenatal care, premature delivery, and maternal use of other substances such as alcohol and cigarette smoke, some children born to heavy cocaine users demonstrate slow development. Nevertheless, teachers and physicians caring for them should be aware that labeling these children as "crack children" does not solve any of the problems they may have. Such stereotyping, in fact, may negatively affect efforts of active intervention to help these children reach their maximum potential (Mayes, Granger, Bornstein, & Zuckerman, 1992).

## Amphetamines and "Look Alikes"

Amphetamines are a group of drugs with chemical structures related to ephedrine and adrenaline. These include *amphetamine* (known as beans, bennies, uppers, and hearts), *dextroamphetamine* (known as Dexedrine), *methamphetamine* (known as speed, ice, crystal, and crystal meth), and *methylphenidate* (known as Ritalin). Modifications of the parent structure contribute to differing effects of these substances. Generally, these drugs affect chemicals in the brain known as dopamine and serotonin to varying degrees. Except for mescaline, the amphetamines are not hallucinogenic as much as stimulants. They have medical uses in the treatment of narcolepsy (uncontrollable periodic attacks of sleepiness) and attention-deficit/ hyperactivity disorder. They are abused orally or intravenously. Over-the-counter weight-reduction medications (or mail-order drugs) containing phenylpropanolamine and caffeine also are used in sufficiently high doses to gain stimulant effects similar to those of amphetamines. These "look-alike" drugs are easily available.

Abuse problems with amphetamines include use for weight reduction (not medically indicated), stress, and binges for pleasure. Similar to cocaine, amphetamines are stimulants that produce mood elevation, a sense of well-being and filled-up energy, and decreased appetite. At the same time, some users experience anxiety, irritability, and sleeplessness. The agitated mood is usually followed by anxiety, fatigue, and sustained feelings of depression. In contrast to cocaine, with its short half-life of 1 hour, it takes 5 to 10 hours to eliminate half of the amphetamine in the bloodstream.

Overdosing results in confusion, assaultiveness, restlessness, hallucinations, excessive sweating, palpitations, and collapse. Suicidal or homicidal tendencies may appear. Convulsions and coma occur in fatal intoxication. Chronic toxicities include hallucinations, paranoid behaviors, and delusions, resembling schizophrenia. These psychotic reactions usually subside after cessation of the drugs but may not disappear in some individuals.

Two chemically modified amphetamines—MDMA (3,4-methylenedioxymethamphetamine, or Ecstasy) and MDEA (3,4-methylenedioxyethamphetamine, or Eve)—are sold on the illicit drug market. Designed and manufactured in unauthorized laboratories, they are called designer drugs. They produce elated feelings without inducing hallucinations or alterations of visual images. Ecstasy has the unique property of causing spasm of the jaw muscles; to prevent tooth damage, the user is often seen carrying a baby pacifier for use during intoxication. In the United States in the year 2000, over 9% of adolescents in Grade 12, over 6% in Grade 10, and over 3.5% in Grade 8 admitted to having used Ecstasy in the past year (Johnston et al., 2001). In the setting of increased physical activity (e.g., dancing all night), dehydration (inadequate replacement of water loss), and warm external environments (inadequately ventilated settings), individuals may be more susceptible to the adverse effects of Ecstasy. Some individuals also have a predisposition to the adverse effects of Ecstasy. These factors may contribute to the increasing number of Ecstasy deaths.

Particularly potent amphetamines have also been introduced in the recent past. One of these, PMA (para-methoxy-amphetamine), is also known as "death" on the streets. Not surprisingly, there is no quality control in the illicit drug world. It is possible that what is sold as one product may be contaminated with or substituted with another.

## Sedatives–Hypnotics

### Alcohol

Alcoholic beverages have been part of human culture for more than 8,000 years and generally are considered socially compatible. Many current societies view drinking alcohol as an acceptable behavior in adulthood. In the United States, about 60% of all adults drink alcohol at least occasionally, and 10% are considered heavy drinkers. Although it is illegal in most countries for minors to consume alcoholic beverages, enormous numbers of adolescents do drink. In a 2000 U.S. survey, 50% of high school seniors, 41% of 10th graders, and 22% of 8th graders said they had used alcohol in the past month (Johnston et al., 2001).

The main component of alcoholic beverages is ethyl alcohol (or ethanol), concentrations of which range from 4% to 5% in regular beer, 11% to 15% in wine, and 45% in liquor. As the concentrations of ethanol increase in one's blood, toxic effects occur proportional to concentration, although sensitivity can differ considerably among individuals. The most imminent health hazards to young drinkers are impaired judgment and motor skills, which often lead to various forms of accidents and suicide attempts. As blood alcohol levels rise into the toxic range, death can occur as a result of inability to protect one's airway and the vomiting of stomach contents into one's lungs.

Although ethanol is metabolized (or broken down by the body) relatively quickly, because the liver has a finite amount of enzyme available to detoxify it, only a fixed amount per unit of time can be eliminated; hence, the greater the amount ingested, the greater the time required for elimination. Consider that an average adult male is able to break down approximately 10 g of alcohol per hour, and that one bottle of 5% beer contains 13.4 g of ethyl alcohol per bottle. At the rate of one beer per hour, after

3 hours, 10 g of alcohol will remain in the body and require a further hour to be eliminated, even if consumption is stopped. Activity levels of the enzymes responsible for ethanol detoxification can differ significantly among people. In general, younger children have slower alcohol metabolism. This translates into prolonged intoxication or influence of alcohol from equivalent amounts.

Tolerance develops when one is exposed to ethyl alcohol repeatedly. The chronic drinker is not as impaired as a naive drinker with any particular blood alcohol concentration, to a limit. Greater amounts of alcohol are required to achieve the same intoxicating effect, setting the stage for dependence. One cannot become tolerant to the lethal concentrations of alcohol, however. Alcohol withdrawal syndrome, which occurs in ethanol-dependent persons 1 to 3 days after stopping drinking, can be life threatening, although a case has not been reported in adolescents.

Many chronic diseases develop in adults who regularly use high amounts of ethanol for a long period. Liver and brain damage are well-known adverse effects of alcohol drinking. These changes are not usually seen in young drinkers because of their relatively brief history of exposure.

Alcohol is a potent toxin for the unborn child. If the mother drinks significant amounts of alcohol (2 g/kg ethanol per day, corresponding to about six to eight drinks per day) during pregnancy, the fetus is often permanently damaged. *Fetal alcohol syndrome* is characterized by mental retardation, delayed growth and development, birth defects, and various behavioral problems such as hyperactivity and learning disabilities (see Chapter 2). In women who drink regularly but to a lesser extent, the fetus may be less severely affected, suffering mainly from behavioral problems, with no obvious physical characteristics of the syndrome. This condition is referred to as *fetal alcohol effects*. Although occasional mild drinking during pregnancy does not seem to pose these risks, safety levels concerning amount of consumption and the mode of drinking during pregnancy (e.g., whether to drink a large amount occasionally or a small quantity constantly) have not been defined clearly. Pregnant women who have a drinking problem need thorough medical consultation.

## Marijuana

In Johnston et al.'s (2001) survey, 18% of 8th graders reported use of marijuana in the past year, and 1.3% admitted to daily use; 35% of 10th graders and 39% of 12th graders had used marijuana in the last year, with 6% of the latter reporting daily use. This compares to 17% of 10th graders in Europe (Hibell et al., 1999) and 36.4% of 10th graders in Ontario, Canada (Adalf, Paglia, & Ivis, 1999), who have used marijuana at some time in their life.

The term *marijuana* (street names include MJ, Mary Jane, weed, joint, ganja, grass, jay, and pot) refers to any part of the hemp plant (*Cannabis sativa*) or its extract prepared for illicit use. Cannabis, obtained from the flowering tops of the hemp plant, is one of the oldest and most widely used psychoactive substances. Recorded use of cannabis goes back thousands of years in China and India. The hemp plant produces more than 60 related compounds called cannabinoids, of which *l*-delta-9-tetrahydrocannabinol ($\Delta^9$-THC) is the main active substance. Currently, $\Delta^9$-THC is used medically as a drug to control nausea and vomiting that are unresponsive to other drugs. Because marijuana is commonly smoked rather than ingested, toxic combustion substances may be clinically important in the development of long-term toxicity, as is the case in tobacco.

$\Delta^9$-THC contents of marijuana vary substantially, ranging from 0.5% to more than 30%. Also, the smoking technique and the effects of *pyrolysis* (the chemical reaction caused by the high temperature of burning) influence the amount of $\Delta^9$-THC that may reach important body organs. In addition, possibilities for contamination by herbicides, fungi, and, in some regions, mercury, also exist.

Marijuana usually causes an enhanced sense of well-being, a subjective feeling of relaxation, talkativeness, spontaneous laughter, and altered perception of time. Slowed thinking (often inaccurate and irrelevant) and sleepiness are also common, and emotional control becomes fragile. These conditions resemble mild ethanol intoxication. High doses of $\Delta^9$-THC may result in acute toxic psychosis, characterized by hallucinations, delusions, and panic reactions, which often need to be handled as psychiatric emergencies. Effects of $\Delta^9$-THC include an increase in heart rate, a fall in the standing blood pressure, and congestion of the blood vessels of the eyes, resulting in redness.

Heavy marijuana users develop many chronic health problems. It is difficult to distinguish chronic effects of cigarette smoking from those of marijuana smoking because both behaviors often go together. However, chronic bronchitis has been observed in heavy marijuana users, which may be partly due to a much higher tar content in marijuana smoke than in tobacco smoke.

Chronic heavy users of marijuana also may display altered mental conditions, such as apathy (extreme indifference), mental slowing, memory loss, impairment of judgment, loss of drive, and emotional flatness (i.e., amotivational syndrome). Although this condition may be due partly to other risky behaviors (e.g., other drug use, malnutrition) or be a result of pre-existing behavioral problems, experiments in rats have shown that heavy chronic exposure to $\Delta^9$-THC can cause structural changes in the brain (Landfield, Cadwallader, & Vinsant, 1988).

Despite the reported adverse effects of high doses of cannabis on fetal development in experimental animals, no data on humans have suggested similar problems and no fetal marijuana syndrome has been described. Recent studies suggest that subtle neurobehavioral adverse effects may result, including hyperactivity, sleep disturbances, and decreased attentiveness (Fried & Watkinson, 2001).

## Organic Solvents

*Organic solvents* is a collective term denoting a volatile liquid that may dissolve water-insoluble organic compounds. Examples are toluene, xylene, various forms of alcohol, acetone, ether, trichloroethylene, trichloromethane, and other petroleum-derived compounds or mixtures such as gasoline. These are part of many household products, including some types of glue, spray paints, lacquer thinners, cleaning fluids, and typewriter correction fluids. They are relatively inexpensive and easy to obtain. Sniffing of these substances has been a substance abuse problem for decades because they create a high that is quite similar to that produced by alcohol drinking. In North America, gasoline sniffing is more prevalent in communities of Native American and Canadian populations than in other ethnic groups; this does not necessarily indicate the existence of a genetic or biologic predisposing factor toward gasoline sniffing in this particular ethnic group. Rather, the social and economic environment appears to be the crucial factor. Overall, about 15% of U.S. high school seniors reported an experience with inhalant abuse (Johnston et al., 2001).

*Organic nitrites* (isobutyl, butyl, or amyl nitrite), another group of volatile compounds, have been abused as aphrodisiacs (to enhance sexual experiences), primarily in the male homosexual community. These compounds are available in pornography or "head" shops and from mail-order stores. Amyl nitrite is used clinically to treat acute angina. In Johnston et al.'s (2001) survey, approximately 1% of U.S. high school seniors said they had used nitrites at least once in the previous year.

Almost immediately after inhalation, these volatile substances exert effects lasting for 5 to 10 minutes. Sudden death, probably due to acute heart failure, is not uncommon because lethal *arrhythmias* (severe forms of irregular heartbeat) can be induced by the organic solvents. Chronic detrimental effects include liver and kidney dysfunction, brain damage, and peripheral nerve toxicity. In the past, gasoline contained various amounts of lead, which is a toxic heavy metal. Gasoline sniffers may have had brain and nerve damage caused by lead intoxication. Children born to heavy organic solvent abusers show health problems similar to the fetal alcohol syndrome effects (see the previous section on alcohol).

The nitrites can cause lowered blood pressure, headaches, and fainting. They may also alter the hemoglobin (an oxygen-carrying protein) in red blood cells, resulting in decreased ability of the blood to carry oxygen.

## Tranquilizers

The term *tranquilizers* implies a therapeutic endpoint rather than overall clinical effects. This category of drugs, which are widely used in clinical medicine, includes antipsychotic drugs with little reinforcing or addictive propensity. Drugs discussed in this section include minor tranquilizers with habit-forming characteristics. The two main groups of addictive drugs in this category are *barbiturates* (phenobarbital, pentobarbital, amobarbital, and secobarbital) and *benzodiazepines* (diazepam [Valium] and lorazepam [Ativan]).

Most abusers take these drugs orally, with the exception of barbiturates, which also can be injected intravenously or intramuscularly. An estimated 5% to 10% of high school students have had an experience with sedative or hypnotic abuse (Johnston et al., 2001). These groups of drugs are often taken with opioids and alcohol by polysubstance abusers to enhance the experience. Another form of sedative or hypnotic abuse is seen in individuals who initially were prescribed these drugs (e.g., for the treatment of anxiety) and who later unknowingly developed dependence on them.

Sedation is a common effect of this group of drugs. Although these drugs are not particularly reinforcing to many people, some individuals find them pleasurable. Acute intoxication leads to mental confusion, slurred speech, *ataxia* (impaired balance and coordination of movement), slow respiration, coma, low body temperature, and death. Concurrent alcohol ingestion is often seen with tranquilizer overdose in a suicide attempt. Because of variations in elimination from the body, duration of effects differs among these sedatives. Intoxication due to most benzodiazepines and barbiturates (pentobarbital, secobarbital, and amobarbital) may last for 2 days, whereas phenobarbital intoxication may cause weeklong coma.

The effects of chronically taken sedatives or hypnotics may not necessarily be evident. Regular use of these drugs as sleeping pills may cause sleeping difficulties and anxiety when the drugs are discontinued. Heavier use may lead to a chronic intoxicated state resembling ethanol intoxication. The withdrawal syndrome following dependence may result in seizures and *delirium* (i.e., visual hallucinations, disorientation, and mental confusion), which can be a medical emergency.

## Gamma Hydroxybutyrate

Gamma hydroxybutyrate (GHB; street names include G, Grievous Bodily Harm, and liquid E) is one of three chemicals—the other two being gamma butyrolactone (GBL) and 1,4 butanediol (both of which are metabolized in the body to GBH)—that have been implicated as "date rape" drugs. GHB is a naturally occurring substance in the body that affects the release of dopamine in the brain. Intoxication with GHB results in effects similar to that of alcohol. At lower doses, relaxation occurs, loss of inhibition, increased appreciation for music, and mood elevation. At increasing doses, coordination is impaired, consciousness is depressed, and breathing is slowed. Deaths due to intoxication with GHB are usually in the setting of large recreational doses (GHB is a liquid sold in varying concentrations) or in combination with some other sedative, such as alcohol.

GHB was first developed as an anesthetic. Side effects limited its use. It then became available as an over-the-counter sleeping aid and as a dietary supplement to enhance muscle bulk. Although illegal to possess or sell in most countries, recipes of the product are available over the Internet. With increased use, one does develop tolerance to its effects. Similarly, once tolerant, if use ceases abruptly, withdrawal syndromes have been described. This state can result in severe symptoms with hallucinations, paranoia, and blood pressure and heart rate abnormalities requiring urgent medical intervention (Sivilotti, Burns, Aaron, & Greenberg, 2001).

## Narcotics

There are several terms, including *narcotic, opioid,* and *opiate,* used to designate a group of chemicals with characteristic effects on brain function; the main effect is a decrease in one's perception of pain. The word *opium* stems from the Greek word for *juice* because historically the source of opium was the milky juice derived from the unripe seed capsules of the poppy plant (*Papaver somniferum*). In the early 19th century, one of the compounds isolated from opium was called *morphine* after Morpheus, the Greek god of dreams. Soon after the discovery of morphine, other biologically active compounds, such as codeine, were isolated from crude opium as well. The relatively obsolete term *opiate* designates such drugs obtained from opium (e.g., morphine and codeine) and those obtained by chemical modification of morphine (e.g., heroin). Both chemically modified opium extracts and synthetic compounds with morphine-like actions (e.g., methadone and meperidine) soon became available. It is now widely known that the human body also synthesizes proteins that produce morphine-like activities by operating on the same brain cell sites as do morphine and related drugs. The term *opioid* denotes all the naturally occurring compounds, including chemically modified ones, and the synthetic drugs that exert morphine-like effects. Opioid use often leads to a habit (i.e., addiction), but clinical use for pain control under appropriate medical supervision rarely does so.

Conventional use of the term *narcotics* may create confusion because it may mean any of the following: (a) a morphine-like potent drug, (b) any drug capable of inducing sleep, (c) any substance causing dependence, or (d) a substance designated in certain legal contexts. Although still widely used at large, the word is being replaced by more strictly defined terms.

Heroin, the most commonly abused opioid, is snorted or injected. Heroin abuse reached a peak in the 1960s and 1970s and then decreased. An accurate estimation of the rate of heroin abuse in adolescents is difficult to determine because heroin addicts are most likely to have dropped out of the school system and are therefore unavailable to answer school surveys. Intravenous heroin abuse also poses risks of various serious infections such as hepatitis viruses and HIV (human immunodeficiency virus), due to the lack of hygienic procedures and the sharing of needles; this risk is common in any injectable substances of abuse.

Opioids, which are sought due to their euphoric effects, depress brain function, resulting in drowsiness, reduced pain sensation, and decreased behavioral and motivational drive. These drugs often cause nausea and vomiting by activating the center in the brain that controls nauseous sensation. Various degrees of tolerance develop to these effects. Because the tolerance usually disappears upon withdrawal, restarting opioid use at the same dose often results in fatality.

Acute intoxication with opioids is usually characterized by small pupils; coma; slow and irregular breathing; cool, moist skin; slow heart rate; and potentially death. Overdosing is always a possibility for heroin addicts because the strength of the heroin formulation in the illegal market varies significantly. Opioid overdose is a medical emergency that should be managed by intensive supportive care and administration of opioid antagonists to counteract the effects.

Upon discontinuing chronic use of opioids, the user will develop a withdrawal (abstinence) syndrome characterized by anxiety, restlessness, insomnia (inability to sleep), muscle pain, gooseflesh, sneezing, tearing, yawning, nasal congestion, vomiting, diarrhea, and rapid heart rate. Because heroin is eliminated from the body relatively quickly, the withdrawal syndrome tends to be intense, although rarely life threatening. Because methadone has less sedative effects and longer elimination time from the body, it is substituted for heroin or morphine to circumvent an opioid withdrawal syndrome in the long-term medical management of opioid addicts.

Unauthorized production of chemically modified opioid drugs has increased the number of opioids introduced into the illicit drug market. There have been reports of deaths due to overdose of potent opioids such as α-methylfentanyl and 3-methylfentanyl, both of which are obtained by chemical modification of a potent anesthetic, fentanyl. Another tragic example is 4-phenyl-4-propionoxy-piperidine (MPPP), which is produced by chemical modification of a synthetic opiate, meperidine. A group of young drug addicts in California had some MPPP that was contaminated with a compound used as a catalyst in the chemical reaction that happened to be toxic to a specific part of the brain. This toxic chemical destroyed a group of brain cells called *substantia nigra,* resulting in a severe brain disorder known as Parkinson's disease (Langston, Ballard, Tetrud, & Irwin, 1983). These drugs, designed and produced in unauthorized laboratories (i.e., designer drugs) will probably continue posing a serious challenge to our society.

## HALLUCINOGENS

### Mescaline

The prototype hallucinogen is mescaline (street names include mesc and button), derived from the cactus plant peyote, which grows in the deserts of Mexico and the Southwestern United States. Typically the plant is dried and smoked to produce physical, visual, and perceptual hallucinations. Its use probably dates back thousands of years to the natives of Mexico. Because it takes years for the plant to mature, it is relatively unavailable and very expensive to purchase. It is probable that anything sold on the streets as mescaline is actually LSD or PCP, discussed next.

## LSD (Lysergic Acid Diethylamide)

LSD (street names include acid and blotter) is a chemical derived from the fungus or mold called ergot that grows on rye. It and similar naturally occurring compounds, such as those found in the seeds of the morning glory plant (LSA, or lysergic acid amide) and nutmeg, are hallucinogens or psychedelics. LSD is made as a liquid; blotting paper is soaked in the liquid and dried. A dose (50–150 μg) is sold as a 1-cm-square "blotter" for $5 to $10. The blotter is placed on the tongue and sucked for release of the hallucinogen. In the survey by Johnston et al. (2001), 3.9% of 8th graders, 7.6% of 10th graders, and 11.1% of seniors admitted to having used LSD at some time in their life.

LSD is the most potent of all hallucinogens. After minute doses of the drug, LSD alters perception of time and space, visual images, and sound. Visual information is often perceived as sound images, and sound provokes colorful visual images. Mood may fluctuate, although pleasurable feelings tend to dominate. Because most, if not all, users correctly recognize these effects as drug induced, the psychological boundary between reality and fantasy appears to be somehow maintained, despite the vivid illusions; strictly speaking, therefore, these are not hallucinations, because they are not confused with reality. These effects occur over 3 to 4 hours and are called a "trip." The illegal use of LSD is typically repeated in weeks or months to reexperience the trip. However, unpredictable episodes of panic ("bad trips") can occur with use of the drug. Moreover, in more than 15% of users, a disturbing phenomenon occurs that is called "flashbacks," which is an unexpected repetition of the drug experience in the absence of the drug, even several years after the last dose of LSD.

## Phencyclidine (PCP)

Although no longer in use medically, PCP (street names include angel dust) originally was developed as an anesthetic for human and animal use in the

1950s. Phencyclidine began to be abused in the late 1960s. Statistics about PCP use are unreliable because it is sometimes contaminated with or mistaken for LSD, mescaline, or marijuana. In general, it is now rare to find PCP available on the streets.

PCP can be injected intravenously, snorted, ingested, or smoked. The effects, lasting 12 hours or more, include an elated feeling, emotional instability, staggering gait, slurred speech, muscle stiffness, confusion, and drowsiness. Higher doses may cause panic reactions, anesthetic effects, auditory hallucinations, coma, and seizures. Disturbed memory and speech and altered personality may be observed in chronic users.

## Ketamine

A synthetic analogue of phencyclidine, ketamine (street names include K, special K, and vitamin K), was developed and is currently used in the medical profession as a dissociative anesthetic, especially in children. Emerging from a ketamine anesthetic has the common side effects of nausea, vomiting, and paranoid delusions. Despite this, however, ketamine has found its place as a drug of abuse. At low doses, it causes a sense of euphoria, increased sociability, and pleasant perceptual distortions. At higher doses, complete dissociation from one's surroundings and near-death experiences have been described.

## Anabolic Steroids

*Steroids* denote compounds that have a specific chemical structure in common. Several of them are important hormones that are synthesized in the human body. *Anabolic steroids* designate those steroids with enhancing actions on protein synthesis and accumulation, possibly leading to an increase in functional muscle mass in some populations. This group of steroids is abused largely for the muscle-enhancing effects. However, a pure anabolic steroid without other effects, such as androgenic effects (see below), has not been, and probably never will be, discovered.

Some athletes, both women and men, use anabolic steroids because they expect them to increase physical competence. Since weight lifters and bodybuilders began using these drugs in the 1950s, the trend has become widespread, from professional to college and high school athletes. Anabolic steroids are not addictive in the same sense as are psychoactive drugs such as cocaine and heroin, but the expectation of becoming more physically fit is reinforcing. It has never been proven that anabolic steroids in medically used doses actually promote muscle growth over the levels achieved by normal levels of naturally occurring male sex hormones in the mature man. In women and sexually immature men, muscle growth is promoted by use of these steroids. The doses of anabolic steroids used for muscle-increasing purposes are 10 to 100 times higher than those used for medical indications.

In 2000, about 2% of students in Grade 12 reported at least one use of an anabolic steroid (Johnston et al., 2001). In a study conducted in Georgia among 9th-grade students, 5.4% of boys and 1.5% of girls had tried anabolic steroids (DuRant, Rickert, Ashworth, Newman, & Slavens, 1993). Importantly, the more often they used anabolic steroids, the more likely they were to abuse cocaine, smokeless tobacco, marijuana, cigarettes, or alcohol. Sharing needles to inject anabolic steroids is a common phenomenon, posing risks of life-threatening infections.

*Testosterone,* a naturally occurring male sex hormone (women also produce testosterone in smaller amounts), is a prototypical anabolic steroid used for muscle-increasing potential, although it has other natural androgenic (male) effects, such as the growth of body hair and coarsening of the voice. Many other synthetic anabolic steroids exist. These synthetic drugs were designed to be purely anabolic, although other androgenic effects are unavoidable. Many anabolic steroids used for "doping" purposes lack human safety data, as they are designated for animal use. Adverse effects of the anabolic steroids are mental changes; liver diseases, including hepatitis and tumors; damages to the testes; and menstrual changes.

# CONCLUSION

Substance-abuse problems in children and adolescents range from experimentation with gateway substances to full-blown addiction to potent drugs. The younger the experimenting child, the more serious the consequences. Whereas many experimenters do not go on to abuse more potent substances, some eventually become fully addicted despite initial confidence in their ability to control such behavior. These victims of substance abuse should be identified immediately, supported, and treated through appropriate medical and behavioral programs. Commitment of the family is essential. It is important for teachers to educate students to promote the prevention of drug use, to intervene in early-stage substance-abusing behavior, and to take immediate actions on emergent situations of advanced substance abuse. Continuous anti–drug-abuse activities in school settings, combined with more broad-based community models, should help create an atmosphere that makes vulnerable minors more resistant to substance abuse.

# APPENDIX 20.A

# Web Sites for Statistics on the Use of Substances of Abuse

Full text of Monitoring the Future (2000–2001) online. (U.S. Department of Health and Human Services, National Institutes of Health)
> http://monitoringthefuture.org

Table of all drug use surveys done in the United States, descriptions of the populations surveyed, and links to the same. (Center for Substance Abuse Research)
> http://www.cesar.umd.edu/cesar/fedsources.asp#prevalence

Links to numerous global and country reports on availability and use of selected drugs of abuse. (United Nations Office on Drugs and Crime)
> http://www.unodc.org/unodc/research.html

*PulseCheck* is a U.S. government publication that identifies trends in substance abuse in 21 selected U.S. centers. Information is gathered and published on a semiannual basis and addresses use of cocaine, heroin, marijuana, club drugs, and methamphetamines. (Office of National Drug Control Policy)
> http://www.whitehousedrugpolicy.gov/publications/drugfact/pulsecheck/
> fall2001/index.html

Canadian National report on use of selected drugs and issues in selected Canadian sites addressing heroin, cocaine, marijuana, HIV, needle exchange, alcohol, stimulants, and so on. (Canadian Community Epidemiology Network on Drug Use)
> http://www.ccsa.ca

Specific resources and statistics on drug abuse in Canadian and U.S. youth. (Canadian Centre on Substance Abuse)
> http://www.ccsa.ca/youthgen.htm

Results of Ontario Student Drug Use Survey, 2001. (Center for Addiction and Mental Health, Ontario, Canada)

> **http://www.camh.net/research/population_life_course.html#
> osdusquestionaires**

Statistics on Drug Use in Toronto, Canada, 2000. (City of Toronto, Ontario, Canada)

> **http://www.city.toronto.on.ca/drugcentre/rgdu00/rgdu1.htm**

# APPENDIX 20.B

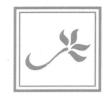

# Web Sites Listing Street Drug Names

Table with substance, common street names, and drug effects. (National Institute on Drug Abuse)
http://www.nida.nih.gov/DrugsofAbuse.html

Searchable site for common street names of drugs of abuse. (Center for Substance Abuse Research)
http://www.cesar.umd.edu/cesar/streetterms.asp

Extensive searchable site for street names of drugs of abuse, both alphabetically and by drug class. (The Office of the National Drug Control Policy)
http://www.whitehousedrugpolicy.gov/streetterms/

Alphabetically organized dictionary of street drug terms.
http://www.erowid.org/psychoactives/slang/slang.shtml

Dictionary, alphabetically organized, containing definitions that relate to both drugs of abuse and addiction. (Center for Addiction and Mental Health)
http://sano.camh.net/curricul/gloss.htm

Searches for slang drug names and matches with terms and explanations. (Indiana Prevention Resource Center)
http://www.drugs.indiana.edu/slang/home.html

# APPENDIX 20.C

# Web Sites for Drug Education Materials and Resources

Follow links to Science Education Resources/For Teachers/Curriculum Supplements/Drug Abuse and Addiction. (National Institute of Health)
**http://science-education.nih.gov/homepage.nsf**

Follow links to Alcohol and Drug Facts for succinct information about many drugs of abuse.

Follow links to For Kids Only for educational activities for grade school children. (National Clearinghouse for Drug and Alcohol Information)
**http://www.health.org/**

*Mind Over Matter* is an eight-part series directed at children in Grades 5 to 9 regarding the brain's response to common drugs of abuse, complete with teacher's guide with activities, word finds, and so on. (National Institute on Drugs of Abuse)
**http://www.nida.nih.gov/MOM/MOMIndex.html**

Follow links to Teacher Information/Slide Teaching Packets for downloadable slides for classroom use.

Follow links to Sarah's Quest for interactive package on effects of common drugs of abuse. Requires "Flash" movie connection. (National Institute on Drugs of Abuse)
**http://www.nida.nih.gov/GoestoSchool/NIDAg2s.html**

Follow links to Drug Facts for web casts on "the rave," heroin, methamphetamine, and others. (Substance Abuse and Mental Health Services Administration)
**http://www.samhsa.gov/**

Lesson plans and curriculum guide for teachers of Grades 1 through 8. (Centre for Addiction and Mental Health, Ontario, Canada)
   **http://sano.camh.net/guide.htm**

Multiple other resources for teachers are listed and explained. Includes Web addresses, phone numbers, and e-mail addresses for obtaining these resources. All school-age groups are identified. (Centre for Addiction and Mental Health)
   **http://sano.camh.net/curricul/add.htm**

"Your Life: Your Choice" educational program for teaching young teens (13- and 14-year-olds) about the use of alcohol. Resource center, teacher's guide, and glossary included.
   **http://www.schoolnet.ca/alcohol/e/MainMenu/Index.html**

Web-based educational program for elementary school drug prevention (aimed primarily at prevention of smoking).
   **http://www.worldsfastestclown.com/**

Extensive links to resources and educational programs in many languages and countries. (Virtual Clearinghouse on Alcohol, Tobacco and Other Drugs)
   **http://www.atod.org/english/home.asp**

# APPENDIX 20.D

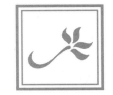

# Web Sites with General Information on Drugs of Abuse

Gives pertinent links for common drugs of abuse. Follow, as well, links to NIDA Research Report Series for pictures, information, and statistics regarding use of selected drugs of abuse. (National Institute on Drugs of Abuse)

  http://www.nida.nih.gov/DrugAbuse.html

Specific information and photographs on selected drugs of abuse. (Center for Substance Abuse Research)

  http://www.cesar.umd.edu/cesar/druginfo.asp

Links to resources and publications on a number of drugs of abuse, populations, topics, and so on. (Office of the National Drug Control Policy)

  http://www.whitehousedrugpolicy.gov/publications/index.html

Valuable information and pictures on numerous drugs of abuse. Follow particularly the links to Plants and Drugs. Links to Experiences are subjective users' accounts of using the particular substance.

  http://www.erowid.org/

Follow a variety of links for information and photographs about some drugs of abuse not included in other Web sites. (State of California Department of Justice)

  http://www.stopdrugs.org/

Information publications on a variety of drugs of abuse and trends in substance abuse. (City of Toronto, Ontario)

  http://www.city.toronto.on.ca/drugcentre/faxdrugs.htm

Excellent printable booklet with definitions and explanations of common terms used in addiction, law, and on the street. Chart of available substances of abuse, legal status, forms, effects, and so on. (Government of Canada)

  http://www.hc-sc.gc.ca

# SUGGESTED READING

Kieber, H. D. (1994). Our current approach to drug abuse—Progress, problems, proposals. *New England Journal of Medicine, 330,* 361–365.

Hogan, M. J. (2000). Diagnosis and treatment of teen drug use. *Medical Clinics of North America, 84*(4), 927–966.

Nelson, R. P., Brown, J. M., Brown, W. D., Koops, B. L., McInerny, T. K., Meurer, J. R., Minon, M. E., Werner, M. J., & Wright, J. A. (2001). Improving substance abuse prevention, assessment and treatment financing for children and adolescents. *Pediatrics, 108*(4), 794–798.

Schonberg, S. K. (Ed.). (1988). *Substance abuse: A guide for health professionals.* Elk Grove Village, IL: American Academy of Pediatrics, and Center for Advanced Health Studies.

U.S. National Institute on Drug Abuse. Statistical data on drug abuse among youth are updated and reported in various publications. The information can be obtained from the National Clearinghouse for Drug Abuse Information, P.O. Box 416, Kensington, MD 20795; 301/468-2600.

# REFERENCES

Adalf, E. M., Paglia, A., & Ivis, F. J. (1999). Drug use among Ontario students, 1977–1999. Toronto, Ontario: Centre for Addiction and Mental Health.

American Psychiatric Association. (2000). *Diagnostic and statistical manual of mental disorders* (4th ed.; text rev.). Washington, DC: Author.

Cloninger, C. R., Dinwiddie, S. H., & Reich, T. (1989). Epidemiology and genetics of alcoholism. *Annual Review of Psychiatry, 8,* 331–346.

Cox, B. M., Goldstein, A., & Nelson, W. T. (1984). Nicotine self-administration in rats. *British Journal of Pharmacology, 83,* 49–55.

DuRant, R. H., Rickert, V. I., Ashworth, C. S., Newman, C., & Slavens, G. (1993). Use of multiple drugs among adolescents who use anabolic steroids. *New England Journal of Medicine, 328,* 922–926.

Felts, W. M., Chenier, T., & Barnes, R. (1992). Drug use and suicide ideation and behavior among North Carolina public school students. *American Journal of Public Health, 82,* 870–872.

Fried, P. A., & Watkinson, B. (2001). Differential effects on facets of attention in adolescents prenatally exposed to cigarettes and marihuana. *Neurotoxicology and Teratology, 23,* 421–430.

Hibell, B., Andersson, B., Ahlström, S., Balakireva, O., Bjarnasson, T., Kokkevi, A., & Morgan, M. (1999). *The 1999 ESPAD report (European School Survey Project on Alcohol and Other Drugs): Alcohol and other drug use among students in 30 European countries.*

Stockholm: The Swedish Council for Information and Other Drugs, CAN Council of Europe, Cooperative Group to Combat Drug Abuse and Illicit Trafficking in Drugs.

Holden, C. (1991). Probing the complex genetics of alcoholism. *Science, 251,* 163–164.

Jacobs, E. A., Joffe, A., Knight, J. R., Kulig, J., Rogers, P. D., Boyd, G. M., Czechowicz, D., Simkin, D., Heyman, R. B., & Smith, K. (2001). Tobacco's toll: Implications for the pediatrician. *Pediatrics, 107*(4), 1025–1029.

Johnston, L. D., O'Malley, P. M., & Bachman, J. G. (2001). *Monitoring the Future national survey results on drug use: 1975–2000—Volume 1. Secondary School Students* (NIH Publication No. 01-4924). Bethesda, MD: National Institute on Drug Abuse. Available on-line at http://www.monitoringthefuture.org

Kandel, D., & Yamaguchi, K. (1993). From beer to crack: Developmental patterns of drug involvement. *American Journal of Public Health, 83,* 851–855.

Landfield, P. W., Cadwallader, L. B., & Vinsant, S. (1988). Quantitative changes in hippocampal structure following long-term exposure to delta 9-tetrahydrocannabinol: Possible mediation by glucocorticoid systems. *Brain Research, 443,* 47–62.

Langston, J. W., Ballard, P., Tetrud, J. W., & Irwin, I. (1983). Chronic parkinsonism in humans due to product of meperidine-analog synthesis. *Science, 219,* 979–980.

Lillie-Blanton, M., Anthony, J. C., & Schuster, C. (1993). Probing the meaning of racial/ethnic group comparisons in crack cocaine smoking. *Journal of the American Medical Association, 269,* 993–997.

Marzuk, P. M., Tardiff, K., Smyth, D., Stajic, M., & Leon, A. C. (1992). Cocaine use, risk taking, and fatal Russian roulette. *Journal of the American Medical Association, 267,* 2635–2637.

Mayes, L. C., Granger, R. H., Bornstein, M. H., & Zuckerman, B. (1992). The problem of prenatal cocaine exposure: A rush to judgment. *Journal of the American Medical Association, 267,* 406–408.

Myers, M. G., & Brown, S. A. (1994). Smoking and health in substance abusing adolescents: A two-year follow-up. *Pediatrics, 93,* 561–566.

Sivilotti, M. L. A., Burns, M. J., Aaron, C. K., & Greenberg, M. J. (2001). Pentobarbital for severe gamma-butyrolactone withdrawal. *Annals of Emergency Medicine, 38*(6), 660–665.

Substance Abuse and Mental Health Services Administration. (2000). Summary of findings from the 2000 National Household Survey on Drug Abuse. Retrieved from http://www.health.org/govstudy/nhsda2000/

United Nations Office for Drug Control and Crime Prevention (2000). World Drug Report 2000. Retrieved from http://www.undcp.org/world_drug_report.html

# CHAPTER 21

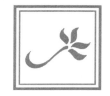

# Sexual Development, Function, and Consequences

## George D. Carson and Sheila L. Carson

During their school years, boys and girls will grow to sexual maturity. They must accept and adapt to these enormous physical changes while developing the attitudes and emotional maturity necessary for adult sexual functioning. Unfortunately, a large majority of these young people must accomplish these major tasks with a distressing lack of knowledge to prepare and help them. For example, the sources that teenage girls rely on for information are as follows: girlfriends, boyfriends, or sister (56%); mass media (51%); sex education classes (25%); and mother (15%) (King et al., 1989). Without even considering disease, it is obvious that much education is needed to allow the normal child to achieve a successful, realistic adult sexual role.

The range of normal variation in development is greater during adolescence than at any other time of life (Tanner, 1962), yet adolescents have a great desire and need to conform to their peers. Tolerance of normal variations is thus low and departures from average may arouse intense concern. The problem is accentuated by the necessity to undress in front of classmates before and after physical education classes, when comparisons of development will be made. Such disrobing often starts at the particularly sensitive time of adolescence. In boys or girls who will eventually be of identical development, a delay of a year or two in the initiation of puberty can be devastating at the time. Knowledge made available from an authoritative, sympathetic source can be invaluable (Grant, 2001). Schools might consider having disrobing become part of the school routine at an earlier, less sensitive age.

Although the preparation of girls for pubertal changes may be poor, it is generally better than that of boys. Because menstruation is a dramatic milestone of maturity, girls usually receive some sex education in school.

Despite concerns about teenage pregnancy, schools and parents may not be giving boys the sex education they need to make them equally responsible. Boys not only may be ignorant about their own development, but may be totally lacking in information about female development. In seeking information, they are likely to receive and incorporate misinformation. Those who advise students should remember that behaviors considered appropriate for the present generation may be different than for previous generations. The factors enumerated by Vincent in 1970 remain valid: (a) our society is undergoing rapid social change, (b) parents and their children are never born at the same time (this is also true, of course, for teachers and students), and (c) the behavior appropriate for a given age is usually learned at that age.

The text that follows outlines normal sexual development and function, some common disorders and their management, and the consequences of sexual activity. It includes a consideration of appropriate roles for teachers and schools in assisting students to learn about their sexuality. A Suggested Reading list is provided at the end of the chapter for readers who want to read more on the topic.

# SEXUAL DIFFERENTIATION

Physiologically speaking, there are at least three mechanisms by which sexual differentiation is expressed: chromosomal, gonadal, and phenotypic (or body appearance). At the time of conception, each human receives 23 chromosomes from each parent, consisting of one of each of the 22 pairs of ordinary chromosomes (called autosomes) and one from the single pair of sex chromosomes, X or Y, which together make up the adult complement of chromosomes (see Chapter 7). All normal females have two Xs and all normal males have an X and a Y. Gender is determined by the sex chromosome received from the father—an X for a female and a Y for a male. From the creation of the fertilized egg, the chromosomal sex thus is determined. Very early in the development of the embryo, a few cells are segregated to become the entire stock of germ cells—those that will give origin to all the eggs or all the sperms—for that individual. These cells migrate into the gonad on the back wall of the developing embryo and direct the gonads to become ovaries if the germ cells are XX or testes if the germ cells are XY. In the male fetus, the testes are stimulated to function and produce both the male sex hormone testosterone and a locally acting substance that causes regression of the structures that otherwise would give origin to the uterus, fallopian tubes, and upper vagina. The testosterone causes the external phallus and labial–scrotal folds to form a penis, scrotum, and other male structures. In the absence of fetal testicular function, development is that of a normal female. The result of the chromosomal sex–causing male or female gonadal development is the direction of subsequent development of the internal and external genitalia as male or female.

Puberty is a process of activation of sexual functioning by an increase in hormone production by the pituitary gland, which stimulates the gonads and causes an increase in estrogen and progesterone from the ovaries or testosterone from the testes. The hormonal stimulation of the gonads also causes ovulation or spermatogenesis.

A control axis exists in men and women that involves the hypothalamus (a part of the brain that forms the floor and lateral wall of the third ventricle), the pituitary gland, and the gonad (ovaries or testes). Gonadal hormones feed back upon the controlling axis and exert other diverse effects. The hypothalamus makes a substance called *gonadotrophin releasing hormone* (GnRH) that travels by local blood vessels to the pituitary gland at the base of the brain. Stimulated by GnRH, the pituitary manufactures two gonadotrophins (*trophine* means "stimulus" in Greek) that act upon the ovary or testes. These gonadotrophins are *luteinizing hormone* (LH), which causes production of hormones, and *follicular stimulating hormone* (FSH), which activates germ cell development. In the ovary, the eggs exist in small cysts called *follicles*—thus the name of the hormone that stimulates them. FSH also acts on the cells in the tubules of the testes that produce sperm.

## Female

In the female, the ovary is a source of the female hormones estrogen and progesterone, as well as the source of eggs. The primordial germ cells divide to produce the entire stock of eggs that a woman will ever have by age 5 months of fetal life. Each egg within the ovary is surrounded by cells able to produce hormones, and the combination is a *follicle unit.* These units lie dormant until activated at puberty by rising gonadotrophins. Thereafter, every day a cohort of follicle units start development. If the correct pattern (described later) of gonadotrophins is encountered, one of these follicles proceeds to ovulation and the possibility of fertilization. In any case, a number of eggs in their follicular units are used up daily. Efficient hormone production can occur only if the hormone-producing cells are arranged around a potential egg in a follicle. When all the follicles are expended, pregnancy can no longer occur and hormone production is also reduced; this time of decline of ovarian function is the *climacteric*, and the cessation of menstruation at that time is known as *menopause*.

An egg will develop to be ready for ovulation only if it is stimulated by FSH. When gonadotrophins rise, FSH causes follicles to develop. An egg prepares for ovulation while the surrounding cells under the influence of LH make ever-increasing amounts of estrogen, the female hormone that stimulates the uterine lining. Although a constant secretion of estrogen would suppress GnRH, if the hypothalamus perceives a sufficiently great concentration of estrogen in a rising pattern, there is an overriding secretion of GnRH that results in a surge of LH, which causes ovulation. Sufficient maturity of the hypothalamus is necessary for this to occur. The released egg now is fertilizable by sperm and survives for 24 hours. After ovulation, the cells remaining from the follicle continue to make estrogen and also release into the circulation the other female hormone, progesterone. Progesterone also acts on the uterine lining to cause it to be ready for implantation of the egg, if it is fertilized. The new hormone-producing structure formed from the follicle after ovulation is called a *corpus luteum*. Unless there is a pregnancy, the corpus luteum functions for a very predictable 14 days and then stops functioning. The resulting decline in the hormone levels leads to the death of the superficial layers of uterine lining, which slough off and are expelled as the menstrual discharge. The cycle then repeats, with an average length between bleeding episodes of 28 days. Several implications follow from these facts about the menstrual cycle:

1. A woman is most fertile during the 24 hours just after the egg has been released. This is always 14 days before menstruation (i.e., Day 14 of a 28-day cycle, counting Day 1 as the first day of menstruation). Many women normally have cycles of quite constant length that may be shorter or longer than 28 days. This difference is always the result of variation in the time spent in follicular development; the period of 14 days from ovulation to menstruation remains constant. In a regular 34-day cycle, for example, the day of ovulation would be Day 20. Because sperm may survive for up to 3 days in the woman after intercourse, the time when a pregnancy is most likely to occur after intercourse extends from 3 days before ovulation to 1 day after. In women who ovulate but have an irregular cycle, the day that is 14 days before bleeding cannot be reliably predicted.

2. In cycles where ovulation does not occur, there is no formation of a corpus luteum and therefore no progesterone. The uterine lining does not receive the normal hormone effect. The interval between bleeds and the amount of bleeding on any one occasion are unpredictable and irregular, but the uterine lining still breaks down. These anovulatory cycles happen when some part of the hypothalamus–pituitary–ovarian axis fails to function normally. The abnormal bleeding is merely a manifestation of the endocrine abnormality; there is nothing intrinsically wrong with the uterus. Malfunction of the axis is most likely to occur just after puberty or before menopause. The hypothalamus takes a little time to mature and become capable of sending out the correct signals. The first few cycles after menarche (the first vaginal bleeding) are commonly anovulatory and irregular. Ovulation and cycle regularity usually follow menarche after a few months, but some teenagers continue to have anovulation and irregular (called *dysfunctional*) bleeding. Regular hormone administration, most conveniently given as the estrogen and progesterone in a birth control pill, will almost always regulate the cycle and control the bleeding.

3. Release of substances called prostaglandins when the endometrium is breaking down can cause uterine contractions, which can cause painful cramps (i.e., *dysmenorrhea*). Drugs called prostaglandin synthetase inhibitors (e.g., indomethacin or ibuprofen) can block prostaglandin production and substantially reduce the pain. Use of birth control pills also substantially reduces dysmenorrhea in most users.

4. The administration of a constant amount of hormones—for example, through birth control pills—will feed back on the hypothalamus and suppress GnRH, which in turn means there will be little FSH or LH and no stimulation of hormone production by the ovary. Because hormone production and egg production are inextricably linked in the ovary, ovulation does not occur either, so conception cannot happen. The administered hormones will cause the uterine lining to grow, however. When the pill is discontinued at the end of a cycle, the hormones are withdrawn and bleeding occurs. Because the hormone effect of the pill upon the uterine lining is usually a little less than that of the hormones produced by the ovary, the bleeding is often scantier than in spontaneous cycling.

## Male

In the male, the sex hormone testosterone is produced when cells scattered through the testes are stimulated by LH. Rising levels of testosterone inhibit the hypothalamus and, thus, the pituitary LH production, so a steady state with a fairly constant amount of testosterone is achieved. This steady state is similar to the constant temperature in a home with a furnace regulated by a thermostat. Sperm are produced by cells in a very large number of small tubules, called *semeniferous tubules,* that make up most of the substance of the testes. The exact regulation of sperm production is unclear but appears to involve stimulation by FSH. The sperm-producing cells continually renew themselves and produce millions of sperm each day after the hormones rise at puberty. The sperm mature over about 60 days in the tubes within the testes and in a complex coiled tube beside the testes called the *epididymis.* Sperm development requires a temperature lower than internal body temperatures; thus the testes must be in the scrotum. Sperm travel to the outside along a tube called the *vas deferens,* which runs from the epididymis to the urethra just below the bladder. Several glands, the function of which is stimulated by testosterone, empty into the vas deferens. Their secretions, together with the sperm, make up the seminal fluid. An implication of the separate localization and regulation of sperm and testosterone production in the testes is that hormone administration by pills to men will not entirely stop sperm production. Therefore, a "pill" for men has not been feasible so far.

# SEXUAL MATURATION—PUBERTY

Although sexual development is continuous starting in infancy, the most dramatic events occur at puberty. Puberty is a process spanning several years during which the child achieves adult mature physical capability and must develop the emotional and attitudinal changes to correspond. In childhood, the hypothalamus is very sensitive to tiny quantities of the sex hormones estrogen or testosterone, which inhibit GnRH effectively. Thus, the pituitary is not stimulated and neither are the gonads. Puberty occurs when the sensitivity of the hypothalamus is markedly reduced. GnRH rises, FSH and LH are stimulated, and the ovaries or testes are driven to produce increased quantities of hormones. These hormones produce effects on all the body tissues with a capacity to respond to them in a predictable sequence according to the relative sensitivity of these tissues. The changes include actions upon specific parts of the reproductive tract, such as the uterus or the penis, as well as parts of the body not specifically connected with reproduction, such as subcutaneous fat in women or the larynx (thus affecting the voice) in men.

The cause of the reduction in hypothalamic sensitivity that initiates sexual maturity is not known. A persuasive theory relates the onset of puberty to the attainment of a critical body weight or, more particularly, a critical body fat mass. Because unregulated hormone metabolism does occur in fat, the achievement of a sufficient amount of fat would raise the body hormone concentration and change the environment of the hypothalamus, perhaps activating it. Menarche, or the first menstrual bleeding, is a remarkable single event marking a stage of sexual maturity in women. The mean age of menarche has fallen significantly, from about age 16 in the early 1800s to 12.5 years at present in North America and Western Europe (Anderson, Dallal, & Must, 2003). This change has coincided with an equally remarkable increase in mean body weight, attributed to improved nutrition, and thus a reduction in the age at which the critical body mass is attained.

No single dramatic event like menarche serves as a marker and facilitates studies of males. However, a recent study suggests that the early stages of pubertal development are commencing at increasingly young ages and that boys are bigger and heavier than previously. On the other hand, the attainment of completion of the pubertal process appears to be staying at the same age as previously (Reiter & Lee, 2001).

## Female

The rising levels of estrogen cause changes as outlined in Table 21.1. The extreme sensitivity of the breast to small amounts of estrogen causes it to be almost invariably the first tissue to respond. An action by estrogen upon the adrenal gland causes it to make more androgen (male sex hormone), which is responsible for some of the effects on hair growth and skin, including secretions from the sebaceous glands, which often result in acne. After several years, the process of sexual maturation is complete and regular ovulatory cycles occur.

## Male

Activation of testosterone production by the testes begins about 8 to 10 years of age and, as in females, the rising concentrations of sex steroids produce a reliable sequence of changes, according to the relative sensitivity of the various target tissues. Some of these effects are outlined in Table 21.2. Body

**TABLE 21.1**
Events at Puberty in Females

| Event | Age (in Years) |
| --- | --- |
| Breast development | 8–13, average 11 (precedes pubic hair by 2–3 months) |
| Pubic hair | 8–14, taking 4 years to complete |
| Growth in height | Growth spurt starts: 9–11<br>Adult height attained: 17–18 |
| Axillary hair | 12–14 |
| Subcutaneous fat deposition | 11–16 |
| Menarche | Average: 12.8<br>Range: 10–15 |

Note. From *Growth of Adolescents*, by J. N. Tanner, 1962, Oxford, England: Blackwell.

**TABLE 21.2**
Events at Puberty in Males

| Event | Age (in Years) |
| --- | --- |
| Penile enlargement | 8–12 |
| Scrotal and testicular enlargement | 10–14 |
| Pubic hair | 10–14 |
| Axillary hair | 12–16 |
| Facial hair | 15–18 |
| Growth spurt begins | 12–15 |
| Adult height attained | 18–21 |
| Mature spermatozoa | 14 |
| First ejaculate | 11–16, average 14 |
| Nocturnal emissions | 11–16 |

Note. From *Growth of Adolescents*, by J. N. Tanner, 1962, Oxford, England: Blackwell.

configuration changes markedly but unevenly. This results in the awkwardness of adolescence as the arms and legs grow faster than the trunk, and facial features change. Muscle mass increases, and the larynx grows and changes the pitch of the voice, but often with embarrassing inconsistency during the transition. Wide variation exists in the age of onset of the changes in size and secondary sexual manifestations, even in those who eventually attain identical adult height and weight. Enlargement of and the size of the penis are often of concern, and several myths exist. In fact, total body size and size of the genitalia do not correlate. Further, the size of the flaccid penis (normally 2.9 to 4.5 in. long) correlates poorly with erect size. In any case, sexual proficiency is not related to penile size, since the vagina accommodates to the size of the penis. However fallacious, the myths and their consequences persist, may be worrisome, and should be dispelled.

## SEXUAL RESPONSE

In both genders, the essential elements of the response to sexual stimulation are similar, and are described by Masters and Johnson (1966) in four stages; excitement, plateau, orgasmic, and resolution. In women, either psychic or physical stimuli initiate excitement, manifested by vascular engorgement of the labia and clitoris, with congestion and enlargement, and passage of fluid across the vaginal skin. Lubrication due to secretion of local glands also occurs. Similar congestion in the internal pelvic organs occurs. The changes are accentuated in the plateau stage. Local physical stimulation then activates a reflex with a series of contractions of the pelvic muscles in the orgasmic phase, so that single or multiple orgasms may normally be realized. Resolution of the congestion then follows, although this may take 2 or 3 hours. In the absence of orgasm, the process is slower and some generalized ache in the pelvis may occur after sexual arousal.

In the male, psychic or tactile stimulation also leads to the excitement stage, resulting in distention with blood (about 30 ml) of the spongy tissue making up the penis, and thus erection occurs. Congestion of pelvic organs and testes accompany this stage and, if prolonged, result in local aching and discomfort, but with no long-term damaging result. Further stimulation leads to the plateau phase, with additional penile enlargement and secretion of a few drops of material from the urethra. This may contain active sperm capable of fertilization and accounts for the failure of attempted contraception by withdrawal or by placement of a condom just before ejaculation. Additional local stimulation leads to secretions into the urethra. Waves of contraction of pelvic muscles then cause expulsion of the semen, which is ejaculation. (In sleep, secreted semen may simply flow out as a nocturnal emission, or "wet dream," without the local stimulation and contractions of ejaculation.) In the final phase of resolution, blood flow to the penis is constricted and loss of erection occurs.

# SEXUAL FUNCTION ABNORMALITIES

## Timing

Variations in timing of the pubertal events previously described are the most commonly perceived abnormalities. Usually the variations are all within the range of normal, but they may cause an individual to look and feel different from his or her peers. Sexual development before age 8 in girls or 10 in boys, or delay of such development until after age 15, is clearly abnormal and requires evaluation by a physician (see Chapter 4).

## Gender Growth Differences

As Tables 21.1 and 21.2 show, growth in body size begins earlier and stops earlier in girls than in boys. Failure to recognize their young chronological age may lead others to have inappropriate expectations of physically large and sexually mature young girls. Girls and boys in their early teens vary markedly in physical maturity; at 13 or 14 years of age, girls are usually larger than boys. By age 15, the heights are about equal, and by 20, the average male is 5 inches taller than the average female. This may be little consolation to a 13- or 14-year-old boy, however.

## Dysmenorrhea

At least half of all girls have significant pain associated with menstruation, and a quarter may be temporarily disabled by the pain. Many myths surround dysmenorrhea, but the cause is now known. When ovulatory periods are established (which explains why the first few anovulatory periods are usually painless), the breakdown of the uterine lining causes production of prostaglandins. These powerful substances may cause intense, painful contractions of the uterus, as well as stimulation of the gastrointestinal tract, producing nausea, cramps, diarrhea, or a combination of these. One should evaluate the intensity of the pain by its effect on the girl's behavior. If she misses activities in which she would ordinarily participate, it is certainly serious. Therapy can include drugs taken just before menstruation to inhibit the formation of prostaglandins. For sexually active teenagers, the birth control pill, which inhibits ovulation, is also effective therapy, with obvious additional benefits.

## Anovulatory Bleeding

In the years just after puberty, immaturity of the hypothalamus results in failure to attain regular ovulatory cycles, as discussed earlier. The irregular, unpredictable bleeding is both troublesome and worrisome for many girls. The affected girls can and should be reassured that regular cycling will soon be attained and that normal adult reproductive capability can be expected. Less than 2% of women fail to attain ovulatory cycles. Some girls will need medical treatment, however, to limit blood loss and regularize the cycle for a short time. For them, medical therapy to cause ovulation to occur is usually simple and effective.

## Psychogenic Amenorrhea

A variety of emotional stresses may interfere with the normal regulation of ovarian function by suppressing the release of hormones from the hypothalamus. Delay or absence of menstruation (amenorrhea) will result, and worry about this will compound the problem. If an obvious transient stress, such as an upcoming examination, can be identified, reassurance can be offered. Of course, one must consider the possibility of pregnancy.

## Athletes and Amenorrhea

Many females who participate in strenuous exercise programs will be amenorrheic. This may be the result of a reduction in body weight, in particular body fat, below the levels that initiated puberty. Vigorous exercise also increases stress-related hormones and suppresses gonadotrophins, causing amenorrhea. Whatever the cause, the condition is temporary. Menstruation will resume when the degree of training lessens, and fertility is not impaired. Explanations are usually sufficient, and lack of periods may be regarded as a benefit by some. Parenthetically, amenorrhea is not a contraindication to physical activity and does not reduce performance capability.

## Anorexia Nervosa

Anorexia nervosa, a complex emotional disorder, is characterized by strong aversion to food, with lack of eating and sometimes self-induced vomiting. Accompanying the marked weight loss is a cessation of menstruation. The affected individuals often are concerned about being obese, although their initial weight is most often not excessive. The emotional impetus appears to be a desire to control their bodies or to eliminate the frightening (to them) changes of sexual maturity. Extensive professional treatment is needed (see Chapter 19).

## Gynecomastia

About one third of pubertal males have some degree of breast enlargement involving one or both breasts, known as gynecomastia. Increasing estrogen, the result of stimulation of the gonads, results in a firm, tender plaque of 0.5 to 1 in. in diameter, which lasts 1 to 2 years. This almost always subsides spontaneously.

## Acne

At puberty, the increased androgens in males and females stimulate the sebaceous glands to produce sebum. This supports a bacterium, the products of which can be locally irritating and may produce visible lesions, called acne. About 85% of high school students will be afflicted, although the spectrum of the lesions is very wide. The hormonal changes cannot be eliminated (and one would not want to do so); therefore, treatment, if any, must be local. In females, use of a birth control pill causes favorable hormonal changes and usually reduces acne. Reassurance may be found from the fact that, by their 20s, the condition will have spontaneously resolved in 90% of affected adults.

# SEXUAL BEHAVIOR

## Abstinence

Many teenagers, pressured by peers or their own expectations toward a sexual relationship, need to know that it is okay to say no. No physical or emotional harm has come to anyone by choosing not to have teenage intercourse. In our concern about teenage sexuality and its consequences, the large numbers of teens not having intercourse have been neglected. Because nearly half of high school students are having intercourse, it follows that half are not. A student can be reassured that he or she is not the only virgin in the class. Only abstinence is 100% effective for the avoidance of both pregnancy and sexually transmissible disease.

Having long-term educational or vocational aspirations is the most common characteristic associated with abstinence. Practice of abstinence need not preclude the establishment of relations with peers that acknowledge sexuality. Activities that do not include vaginal intercourse and alternatives such as "outercourse" may be advocated not as activities necessarily leading to intercourse, but rather as alternatives that can provide sexual satisfaction while permitting and indeed contributing to a delay in the initiation of sexual intercourse.

Teenage girls are often pressured to declare their independence and maturity by engaging in intercourse. In fact, it may be much more independent and liberated to conclude and state, "I am not ready for a sexual component of a relationship and I shall say no." This kind of thinking and decision should be supported. Failure to maintain abstinence, failure to use contraception, and exploitive sex often occur during alcohol or drug use. Teenagers must be made aware of these possibilities.

In support of abstinence, each teenager should be urged to determine his or her limits and, if there is a partner, to discuss these limits in advance. The teenager must say "no" emphatically so that the partner is clear about the decision. High-risk sexual situations should be avoided. In case of a change of mind, the teenager needs to have previous knowledge about contraception, and access to condoms or other protection. Abstinence should be welcomed as normal, common, and acceptable.

## Heterosexual Intercourse

Increasing numbers of teenagers are using their normal physical capabilities and engaging in sexual intercourse. The occurrence of sexual activity at younger ages is increasing, particularly in middle-class teenagers. The average age at which Americans first have sex has been declining, with sex before marriage becoming the norm (National Institute of Child Health and Human Development [NICHHD], 1993; O'Donnell, M'yint-U, O'Donnell, & Stueve, 2003). Perspective may be gained, however, from the fact that 200 years ago, fully one third of brides in Massachusetts confessed "fornication" to their ministers.

All students pass through puberty and the attainment of physical sexual maturity during the ages when they are in school. Many begin their sexual activity, and many of these do not—or at least do not consistently—protect themselves against the consequences of unintended pregnancy or sexually transmitted diseases. King et al. (1989) found that 31% of males and 21% of females in Grade 9 had had intercourse at least once (7% and 6%, respectively, did so "often") and 49% of males and 46% of females had had intercourse by Grade 11 (16% and 21%, respectively, did so "often"). Curiosity (19%), love (17%), and physical attraction (28%) were the reasons for first intercourse given by males, whereas love, at 52%, was the principal reason given by females, followed by curiosity (15%) and physical attraction (9%). For 6% of males and females, drugs and alcohol were a reason for first intercourse. The higher the educational aspirations of the high school respondents, the less likely they were to have engaged in sexual intercourse. Of those who had intercourse often, only 14% always used a condom and more than a quarter never used a condom.

In the United States (Henshaw & VanVort, 1989), 45% of female teenagers have premarital sexual intercourse and most are not consistent contraceptive users. Therefore, about 40% of female adolescents become pregnant at least once and 20% bear a child. Fewer than 5% of these give the child up for adoption. More than 80% of the children in families headed by 15- to 21-year-old females are poor. Rates of adolescent premarital sexual activity are higher among African Americans than Hispanics or Whites,

**TABLE 21.3**

Reasons for First Teenage Intercourse

| Reasons | Male | Female |
|---------|------|--------|
| Sexual drive | 48% | 16% |
| Love | 10% | 42% |
| Curiosity | 25% | 13% |

particularly under age 18. African American and Hispanic teens are less likely to use contraception or to have abortions, so adolescent childbearing is 2.5 times higher among African Americans and twice as high in Hispanics as in Whites (Lawson & Rhode, 1993).

For both males and females, the motivation for engaging in intercourse may be broadly defined as "permissiveness with affection." Teenagers believe (with considerable justice) that adults envisage that they are having intercourse solely for physical pleasure; teens themselves are likely to believe that the whole relationship is important. Significant differences between male and female attitudes remain, however. Frequently, each gender does not understand the motivation of the other. The difference is obvious in the reasons for the first teenage intercourse as listed in Table 21.3.

The male has learned to experience physical sexual pleasure and has probably ejaculated since shortly after puberty, by masturbation. His sex drive is high, and his lifetime peak is at age 16 to 18 years. His interest, therefore, is largely physical. The female usually initially experiences orgasm with intercourse or noncoital sex. She more often requires a belief in a relationship and perhaps an aura of fantasy to achieve sexual response. Her capabilities will continue to develop, not peaking until her mid-20s. As a teenager, she may be "in love with love" and may have uninformed ideas of all this implies; however, her earlier age of physical development conveys the impression of an emotional maturity that she may not yet have attained. The code of permissible behavior for their peers in general is more liberal than that which individuals or couples hold for themselves. Teens often practice serial monogamy. A relationship may be regarded by them as long term, established, and warranting sexual activity after a few weeks or a month.

Sexual expression is a part of normal development. Surrounded as they are by the blatant sexuality of our society in advertising and public entertainment, and given their own physical capabilities, some sexual activity by teenagers is almost inevitable. A survey by Whitehead (1994) found that sexual expression is common in serial monogamous relationships, with some emotional commitment and affection in most of these relationships. In at least some cases, the nonmarital sexual experience confers benefit by meeting physical demands while allowing continued emotional and intellectual growth until each individual is ready for a long-term relationship with someone. Others benefit from practicing restraint. No one answer serves all.

For a teenager to engage in sexual activity and avoid an unintended pregnancy or a sexually transmitted disease, several things must be accomplished. He or she must accept being sexual, must want to and know how to reduce the risk of the adverse consequences, and must be able to put the plan into effect. This includes planning for abstinence or noncontact sexual activity, or intercourse. This must be negotiated and agreed upon with a partner. If intercourse is going to occur, the preventive activities (e.g., birth control pill use, use of a condom) must be performed both in preparation for intercourse and at the time.

Sexual interest is heightened by the pervasive use of positive sexual images in advertising and in movies and television. The latter rarely show adverse consequences or the use of prevention methods. In North America, ambivalence results from persisting attitudes that sexual activity is wrong or inappropriate for teenagers. Many teenagers thus are uncomfortable about sex. They are too uncomfortable to prepare for it, but often not uncomfortable enough not to do it. Clearly, acceptance of the widely prevalent adolescent sexual activity (which is not going to stop) must precede consideration of how to increase the probability that the participants will avoid adverse consequences.

## Sexual Dysfunction

With increasing public knowledge that many teenagers are sexually active comes the recognition of problems associated with that activity. Sexual activity conducted with immaturity or ignorance is unlikely to be pleasurable. Forty-eight percent of males and 30% of females reported that their first coitus was pleasurable, but 25% of females and 10% of males reported shame or guilt following that experience (Sprecher, Barbee, & Schwartz, 1995).

The partners must be able to communicate and must have realistic expectations. Males with unrealistic ideas about the female orgasm, for example, will not have these expectations met and will be dissatisfied with the experience. When questioned, many teenage females define *virility* as "caring" and "decent" and not as a capacity for genital prowess; however, teenage males often think that prowess is what is wanted and expected of them. Obviously, these teens should talk to each other and should be encouraged to do so.

In males, premature ejaculation is the most common dysfunction. It may be related to hurried teen sex, but if it continues, it represents a disregard for the partner's needs. Discussion about, recognition of, and accommodation to the pace of each partner's sexual response should resolve the difficulty. Impotence is rare in teen males but may result from anxiety, guilt, or unrealistic expectations about performance. In females, there may be lack of orgasm. In fact, some teenage females are orgasmic but do not realize it because their experience does not conform to sensational expectations. Accusations between the partners then worsen the situation. Teenagers, like everyone else, need to know that mutually pleasurable sexual functioning is learned behavior and it takes time and practice to learn. With elimination of fears of inadequacy and enhanced confidence, and partners who can communicate, this difficulty can be resolved.

## Noncoital Sex

There is a succession of actions tending toward intercourse, including kissing, breast fondling, active and passive genital stimulation, and genital apposition. Carried to the extent of orgasm, or petting to climax, these activities can afford enjoyment without coitus. Only if one regards the only acceptable sexual expression as vaginal intercourse for procreation can these activities not find a role. By age 18 years, well over half of males will have experienced active and passive genital stimulation with a partner, whereas half of females will have had passive genital stimulation and nearly half will have had active genital stimulation. In the progression of a couple's sexual expression, it most commonly is the female who sets the limits, and the male accepts them because he "respects his partner" or believes she will refuse further advances.

It has been argued that noncoital sex will encourage intercourse. The alternative viewpoint is that if noncoital activity is carried to orgasm, it may be sufficiently satisfying for intercourse to be avoided. The couple does need to know that semen deposited near the vaginal opening may, in rare cases, cause a pregnancy. Mutual masturbation or petting to orgasm may beneficially avoid the risk of pregnancy and sexually transmitted disease; thus, such activities may have a useful role in adolescent sexual expression.

## Masturbation

Probably no activity has been as uniformly condemned—and as uniformly practiced—as masturbation. Physical, mental, and moral degeneracies all have been claimed to result from this behavior, and biblical prohibitions have been widely proclaimed. In fact, even where there are enormous pressures against the act, nearly all males (more than 98%) and more than three quarters of women masturbated, according to Semmens and Krantz (1970; see also Gates & Sonenstein, 2000). It is now known that masturbation itself does no harm, although fear or worry about it may be detrimental.

Because masturbation was not discussed with the healthy population, studies were once done in which only those who were institutionalized were observed. Many of them masturbated, sometimes openly, and it was concluded that masturbation caused their diseases. Now we know that, although disturbed persons may masturbate frequently, it is a result, not a cause, of their condition.

It is not physiologically possible to masturbate too much. The actual frequency varies widely, and some males may masturbate more in a week than others do in a year. Most people do not consider their own frequency—whether it is once a week or four times a day—excessive but believe any frequency greater than their own may have ill effects. The age of beginning to masturbate varies. Infants, exploring their own bodies, may masturbate, and boys can have pleasurable sensations without ejaculation before puberty.

Most males will have experienced their first ejaculation through masturbation. They learn how to produce their own sexual pleasure through this means but may acquire expectations about a rapid pace of sexual response that are inappropriate when they attempt heterosexual intercourse. Although there have been concerns that the solitary nature of masturbation may adversely affect sexual function of a couple, women who have masturbated are in fact more likely to achieve orgasm from intercourse during the first year after beginning intercourse than those who did not masturbate. Masturbation is now recognized as a common, harmless, and pleasurable part of sexual expression.

## Homosexuality

The determination of sexual orientation is complex and multifactorial. With the rise in hormones and consequently of sexual interest in adolescence, the expression of sexual orientation is one of the critical developmental tasks. When that orientation is toward the same sex or when an adolescent is uncertain about his or her sexual orientation, there are significant additional stressors.

Sexual orientation is the persistent pattern of physical and emotional attraction to members of the same or opposite sex. It includes sexual fantasy, emotional attraction, and sexual behavior, as well as self-identification and self-affiliation. Homosexuality is a persistent pattern of same-sex arousal. *Gay* is a term referring to homosexual males and *lesbian* a term for homosexual females. *Bisexuality* refers to attraction to both genders.

Estimates of the prevalence of homosexuality were provided in the 1940s and 1950s by Kinsey and others, who reported that 37% of adult men and 13% of adult women had at least one homosexual experience resulting in orgasm. These studies have been criticized as being nonrepresentative, and more recent studies are considered more accurate. In samples from the United States, the United Kingdom, and France, between 16% and 21% of men and about 18% of women reported homosexual attraction or behavior after the age of 15 years. In the same study in the same countries, same-sex sexual behavior in the preceding 5 years had occurred in 4.5% to 10.7% of men and 2.1% to 3.6% of women. Adolescent sexual orientation was studied in a large sample of junior and senior high school students. Only 1.1% of these students considered themselves predominantly homosexual or bisexual. Homosexual experiences increased in prevalence from 0.4% of 12-year-old boys to 2.8% of 18-year-old boys and was constant at 0.9% among girls. About one quarter of 12-year-olds were uncertain about their sexual orientation. This uncertainty declined with increasing age and increasing sexual experience to be only 5% among 18-year-olds. As the students became more certain of their sexual orientation, either homosexual or heterosexual, most reported that, in restrospect, they had felt that orientation from an age before puberty (Telljohann & Price, 1993).

*Heterosexism* is the assumption that heterosexuality is the only norm. *Homophobia*, a perception of homosexuality characterized by fear or hatred, may be manifested by stereotyping, prejudice, or discomfort. Some individuals with homophobia overtly express their negative attitudes. Exposure to such negative attitudes can lead to an internalized homophobia in gay or lesbian youth. Such attitudes among homosexual adolescents impair social, emotional, and physical health and lead to risk-taking in sexual and other behavior.

The cause or causes of homosexuality have been extensively debated. Whether the origins of this behavior are biological or social is much contested, and the origin of homosexuality in which one believes may serve to create or sustain attitudes toward homosexual individuals. Human behavior, of course, is complicated, and a single cause for any behavior is unlikely.

Homosexuality is clustered in some families. Twin studies show greater concordance of homosexuality among identical (monozygotic) twins than fraternal (dizygotic) twins, with concordant rates about 50% for monozygotic twins and 20% for dizygotic twins (Kendler, Thorton, Gilman, & Kessler, 2000). Some markers on the X chromosome have been identified; however, because many homosexual identical twins have heterosexual identical twins, sexual orientation cannot be directed exclusively by genetic factors, although they are powerful. After developing the ability to measure sex hormone levels, researchers turned to speculation that these might determine sexual orientation. In fact, there is no difference in sex steroid levels between heterosexual and homosexual adults (Banks & Gartrell, 1995). Lowering sex hormone levels results in reduced sexual drive and raising the levels results in increased sexual drive, but the direction of sexual orientation is unchanged. Researchers also have sought evidence of differences in brain structure or function of homosexual and heterosexual individuals. Preliminary work suggests that there may be differences in the size of one of the nuclei in the hypothalamus. Differences in brain organization also have been postulated, but researchers have not established whether such differences clearly exist and, if they do, whether they are the cause or the effect of sexual orientation (Zhou, Hofman, Gooren, & Swaab, 1995).

No differences have been found in the family or socioeconomic backgrounds of homosexual versus heterosexual men or women (Bell, Weinberg, & Hammersmith, 1991). Although biological differences are established, the expression of homosexual orientation must reflect interaction of the individual with experience in his or her environment. Thus, an integrated model recognizing a biological basis and many determining factors of sexual orientation and behaviors seems most plausible.

External homophobia, as expressed by groups within the school, may be internalized by individuals with either homosexual orientation or uncertainty about their orientation. Therefore, the school should include as a goal the support of normal development, which means acceptance of the integration of each adolescent's own sexual orientation, achievement of social and emotional well-being, and physical health. The best way to prevent adverse outcomes is to maintain a supportive environment, because rejection poses the greatest damage to the adolescent. The adolescents also need to accept their own beliefs and values, and have acceptance of parents and friends. Parents and others may receive support from the National Federation of Parents and Friends of Lesbians and Gays (P-FLAG; http://www.pflag.org).

A study of high school students in a northern California school district found that 6% identified themselves as gay, lesbian, or bisexual, and an additional 13% were unsure of their sexual orientation. Both of these groups were more likely than heterosexual teens to be uncomfortable with their sexual orientation. More general and mental health problems are encountered with minority sexual orientation, especially when individuals are uncomfortable with their orientation. The occurrence of significant problems in gay and lesbian students relates not to inherent psychopathology, but to their reaction to homophobia. Homosexual youth are more likely than heterosexual youth to attempt and complete suicide. Students may fear discovery, assault, and humiliation in school, which can make it a punishing environment that contributes to their dropping out and underachieving. With an increased likelihood of family rejection after revealing their sexual orientation, homosexual youth are at risk of running away and living in the streets. This results in increased high-risk behaviors, such as substance abuse, sexual abuse, theft, and prostitution (Lock & Steiner, 1999).

High-risk sexual behavior is unfortunately common among homosexual adolescents. After a decline attributed to practice of safe sex techniques, there has been a recent increase in the prevalence in human immunodeficiency virus (HIV) and acquired immunodeficiency syndrome (AIDS) (Hogg et al., 2001). Unprotected receptive anal intercourse is the most dangerous practice for males. Lesbians who only have homosexual behavior are less likely than other sexually active teenagers to acquire sexually transmitted diseases (STDs). For those who have heterosexual relations as a result of being uncertain about orientation or in stages of denial of homosexual orientation, pregnancy and STD prevention must be considered.

The overall goals and aspirations for the development of homosexual individuals is the same as for those who are heterosexual. Adults strongly influence the environments in which this development occurs, including at school, which is such a significant part of the environment for adolescents. All of those adults, and certainly the teachers, should promote normal adolescent development. For the successful assumption of adult identity, there must be integration of sexual orientation and personality. This requires the understanding and acceptance of each individual's sexuality. The homosexual adolescent's perception of being different emerges with awareness of arousal when with members of the same sex. Such beginning awareness may lead to denial or avoidance of situations that might establish or demonstrate homosexuality. Eventually, the individual needs to accept his or her own orientation and then begin the process of disclosure to others, called "coming out." Such disclosure may be difficult and may not elicit the support of parents or others who are important to the adolescent. The best way for adults to prevent difficulties is to maintain a supportive environment; rejection poses the greatest damage to the adolescent. This critical developmental task of integrating sexual orientation with other aspects of life is most likely to be achieved successfully if the individual is given access to information and support (Stronski Huwiler & Remafedi, 1998).

The provision of support and of education about sexuality, especially about sexual orientation, may not be achieved well in schools. Several studies found that teachers have little knowledge about homosexuality, accepting many of the myths and avoiding the topic as much as possible (Mathison, 1998). Sexuality is commonly taught in health classes, and the teachers may not be well prepared. Even though sexuality is a natural and essential part of healthy development and functioning, courses in human sexuality are typically not included as part of the academic preparation of teachers, even for those who are required to teach sexuality education. The relatively safe topics of anatomy and physiology are taught, including the biological basis of sexuality, which is necessary but insufficient. Teachers of human sexuality may have to rely on their own experiences, which may not have included an unbiased discussion of homosexuality or the definition of the range of normalcy in sexual expression and orientation.

Teachers, parents, and students may question the acceptability of discussions of homosexuality in the school and the compatibility of such discussions with what may be perceived as being school policy for providing support for homosexual individuals. In the United States, an estimated quarter of a million homosexual teachers work in public schools, an average of 2 to 3 per school. That these individuals themselves may encounter significant difficulties trying to cope with a cultural aversion to homosexuality will make it more difficult to create an environment in which successful adolescent development can occur. The school should play a valuable role in supporting each person's responsible sexual expression.

One reason for lack of institutional support for acceptance of homosexuality may be the fear that this implies an acceptance of *pedophilia* (sexual desire for children). Pedophilia has been used as an excuse for the exclusion of homosexuals from being teachers, but most pedophiles are predominantly heterosexual (Cameron & Cameron, 1996).

Many adolescents experience fears about homosexuality. About a third of teenage boys will have a homosexual experience leading to orgasm and half will experience sexual arousal by a male. Society's persisting condemnation of homosexuality and the strong desire of teenagers to conform can cause intense anxiety in those who have had homosexual experiences or feelings. Peers (half of whom will also have had such feelings) will denounce "queers" and ridicule such behavior. Those teenage males who are awkward in establishing relationships with girls may feel permanently assigned to a homosexual life. Premature labeling must be avoided and fears dispelled because most adolescents establish successful sexual function with heterosexual orientation. A single experience or thought does not fix the teenager's sexual preference for life.

On the other hand, sexual orientation may be established by the middle to late teens. Change of sexual preference is rarely desired by someone who is homosexual and almost never occurs. In the context of negative peer and societal attitudes, the individual needs to accept his or her sexuality. Parents must be informed and some sort of relationship maintained with them. It rarely is possible to live a life successfully with deceit and lies. Parents have almost nothing to do with their child's homosexual orientation so they have not failed in any way if they have a homosexual son or daughter; however, this rational conclusion may be at odds with the parents' conventional values and expectations.

## Rape and Incest

Rape and incest are acts of violence against children and adolescents that exploit their sexuality. These acts are discussed in more detail in Chapter 23.

## Risky Behaviors and Sex

Taking risks is a characteristic of adolescence. Indeed, risk taking is an essential part of the development of identity and autonomy. However, risks can be excessive and multiple, with unprotected sex as part of the behavior pattern (Lawson & Rhode, 1993). Alcohol and drug use impairs judgment and results in failure to say or implement "no" to sex or to use safer sexual practices. Increased alcohol and drug use is clearly found in those having sexual intercourse often. King et al. (1989) found that more students in Grade 9 who had had sexual intercourse, compared to those who had not, smoked cigarettes, avoided seat-belt use, and traveled in cars driven by those who had been drinking heavily. Fewer sexually active students in Grade 11 expected to attend a university than those who had not had intercourse. Because risk-taking activities are interrelated, interventions must be comprehensive to meet heterogenous needs and problems.

## Sexual Exploitation and the Internet

As technology develops, there are gains and risks. The world that is accessible on the Internet offers interest and benefit, and teens are frequent users of the technology. Unfortunately, this has provided a new territory for predators. A survey of young regular users of the Internet found that 19% of them had received unwanted sexual solicitation, sometimes quite aggressive, and that one quarter of those who were solicited experienced significant distress (Mitchell, Finkelhor, & Wolak, 2001). This is another peril about which youth need to be alerted.

# CONTRACEPTION

For the sexually active teenager, any method of contraception is better than no method. Unfortunately, both the use of contraception and the correct use of the chosen method are uncommon. Only 15% to 20% of teens regularly use contraception, whereas 20% never do and 60% do so occasionally (Lawson & Rhode, 1993). Although 3 of 4 pregnant teenagers did not want to be pregnant, only 13% were using contraception when they conceived, and most often the method was one of low effectiveness, such as with-drawal or condoms used inconsistently.

Several reasons account for nonuse of contraception, including the thinking that "It can't happen to me." Many teens have a vague faith that fate will protect them, or an illusion of invulnerability (King et al., 1989), even if they know about the relationship between coitus and conception. Such beliefs were held by 83% of nonvirgin females and 60% of nonvirgin males.

## Ignorance About the Need

Although most sexually active teenagers and their partners have had some sex education, they still are surprisingly ignorant about preventing pregnancy. Many do not know when the woman is most fertile, that preejaculatory penile secretions contain sperm, and other essentials. Faith in myths such as use of plastic food wrap or douching with colas persists. Many teenagers believe in serious side effects of contraceptives, especially the pill, far above the actual incidence and severity, which deters use.

## Ignorance About Getting and Using Contraception

Even when they know about and want contraceptives, many teens are un-sure about how to get them, where to go, or what would be required in terms of medical examination or cost. Some believe that prescriptions for the pill would be given only to married women or only to individuals above a certain age limit.

Oral contraceptives are highly effective at preventing pregnancy, with a failure rate of about 0.1% of women per year becoming pregnant if all women took the pills consistently and correctly. Unfortunately, the actual failure rate is between 3% and 20% because users either stop the pill or take it incorrectly. Stopping can be due to forgetting and relates to the motivation for having effective contraception. Stopping also can relate to side effects of the pill or the fact that the user believes the horror stories (nearly always completely false) that abound about the pill.

Knowledge about reproductive function and the effects that contraceptive methods have on it is a necessary condition for successful use of such methods. For teenagers, however, knowledge alone is not a sufficient condition, and services must also be available. Although the health care provider has a clear obligation to provide information, this is easier to do when background knowledge already exists as a result of education. This knowledge will be needed by some teens, and if not used then, it will almost certainly be used later in life for adult sexuality. Furthermore, the health care provider can provide services only for those who come for them. If ignorance keeps the teenager away from health care, he or she cannot be helped by whatever information or services would have been provided.

## Concern About Confidentiality

Many teenagers are afraid that laws or regulations require their parents to be informed about their seeking contraceptives, or that their family doctor will tell their parents. Also, many teenagers cannot afford to pay for services without using parents' health insurance. Charges for services would then appear on their insurance statements. Although it is desirable that teenagers be able to communicate freely and openly about their sexuality with their parents, it is unrealistic to expect this for many of them. Requirements that parents be informed will not likely deter many teens from engaging in intercourse but will deter them from being responsible about it. Teens should be assured that breaches of confidentiality by the physician and health care provider, most often inadvertent, are very rare.

## Acceptance of Sexuality

If teenagers take the pill or carry condoms, they must admit to themselves that they are intending to have intercourse. This preparedness requires a mature acceptance of their own sexuality, as well as a risk of the items being discovered by parents or others. Teenagers with feelings of guilt or discomfort about their sexual activity may not want to admit by prior preparation that intercourse may occur and prefer to have it "just happen."

Avoiding unintended pregnancy requires a series of beliefs and performances. The teenager must accept that he or she is sexual and wants to have intercourse but wants to avoid pregnancy. He or she then must acquire the means to do so, which may require public purchase of condoms or visits to clinics or physicians' offices. Use of a contraceptive, particularly a condom, must be negotiated and agreed upon with the partner. The motivation to avoid pregnancy is substantiated by the apparent benefits for the teenager in delaying being a parent. This motivation is affected by the individual's present circumstances, hopes and aspirations for the future, and belief that they can be attained. For those teenagers who feel hopeless or helpless, the motivation for abstinence or for use of contraceptives unfortunately but realistically will be scant.

## Desire for Pregnancy

Teenage pregnancy is not necessarily synonymous with unintended pregnancy. A considerable proportion of teenagers who get pregnant want to do so. Furthermore, many potentially adverse consequences of the pregnancy, such as lack of hope for the future, poor performance in school, or dropping out, are reasons why these young women want to get pregnant in the first place. Pregnant teens achieve a status and recognition that, at least in the short term, may seem beneficial to many of them. Childbearing may seem to satisfy needs to love and be loved (Lawson & Rhode, 1993). Conceiving a child may be "proof" of adulthood for the teenager. It may attract attention, declare independence, or allow a teenager out of a difficult family situation. Either partner may try to use a pregnancy to trap the other. Seldom do the teenagers connect pregnancy with the reality and responsibilities of parenthood. As an attempt to resolve conflict or act out fantasies, such a method will backfire.

## Contraception Methods

Many choices exist for pregnancy prevention (Greydanus, Patel, & Rimsza, 2001). Some of these methods also reduce the risk of acquiring STDs. Table 21.4 lists the available methods and their effectiveness (Hatcher et al., 1998). Specific comments on various methods (some not listed in the table) follow.

### Withdrawal

The withdrawal method is cheap and available, and that is all that is good about it. Emission of secretions before ejaculation can cause failure even if the withdrawal is carried out. This method, therefore, does not protect against pregnancy or STDs.

**TABLE 21.4**

Effectiveness of Various Contraception Methods

| Method | Theoretic Effectiveness (%)[a] | Use Effectiveness (%)[b] |
|---|---|---|
| Birth control pill | 0.5 | 2 |
| Intrauterine device | 1.5 | 5 |
| Condoms | 2 | 10 |
| Diaphragm with spermicide | 2 | 19 |
| Spermicidal foams, creams, etc. | 3–5 | 15–20 |
| Sponge | not known | 10–20 |
| Coitus interruptus | 2–20 | 20–30 |
| Douche | — | 40 |
| Injectable progestin (Depo-provera) | 1 | 10 |
| Subcutaneous progestin (Norplant) | 0.5 | 0.5 |
| No method | 90 | 90 |

[a] Theoretic effectiveness is the number out of 100 women who will get pregnant in 1 year, using a given method correctly and consistently every time they have intercourse.

[b] Use effectiveness is the number out of 100 women who will get pregnant in 1 year with typical use of a given method.

Adapted from *Contraceptive Technology* (17th ed.), by R. A. Hatcher et al., 1998, New York: Ardent Media.

## Condoms

There is a myth that all males instinctively know how to use condoms. Many do not know, however, and this reduces the effectiveness. Used correctly, condoms are a good method and appropriate for those having occasional intercourse. They are readily available, and also offer some protection against venereal disease. Ideally, the condom should be used simultaneously with a spermicidal foam. The condom must be put on after a full erection is attained and before vaginal penetration. The terminal portion must be squeezed free of air and left as a receptacle for the ejaculate. The penis must be withdrawn after ejaculation before loss of erection allows semen to spill from the condom into the vagina.

## The Birth Control Pill

The birth control pill is an effective and popular method. The pill is taken starting on the first day of vaginal bleeding or on the first Sunday after the first day of vaginal bleeding, for a total of 21 days, followed by 7 pill-free days. It contains the hormones estrogen and progesterone, each modified to allow oral administration. These hormones suppress the release of pituitary gonadotrophins, so the ovary is not stimulated, ovulation does not occur, and hence there cannot be a pregnancy. The uterine lining is stimulated by these hormones, although a little less than in a spontaneous cycle, so when the pill is stopped that lining will break down. Vaginal bleeding, often a little lighter than when a woman is not on the pill, will occur a day or two later. The cycle is then repeated every 28 days. Some pill preparations contain 28 pills, of which the last 7 contain no hormone, and are taken continuously. Bleeding occurs while the woman is taking the 7 inactive pills. The 28-day preparation is convenient for many users because it maintains the habit of taking a pill daily and properly spaces out the active medicine–containing pills. It may be particularly useful for teenagers, who have more problems with compliance than most older users.

Many teenagers believe side effects will occur. For example, 51% think there will be weight gain, 23% have heard about nausea, 17% have heard about blood clotting and strokes, and 15% think the pill causes cancer. In fact, mild nausea and breast tenderness occur in about 15% to 20% of women during the first cycle on the pill, but these problems resolve spontaneously in nearly all women by the third cycle. Some women will have menstrual irregularities after stopping the pill, but most have already had such irregularities before going on the pill. Similarly, 10% of couples with no prior pregnancies will be infertile after using the pill, but so are 10% of couples who never used the pill. Stopping for a "rest period" is a frequent error; it confers no benefit and only results in confusion and possibly pregnancy. If the pill is well tolerated medically, it may be used continuously for years with no increased risk. The pill does not cause cervical, breast, or any other cancer. Severe clotting disorders are a rare but serious complication of the pill, and strokes or blood clots to the lungs may occur. The incidence of this problem is increased in pill users, but to a very small extent in teenagers, who have a very low risk for all blood vessel disorders. Furthermore, such vascular and clotting complications also occur in pregnancy, often the alternative to the pill, but at a rate much higher than for women on the pill.

Not only does the pill have few side effects, but it confers several benefits in addition to very effective, convenient contraception. Iron-deficiency anemia due to excessive menstrual bleeding is reduced and cycles are regular. The risk of cancer of the uterine lining and of the ovary, functional cysts of the ovary, and benign breast disease are reduced.

To be effective, the pill must be taken daily. If a pill is forgotten, it should be taken as soon as the omission is recognized. If vaginal spotting occurs, the pill should still be administered because it provides effective contraception while the problem is being resolved. A medical examination is necessary before prescribing the pill, to avoid giving it to the very few women who have risk factors and should not take it, and periodic medical supervision should be maintained during pill use. It takes motivation and an acceptance of one's sexuality to regularly take the pill, and it should not be used by those who will not be compliant in its use. Because the birth control pill does not protect against STDs, condom use is still necessary for this purpose.

### The Patch

The hormones of the birth control pill can also be given in a contraceptive patch. The estrogen and progestin are absorbed across the skin of the user. Each patch is worn for a week, and three patches are used in succession in one cycle. One patch maintains hormone levels for a week. The steady hormone levels may produce better control of the uterine lining with less breakthrough bleeding. The lack of oral administration may be associated with less nausea. Apart from these indications, the indications and contraindications for and side effects of the contraceptive patch are the same as those for the birth control pill. Using hormonal contraceptive administered by a patch may enhance compliance because usage is simpler; the user needs only to apply a patch once a week. This avoids requiring the consistency of taking a pill each day and may fit better into the life of a teenager. Also the method, or at least the route of administration, is new and currently trendy, and it may therefore be more attractive to some users.

### "Morning After" Contraception

A variety of hormone medications are available that rapidly interfere with the preparation of the uterine lining for implantation. The most recent, which is highly effective and has few side effects, is called Plan B. If unprotected intercourse at midcycle has occurred and such medication is taken, ovulation is blocked. Even if fertilization has happened, there is a very high likelihood that the pregnancy can still be prevented. This method prevents the establishment of pregnancy; it is not an abortifacient. The hormone effect disrupts the cycle. A medication with a high dose of estrogen often causes transient nausea, so this method cannot be used on a regular basis. It may be used to deal with an acute situation, however, if the woman is seen promptly. The opportunity may then be taken to institute an ongoing method of contraception.

Postcoital contraception is very effective if this medication is taken within 48 hours of unprotected intercourse or intercourse with breakage or slippage of a condom. Most Planned Parenthood or community health units and most physicians can provide these pills. This underutilized method has the potential to significantly reduce the occurrence of unintended pregnancies and requests for pregnancy termination. Persons to whom teenagers may turn for advice when concerned about pregnancy risk should provide information about this option. Throughout North America, information about providers of emergency or postcoital contraception may be obtained by calling 888/NOT-2-LATE.

## Spermicides

Spermicides are foams (the most effective), creams, or jellies that must be inserted in the vagina just before intercourse. The formulations are improving, leading to increased ease of carriage and insertion of these agents. A spermicidal sponge is available that may be inserted well before intercourse and remains effective for 24 hours. Spermicides are readily available without prescription, and may slightly reduce the risk of gonorrhea or HIV infection. Ideally, spermicides would be used together with a condom by the male. These methods are reliable if regularly used together. Spermicide use is somewhat messy, however, and it requires that the act of contraception be undertaken at the same time as the act of intercourse. There are no significant side effects, but occasionally the spermicidal chemicals cause local irritation.

## Diaphragm

The diaphragm is a barrier method that consists of a shallow, concave, thin sheet of rubber on a flexible, firm rim. It is used with a spermicidal jelly applied uniformly around the edge. The diaphragm must be inserted correctly into the vagina prior to intercourse, but this may be done up to 6 hours before, so the acts of contraception and of intercourse may be separated in time, which is an attraction to many users. It must be left in place for 6 hours following intercourse before removal. Fitting must be done by a competent health care professional, and correct fitting of the diaphragm is essential. No health risks are associated with its use, except rare local irritation by the spermicide. This method does not protect against STDs.

## Rhythm Method

The regulation of the cycle with the fertile interval has been previously explained. Avoiding intercourse at this time is relatively safe. Cycle irregularity can occur, however, particularly in adolescents. Therefore, the rhythm method calls for considerable calculation and restraint. This method does not protect against STDs.

## Intrauterine Device

Available in a variety of shapes and constructions, all intrauterine devices (IUDs) act to prevent implantation of the egg into the uterine wall. They must be inserted by a physician. Once inserted, no further action need be taken to prevent conception, and the menstrual cycle continues spontaneously. Because no action needs to be taken by the woman to prepare for coitus, doubt about compliance is not important. There is increased efficacy in smaller sized copper-wound devices, which may therefore be used in women who have never been pregnant. The foreign body in the uterus, however, may cause pain with menstruation or increased blood loss, and in 15% of women the device must be removed. In another 15% there will be unrecognized expulsion. Infection in the uterus or the fallopian tubes may occur for the user of an IUD, particularly if she has multiple partners. The prescription of an IUD to teenagers who require passive contraception should be limited to the method of last resort. As with many other methods, IUDs do not prevent STDs and should be used in conjunction with condoms if STDs are a concern.

## Injectable Progestin

Some females choose to receive injections of a progesterone-like hormone, such as Depo-Provera, every 3 months. This method is highly effective and requires no action between injections, but of course the woman must return to the doctor as required every 3 months. Menstrual disturbance or eventual amenorrhea are common and must be acceptable possibilities to the woman if she is to use this method. Normal fertility is resumed by 6 months after the last injection. No protection against STDs is provided by this method.

## Subcutaneous Implanted Progestin

A preparation called Norplant is available for subcutaneous implantation. It consists of six silastic capsules that release a progesterone-like compound in a slow, sustained way for 5 years. The insertion is a minor surgical procedure. This method blocks ovulation and produces a thick cervical mucus that is not readily penetrable by sperm. It is 99.8% effective, and there is no problem with compliance because the method cannot be forgotten or omitted. It may cause menstrual irregularity, with light but unpredictable spotting. It is expensive initially, although the cost is about half of that for birth control pills for 5 years. An appropriate candidate for this method must know that she does not want to be pregnant for the next 5 years and be able to accept cycle irregularity. At the end of 5 years, or when pregnancy is wanted, the implants must be removed through another minor surgical procedure. This device, like many others, provides no protection against STDs.

## Safety

Safety of birth control methods is a very important issue, but concerns are exaggerated. For example, consider the risk of death per 100,000 women per year for several methods of contraception (Kost, Forrest, & Harlap, 1991). For any method, the risk consists of that due to the method itself and that due to the pregnancies not prevented by the method. For birth control pill users, the risks of vascular complications are additive if there are other risk factors; smoking is one example. Comparison is made at each age with the risk of death due to the pregnancies that would occur if no method was used. Many sexually active women object to contraception due to perceived risks. Because they are unlikely to give up sexual activity, their choice is not really risk versus no risk, but which risk they would choose. The risk of no method far exceeds that of any method, and this risk does not take into account all of the other advantages of effective contraception.

# SEXUALLY TRANSMITTED DISEASES

An unhappy but inevitable consequence of the growing sexual activity of teenagers is the increased incidence of STDs, including HIV and AIDS. Except for the common cold and flu, STDs are the most common infectious diseases in the United States. Transmission is invariably by sexual intercourse or contact between the sex organs and the mouth or rectum. STDs and their prevention are discussed fully in Chapter 22. Because the strategies for contraception and STD prevention are similar, the provision of education and services must be linked in an approach to both these problems.

# ABORTION

Substantial numbers of pregnant teenagers will seek termination of their pregnancies. When the U.S. Supreme Court legalized abortion in 1973, the number of procedures performed for teenagers doubled, representing not an increased need for the service, but increased availability of the service to meet a preexisting demand.

The available methods of abortion include dilatation of the cervix and evacuation of the uterus by suction, before 12 weeks; cervical dilatation and extraction of the fetus by instruments, up to 20 to 24 weeks; and instillation into the uterus of substances (e.g., saline or prostaglandins) to cause uterine contractions and abortion, up to 20 weeks in Canada and 24 weeks in the United States. The suction methods are much safer than the others, and even for this method, the earlier the procedure is done, the safer it is. The risk of death is very small if abortion only is used as a method of birth control or if abortion is used as a backup to barrier contraception, and therefore is required much less often. For any single suction abortion, the risk of maternal death is less than 1 in 100,000. If abortion is to be done, it should be accomplished as early in pregnancy as possible to minimize risks. However, because of delay in recognizing a pregnancy, reluctance to reveal the existence of the pregnancy, and inaccessibility of services, all too many women come late for pregnancy termination and undergo the physically more risky and psychologically more traumatic procedures. Physical complications include bleeding and infection, and individuals may experience problems of emotional acceptance of the pregnancy and then its termination. Despite concerns about subsequent emotional or psychological sequelae, women with unintended pregnancies who choose abortion show no increase, and perhaps a decrease, in psychological difficulties after the procedure as compared to those who continue the pregnancy. They are also more likely to make subsequent progress in school (Alder et al., 1990).

The need for abortion represents contraception failure, and the pregnancy termination must be associated with teaching about contraception. Despite any claims to the contrary, sexual activity is soon reestablished in most teenagers who have had an abortion. Although he often is not involved, and indeed may be actively excluded from the situation, the male partner should be considered as well. He should be helped to accept his responsibility for the situation; allowed to be supportive, if reasonable, in the relationship; and instructed in contraception and responsible sexuality.

## TEENAGE PREGNANCY

Teenage pregnancy, whether intended or not, is the most dramatic manifestation of teenage intercourse, and one of the most devastating in its immediate and long-term effects. There are serious consequences for the women, the men, and the children who are born. The children are at increased risk of being neglected or abused and of themselves becoming teenage parents.

The number of pregnancies in teenagers proceeding to delivery of the baby is determined by the number of teenage women; the percentage who are sexually active and, of them, the proportion not using effective contraception; and the proportion of pregnant teenagers who choose elective abortion. It is apparent that sexual activity is increasing and that contraceptive efficacy is not changing (as the rate of conceptions is about constant), but because increasing numbers of pregnant teenagers are having abortions, the number of births to teenage mothers is decreasing slightly

(Martin et al., 2002). Group figures for all teenagers, however, obscure significant events within subgroups. The number of births to young, White, middle-class teenagers was increasing until recently, whereas the number to older teens was decreasing. There have been more births to unwed mothers than in the past (NICHHD, 1993). More recently the number of pregnancies for U.S. females ages 15 to 19 has fallen a little from 116 per 1,000 to 90.7 per 1,000. For those younger than 15, the rate also has fallen from 3.5 per 1,000 to 2.6 per 1,000, with higher rates in both groups for African Americans than Whites. Although encouraging, these rates remain four to five times higher than in France and Germany and nine times higher than in the Netherlands.

These younger mothers are most likely to have unwanted, illegitimate pregnancies requiring a great deal of support. In the United States, almost 1 in 10 women ages 15 to 19 years becomes pregnant, so there were 800,000 to 900,000 pregnancies and, in 2001, 497,367 births (American College of Obstetricians and Gynecologists, 2003; Freijoo, 2001). Rates in Canada are about equal for having had sexual intercourse but half as high for pregnancies and births. More than three quarters of all teenage pregnancies are unintended. For more than half of these pregnancies, induced abortion is performed. About 75% of teenage pregnancies are conceived while the parents are unwed. Of the unmarried teenagers bearing a child, 93% keep their babies, reflecting an increased acceptance of a single mother raising a child. Placement for adoption was a last resort before abortion became available as an option.

When unintended pregnancy occurs in a teenager, there is often considerable delay before confirmation. This is partly due to the teenager's physiologic cycle irregularity, but mostly to denial or to fantasies, for example, that her boyfriend will marry her and take her out of the situation. Eventually decisions must be made. These are nearly always done in an atmosphere of enormous emotional upheaval involving the girl and her family and perhaps the boy and his family. Anger and then shame are the common family reactions. These often lead to rejection of the teenager at a time of great need.

Abortion may be one realistic option. Those who make this choice usually resolve their psychological difficulties promptly, continue their education, and achieve their life's goals (Zabin & Sedivy, 1992). Women who place their babies for adoption demonstrate more personality difficulty than those who receive an abortion, and their families often experience continuing guilt and grief. Those who continue the pregnancy must face major problems (Maynard, 1997).

Pregnancy in a teenager is associated with a 3 to 4 times greater risk of death or injury to the mother or baby (Baldwin, 1981). Complications include preterm delivery, pregnancy-induced high blood pressure, poor fetal growth, and both increased incidence and decreased tolerance by the teenager of common pregnancy complaints such as nausea and vomiting. Coexisting drug or alcohol abuse and venereal disease might complicate the situation.

The teenagers who conceive are likely to be poor academic performers before conception (Maynard, 1997). Once pregnant, they are often effectively excluded from school for long periods or perhaps permanently by many personal, family, and social pressures. Teenagers who have babies are much more likely to drop out of school, have more children, and require welfare support than otherwise comparable peers. Schools are increasingly and desirably developing programs for pregnant teens to stay in school. Participants are a selected and perhaps more motivated group. Arrangements also are needed for child care after delivery so schooling can be completed or a mother can return to school. These arrangements provide benefits of further education and eventual greater range of choices.

Teenage fathers also face many stresses but have less attention paid to their needs. Although there is often an established relationship between the father and his pregnant girlfriend, the boyfriend stays involved after pregnancy in only 20% of couples (Lawson & Rhode, 1993). Education attainment will be more limited and jobs will be less personally or financially rewarding for teenagers who father a child. If the couple marries, the divorce rate is very high and many of the marriages are unsuccessful with, for example, an 80% incidence of sexual dysfunction (Elster & Panzarine, 1981). The number of children is greater. Forced early and without completed education into the labor market, the fathers are considerably disadvantaged. Often there is hostility and rejection, particularly by the girl's parents. Previously, the boy may have depended predominantly on his girlfriend for social support and is now isolated. Lack of knowledge about pregnancy and exclusion from the care provided for the pregnant teen accentuate anxieties. After delivery, ignorance and inappropriate expectations of child development and low levels of frustration tolerance lead to teenage fathers' poor performance as parents.

Normal teenage development imposes stresses. Added situational stresses surrounding pregnancy may overwhelm the pregnant adolescent and the teenage father. Social and emotional support from significant people in their environment, including teachers, will increase the teenagers' ability to cope with stresses.

# THE SCHOOLS AND SEX

## Provision of Education

A survey by the Global Program on AIDS of the World Health Organization showed no evidence that sex education leads to earlier or increased sexual activity among adolescents. Sex education only increased the adoption of safer sexual practices (Senanayake & Ladjall, 1994). Nevertheless, controversy exists about whether education about sex, or family life as it is often called, should be in the curriculum at all, and if so with what content. Some argue that if sex is to be taught at all, it must be with a clear and exclusive abstinence message. Mention of contraception, they say, implicitly condones sexual activity. Others say that teenage sexual activity and a high incidence of adverse consequences, including unintended pregnancy and STDs, are realities. Comprehensive sex education should be provided in the schools so students may make appropriate and healthy choices. Although complete abstinence is an ideal prevention for both pregnancy and STDs, it is not practiced by many teens. Furthermore, monogamy is unusual for those who are sexually active. Dr. Jocelyn Elder, the former Surgeon General of the United States, once said, "Everyone in the world is opposed to sex outside of marriage, and yet everybody does it. I'm saying 'Get real'" (Whitehead, 1994, p. 56).

Abstinence-only courses tend to be ineffective and also may be academically deficient because they preclude consideration of the full range of options that can be learned about sexuality. Furthermore, they do not address the needs of the students who are now sexually active or who may become so later. Evaluation of such programs is often flawed because the participants are self-selected and therefore may be those who are more likely to postpone the initiation of sexual activity.

An example of a clearly focused and short-duration course with the objective of helping adolescents defer sexual activity is that of Grady Memorial Hospital and Emory University in Atlanta (Lawson & Rhode, 1993). It is effective in postponing the initiation of sexual activity in those who were virgins at the time they received the course, and these teens were more likely to use contraception when they did begin sexual activity. However, there was no change in the behavior of adolescents who were already sexually active. These results suggest that such courses should be provided to children young enough that they have not already begun voluntary sexual activity, which means probably in Grade 6 or 7. (Younger children who are sexually active are often exploited and victims of abuse. For these children, teaching refusal skills is irrelevant.) Other interventions are needed as described in Chapter 23.

Postponement of pregnancy by postponing intercourse, using noncoital sex, or using effective contraception is an objective of comprehensive sex education curricula. To be successful, such programs need to be part of a package addressing other aspects of an adolescent's needs (Dryfoos, 1985). A comprehensive program in New Jersey exemplifies mandatory family life education. It includes classes from kindergarten to Grade 12 for every public school student. Courses offered by most other states or provinces are not as inclusive or sustained. An already declining adolescent pregnancy rate in Ontario continued downward after the establishment of a provincial policy that provided sex education in schools and contraceptive services in public health units (Orton & Rosenblatt, 1986). The provincial policy had particular impact in lower socioeconomic status communities, where there are presumably lower life expectations by both adults and children, and less access to other resources for information.

The education of teachers who will provide sex education is a problem in all developed countries, even those with centrally mandated and comprehensive curricula such as Sweden or the Netherlands. Universities do not adequately include such preparation in teacher education courses, and it is left to in-service sessions or workshops (Dryfoos, 1985). Education of teachers is necessary not only to provide knowledge of the curriculum content but also so that teachers can be comfortable with teaching about sex.

Parental opposition to the provision of sex education by the schools is widespread and vociferous and occurs in most developed countries with or without mandated sex education. But public opinion polls in all these countries, including the United States, support sex education. A poll by Rutgers University found that 61% of parents with school-age children would permit their children to obtain condoms in the schools (Whitehead, 1994). The schools can play a complementary role with sex education in the home, from the church, and from other community resources. The importance of the schools becomes greater when one or more of these other sources of information is absent or unwilling to provide instruction.

Similar levels of adolescent sexual activity exist in Denmark, the Netherlands, Canada, and the United States, but the birth rate for teens in the United States is 5 times higher than in Denmark and 10 times higher than in the Netherlands (NICHHD, 1993). In both Denmark and the Netherlands, sex is accepted as part of a normal, healthy life but only when accompanied by a strong responsibility to prevent unwanted pregnancy and STDs. Both countries offer comprehensive programs in sex education beginning in the primary years, along with counseling and contraceptive services. As public programs of prevention become accessible, adolescents choose to avoid pregnancy (Orton & Rosenblatt, 1986). Sex education in the schools alone is biased to a greater effect in higher socioeconomic areas, perhaps due to parental and social reinforcement, and also to greater alternative access to services. The combination of sex education in schools and clinic contraception services is a minimum strategy for prevention of adolescent pregnancy. A U.S. study also strongly supports the connection between the school and the clinic (Dryfoos, 1985). Sex education does not mean more sex; it can mean a reduction in the rates of STDs and teenage pregnancy ("Sex Education in Schools," 1994).

## Provision of Services

Many people express the worry that making contraception available to teenagers will encourage intercourse and promote promiscuity. In fact, most teenagers seek contraceptive services only after they have been sexually active for at least 3 to 6 months and often when they are afraid they are pregnant. Only 4 of 250 teenage women coming to one birth control clinic were sexually inactive (Roberts, 1979; see also French, 2002). Half of initial nonmarital pregnancies occur within the first 6 months of sexual activity, and 20% in the first month. It follows that providing contraception does not initiate sexual activity and denying it will not eliminate such activity. Furthermore, directing birth control education and services only to those already sexually active will not reduce the incidence of unintended pregnancies.

The benefits of the provision of services with education is apparent in the low pregnancy, birth, and abortion rates in Sweden, Denmark, and the Netherlands. It also has been shown in a carefully evaluated project for urban teenagers in Baltimore (Zabin, Hersch, Smith, Street, & Hardy, 1986). Education and services were provided over 3 years to students in a junior and a senior high school, and the students' knowledge and behavior were compared with those of students from matched schools. High levels of sexual activity were found at all the schools before the program. An increase in knowledge (e.g., about the time in the menstrual cycle when conception is likely to occur) and a decrease in misinformation occurred. There was a rapid uptake of clinic use, however, which suggested that it was the accessibility of the staff and the clinic and not new information that encouraged students to obtain services. Behavioral change occurred so that the age at first intercourse was delayed by 7 months among students exposed to the program for 3 years. A much higher proportion of both male and female students attended a clinic for contraception within a month of first intercourse or before intercourse. Methods of contraception requiring forethought and planning were more likely to be used. Finally, the cumulative pregnancy rate over 2 years of the program, compared to no program, declined by 30% for those with education and contraceptive services provided and rose by 57% for those without a pregnancy prevention program.

The schools are not the cause of adolescent pregnancy and they cannot be restructured to cure the problem in the absence of other efforts (Hatcher et al., 1998). However, teenagers may translate their attitudes, resulting in part from sex or family life education in schools, into constructive preventive behavior when they also have access to services.

## Results of School-Based Programs

School programs have clearly and consistently demonstrated a small delay in the age of onset of sexual activity and a substantial decrease in the occurrence of unintended pregnancy and STDs. Those programs that include contraception as an option rather than those that promote abstinence only have a more persistent effect.

Financial issues are critical for access to care and use of contraceptives. The availability of subsidized clinics and facilitated access to condoms and other contraceptives is cost effective. Benefits include a reduction of the immediate and long-term costs of pregnancy and the care of children of adolescents, as well as a reduction of STDs.

# SUMMARY

Growing to successful maturity must include attaining adult sexual function. The turbulent transition occurs during years of school attendance, and many problems lie in wait for any teenager. If adverse consequences of their developing sexual nature and function are to be dealt with or, much better, avoided, then all teenagers need a sympathetic, authoritative (but not authoritarian), accurate source of information. An apparently judgmental approach will be counterproductive, but it should be clear that in sexual matters, as in all areas of human functioning, there are standards of responsible behavior toward oneself and others. Difficulty communicating with parents is one of the normal characteristics of all adolescents. Teachers therefore will assume an important complementary role to other sources of information and standards of behavior in all cases, and an essential role in many. We hope that this chapter will be of assistance in meeting that responsibility.

## SUGGESTED READING

Austin, C. R., & Short, R. V. (1980). *Human sexuality*. Cambridge, MA: Cambridge University Press.

Franklin, C., & Corcoran, J. (2000). Preventing adolescent pregnancy: A review of programs and practices. *Social Work, 45,* 40–52.

Hatcher, R. A. (1999). *Safely sexual.* New York: Ardent Media.

National Institutes of Health, Center for Population Research, National Institute of Child Health and Human Development. (1993). *Negotiating the paths of parenthood* (Workshop Report).

Semmens, J. P., & Krantz, K. E. (1970). *The adolescent experience: A counseling guide to social and sexual behavior.* New York: Macmillan.

## REFERENCES

Alder, N. E., David, H. P., Major, B. N., Roth, S. H., Russo, N. F., & Wyatt C. E. (1990). Psychological responses after abortion. *Science, 268,* 41–44.

American College of Obstetricians and Gynecologists. (2003). *Adolescent pregnancy facts.* Washington, DC: Author.

Anderson, S. E., Dallal, G. E., & Must, A. (2003). Relative weight and race influence average age at menarche: Youth from two nationally representative surveys of U.S. girls studied 25 years apart. *Pediatrics, 111,* 844–850.

Baldwin, W. (1981). Adolescent pregnancy and child-bearing—An overview. *Seminars in Perinatology, 5*(1), 1–8.

Banks, A., & Gartrell, N. K. (1995). Hormones and sexual orientation: A questionable link. *Journal of Homosexuality, 28*(3–4), 247–268.

Bell, P., Weinberg, M. S., & Hammersmith, S. K. (1991). *Sexual preference: Its development in men and women.* Bloomington: Indiana University Press.

Cameron, P., & Cameron, K. (1996). Do homosexual teachers pose a risk to pupils? *Journal of Psychology, 130*(6), 603–613.

Dryfoos, J. (1985). What the United States can learn about prevention of teenage pregnancy from other developed countries. *SIECUS Report, 14*(2), 1–7.

Elster, A. B., & Panzarine, S. (1981). The adolescent father. *Seminars in Perinatology, 5,* 39–51.

Freijoo, A. N. (2001). *Adolescent sexual health in Europe and the U.S.—Why the difference?* (2nd ed.). Washington, DC: Advocates for Youth.

French, R. S. (2002). The experience of young people with contraceptive consultations and health care workers. *International Journal of Adolescent Medical Health, 14*(2), 131–138.

Gates, G. J., & Sonenstein, F. L. (2000). Heterosexual genital sexual activity among adolescent males: 1998 and 1995. *Family Planning Perspectives, 32*(6), 295–297.

Grant, L. J. (2001). Caring for the adolescent patient. *Journal of the Society of Obstetrics and Gynecology of Canada, 23,* 231–234.

Greydanus, D. E., Patel, D. R., & Rimsza, M. E. (2001). Contraception in the adolescent. *Pediatrics, 107,* 562–573.

Hatcher, R. A., Trussell, J., Stewart, F., Cates, W., Stewart, G. K., Guest, F., & Kowal, D. (1998). *Contraceptive technology* (17th ed.). New York: Ardent Media.

Henshaw, S. K., & VanVort, J. (1989). Teenage abortion, birth and pregnancy statistics: An update. *Family Planning Perspectives, 21,* 85.

Hogg, R. S., Weber, A. E., Chan, K., Martindale, S., Cook, D., Miller, M. L., & Craib, K. J. (2001). Increasing incidence of HIV infections among young gay and bisexual men in Vancouver. *AIDS, 15*(10), 1321–1322.

Kendler, K. S., Thorton, L., Gilman, S. E., & Kessler, R. C. (2000). Sexual orientation in a U.S. national sample of twin and nontwin sibling pairs. *American Journal of Psychiatry, 157*(11), 1843–1846.

King, A. J. C., Beazley, R. P., Warren, W. K., Hankins, C. A., Robersson, A. S., & Redford, J. L. (1989). *Canada youth and AIDS study.* Kingston, Ontario: Queen's University at Kingston, Social Program Evaluation Group.

Kost, K., Forrest, J. D., & Harlap, S. (1991). Comparing the health risks and benefits of contraceptive choices. *Family Planning Perspectives, 23,* 54–61.

Lawson, A., & Rhode, D. L. (1993). *The politics of pregnancy.* New Haven, CT: Yale University Press.

Lock, J., & Steiner, H. (1999). Gay, lesbian, and bisexual youth risks for emotional, physical, and social problems: Results from a community based survey. *Journal of the American Academy of Child and Adolescent Psychiatry, 38,* 297–304.

Martin, J. A., Hamilton, B. E., Ventura, S. J., Menacker, F., Park, M. M., & Sutton, P. D. (2002). Births: Final data for 2001. *National Vital Statistics Report, 51*(2), 1–102.

Masters, W. H., & Johnson, V. E. (1966). *Human sexual response.* Boston: Little Brown.

Mathison, C. (1998). The invisible minority: Preparing teachers to meet the needs of gay and lesbian youth. *Journal of Teacher Education, 49,* 151–156.

Maynard, R. A. (Ed.). (1997). *Kids having kids: Economic costs and social consequences of teen pregnancy.* Washington, DC: Urban Institute Press.

Mitchell, K. J., Finkelhor, D., & Wolak, J. (2001). Risk factors for and impact of online sexual solicitation of youth. *Journal of the American Medical Association, 285,* 3011–3014.

National Institute of Child Health and Human Development. (1993). Behavioral determinants of unintended pregnancy. In *Conference of the Center for Population Research at the Rockefeller Foundation.* Bethesda, MD: Author.

O'Donnell, L., M'yint-U, A., O'Donnell, C. R., & Stueve, A. (2003). Long-term influence of sexual norms and attitudes of sexual initiation among urban minority youth. *Journal of School Health, 73*(2), 68–75.

Orton, M. J., & Rosenblatt, E. (1986). *Adolescent pregnancy in Ontario: Progress in prevention.* Ontario: Planned Parenthood.

Reiter, E. O., & Lee, P. A. (2001). Have the onset and tempo of puberty changed? *Archives of Pediatrics and Adolescent Medicine, 155,* 1001–1003.

Roberts, L. (1979). Female teenagers and contraception. In B. Schlessenger (Ed.), *Sexual behavior in Canada: Patterns and problems* (pp. 35–44). Toronto: University of Toronto Press.

Semmens, J. P., & Krantz, K. E. (1970). *The adolescent experience: A counseling guide to social and sexual behavior.* New York: Macmillan.

Senanayake, P., & Ladjall, M. (1994). Adolescent health: Changing needs. *International Journal of Gynecology and Obstetrics, 46,* 137–143.

Sex education in schools: Peers to the rescue? (1994). *Lancet, 344,* 899–900.

Sprecher, R., Barbee, A., & Schwartz, P. (1995). Was it good for you too? Gender differences in first sexual intercourse experiences. *Journal of Sex Research, 32,* 3–15.

Stronski Huwiler, S. M., & Remafedi, G. (1998). Adolescent homosexuality. *Advances in Pediatrics, 45,* 107–144.

Tanner, J. N. (1962). *Growth of adolescents.* Oxford, England: Blackwell.

Telljohann, S. K., & Price, J. H. (1993). A qualitative examination of adolescent homosexuals' life experiences: Ramifications for secondary school personnel. *Journal of Homosexuality, 26*(1), 41–56.

Vincent, C. E. (1970). The social horns of youth's dilemmas. In J. P. Semmens & K. E. Krantz (Eds.), *The adolescent experience: A counseling guide to social and sexual behavior* (pp. 18–22). New York: Macmillan.

Whitehead, B. D. (1994, September). The failure of sex education. *Atlantic Monthly,* pp. 55–80.

Zabin, L. S., Hersch, M. B., Smith, E. A., Street, R., & Hardy, J. B. (1986). Evaluation of a pregnancy prevention program for urban teenagers. *Family Planning Perspectives, 18,* 119–126.

Zabin, L. S., & Sedivy, V. (1992). Abortion among adolescents: Research findings and the current debate. *Journal of School Health, 62*(7), 319–324.

Zhou, J. N., Hofman, M. A., Gooren, L. J., & Swaab, D. F. (1995). A sex difference in the human brain and its relation to transsexuality. *Nature, 378*(6552), 68–70.

# CHAPTER 22

# Sexually Transmitted Diseases

Susan M. King

**M**any infections can be transmitted during sexual contact. The term *sexually transmitted disease* (STD) has replaced the term *venereal disease* for referring to these infections. Except for the common cold or flu, STDs are the most common infectious diseases in the United States. The spectrum of illness caused by these infections ranges from mild symptoms that can be cured with a short course of antibiotics to the incurable, fatal disease of acquired immunodeficiency syndrome (AIDS). More than ever before, education of youth so as to promote prevention of STDs is essential. Teachers can help in this educational process. For those readers who would like more information on STDs, a Suggested Reading list is included at the end of the chapter.

The rates of many STDs are higher among adolescents than other age groups. For example, the rate of gonorrhea is highest for females 15 to 19 years of age, the prevalence of chlamydial infections is highest among adolescents, and half of all new human immunodeficiency virus (HIV) infections in the United States occur in young people between 13 and 24 years of age (Centers for Disease Control [CDC], 2002).

Prevention of STDs requires that there be acceptance by society of human sexuality. Although abstinence prevents acquisition of STDs, it clearly is unacceptable for many adolescents. Monogamy is not an adequate method of prevention, because serial monogamy leads to multiple sexual partners over time. Consistent condom use should be promoted for "safer sex"; there is no evidence that promotion of condom use increases promiscuity. Although condoms are readily available, the skills to purchase them, have them available at the right time, negotiate their use, and use them correctly need to be learned (see Chapter 21).

# HIV INFECTION

HIV is the virus that causes AIDS. In the United States, an estimated 800,000 to 900,000 people are currently infected with HIV and about 40,000 new HIV infections occur every year (CDC, 2002). Sexual transmission accounts for most of the cases of HIV infection during adolescence. More than half of the new cases in adolescents are female. Because the median time from infection to the development of symptoms and progression to AIDS is 10 years, those who die as young adults may have become infected as adolescents (Kuo, Taylor, & Detels, 1991). There is no cure for AIDS, and, as far as we know, everyone infected with HIV will eventually develop AIDS. Prevention is therefore crucial.

The chronic viral infection of HIV can be associated with symptoms such as recurrent fevers, fatigue, diarrhea, and weight loss. Over a period of several years, there is progressive decline of the immune defenses so that infections occur with unusual organisms such as *Pneumocystis carinii* (PCP). This stage of severe dysfunction of the immune system is called AIDS. Adolescents who become HIV positive likely will have no symptoms because they are at an early stage in their disease. However, some younger children at school may have been infected with HIV since birth. Some of these children may have developed symptoms before they started school, although many being treated for HIV infection may have no symptoms. The signs of HIV are quite variable. Many children have enlarged lymph nodes (e.g., in the neck); some have an increased frequency of common childhood infections, such as ear infections; others have a chronic cough or persistent diarrhea; and many do not grow well. The virus also affects the brain, and infected children may develop motor problems with spasticity and cognitive abnormalities, especially memory difficulties.

Therapies for the management of HIV infection have evolved rapidly over the last decade. These medications (antiretroviral agents) can usually control the HIV infection but cannot eradicate it. Medications for HIV infection are almost always used in combinations of three or four drugs. Side effects are not uncommon with these drugs, and children taking them are usually monitored monthly, including having their blood checked for any effects on the bone marrow, liver, or pancreas. Medications also are given to prevent some of the complications associated with a waning immune system, such as pneumonia caused by PCP infection. In children and adolescents, early diagnosis and treatment are of benefit.

Although HIV is predominantly transmitted by sexual contact, adolescents may be infected through other routes, for example, via their infected mother, from unscreened blood transfusions (before 1985 for transfusions in North America), or from sharing injection drugs and contacting the blood of an HIV-positive drug user. Because most infected adolescents will have no HIV-associated symptoms, all adolescents should consider every partner as potentially infected. The most effective way to prevent infection with HIV is to avoid sexual intercourse with an infected partner. Condom use is the next best method of prevention; although it is not 100% effective, it is more realistic than abstinence. The risk of transmission from men to women apparently is higher than from women to men, and the risk of transmission is much higher for anal intercourse than vaginal intercourse (Royce, Seña, Cates, & Cohen, 1997). This information is important to heterosexual as well as gay youth, because some youth use anal sex as a form of birth control. The risk of transmission of HIV through oral sex is probably very low; however, the risk is increased when there is contact between semen and the oral mucosa, and when the recipient has bleeding gums or mouth ulcers. The chance that HIV will be transmitted from an HIV-infected woman to her baby, even if the mother has no symptoms, is about 1 in 4. With appropriate therapy for HIV during pregnancy, the risk of infection in the baby can be reduced to about 1 in 100 (Cooper et al., 2002). It is therefore recommended that HIV testing should be routinely performed in pregnancy. Most adolescents have knowledge about HIV, including prevention of transmission, but many do not apply that information to themselves, and condom use may be inconsistent. Youth may need help to acquire the skills to negotiate with their partners for consistent use of condoms and information on the correct use of condoms. Education is the only means to reduce the stigma of HIV and AIDS and increase the acceptance of safer sex practices for adolescents.

In the absence of blood exposure, HIV infection is not transmitted through the types of contact that usually occur in a school setting; therefore, children and adolescents with HIV infection should not be excluded from school for the protection of other children or personnel, unless the child poses an increased risk to others, for example, by aggressive biting. All schools should adopt routine procedures for handling blood or blood-contaminated fluids, regardless of whether there are known to be students with HIV infection at the school.

The family of a child with HIV has the right to choose whether they inform the school. The number of people informed should be kept to the minimum needed to ensure proper care of the student. Everyone involved in the care and education of the student must respect the student's right to privacy. Unfortunately, stigma is associated with this disease, making it essential that confidentiality be maintained. Disclosures of information should occur only with consent from the family.

# GONORRHEA

The highest reported rates of gonorrhea are in young men 15 to 24 years of age and women 15 to 19 years of age (CDC, 2001). Symptoms develop 2 to 7 days following intercourse with an infected partner. Men usually develop a penile discharge and burning with urination. Women may have a vaginal discharge or irritation, but 80% have no symptoms. Even in asymptomatic infection, it can be spread to other sites, for example, to the tubes going to the testes in men and the tubes going to the ovaries in women. Lower abdominal pain or *dyspareunia* (painful intercourse) may be a sign of spreading infection with *pelvic inflammatory disease* (PID). PID may lead to chronic pain with tubal scarring, causing ectopic pregnancies or infertility. In both sexes, skin lesions or arthritis may occur. Culture of the cervix in women or the throat or rectum in either sex, and microscopic examination of the discharge from the penis in men, allows the diagnosis to be made. Antibiotic treatment will cure the condition, but all sexual partners must be treated or reinfection will occur. Because more than one STD can be picked up at the same time, if gonorrhea is found, then tests for other STDs should be done and treatment given for presumptive chlamydia infection.

# CHLAMYDIA INFECTIONS
# OF THE GENITAL TRACT

Chlamydia is more common than gonorrhea and is particularly common in sexually active adolescents. Chlamydial organisms are intracellular parasites that share many properties with bacteria. As with gonorrhea, the male partner who is infected with chlamydia may complain of burning or discomfort during urination and probably will note a purulent discharge at the tip of the penis. Fifty percent of females may be asymptomatic, although some may have an abnormal vaginal discharge, lower abdominal pain, abnormal vaginal bleeding, or dyspareunia. This infection may also lead to the long-term problems of chronic pelvic pain, infertility, and ectopic pregnancy. Infants born to infected mothers can develop an eye infection or pneumonia due to exposure to the organism in the vagina during delivery. The diagnosis is made when the organism is identified in the cells on a swab of the affected site, that is, the urethra in men and the cervix in women. Antibiotics will cure most acute chlamydial infections. Because gonorrhea and chlamydia frequently occur together, treatment for both is given at the same time. For both of these STDs, sexual partners should be tested and treated as appropriate.

# SYPHILIS

Syphilis is not a disease of the past. The local lesion is a *chancre,* a shallow painless ulcer, usually on the penis or in the vagina, where it is not frequently noticed. This lesion appears about 3 weeks after exposure and lasts for 1 to 5 weeks, during which time the person is highly infectious. The chancre then disappears even without treatment. Later, there is a transient rash. Untreated, the disease can persist for years without causing symptoms. Ten to 30 years later, damage to the heart, blood vessels, or nervous system may become evident. The organism, *Treponema pallidum,* may be passed across the placenta in pregnant women, whatever the stage of the disease. Abortion or stillbirth may result, or infants may be born with congenital syphilis affecting the brain, skin, bones, and other organs. The diagnosis of syphilis is made by examining fluid from the chancre, if one is present, or by a specific blood test. Treatment is by injection of penicillin.

# GENITAL HERPES

The same virus that causes cold sores or fever blisters causes genital herpes. Once infected, a person carries this virus forever, and genital lesions may recur at any time. There is no cure. The first episode of genital herpes usually is the most painful. It occurs 2 to 21 days after exposure to an infected partner. Blisters develop on or near the site of contact and may be external or internal (i.e., penis or urethra, vulva or cervix, perianal or anal). The blisters become ulcers, which are usually painful and often associated with fever and swelling of the lymph glands in the groin. Sometimes this infection also makes urination painful. If the lesions recur, they usually do so near the site of the first ulcers but heal faster and are less painful. The virus is most likely to be transmitted when there are lesions, but it can be transmitted even when there are no symptoms; therefore, sexual partners should be informed of a history of genital herpes and safer sex practices encouraged. Infection at the time of vaginal delivery may lead to a serious, sometimes fatal infection in the baby. Delivery by cesarean section protects the baby from exposure to the herpes virus if there are lesions at the time of delivery. The diagnosis of genital herpes can be confirmed by a culture from a lesion. Acyclovir tablets, if started early, can be useful in reducing the symptoms and shortening an episode of genital herpes. For those who have frequent recurrence, defined as six or more episodes per year, taking acyclovir tablets continuously may help reduce the frequency of episodes. Topical acyclovir provides little or no benefit.

## HEPATITIS

Several types of viruses can infect the liver, causing hepatitis. Hepatitis may be transient, may or may not cause symptoms, and may be persistent, leading to cirrhosis or cancer. Several of the viruses (hepatitis A to G, cytomegalovirus, and Epstein-Barr virus) that cause hepatitis can be transmitted by sexual contact. Hepatitis B (HBV) is the most common STD causing hepatitis. All children should have been immunized with hepatitis B vaccine in infancy, and any child or adolescent who did not receive the vaccine in infancy should be immunized (see Chapter 3).

## HUMAN PAPILLOMAVIRUS (HPV)

There are over 70 types of human papillomavirus (HPV). HPV produces warts on the skin and mucous membranes. The types of HPV that cause nongenital warts are different from those that cause anogenital infections. Some of the types causing genital warts may also cause cervical cancer. Warts can be removed by treatment with topical chemicals or by surgery. Because HPV infection of the cervix is common in sexually active adolescents and can lead to cervical cancer, it is recommended that all sexually active adolescent females have an annual *Papanicolaou* (PAP) smear to screen for cervical *dyspasia* (abnormal cells).

## SUSPECTED STD

Teenagers should be able to talk to their sexual partners about the risks of STDs. Because some STDs may have periods with no symptoms, it is always safer to use a condom with a new sexual partner. The risks of transmitting an infection are high during the time of symptoms, and sexual contact should be avoided until treated.

## REPORTING AND CONFIDENTIALITY

When someone is diagnosed with an STD, the treating physician will ask that any recent sex partners be referred to make sure that others who may have the same infection also get treatment. Notification of partners may be done personally or anonymously through the local public health authorities. There are laws requiring reporting to health authorities and notification of sex partners for certain STDs, including HIV, syphilis, and gonorrhea. These reports on STDs are held in strict confidence.

## SUGGESTED READING

Gordon, S. (1987). *Seduction lines heard around the world and answers you can give: A world book of lines.* Buffalo, NY: Prometheus Books.

Hein, K., Foy DiGeronimo, T., & Editors of *Consumer Report* Books. (1994). *AIDS: Trading fears for facts: A guide for teens* (3rd ed.). Mount Vernon, NY: Consumers Union.

Kirby, D. (1999). Sexuality and sex education at home and school. *Adolescent Medicine, 10*(2), 195–209.

# REFERENCES

Centers for Disease Control. (2002). Sexually transmitted diseases treatment guidelines. *Morbidity and Mortality Weekly Report, 52*(RR-6), 1–80.

Cooper, E. R., Charurat, M., Mofenson, L., Hanson, I. C., Pitt, J., Diaz, C., Hayani, K., Handelsman, E., Smeriglio, V., Hoff, R., Blattner, W., & Women and Infants' Transmission Study Group. (2002). Combination antiretroviral strategies for the treatment of pregnant HIV-1–infected women and prevention of perinatal HIV-1 transmission. *Journal of Acquired Immune Deficiency Syndrome, 29,* 484–494.

Kuo, J. M., Taylor, J. M. G., & Detels, K. (1991). Estimating the AIDS incubation period from a prevalent cohort. *American Journal of Epidemiology, 133,* 1050–1057.

Royce, R. A., Seña, A., Cates, W., & Cohen, M. S. (1997). Current concepts: Sexual transmission of HIV. *New England Journal of Medicine, 336,* 1072–1078.

# CHAPTER 23

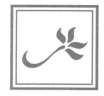

# Child Maltreatment

Marcellina Mian

**C**hild maltreatment of any type can interfere with a child's well-being and development, including school performance. By virtue of their close contact with children, educators are in a unique position to detect the early signs of maltreatment and to intervene on the child's behalf. Thus, their contribution is invaluable in providing a coordinated multidisciplinary approach to the prevention, detection, and management of child abuse and neglect and their effects. Professionals from the fields of education, health, social sciences, law, and law enforcement must work cooperatively to contribute their particular expertise and perspective to this complex problem. This chapter covers the role of school personnel in the prevention of child maltreatment and identification of child abuse or neglect and guidelines on management of cases.

## DEFINITIONS

According to a definition that was written by consensus in the course of a World Health Organization (WHO; 1999) expert consultation,

> child abuse or maltreatment constitutes all forms of physical and/or emotional ill-treatment, sexual abuse, neglect or negligent treatment or commercial or other exploitation, resulting in actual or potential harm to the child's health, survival, development or dignity in the context of a relationship of responsibility, trust or power.

Maltreatment is generally categorized into four types: physical, sexual, and emotional abuse, and neglect. The following are practical definitions of these categories.

*Physical abuse* of a child results in actual or potential harm from an interaction or lack of interaction that is reasonably within the control of a parent or person in a position of responsibility, power, or trust (WHO, 1999). It may include bruises, welts, cuts, burns, fractures, head injuries, internal injuries, or even death. Injury is caused by beating, shaking, pulling, twisting, burning, penetration, suffocation, or any other force used against the child. Physical discipline becomes abuse when it leaves a mark or causes physical or emotional harm.

*Sexual abuse* is the involvement of a child in sexual activity that he or she does not fully comprehend, to which the child is unable to give informed consent, or for which the child is not developmentally prepared and cannot give consent, or that violates the laws or social taboos of society. Child sexual abuse is evidenced by this activity between a child and an adult or another child who by age or development is in a relationship of responsibility, trust, or power, and the activity is intended to gratify or satisfy the needs of the other person (WHO, 1999). Sexual abuse covers a range of activities from exposure of the genitals with no physical contact to full vaginal or anal intercourse and includes oral–genital contact and fondling. It also covers situations where the child is invited to touch the perpetrator (e.g., fellatio) rather than the perpetrator being the active partner. Sexual abuse may or may not involve physical force. When the participants have a familial relationship to each other, the sexual abuse is termed *intrafamilial* or *incestuous* (Sgroi, Blick, & Porter, 1982).

*Emotional abuse* is defined as adverse parental behaviors occurring in a sustained pattern of interaction which impacts on a vulnerable child and produces damage to the child's emotional and psychological functioning (Thompson & Kaplan, 1996). Adverse parental behaviors include rejecting, ignoring, terrorizing, isolating, exploiting, or missocializing a child. Terrorizing includes exposure of the child to family violence. Emotional abuse often exists concurrently with physical and sexual abuse (Wolfe, 1991a).

*Neglect* "occurs when basic needs of children are not met regardless of cause" (Dubowitz, Black, Starr, & Zuravin, 1993, p. 12). It includes the failure to provide adequate shelter, food, clothing, health care, and nurture to a child, as well as adequate supervision to ensure the child's safety. Mild or occasional inadequacies may not have any discernible results and do not usually fit the criterion for protective intervention, whereas more severe or consistent inadequacies can result in impaired growth, development, or overall health, and gross inadequacies can result in death. Inadequate caloric intake may lead to failure-to-thrive, a condition of neglect wherein a child fails to grow according to expected norms (Ludwig, 1992).

# EXTENT OF THE PROBLEM

According to Canadian figures for 1998, the estimated incidence rate for investigations of child maltreatment was 21.52 per 1,000 children (Trocmé et al., 2001). Of these, 9.71 per 1,000 were substantiated, 4.71 were suspected to involve abuse but lacked sufficient evidence to substantiate them, and 7.09 were felt not to involve child maltreatment. One must remember that these figures represent only the tip of the child maltreatment iceberg because they do not include those cases where abuse is known but not reported or cases of abuse that are unknown. Substantiated cases were divided approximately as follows: 37.7% neglect, 23.0% physical abuse, 8.9% sexual abuse, and 22.7% emotional abuse. The remaining 7.7% had undergone a form of abuse substantiated as different from the primary reason of investigation.

A nationwide random survey of teachers in the United States indicated that almost three quarters had suspected that a child had been abused or neglected at one time or another (Abrahams, Casey, & Daro, 1992). Ninety percent of these teachers indicated that they had reported their suspicion within the school system, but only 23% had reported to child protection authorities directly. This same survey found that the majority of teachers received insufficient education on the skills required to identify, report, and intervene in cases of suspected child abuse and neglect.

In the Canadian Incidence Study of Reported Child Abuse and Neglect (Trocmé et al., 2001), the following selected information about referral sources is noteworthy: Professionals made 59% of the reports to the child welfare agencies. School personnel referred 21% of all investigations, compared with 12% by police, 5% by health personnel, and 34% by nonprofessionals in the community. The school referrals were substantiated in 39% of cases; cases referred by police had the highest substantiation rate, at 57%; and referrals by other child welfare agencies and mental health professionals were substantiated in 50% and 47% of cases, respectively. Of nonprofessional referrals, 50% of those made by children, 45% of those made by parents, 34% made by relatives and friends, and 13% of those made anonymously were substantiated. School personnel referred over one third of physical abuse cases, and 39% of these were substantiated. They also referred 16% of neglect and sexual abuse cases, and 15% of emotional maltreatment.

# CAUSES OF MALTREATMENT

The causes of child abuse and neglect are not well understood. The current perspective views "child abuse along a continuum ranging from normal and acceptable forms of parenting at one end, to more extreme and violent forms of child care at the other" (Wolfe, 1991a, p. 5). Child neglect also begins somewhere along the continuum from optimal care to grossly inadequate care (Dubowitz et al., 1993). Although certain risk indicators or factors have been identified as being associated with an increased risk of child maltreatment, it is not known what the *causal* risk factors are—that is, which factors would make the difference between maltreatment occurring or not. Therefore, risk factors need to be interpreted cautiously in specific cases and should be used only to enhance services and not to stigmatize children.

Societal factors play a significant role. Poverty is highly associated with child abuse, essentially through its impact on the behavior of caregivers and community resources (Krug, Dahlberg, Mercy, Zwi, & Lozano, 2002). In the Canadian survey (Trocmé et al., 2001), emotional abuse and neglect were more likely in families that relied on social assistance or some other form of benefit for their income, in comparison to cases of physical or sexual abuse, which were more likely in families that relied on full-time employment. Several other societal factors have an impact on child maltreatment but have not yet been well studied. Among these are cultural values and economic forces, gender roles, and child and family policies that provide support for the families (Krug et al., 2002). There is a strong relationship between domestic violence and child abuse. Substance abuse, so prevalent in society today, is also associated with child abuse, but its effect is entangled with those of poverty, overcrowding, and mental disorders (Krug et al., 2002).

Within this societal framework, there are risk indicators associated with an increase in the probability that some families will abuse their children. The following risk indicators (MacMillan, 2000a, 2000b) have been identified for parents who engage in physical abuse: youth, psychiatric impairment, or low education of the mother; single parenthood; history of physical abuse as a child; spousal violence; unwanted pregnancy; nonattendance at prenatal classes; substance abuse; limited religious participation; large family size; and recent life stresses. For parents who engage in sexual abuse, risk indicators include parental death, absence of a natural parent in the family, presence of a stepfather, poor relations between the parents and between parent and child, and low education in the mother. For parents who neglect their children, these indicators include sociopathic behavior and substance abuse by the parents.

There are risk factors for children as well. More physically abused children are male, and more sexually abused children are female (MacMillan, 2000a). Girls are more likely to be neglected, whereas boys are at greater risk of harsh physical punishment (Krug et al., 2002). In the United States, nonfatal physical abuse is highest in children ages 6 to 12 years. Sexual abuse is highest in adolescence (Krug et al., 2002). Other factors, including being born prematurely, having a congenital deformity or illness, being temperamentally difficult, being or having undesirable physical attributes (e.g., looking like someone the parent detests), also render children vulnerable. Sometimes the child's behavior—taunting, aggressive or seductive—is said to invite abuse (Christian, 1992).

The high-risk factors associated with maltreatment can be mitigated by compensatory factors, which include community connections and social networks (Krug et al., 2002). One intervention that has definitely been shown to be of assistance in preventing child maltreatment is a program of home visitation by nurses to first-time disadvantaged mothers around the time of the child's birth and through the infancy period (MacMillan, 2000b). However, community resources to cope with the basic needs of all of its members and the special needs of some of its members are limited, and this difficulty has increased with the economic downturn of recent years.

# EFFECTS OF ABUSE

The physical injuries of abuse will have effects that depend on the site and severity of the injury. These can vary from transient injuries that heal completely to serious injuries that can disfigure or maim or that, in some cases, even result in death. Data now indicate that the effects of abuse on children can result in major adult illnesses, including heart disease, chronic lung disease, and cancer (Krug et al., 2002). Much more difficult to identify and to correct than the physical sequelae of abuse and neglect are psychological short- and long-term effects associated with that maltreatment.

The psychological (i.e., emotional, cognitive, and developmental) effects of maltreatment depend on the age and developmental level of the child at the time of its occurrence; the severity, frequency, and duration of abuse; and the presence or absence of mediating factors (Blount, 1992; Krug et al., 2002). Maltreatment can interfere with the child's accomplishment of normal developmental tasks, such as the acquisition of language. Data indicate that the school performance of maltreated children may be adversely affected and that victims may underachieve relative to their ability. Maltreated children have been found to have lower intelligence quotient scores and more learning disabilities, and have consistently been rated by teachers as being less competent academically and socially and as having greater behavioral problems than nonabused children. Unless corrective steps are taken, this failure in school will result in failure in later life.

Abuse and the abusive environment interfere with nurturance of the child by the caregiver. Thus, the formation of attachment, one of the most critical tasks of early development, is impaired (Wolfe, 1991b). The child's ability to form relationships with anyone is affected. Abused children tend to have fewer friends and to be more shy and inhibited in social contacts. They exhibit more aggressive and oppositional behavior. Their behavior also may be impulsive, exploitive, and manipulative (Blount, 1992). Not surprisingly, given their limited competence and social success, abused children often have lowered self-esteem and ambition, with greater feelings of depression and hopelessness (Blount, 1992; Wolfe, 1991b). Studies have shown an increased likelihood of a psychiatric disorder in children who have been maltreated (MacMillan, 2000a). Some abused children may develop multiple personalities or other forms of dissociation; these children may suffer from acute or chronic anxiety (Blount, 1992).

Abused children may develop degrees of dissociation, at times as severe as *multiple personality disorder* (MPD). A clinical profile of this continuum is provided by Putnam (1989). The incidence of MPD has not been established, but it may be more common than is generally recognized. Dissociation is believed to originate as a defense mechanism against the trauma of abuse and isolation. Children learn to separate their minds from their bodies so that the mind can wander away from the misery into another time, place, or person. Children have described themselves as flying up to the ceiling from where they have observed their body being abused, without being affected. If the need for this dissociation persists too long, the child may lose the ability to control it, and it becomes maladaptive. Separate personalities may become well established. Each may have a separate function with different characteristics and abilities. These differences may even be physical, so that one personality may be myopic or allergic although the host child is not. One personality may have learning problems and poor impulse control, whereas another is docile and academically gifted. This disorder may account for markedly erratic performance in a student. Careful assessment is required to diagnose MPD.

All this does not mean that children who are abused are uniformly and inexorably doomed to continue suffering. Indeed, children are extremely resilient and many do recover from their abuse to become functioning adults and contributing members of society. The factor that is most helpful to a child's recovery is the presence of an adult whom they can trust and on whom they can rely. Thus, the teacher is in an ideal position to sustain a child and help in the healing process.

# DISCLOSURES OF MALTREATMENT

It is often surprising for the public to realize that children can be maltreated and not tell anyone about it. They expect children to reveal that they have been abused at the earliest opportunity. In fact, data on sexually abused children, whose abuse has been confirmed by the perpetrators' confessions or their conviction in court, indicate that the majority do not disclose it (Sorensen & Snow, 1991). In 75% of cases, the identification of abuse is often accidental and is not intended by the child to be a disclosure. How does this happen? The child says or does something that prompts someone else to suspect that he or she has been abused, or the child confides in a friend who breaks this confidence and informs an adult. Alternately, the child may be found to have a sexually transmitted disease. Preschool children (3 to 5 years of age) are least likely to disclose purposefully; adolescents (13 to 17 years of age) are most likely to do so. School-age children, taken as a whole, show no real propensity either way.

In most cases, children who are confronted with a suspicion of sexual abuse will deny the abuse initially, sometimes even when it includes "hard evidence," such as a pornographic photograph of themselves or a perpetrator's confession. Tentative disclosures, in which the abuse is minimized, is distanced, or shows features of dissociation, is the usual next step. Most children then go into active disclosure and can give age-appropriate detailed accounts of their abuse. Depending on the parental and societal response, some children then recant their allegations, denying responsibility for their previous allegations and saying someone else made them do it. Of these children, the majority then reaffirm their allegations and return to active disclosure.

The above dynamics can be explained by the child sexual abuse accommodation syndrome (Summit, 1983), wherein it is physically more comfortable for the child to accommodate to the abuse and participate in the secrecy. It therefore is not surprising that the public is confused by sexual abuse allegations and about whether the alleged victims are telling the truth or which part of what they have said is the truth. Every disclosure of abuse must be evaluated carefully so that no child who is truly abused is left unprotected and false allegations are not allowed to ruin the lives of innocent people, including the children.

Some children disclose physical abuse. Few disclose neglect because the latter is more of an ongoing condition than one or a series of recognizable events. Physical abuse and neglect are most often recognized by their physical and developmental effects. Bruises, burns, fractured bones, and strange marks and symptoms are detected, and a satisfactory explanation for them cannot be found. The child may or may not be able or ready to disclose the cause of the injuries or behaviors, and further action depends on the strength of the medical information that originally raised the concerns.

Emotional abuse is least likely to be disclosed and the most difficult to detect. Children are unlikely to complain about the belittling or anxiety-provoking behavior of the caregiver, and the cause of a child's anxiety, nervousness, low self-esteem, and poor performance may be difficult to determine. In fact, the caregivers may describe their own conduct as being a consequence of the children's behavior problems and may feel quite justified. Further, the very effect of the abuse renders the children less likable and may incline others to identify them as the cause of the problem. This difficulty is compounded when caregivers, apparently acting in the child's best interest, take their child to professionals for counseling yet are unable or unwilling to comply with recommendations and withdraw from therapy. This cycle may be repeated again and again, unless some protective action can be taken.

"False memory syndrome" is the alleged recollection by adults of childhood abuse that, in fact, never occurred. It is claimed that these false memories are the result of the influence of therapists, incest recovery books, or self-help groups. The debate about the validity of this syndrome continues, as legitimate victims continue to speak up and society continues to want to believe that horrors like child sexual abuse do not exist (Bass & Davis, 1994). In the Canadian Incidence Study (Trocmé et al., 2001), 38% of sexual abuse reports were substantiated and another 22% were suspected but with insufficient evidence to substantiate, leaving 40% unsubstantiated. Even if all of these unsubstantiated cases represent no abuse, because the majority of the referrals were made by parents in this study and none from the child directly, the source of untrue allegations remains unclear.

Questions also have been raised about the reliability of children's statements based on their memory and suggestibility. A review of the available literature indicates that the ability to provide information about an experience increases with age and that young children are often more suggestible than older children and adults (Saywitz, Goodman, & Lyon, 2002). Suggestibility can be affected by cognitive factors as well as social factors, such as a child's prior experience; the context and dynamics of the interview, including the props used; the knowledge and belief of the interviewer; and the emotional tone of the questioning. Also, some children and youth deliberately lie. As for adults, the motivation includes the avoidance of punishment, the achievement of personal gain, or the protection of others.

What is currently known about children indicates that even the very young can reliably recall traumatic events (Saywitz et al., 2002). This is particularly true for the central events (e.g., the action involved) rather than peripheral events (e.g., what the abuser was wearing). Evidence indicates that free recall produces fewer factual errors than responses to leading questions, but it also provides less information. Conversely, more pointed questions result in more information but also more inaccuracies (Saywitz et al., 2002).

The validity of a disclosure can be determined only after careful assessment. Therefore, all disclosures must be believed to the extent that they will result in appropriate, competent, and unbiased investigation of the allegations. Untrained individuals should refrain from asking a child questions about potential abuse because of the possibility of inadvertently contaminating the child's subsequent reports.

# INDICATORS OF ABUSE

Given the previous information, educators need to know what the indicators of abuse are in school-age children. These indicators may be physical or behavioral; some are nonspecific signs of distress in a child's life, which could be the result of any stressful events such as parental separation or the birth of a sibling, and others are more specific to abused children. Some maltreated children may not present any recognizable signs of their experience.

Physical indicators of abuse include injuries that are not consistent with the explanation given for them or for which no explanation is available. In addition, common indicators include the presence of multiple injuries at the same time or over time and injuries that are inconsistent with the child's developmental phase or allegedly sustained in a manner that is out of character for the child's usual range of behavior. Excessive or unusual itching or soreness in the genital area, torn or bloody underwear, and age-inappropriate urinary or stool incontinence may indicate sexual abuse. Frequent psychosomatic complaints; chronic fatigue, with the child frequently falling asleep in class; and inappropriate clothing for the weather, especially concealing clothing in warm weather, also suggest physical or sexual abuse. Specific physical indicators for abuse are injuries whose cause is readily identifiable as nonaccidental. Examples include a bruise in the shape of a belt, a burn in the pattern of a steam iron, and sexually transmitted diseases in children too young to be engaging in consensual sex.

Nonspecific behavioral indicators include the following: unusually noncompliant or aggressive behavior and, conversely, unusually compliant and docile behavior; wariness of adults; watchfulness; and recoil or flinching from being touched or from gestures of affection. In addition, overly affectionate or indiscriminately affectionate behavior; depression; self-destructive behavior, including promiscuity, drug abuse, suicidal ideation or attempts; and running away all point to the possibility of physical or sexual abuse. Also included in this list are poor peer relations, failure to participate in school activities, frequent school absences or late attendance, or, conversely, a child's apparent reluctance to return home at the end of the school day. Poor school performance on a chronic basis or a sudden drop in academic performance should also raise suspicion. Specific behavioral indicators of sexual abuse include age-inappropriate detailed knowledge of sexual activity; bizarre or unusual sexual knowledge; age-inappropriate sexual play with self, toys, or others; seductive behaviors or comments toward others; and age-inappropriate sexually explicit drawings or descriptions.

What is age-inappropriate sexual behavior? When is sexual behavior between peers normative and acceptable and when is it an indicator of sexual abuse? Self-stimulation or masturbation is quite normal and is used by many children at times of stress or for comfort. If done in moderation and with some respect for privacy, it is of no concern. If it is preferred over other activities or involves excessive stimulation or harm, further assessment of the situation is warranted. Generally speaking, normative and appropriate sexual behavior with peers is based on curiosity, is mutually enjoyable and consensual, and does not result in harm to any participant (Haka-Ikse & Mian, 1993). A good example is "playing doctor." The language and behaviors used display age-appropriate knowledge; thus, younger children will be less sophisticated and detailed in their verbal and action knowledge of sexual acts, whereas teenagers will know much more. Worrisome behaviors are ones that involve an unusual degree of sophistication, coercion of another party, or lack of respect for "a time and a place" in which to do them.

Teachers should not be concerned if a developmental stage or event arouses sexual curiosity in a class. For example, pregnancy in a class hamster, the discovery that a schoolmate has been sexually abused, or comments made by older children or a video star may arouse a great deal of talk among the children and some attempts at imitation. However, if a basic explanation and exploration of the topic, such as conception, pregnancy, and delivery in mammals, fails to extinguish the behavior after some reasonable period of time, further assessment of the situation is required. Usually, one child or a group of children are then found to be the instigators. Further exploration of that child's or those children's needs is warranted because sexual abuse may be at the root of the problem.

# REPORTING AND MANAGING SUSPECTED ABUSE

Educators interact with children on a daily basis and, therefore, are able to observe the indicators of abuse or neglect already discussed. A decision to take action in these circumstances may be pivotal in preventing further abuse. When, however, is there sufficient information to warrant taking action? If a child demonstrates some nonspecific indicators, tactful questioning of the family about recent stresses is in order. An older child may be interviewed directly. It is helpful if the teacher informs the youth that any topic can be discussed and that no disclosure would be too embarrassing or dreadful to face. The teacher may explore the nature of the visual or reading material, such as soap operas or pornography, to which the child might have been exposed.

If there are more specific indicators, or if the child makes a disclosure, it is appropriate to have the mandated authorities conduct an interview. However, in some circumstances an educator may be unsure of the significance of what has been observed or heard and may want to ask clarifying questions. It is important to remember that this is a delicate area that requires sensitivity and skill.

The best way to ensure a helpful interview is to have the interviewer enter the process without a preconceived notion of the result. The atmosphere should be nonthreatening and the child should not be made to feel that a certain performance or answer is required. Leading questions—those that can be answered "yes" or "no" or that contain the answer in themselves, such as, "Did he touch your privates?"—should be avoided. Open-ended questions are best, such as, "How did you learn to touch girls like that?" "What happened to your arm?" or "You say you're sad; can you tell me what makes you sad?" Questions should be simple and in language appropriate to the child's age. The same question should not be asked repeatedly because that suggests to the child, especially a young one, that the initial answer was incorrect and that the interviewer expects a different response.

If an educator is unsure of how to proceed in an interview, he or she should seek advice from a specialist who has knowledge of child abuse before continuing, because inappropriate early questioning may jeopardize the subsequent investigation. Child protection authorities or hospital-based child abuse programs generally are willing to consult on the preferred course of action for an educator to take in specific cases.

Most jurisdictions have mandatory reporting of child abuse based on suspicion and not on proof of abuse. Educators are among the professionals bound by those laws. The specifics of how that reporting takes place depend in large part on the individual situation and the local school board policy. Each school should have a clear set of guidelines in place for dealing with child abuse.

Professionals are reluctant to report suspected child abuse or neglect for many reasons. Some teachers feel that a significant obstacle to reporting is the lack of sufficient knowledge concerning how to detect and report cases (Abrahams et al., 1992). They may not be confident that their concerns are valid. They may be afraid of causing more harm than good, be frightened of reprisals and legal repercussions, or simply be loath to become involved. Clearly, reporting child abuse has many ramifications and is unquestionably a difficult decision. However, for legal and ethical reasons, and for the sake of the child, this reluctance must be overcome.

One major area of concern is the timing for informing parents of suspected abuse. A critical factor in making that determination is whether there is reason to believe that the parent is the perpetrator. If that is the case, it is recommended that the child be interviewed by the authorities before the parents have an opportunity to influence the disclosure. On the other hand, parents should not be excluded from the investigative process altogether. They may be able to provide information that may assist in clarifying details provided by the child. Parents usually wish to be present during their child's physical examination, or at least be informed of it.

The interview of the child by the authorities may be conducted on the school premises. Educators may be intimidated by the process, especially if this is their first encounter with a child-abuse situation. Teachers need to realize that if they are a little apprehensive, the child is more so. The teacher must act as the child's support person during this process, which means cooperating with the investigative team during the initial investigation process to ensure that the child's needs are being met in the best possible way. For example, the teacher should consider whether it is appropriate for the interview to be taking place at the school and what measures need to be taken to ensure confidentiality for the child, particularly an adolescent. Issues of confidentiality are concerned not only with the content of the interview, but also with the fact that the interview will arouse curiosity in the school population and will result in discomfort for the youth if steps are not taken to reduce that curiosity. The teacher must assume an air of quiet confidence to guide and reassure the youth through this difficult time. If the proceedings seem unclear or confusing, the teacher can act as the child's advocate, particularly when the student is confronted by strangers. The school may also know the parents well enough to help strategize on the best way to notify them and elicit their cooperation.

School personnel may be asked to participate in case conferences or provide valuable information to understand the abusive situation more clearly. Also, educators may be asked to provide statements to the police and called to appear in court. Although this is an intimidating process, an open and cooperative approach is most helpful in providing the information required to arrive at the best disposition for the child.

Throughout the investigation and any legal proceedings, as well as following them, school personnel need to be aware of the emotional trauma on the pupil and his or her family. Educators may not be cognizant of the particulars of the situation and do not have to be; however, they should be aware that the child and family are under increased stress at this time. Many changes may be taking place in their lives; the child may be removed from the family or the offending parent may be criminally charged. Some extra patience and reassurance may be needed. The rules of the class should not be altered, because, in this time of turmoil, as much stability as possible is needed. Therapists may become involved, and it is wise for the teacher to form an alliance with them to maximize the effectiveness of the therapy.

# THE TEACHER
# AS THE PERPETRATOR

Some situations have occurred in which teachers have been accused, and in some cases convicted, of molesting children (Steed, 1994). How should other educators, the alleged perpetrator's colleagues, react and act in these circumstances? The temptation often is to seek the facts individually so that one can make a determination of guilt and then behave accordingly. Unfortunately, the bias is usually in favor of one's colleague. It is difficult to imagine how someone whom an educator knows on a daily basis and who shares the daily tribulations of the school environment could violate a sacred trust. It is easier to believe that a child would lie or even misunderstand a teacher's innocent actions or remarks.

The most desirable course of action for other teachers to take is one of support for the children. This means providing the children with the opportunity to come forward with whatever feelings they have in the situation, rather than telling them how to respond or react. The feelings of the parents and other teachers, particularly for an accused teacher who is well liked, must not influence the children. Support for the teacher can be expressed in such a way that children who may have personal concerns to bring forward are not silenced. Ultimately, only a proper and thorough investigation will determine the truth of the situation and vindicate the teacher, if appropriate. Taking sides prematurely will only contaminate the process and may result in leaving children at continued risk.

# PREVENTION

Some schools participate in personal safety education courses intended to teach children and adolescents that they have a right to determine what contact others may have with their bodies. Good programs aim at teaching children that people need contact with each other, but that there is a difference between good and bad touch. Most of these programs focus on preventing child sexual abuse. Current evidence shows that these programs increase knowledge and skills in the children, but they do not necessarily reduce abuse (MacMillan, 2000b).

Prevention of maltreatment needs to be seen in a broader sense. This involves changing current societal values to eliminate the root cause of violence and abuse. Some specific programs with this objective have been developed in schools and aimed at different developmental stages (Caring Communities Project, 1993). For example, one provides retreats for secondary school teachers and students that focus on gender, in order to address sex-role stereotyping and increased violence against women. Another aims to teach preadolescent boys how to step out of traditional masculine roles by providing them a course in baby care; the belief is that if young men learn to nurture babies, they will be less likely to harm children.

Patriarchal, sexist, and violent attitudes must be discouraged and replaced with social values that promote mutuality, respect, and optimal development for all members of society (Bagley & King, 1990). Teachers can provide an atmosphere for their students in which mutual respect is fostered, regardless of age, size, and ethnic or racial differences. Educators can teach and model nonviolent conflict resolution and inform children that they are available and willing to provide assistance if students find themselves in difficult situations.

# REFERENCES

Abrahams, N., Casey, K., & Daro, D. (1992). Teachers' knowledge, attitudes, and beliefs. *Child Abuse & Neglect, 16,* 229–238.

Bagley, C., & King, K. (1990). *Child sexual abuse.* London: Tavistock/Routledge.

Bass, E., & Davis, L. (1994). Honoring the truth: A response to the backlash. In E. Bass & L. Davis (Eds.), *The courage to heal* (3rd ed., pp. 475–534). New York: HarperCollins.

Blount, K. (1992). Chronic psychological manifestations. In S. Ludwig & A. E. Kornberg (Eds.), *Child abuse: A medical reference* (2nd ed., pp. 369–381). New York: Churchill Livingstone.

Caring Communities Project. (1993). *Communities preventing child abuse* (Publication No. 71). Toronto: Canadian Institute of Child Health.

Christian, C. W. (1992). Etiology and prevention of child abuse: Individual and family factors. In S. Ludwig & A. E. Kornberg (Eds.), *Child abuse: A medical reference* (2nd ed., pp. 39–47). New York: Churchill Livingstone.

Dubowitz, H., Black, M., Starr, R. H., & Zuravin, S. (1993). A conceptual definition of child neglect. *Criminal Justice & Behavior, 20,* 8–26.

Haka-Ikse, K., & Mian, M. (1993). Sexuality in children. *Pediatrics in Review, 14,* 401–407.

Krug, E. G., Dahlberg, L. L., Mercy, J. A., Zwi, A. B., & Lozano, R. (Eds.). (2002). Child abuse and neglect by parents and other caregivers. In *World report on violence and health.* Geneva, Switzerland: World Health Organization.

Ludwig, S. (1992). Failure-to-thrive/starvation. In S. Ludwig & A. E. Kornberg (Eds.), *Child abuse: A medical reference* (2nd ed., pp. 303–319). New York: Churchill Livingstone.

MacMillan, H. L. (2000a). Child maltreatment: What we know in the year 2000. *Canadian Journal of Psychiatry, 45,* 702–709.

MacMillan, H. L. (2000b). Preventive health care, 2000 update: Prevention of child maltreatment. *Canadian Medical Association Journal, 163,* 1451–1458.

Putnam, F. (1989). *Diagnosis and treatment of multiple personality disorder.* New York: Guilford Press.

Saywitz, K. J., Goodman, G. S., & Lyon, T. D. (2002). Interviewing children in and out of court: Current research and practice implications. In J. E. B. Myers, L. Berliner, J. Briere, C. T. Hendrix, C. Jenny, & T. A. Reid (Eds.), *The APSAC handbook on child maltreatment* (2nd ed., pp. 349–377). Thousand Oaks, CA: Sage.

Sgroi, S. M., Blick, L. C., & Porter, F. S. (1982). A conceptual framework for child sexual abuse. In S. M. Sgroi (Ed.), *Handbook of clinical intervention in child abuse* (p. 10). Lexington, MA: D.C. Heath.

Sorensen, T., & Snow, B. (1991). How children tell: The process of disclosure in child sexual abuse. *Child Welfare, 70,* 3–15.

Steed, J. (1994). *Our little secret.* Toronto, Canada: Random House.

Summit, R. C. (1983). The child sexual abuse accommodation syndrome. *Child Abuse & Neglect, 7,* 177–193.

Thompson, A. E., & Kaplan, C. A. (1996). Childhood emotional abuse. *British Journal of Psychiatry, 168,* 143–148.

Trocmé, N., MacLaurin, B., Fallon, B., Daciuk, J., Billingsley, D., Tourigny, M., Mayer, M., Wright, J., Barter, K., Burford, G., Hornick, J., Sullivan, R., & McKenzie, B. (2001). *Canadian Incidence Study of Reported Child Abuse and Neglect: Final report.* Ottawa, Ontario: Minister of Public Works and Government Services.

Wolfe, D. A. (1991a). Defining physical and emotional abuse. In D. A. Wolfe (Ed.), *Preventing physical and emotional abuse in children* (pp. 1–18). New York: Guilford Press.

Wolfe, D. A. (1991b). Causes and consequences of abusive behavior. In D. A. Wolfe (Ed.), *Preventing physical and emotional abuse of children* (pp. 19–43). New York: Guilford Press.

World Health Organization. (1999). *Report of consultation on child abuse prevention* (Document No. WHO/HSC/PVI/99.1). Geneva, Switzerland: Author.

# CHAPTER 24

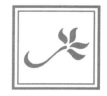

# The Science of Reading and Dyslexia

Sally E. Shaywitz and Bennett A. Shaywitz

**D**yslexia is characterized by an unexpected difficulty in reading for children and adults who otherwise possess the intelligence, motivation, and schooling considered necessary for accurate and fluent reading (S. Shaywitz, 1998). Historically, dyslexia in adults was first noted in the latter half of the 19th century, and developmental dyslexia in children was first reported in 1896. Recent epidemiologic data indicate that, like hypertension and obesity, dyslexia fits a dimensional model. In other words, within the population, reading ability and reading disability occur along a continuum, with reading disability representing the lower tail of a normal distribution of reading ability (Gilger, Borecki, Smith, DeFries, & Pennington, 1996; S. E. Shaywitz, Escobar, Shaywitz, Fletcher, & Makuch, 1992). Dyslexia is perhaps the most common neurobehavioral disorder affecting children, with prevalence rates ranging from 5% to 10% in clinic- and school-identified samples to 17.5% in unselected population-based samples (S. Shaywitz, 1998). Previously, it was believed that dyslexia affected boys primarily (Finucci & Childs, 1981); however, more recent data indicate similar numbers of affected boys and girls (Figure 24.1) (Flynn & Rahbar, 1994; S. E. Shaywitz, Shaywitz, Fletcher, & Escobar, 1990; Wadsworth, DeFries, Stevenson, Gilger, & Pennington, 1992). Longitudinal studies, both prospective (Francis, Shaywitz, Stuebing, Shaywitz, & Fletcher, 1996; B. A. Shaywitz et al., 1995) and retrospective (Bruck, 1992; Felton, Naylor, & Wood, 1990; Scarborough, 1984), indicate that dyslexia is a persistent, chronic condition; it does not represent a transient "developmental

---

Portions of this chapter appeared in and are similar to other reviews by us (B. Shaywitz et al., 2000; S. Shaywitz, 1998; S. Shaywitz & Shaywitz, 1999; S. Shaywitz et al., in press).

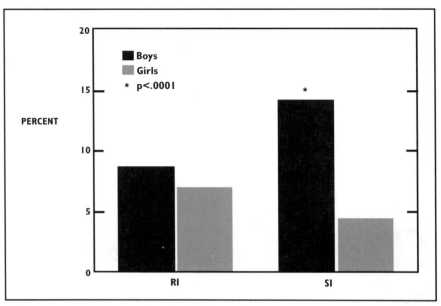

**FIGURE 24.1.** Percentage of reading disability in boys and girls. There is no significant difference in the prevalence of reading disability in research identified (RI) boys and girls. In contrast, school identified (SI) children with a reading disability showed a significant difference between boys and girls. The study suggests that SI samples are subject to referral bias and cautions against relying solely on schools for identification of reading disabled children. *Note.* From "Prevalence of Reading Disability in Boys and Girls: Results of Connecticut Longitudinal Study," by S. E. Shaywitz, B. A. Shaywitz, J. M. Fletcher, and M. D. Escobar, 1990, *Journal of the American Medical Association, 264*(8), pp. 298–1002. Copyright 1990 by S. E. Shaywitz. Reprinted with permission.

lag" (Figure 24.2). Over time, poor readers and good readers tend to maintain their relative positions along the spectrum of reading ability (B. A. Shaywitz et al., 1995).

Dyslexia is both familial and heritable (Pennington & Gilger, 1996). Family history is one of the most important risk factors: 23% to as much as 65% of children who have a parent with dyslexia are reported to have the disorder (Scarborough, 1990). Because the rate of dyslexia among siblings of affected persons is approximately 40% and that for parents ranges from 27% to 49% (Pennington & Gilger, 1996), there is an opportunity for early identification of affected siblings and often for delayed but helpful identification of affected adults. Linkage studies implicate loci on chromosomes 6 and 15 (Cardon et al., 1994, 1995; Grigorenko et al., 1997), chromosome

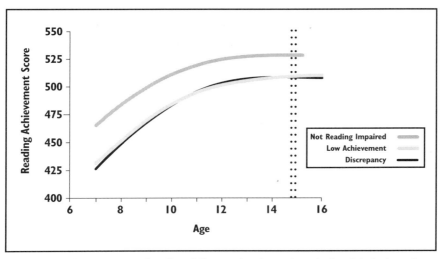

**FIGURE 24.2.** Trajectory of reading skills over time in nonimpaired and dyslexic readers. The ordinate is Rasch scores (W scores) from the *Woodcock-Johnson Reading Test* (Woodcock & Johnson, 1989) and the abscissa is age in years. Both dyslexic and nonimpaired readers improve their reading scores as they get older, but the gap between the dyslexic and nonimpaired readers remains. Thus, dyslexia is a deficit and not a developmental lag. *Note.* From "Developmental Lag Versus Deficit Models of Reading Disability: A Longitudinal, Individual Growth Curves Analysis," by D. J. Francis, S. E. Shaywitz, K. K. Stuebing, B. A. Shaywitz, and J. M. Fletcher, 1996, *Journal of Educational Psychology, 88*(1), pp. 3–17. Copyright 1996 by S. E. Shaywitz. Reprinted with permission.

1 (Rabin et al., 1993), and chromosome 2 (Fagerheim et al., 1999) for the transmission of phonologic awareness deficits and subsequent reading problems. Whether the differences in the genetic loci represent polygenic inheritance, different cognitive paths to the same phenotype, or different types of dyslexia is not clear.

# PATHOPHYSIOLOGY

## Cognitive Influences

### The Phonologic Deficit Hypothesis

There is now a strong consensus among investigators in the field that the central difficulty in dyslexia reflects a deficit within the language system, although other systems and processes also may contribute to the difficulty. The language system is conceptualized as a hierarchical series of components. At higher levels are neural systems engaged in processing (e.g., semantics, syntax, and discourse), and at the lowest level is the phonologic module dedicated to processing the distinctive sound elements that constitute language. The functional unit of the phonologic module is the phoneme, defined as the smallest discernible segment of speech; for example, the word *bat* consists of three phonemes: /b/, /æ/, and /t/ (buh, aah, tuh). To speak a word, the speaker retrieves the word's phonemic constituents from his or her internal lexicon, assembles the phonemes, and then utters the word. Conversely, to read a word, the reader must first segment that word into its underlying phonologic elements. The awareness that all words can be decomposed into these basic elements of language (phonemes) allows the reader to decipher the reading code. In order to read, a child has to develop the insight that spoken words can be pulled apart into phonemes and that the letters in a written word represent these sounds. Results from large and well-studied populations with reading disability confirm that in young school-age children (Fletcher et al., 1994; Stanovich & Siegel, 1994), as well as in adolescents (S. E. Shaywitz et al., 1999), a deficit in phonology represents the most robust and specific (Morris et al., 1998) correlate of reading disability. Such findings form the basis for the most successful and evidence-based interventions designed to improve reading (Report of the National Reading Panel, 2000).

## Implications of the Phonologic Model of Dyslexia

Basically, reading comprises two main processes: decoding and comprehension. In dyslexia, a deficit at the level of the phonologic module impairs the ability to segment the written word into its underlying phonologic elements. As a result, the reader experiences difficulty, first in decoding the word and then in identifying it. The phonologic deficit is domain specific; that is, it is independent of other, nonphonologic linguistic abilities. In particular, the higher-order cognitive and linguistic functions involved in comprehension, such as general intelligence and reasoning, vocabulary, and syntax, are generally intact. This pattern—a deficit in phonologic analysis but intact higher-order cognitive abilities—offers an explanation for the paradox of otherwise intelligent people who experience great difficulty in reading.

According to the model, a circumscribed deficit in a lower-order linguistic (phonologic) function blocks access to higher-order processes and to the ability to draw meaning from text. The problem is that the affected reader cannot use his or her higher-order linguistic skills to access the meaning until the printed word has first been decoded and identified. For example, an individual who knows the precise meaning of the spoken word *apparition* will not be able to use her knowledge of the meaning of the word until she can decode and identify the printed word on the page, and thus will appear not to know the word's meaning.

## The Phonologic Deficit in Adolescence and Adult Life

Deficits in phonologic coding continue to characterize dyslexic readers even in adolescence; performance on phonologic processing measures contributes most to discriminating dyslexic from average readers, as well as average from superior readers (S. E. Shaywitz et al., 1999). Children with dyslexia do not spontaneously remit or demonstrate a lag mechanism for "catching up" in the development of reading skills. However, many dyslexic readers do become quite proficient in reading a finite domain of words that are in their area of special interest, usually words that are important for their careers. For example, an individual who is dyslexic in childhood but becomes interested as an adult in molecular biology can learn to decode words that form a minivocabulary important in molecular biology. Such an individual, although able to decode words in a specific domain, still exhibits evidence of his early reading problems when he has to read unfamiliar words, which he then does accurately but not fluently and automatically (Ben-Dror, Pollatsek, & Scarpati, 1991; Bruck, 1985, 1990, 1992, 1994; Lefly & Pennington, 1991; S. E. Shaywitz et al., 1999). In adolescents, the rate of reading and the facility with spelling may be most useful clinically in differentiating average from poor readers. From a clinical perspective, these data indicate that, as children approach adolescence, a manifestation of dyslexia may be a very slow reading rate; in fact, children may learn to read words accurately, but they will not be fluent or automatic, reflecting the lingering effects of a phonologic deficit (Lefly & Pennington, 1991). Because they are able to read words accurately (albeit very slowly), dyslexic adolescents and young adults may mistakenly be assumed to have "outgrown" their dyslexia.

Data from studies of children with dyslexia who have been followed prospectively support the notion that the rate of reading and facility with spelling may be most useful clinically in differentiating good from poor readers in students in secondary school, as well as in college and even graduate school. It is important to remember that older dyslexic students may be similar to their unimpaired peers on untimed measures of word recognition yet continue to suffer from the phonologic deficit that makes reading less automatic, more effortful, and slow. For these readers with dyslexia, the provision of extra time is an essential accommodation; it allows them to decode each word and to apply their unimpaired higher-order cognitive and linguistic skills to the surrounding context to get at the meaning of words that they cannot entirely or rapidly decode. (More on this topic appears later in the section on management.)

## Neurobiological Influences

To a large degree, these advances in understanding dyslexia have informed and facilitated studies examining the neurobiological underpinnings of reading and dyslexia. Historically, as early as 1891, the French neurologist Dejerine suggested that a portion of the left posterior brain region is critical for reading. Beginning with Dejerine, a large literature on acquired inability to read (*alexia*) describes neuroanatomic lesions most prominently centered in the parietotemporal area (including the angular gyrus, supramarginal gyrus, and posterior portions of the superior temporal gyrus) as a region pivotal in mapping the visual percept of the print onto the phonologic structures of the language system (Damasio & Damasio, 1983; Friedman, Ween, & Albert, 1993; Geschwind, 1965). Another posterior brain region, this more ventral in the occipitotemporal area, was also described by Dejerine (1892) as critical in reading. More recently, a range of neurobiologic investigations using postmortem brain specimens (Galaburda, Sherman, Rosen, Aboitiz, & Geschwind, 1985), brain morphometry (Filipek, 1996), and diffusion tensor magnetic resonance imaging (Klingberg et al., 2000) supports the belief that there are differences in the temporal, parietal, and occipital brain regions between dyslexic and nonimpaired readers.

# FUNCTIONAL BRAIN IMAGING

Rather than being limited to examining the brain in an autopsy specimen, or measuring the size of brain regions using static morphometric indices, functional imaging offers the possibility of examining brain function during performance of a cognitive task. In principle, functional brain imaging is quite simple. When an individual is asked to perform a discrete cognitive task, that task places processing demands on particular neural systems in the brain. Meeting those demands requires activation of neural systems in specific brain regions, and those changes in neural activity are in turn reflected by changes in brain metabolic activity, which in turn are reflected, for example, by changes in cerebral blood flow and in the cerebral utilization of metabolic substrates such as glucose. Functional magnetic resonance imaging (fMRI) promises to supplant other imaging methods (e.g., positron emission tomography) because of its ability to map the individual brain's response to specific cognitive stimuli. Because fMRI is noninvasive and safe, it can be used repeatedly, making it ideal for studying humans, especially children.

Converging evidence using functional brain imaging in adult dyslexic readers shows a failure of left-hemisphere, posterior brain systems to function properly during reading (Brunswick, McCrory, Price, Frith, & Frith, 1999; Helenius, Tarkiainen, Cornelissen, Hansen, & Salmelin, 1999; Horwitz, Rumsey, & Donohue, 1998; Paulesu et al., 2001; Pugh et al., 2000; Rumsey et al., 1992; Rumsey et al., 1997; Salmelin, Service, Kiesila, Uutela, & Salonen, 1996; B. A. Shaywitz et al., 2002; S. E. Shaywitz et al., 1998; Simos, Breier, Fletcher, Bergman, & Papanicolaou, 2000), as well as during nonreading visual processing tasks (Demb, Boynton, & Heeger, 1998; Eden et al., 1996) (see Figure 24.3). In addition, some functional brain imaging studies show differences in brain activation in frontal regions in dyslexic compared to nonimpaired readers; in some studies dyslexic readers are more active in frontal regions (Brunswick et al., 1999; Rumsey et al., 1997; S. E. Shaywitz et al., 1998), and in others nonimpaired readers are more active in frontal regions (Corina et al., 2001; Georgiewa et al., 1999; Gross-Glenn et al., 1991; Paulesu et al., 1996).

Logan (1988, 1997) proposed two systems critical in the development of skilled, automatic processing, one involving word analysis, operating on individual units of words such as phonemes, requiring attentional resources and processing relatively slowly, and the second system operating on the whole word (word form), an obligatory system that processes very rapidly and does not require attention. Converging evidence from a number of lines of investigation indicates that Logan's word analysis system is localized within the parietotemporal region, whereas the automatic, rapidly responding system is localized within the occipitotemporal area, functioning as a visual word form area (Cohen et al., 2000; Cohen et al., 2002; Dehaene et al., 2001; Moore & Price, 1999). The visual word form area appears to respond preferentially to rapidly presented stimuli (Price, Moore, & Frackowiak,

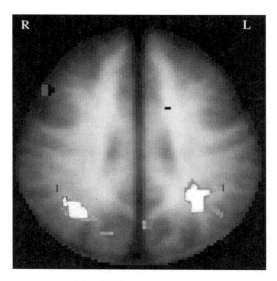

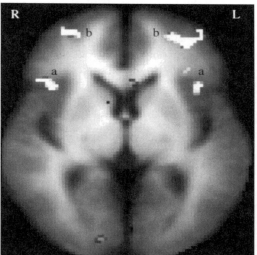

**FIGURE 24.3.** Composite fMRI activation maps in nonimpaired and dyslexic readers engaged in phonological processing during the nonword rhyme task. Nonimpaired readers (top frame) activate a large region involving the angular gyrus (1), supramarginal gyrus, and posterior portions of the superior temporal gyrus. In contrast, dyslexic readers (bottom frame) demonstrate a relative underactivation in this posterior region and an increased activation in the inferior frontal gyrus (a) and middle frontal gyrus (b) bilaterally. *Note.* From "Functional Disruption in the Organization of the Brain for Reading in Dyslexia," by S. E. Shaywitz et al., 1998, *Proceedings of the National Academy of Science USA, 95,* 2636–2641. Copyright 1998 by S. E. Shaywitz. Reprinted with permission.

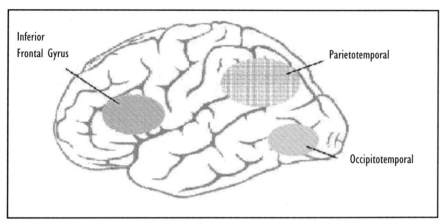

**FIGURE 24.4.** Neural systems for reading. Converging evidence indicates three important systems in reading, all primarily in the left hemisphere. These include an anterior system and two posterior systems: (a) anterior system in the left inferior frontal region; (b) dorsal parietotemporal system involving angular gyrus, supramarginal gyrus, and posterior portions of the superior temporal gyrus; and (c) ventral occipitotemporal system involving portions of the middle temporal gyrus and middle occipital gyrus. For details, see text.

1996) and is engaged even when the word has not been consciously perceived (Dehaene et al., 2001). It is this occipitotemporal system that appears to predominate when a reader has become skilled and has bound together as a unit the orthographic, phonologic, and semantic features of the word (see Figure 24.4).

Recognition of these two systems allows us to suggest an explanation for the brain activation patterns observed in dyslexic children. We suppose that, rather than the smoothly functioning and integrated reading systems observed in nonimpaired children, disruption of the posterior reading systems in dyslexic children results in attempts to compensate by shifting to other, ancillary systems, for example, anterior sites such as the inferior frontal gyrus and right hemisphere sites. The anterior sites, critical in articulation (Brunswick et al., 1999; Fiez & Peterson, 1998; Frackowiak, Friston, Frith, Dolan, & Mazziotta, 1997), may help the child with dyslexia develop an awareness of the sound structure of the word by subvocalizing—that is, forming the word with the lips, tongue, and vocal apparatus—and thus allow the child to read, albeit more slowly and less efficiently than if the fast occipitotemporal word identification system were functioning. The right-hemisphere sites may represent the engagement of brain regions that allow the poor reader to use other perceptual processes to compensate for his or her poor phonologic skills. A number of studies of young adults with childhood histories of dyslexia indicate that, although they may develop some accuracy in reading words, they remain slow, nonautomatic readers (Bruck, 1992; Felton et al., 1990).

# DIAGNOSIS

The diagnosis of dyslexia is basically no different from that for any other medical disorder. Guided by knowledge of the presumed underlying pathophysiology, the clinician seeks to determine through history, observation, and psychometric assessment if there are (a) unexpected difficulties (for age, intelligence, or level of education) in reading and (b) associated linguistic problems at the level of phonologic processing. No single test score is pathognomonic of dyslexia. As with any other medical diagnosis, the diagnosis of dyslexia should reflect a thoughtful synthesis of all the clinical data available. What the clinician is seeking is converging evidence of a phonologically based reading disability as indicated by a disparity between the individual's reading and phonologic skills in contrast to his or her intellectual capabilities, age, or level of education. Dyslexia is distinguished from other disorders that may prominently feature reading difficulties by the unique, circumscribed nature of the phonologic deficit, one not intruding into other linguistic or cognitive domains. How reading and language are assessed will reflect the age and educational level of the patient (Tables 24.1 and 24.2).

## Diagnosis at School Age

Presenting complaints about school-age children who are later found to have dyslexia most commonly relate to school performance (e.g., "She's not doing well in school"), and often parents and teachers do not appreciate that the reason for this is a reading difficulty. Thus, an evaluation for dyslexia should be considered for all children presenting with school difficulties, even if reading difficulty is not the chief complaint. As with most

## TABLE 24.1
### Clues to Dyslexia in School-Age Children [a]

**History**

Delayed language

Problems with the sounds of words (trouble rhyming words, confusion of words that sound alike)

Expressive language difficulties (mispronunciations, hesitations, word finding difficulties)

Difficulty naming (difficulty learning letters of alphabet and the names of numbers)

Difficulty learning to associate sounds with letters

History of reading and spelling difficulties in parents and siblings

**Reading**

Difficulty decoding single words

Particular difficulty reading nonsense or unfamiliar words

Inaccurate and labored oral reading

Slow reading

Comprehension often superior to isolated decoding skills

Poor spelling

**Language**

Relatively poor performance on tests of word retrieval (name the pictured item)

Relatively superior performance on tests of word recognition (point to the pictured item)

Poor performance on tests of phonological awareness

**Clues Most Specific to Young Children At-Risk for Dyslexia**

Difficulty on tests assessing: knowledge of the names of letters, the ability to associate sounds with letters and phonological awareness

**Clues Most Specific to Bright Young Adults with Dyslexia**

Childhood history of reading and spelling difficulties

Accurate but not automatic writing

Very slow performance on timed reading tests (e.g., *Nelson-Denny Reading Test*)

Penalized by multiple choice tests

[a] Clues are based on history, observations, testing, or a combination of the three.

*Note.* From "Current Concepts: Dyslexia," by S. Shaywitz, 1998, *The New England Journal of Medicine, 338*(5), pp. 307–312. Copyright 1998 by *New England Journal of Medicine*. Reprinted with permission.

**TABLE 24.2**

Types of Tests Useful in Identifying Children At Risk for Dyslexia
at the Time of School Entry

---

Letter identification (naming letters of the alphabet)

Letter–sound association (e.g., identifying words that begin with the same letter from a list: *doll, dog, boat*)

Phonological awareness (e.g., identifying the word that would remain if a particular sound was removed: if the /k/ sound was taken away from *cat*)

Verbal memory (e.g., recalling a sentence or a story that was just told)

Rapid naming (rapidly naming a continuous series of familiar objects, digits, letters, or colors)

Expressive vocabulary, or word retrieval (e.g., naming single pictured objects)

---

Note. From "Current Concepts: Dyslexia," by S. Shaywitz, 1998, *The New England Journal of Medicine, 338*(5), pp. 307–312. Copyright 1998 by *New England Journal of Medicine*. Reprinted with permission.

medical disorders, the history is critical to the diagnosis of dyslexia. Clinicians need to develop a sense of the developmental pattern demonstrated by children with dyslexia. Overall, the ontogeny of dyslexia is that of a child who may have had a delay in speaking, does not learn letters during kindergarten, and has not begun to learn to read by the completion of first grade. The child progressively falls behind, with teachers and parents puzzled as to why such an intelligent child may have difficulty learning to read. The reading difficulty is unexpected with respect to the child's ability, age, or grade. Even after acquiring decoding skills, the child generally remains a slow reader. When teachers are not informed, they may unnecessarily pressure or hurry the student. Dysgraphia is often present and accompanied by laborious note taking. Self-esteem is frequently affected, particularly if the disorder has gone undetected for a long period of time. Children with learning disabilities are likely to have encountered negative test-taking experiences where there was a disparity between their knowledge and their test scores, especially on timed tests, and thus tend to exhibit more test anxiety than nondisabled peers. Test scores may thus be artificially depressed as a result of such anxiety. Adults with strong histories of dyslexia who have compensated for their reading disability demonstrate good accuracy in reading but are less automatic than typical readers. These individuals take longer to apply their decoding skills and thus are slower readers; however, given sufficient time, they score very well on tests of reading comprehension.

Reading is assessed by measuring decoding and comprehension. In the school-age child, one important element of the psychometric evaluation is how accurately the child can decode words, that is, read single words in isolation. This is measured with standardized tests of single real-word and pseudoword reading, such as the *Woodcock-Johnson Psycho-Educational Battery–Revised* (Woodcock & Johnson, 1989) and the *Woodcock Reading Mastery Tests–Revised–Normative Update* (Woodcock, 1998). Difficulties also often emerge on tests of spelling, which depend on these same abilities. Reading fluency should be assessed by oral reading aloud, using the *Gray Oral Reading Tests–Fourth Edition* (Wiederholt & Bryant, 2001). This test consists of 14 increasingly difficult passages, each followed by 5 comprehension questions. Word reading efficiency may be assessed using the *Test of Word Reading Efficiency* (Torgesen, Wagner, & Rashotte, 1999), a test of speeded reading of single words. This test measures how many words, from a list that increases gradually in difficulty, the child can read in 45 seconds.

## Diagnosis in Preschool and at School Entry

Currently, most children with a reading disability are not diagnosed until they are in third grade or about 9 years old. Good evidence indicates that it is possible to screen children as young as 4 to 5 years of age and identify those at risk for reading disability, an identification based on poor reading relative to chronological age—that is, poor reading defined solely on the basis of low reading achievement. A history of language delay or of not attending to the sounds of words (trouble playing rhyming games with words, confusing words that sound alike) and a positive family history represent significant risk factors for dyslexia. The most helpful measures in predicting reading difficulties are those designed to assess phonemic awareness and phonologic skills, in general. Normed tests of phonologic analysis for young children are now available, including the *Comprehensive Test of Phonological Processing* (Wagner, Torgesen, & Rashotte, 1999). This test consists of measures of phonologic awareness, phonologic coding and working memory, and rapid naming, and has a national standardization on individuals ranging in age from 5 to adulthood. For example, measures most predictive of later reading ability involve the child's knowledge of letter sounds, the ability to blend sounds into words (done orally), and, at the end of kindergarten, the ability to name letters rapidly. There is growing evidence that early identification and intervention in kindergarten and Grade 1 may substantially reduce the number of children requiring special services for reading disability. These early identification procedures are very sensitive but not very specific, so they tend to overidentify children with dyslexia, but this is reasonable given that the costs of delaying intervention are too great to wait.

## Diagnosis in Adolescents and Young Adults

Dyslexia is persistent; it does not go away. On a practical level, this means that once a person is diagnosed as dyslexic, there is no need for reexamination to reconfirm the diagnosis. Over the course of development, skilled readers become more accurate and more automatic in decoding; they do not need to rely on context for word identification. Dyslexic readers also become more accurate over time, but they do not become automatic in their reading. Residua of the phonological deficit persist so that reading remains effortful and slow, even for the brightest of individuals with childhood histories of dyslexia. Failure to either recognize or measure the lack of automaticity in reading represents, perhaps, the most common error in the diagnosis of dyslexia in accomplished young adults. It is often not appreciated that tests measuring word accuracy are inadequate for the diagnosis of dyslexia in young adults at the level of college, graduate, or professional school, and that, for these individuals, timed measures of reading must be employed in making the diagnosis. However, there are very few standardized tests for adult readers that are administered under timed and untimed conditions; the *Nelson-Denny Reading Test* (Brown, Fishco, & Hanna, 1993) represents an exception. Reading measures commonly used for school-age children may provide misleading data in some adolescents and young adults because these tests assess reading accuracy, not automaticity (speed). In bright young adults, a history of phonologically based reading difficulties, requirements for extra time on tests, and current slow and effortful reading (i.e., signs of a lack of automaticity in reading) are the sine qua non of a diagnosis of dyslexia. *At all ages, and especially in young adults, dyslexia is a clinical diagnosis.*

# MANAGEMENT

Because physicians and educators are frequently asked about various reading programs for individuals with dyslexia, they should understand the principal elements of an effective training program. These elements reflect an understanding of the reading process and of why it is so difficult for children and adults with dyslexia to learn to read. The management of dyslexia demands a life-span perspective: Early on, the focus is on remediation of the reading problem; as a child matures and enters the more time-demanding setting of secondary school, the emphasis shifts to the important role of providing accommodations. The goal of effective intervention programs is to remediate the underlying problem in phonemic awareness, but the standard instruction provided through remediation is frequently too little, too general, and too unsystematic.

According to the Report of the National Reading Panel (2000), evidence-based reading intervention programs have been identified that provide instruction in the most important elements in reading: phonemic awareness, phonics, reading fluency, vocabulary, and reading comprehension strategies. In identifying these programs, the National Reading Panel used the same methodology that has been recognized as the scientific standard and that has been used so successfully in providing evidence-based treatments for many other disorders affecting children. Taking each component of the reading process in turn, the interventions used with younger children and even with older children are programs to improve phonemic awareness (PA), that is, the ability to focus on and manipulate phonemes (speech sounds) in spoken syllables and words. The program elements found to be most effective in enhancing PA, reading, and spelling skills include teaching children to manipulate phonemes with letters; focusing the instruction on one or two, rather than multiple, types of phoneme manipulations; teaching children in small groups; and providing explicit instruction rather than incidental instruction in PA. The next step in teaching reading is to teach phonics, that is, to make sure that the beginning reader understands how letters are linked to sounds (phonemes) to form letter–sound correspondences and spelling patterns. Critical to teaching phonics is making sure that the instruction is explicit and systematic; phonics instruction enhances children's success in learning to read, and systematic phonics instruction is more effective than instruction that teaches little or no phonics. Furthermore, the effects of phonics instruction are substantial in kindergarten and first grade, indicating that systematic phonics programs should be implemented in these early grades. The evidence indicates that kindergartners who receive phonics instruction benefit in their ability to read and spell words, and first graders taught phonics are better able to decode and spell, and show significant improvement in their ability to comprehend text. In contrast, older children receiving phonics instruction are better able to decode and spell words and to read text orally, but their comprehension of text is not significantly improved.

Fluency refers to the ability to read aloud orally with speed, accuracy, and proper expression. Although it is generally recognized that fluency is an important component of skilled reading, it is often neglected in the classroom. The most effective method to build reading fluency is guided oral reading—that is, reading aloud repeatedly to a teacher, an adult, or a peer, and receiving feedback. The evidence indicates that guided oral reading has a clear and positive impact on word recognition, fluency, and comprehension at a variety of grade levels and applies to all students—good readers, as well as those experiencing reading difficulties. Where the evidence is less secure is for programs for struggling readers that encourage large amounts of independent reading, that is, silent reading without any feedback to the student. Thus, even though independent silent reading is intuitively appealing, at this time the evidence does not support the notion that reading fluency improves. No doubt there is a correlation between being a good reader and reading large amounts; however, there is a paucity of evidence indicating that there is a *causal relationship* such that if poor readers read more, they will become more fluent.

Fluency is of critical importance because text reading that is dysfluent is slow and may impair the child's ability to comprehend what he or she has read, and, clearly, comprehending the text is the ultimate goal of reading. In contrast to teaching phonemic awareness, phonics, and fluency, interventions for reading comprehension are not as well established, in large measure because of the nature of the very complex processes influencing reading comprehension. The limited evidence indicates that the most effective methods for teaching reading comprehension involve teaching such components as vocabulary and an active interaction between reader and text, an interaction fostered by teachers who have the knowledge and skills to apply strategies designed to engage the student with the material.

One of the most exciting developments in reading and reading disability is the converging evidence that, in many cases, and if recognized very early (at ages 4 and 5 years), reading difficulties may be prevented. As early as kindergarten, and perhaps even in preschool, it is now possible to identify children who are at risk for word reading difficulties on the basis of their performance on tasks that assess phonemic awareness and naming abilities. Even with the early identification and interventions designed to prevent reading disability, a substantial number of children may need the interventions discussed previously.

Large-scale studies to date have focused on younger children; as yet, few or no data are available on the effect of these training programs on older children. The management of dyslexia in students in secondary school, and especially in college and graduate school, is based on accommodation rather than remediation. College students with a history of childhood dyslexia often present a paradoxical picture; they are similar to their unimpaired peers on measures of word recognition and reading comprehension, yet they continue to suffer from the phonologic deficit that makes reading less automatic, more effortful, and slow. For young adults with dyslexia, the provision of extra time is an essential accommodation; it allows them the time to decode each word and to apply their unimpaired higher-order cognitive and linguistic skills to the surrounding context to get at the meaning of words that they cannot entirely or rapidly decode. Studies comparing performance of students with reading disabilities who are or are not given extra time demonstrate the latent potential of such students that emerges only if they are provided with extra time to compensate for their lack of automaticity. In contrast, additional time makes little to no difference in the performance of nonimpaired readers. Although providing extra time for reading is by far the most common accommodation for people with dyslexia, other helpful accommodations include allowing the use of laptop computers with spelling checkers, tape recorders in the classroom, and recorded books (materials are available from Recording for the Blind and Dyslexic; 800/221-4792), and providing access to syllabi and lecture notes, tutors to "talk through" and review the content of reading material, alternatives to multiple-choice tests (e.g., reports or orally administered tests), and a separate, quiet room for taking tests. With such accommodations, many students with dyslexia are now successfully completing studies in a range of disciplines, including medicine.

People with dyslexia and their families frequently consult their physicians or teachers about unconventional approaches to the remediation of reading difficulties (e.g., optometric training, medication for vestibular dysfunction, chiropractic manipulation, dietary supplementation). In general, there are no credible data to support the claims made for these treatments.

## SUMMARY

There is now convincing scientific evidence (a) to explain why some very smart people have trouble learning to read and (b) to govern the management of children and adults who are dyslexic. Longitudinal, cognitive, and neurobiological studies provide powerful proof of the enduring nature of the phonologic deficit even in the brightest of people with dyslexia, including those who are accurate but not automatic readers. Key factors to keep in mind are that dyslexia is a clinical diagnosis, that in bright young adults developmental history and slow reading are the sine qua non of the diagnosis, and that accommodations are as essential to these individuals as insulin is to a diabetic. There are now at least two Nobel laureates (Niels Bohr and Baruch Benacerref), as well as numerous other distinguished physicians and scientists, who are dyslexic; no doubt, there could be many more if otherwise bright and able dyslexic men and women are provided with the accommodations necessary to access their strengths on tests that serve as gatekeepers. It is the obligation of each physician or educator to ensure that the diagnosis and management of children and adults with dyslexia is now based on science, and not on arbitrary and capricious dogma.

# REFERENCES

Ben-Dror, I., Pollatsek, A., & Scarpati, A. (1991). Word identification in isolation and in context by college dyslexic students. *Brain and Language, 40,* 471–490.

Brown, J. I., Fishco, V. V., & Hanna, G. S. (1993). *Nelson-Denny Reading Test.* Itasca, IL: Riverside.

Bruck, M. (1985). The adult functioning of children with specific learning disabilities: A follow-up study. In I. Siegel (Ed.), *Advances in applied developmental psychology* (pp. 91–129). Norwood, NJ: Ablex.

Bruck, M. (1990). Word-recognition skills of adults with childhood diagnoses of dyslexia. *Developmental Psychology, 26*(3), 439–454.

Bruck, M. (1992). Persistence of dyslexics' phonological awareness deficits. *Developmental Psychology, 28*(5), 874–886.

Bruck, M. (1994). Outcomes of adults with childhood histories of dyslexia. In C. Hulme & R. M. Joshi (Eds.), *Reading and spelling: Development and disorder* (pp. 179–200). Mahwah, NJ: Erlbaum.

Brunswick, N., McCrory, E., Price, C. J., Frith, C. D., & Frith, U. (1999). Explicit and implicit processing of words and pseudowords by adult developmental dyslexics: A search for Wernicke's Wortschatz. *Brain, 122,* 1901–1917.

Cardon, L. R., Smith, S. D., Fulker, D. W., Kimberling, W. J., Pennington, B. F., & DeFries, J. C. (1994). Quantitative trait locus for reading disability on chromosome 6. *Science, 266,* 276–279.

Cardon, L. R., Smith, S. D., Fulker, D. W., Kimberling, W. J., Pennington, B. F., & DeFries, J. C. (1995). Quantitative trait locus for reading disability: Correction. *Science, 268*(5217), 1553.

Cohen, L., Dehaene, S., Naccache, L., Lehéricy, S., Dehaene-Lambertz, G., Henaff, M., & Michel, F. (2000). The visual word form area: Spatial and temporal characterization of an initial stage of reading in normal subjects and posterior split-brain patients. *Brain, 123*, 291–307.

Cohen, L., Lehéricy, S., Chochon, F., Lemer, C., Rivaud, S., & Dehaene, S. (2002). Language-specific tuning of visual cortex? Functional properties of the Visual Word Form Area. *Brain, 125*(PL5), 1054–1069.

Corina, D., Richards, T., Serafini, S., Richards, A., Steury, K., Abbott, R., Echelard, D., Maravilla, K., & Berninger, V. (2001). fMRI auditory language differences between dyslexic and able reading children. *NeuoReport, 12*, 1195–1201.

Damasio, A. R., & Damasio, H. (1983). The anatomic basis of pure alexia. *Neurology, 33*, 1573–1583.

Dehaene, S., Naccache, L., Cohen, L., Le Bihan, D., Mangin, J., Poline, J., & Riviere, D. (2001). Cerebral mechanisms of word masking and unconscious repetition priming. *Nature Neuroscience, 4*, 752–758.

Dejerine, J. (1891). Sur un cas de cécité verbale avec agraphie, suivi d'autopsie. *C. R. Société du Biologie, 43*, 197–201.

Dejerine, J. (1892). Contribution a l'étude anatomo-pathologique et clinique des differentes varietes de cecite verbale. *Memoires de la Société de Biologie, 4*, 61–90.

Demb, J., Boynton, G., & Heeger, D. (1998). Functional magnetic resonance imaging of early visual pathways in dyslexia. *Journal of Neuroscience, 18*, 6939–6951.

Eden, G. F., VanMeter, J. W., Rumsey, J. M., Maisog, J. M., Woods, R. P., & Zeffiro, T. A. (1996). Abnormal processing of visual motion in dyslexia revealed by functional brain imaging. *Nature, 382*, 66–69.

Fagerheim, T., Raeymaekers, P., Tonnessen, F., Pedersen, D., Tranebjaerg, L., & Lubs, H. (1999). A new gene (DYX3) for dyslexia is located on chromosome 2. *Journal of Medical Genetics, 36*, 664–669.

Felton, R. H., Naylor, C. E., & Wood, F. B. (1990). Neuropsychological profile of adult dyslexics. *Brain and Language, 39*, 485–497.

Fiez, J. A., & Peterson, S. E. (1998). Neuroimaging studies of word reading. *Proceedings of the National Academy of Science USA, 95*(3), 914–921.

Filipek, P. (1996). Structural variations in measures in the developmental disorders. In R. Thatcher, G. Lyon, J. Rumsey, & N. Krasnegor (Eds.), *Developmental neuroimaging: Mapping the development of brain and behavior* (pp. 169–186). San Diego, CA: Academic Press.

Finucci, J. M., & Childs, B. (1981). Are there really more dyslexic boys than girls? In A. Ansara, N. Geschwind, M. Albert, & N. Gartrell (Eds.), *Sex differences in dyslexia* (pp. 1–9). Towson, MD: Orton Dyslexia Society.

Fletcher, J. M., Shaywitz, S. E., Shankweiler, D. P., Katz, L., Liberman, I. Y., Stuebing, K. K., Francis, D. J., Fowler, A. E., & Shaywitz, B. A. (1994). Cognitive profiles of reading disability: Comparisons of discrepancy and low achievement definitions. *Journal of Educational Psychology, 86*(1), 6–23.

Flynn, J., & Rahbar, M. (1994). Prevalence of reading failure in boys compared with girls. *Psychology in the Schools, 31*, 66–71.

Frackowiak, R., Friston, K., Frith, C., Dolan, R., & Mazziotta, J. C. (1997). *Human brain function.* New York: Academic Press.

Francis, D. J., Shaywitz, S. E., Stuebing, K. K., Shaywitz, B. A., & Fletcher, J. M. (1996). Developmental lag versus deficit models of reading disability: A longitudinal, individual growth curves analysis. *Journal of Educational Psychology, 88*(1), 3–17.

Friedman, R. F., Ween, J. E., & Albert, M. L. (1993). Alexia. In K. M. Heilman & E. Valenstein (Eds.), *Clinical neuropsychology* (3rd ed., pp. 37–62). New York: Oxford University Press.

Galaburda, A. M., Sherman, G. F., Rosen, G. D., Aboitiz, F., & Geschwind, N. (1985). Developmental dyslexia: Four consecutive patients with cortical anomalies. *Annals of Neurology, 18*(2), 222–233.

Georgiewa, P., Rzanny, R., Hopf, J., Knab, R., Glauche, V., Kaiser, W., & Blanz, B. (1999). fMRI during word processing in dyslexic and normal reading children. *NeuroReport, 10,* 3459–3465.

Geschwind, N. (1965). Disconnection syndromes in animals and man. *Brain, 88,* 237–294.

Gilger, J. W., Borecki, I. B., Smith, S. D., DeFries, J. C., & Pennington, B. F. (1996). The etiology of extreme scores for complex phenotypes: An illustration using reading performance. In C. H. Chase, G. D. Rosen, & G. F. Sherman (Eds.), *Developmental dyslexia: Neural, cognitive, and genetic mechanisms* (pp. 63–85). Baltimore: York Press.

Grigorenko, E. L., Wood, F. B., Meyer, M. S., Hart, L. A., Speed, W. C., Shuster, A., & Pauls, D. L. (1997). Susceptibility loci for distinct components of developmental dyslexia on chromosomes 6 and 15. *American Journal of Human Genetics, 60,* 27–39.

Gross-Glenn, K., Duara, R., Barker, W. W., Loewenstein, D., Chang, J.-Y., Yoshii, F., Apicella, A. M., Pascal, S., Boothe, T., Sevush, S., Jallad, B. J., Novoa, L., & Lubs, H. A. (1991). Positron emission tomographic studies during serial word-reading by normal and dyslexic adults. *Journal of Clinical and Experimental Neuropsychology, 13*(4), 531–544.

Helenius, P., Tarkiainen, A., Cornelissen, P., Hansen, P. C., & Salmelin, R. (1999). Dissociation of normal feature analysis and deficient processing of letter-strings in dyslexic adults. *Cerebral Cortex, 4,* 476–483.

Horwitz, B., Rumsey, J. M., & Donohue, B. C. (1998). Functional connectivity of the angular gyrus in normal reading and dyslexia. *Proceedings of the National Academy of Science USA, 95,* 8939–8944.

Klingberg, T., Hedehus, M., Temple, E., Salz, T., Gabrieli, J., Moseley, M., & Poldrack, R. (2000). Microstructure of temporo-parietal white matter as a basis for reading ability: Evidence from diffusion tensor magnetic resonance imaging. *Neuron, 25,* 493–500.

Lefly, D. L., & Pennington, B. F. (1991). Spelling errors and reading fluency in compensated adult dyslexics. *Annals of Dyslexia, 41,* 143–162.

Logan, G. (1988). Toward an instance theory of automatization. *Psychological Review, 95,* 492–527.

Logan, G. (1997). Automaticity and reading: Perspectives from the instance theory of automatization. *Reading and Writing Quarterly: Overcoming Learning Disabilities, 13,* 123–146.

Moore, C., & Price, C. (1999). Three distinct ventral occipitotemporal regions for reading and object naming. *NeuroImage, 10,* 181–192.

Morris, R. D., Stuebing, K. K., Fletcher, J. M., Shaywitz, S. E., Lyon, G. R., Shankweiler, D. P.,

Katz, L., Francis, D. J., & Shaywitz, B. A. (1998). Subtypes of reading disability: Variability around a phonological core. *Journal of Educational Psychology, 90,* 347–373.

Paulesu, E., Demonet, J.-F., Fazio, F., McCrory, E., Chanoine, V., Brunswick, N., Cappa, S., Cossu, G., Habib, M., Frith, C., & Frith, U. (2001). Dyslexia–cultural diversity and biological unity. *Science, 291,* 2165–2167.

Paulesu, E., Frith, U., Snowling, M., Gallagher, A., Morton, J., Frackowiak, R. S. J., & Frith, C. D. (1996). Is developmental dyslexia a disconnection syndrome? Evidence from PET scanning. *Brain, 119,* 143–157.

Pennington, B. F., & Gilger, J. W. (1996). How is dyslexia transmitted? In C. H. Chase, G. D. Rosen, & G. F. Sherman (Eds.), *Developmental dyslexia: Neural, cognitive, and genetic mechanisms* (pp. 41–61). Baltimore: York Press.

Price, C., Moore, C., & Frackowiak, R. S. J. (1996). The effect of varying stimulus rate and duration on brain activity during reading. *Neuroimage, 3*(1), 40–52.

Pugh, K., Mencl, E. W., Shaywitz, B. A., Shaywitz, S. E., Fulbright, R. K., Skudlarski, P., Constable, R. T., Marchione, K. E., Shankweiler, D. P., Katz, L., Fletcher, J. M., Lacadie, C., & Gore, J. C. (2000). The angular gyrus in developmental dyslexia: Task-specific differences in functional connectivity in posterior cortex. *Psychological Science, 11,* 51–56.

Rabin, M., Wen, X., Hepburn, M., Lubs, H., Feldman, E., & Duara, R. (1993). Suggestive linkage of developmental dyslexia to chromosome 1p34–p36. *Lancet, 342,* 178.

Report of the National Reading Panel. (2000). *Teaching children to read: An evidence-based assessment of the scientific research literature on reading and its implications for reading instruction.* Bethesda, MD: National Institute of Child Health and Human Development, National Institutes of Health.

Rumsey, J. M., Andreason, P., Zametkin, A. J., Aquino, T., King, C., Hamburber, S. D., Pikus, A., Rapoport, J. L., & Cohen, R. M. (1992). Failure to activate the left temporoparietal cortex in dyslexia. *Archives of Neurology, 49,* 527–534.

Rumsey, J. M., Nace, K., Donohue, B., Wise, D., Maisog, J. M., & Andreason, P. (1997). A positron emission tomographic study of impaired word recognition and phonological processing in dyslexic men. *Archives of Neurology, 54,* 562–573.

Salmelin, R., Service, E., Kiesila, P., Uutela, K., & Salonen, O. (1996). Impaired visual word processing in dyslexia revealed with magnetoencephalography. *Annals of Neurology, 40,* 157–162.

Scarborough, H. S. (1984). Continuity between childhood dyslexia and adult reading. *British Journal of Psychology, 75,* 329–348.

Scarborough, H. S. (1990). Very early language deficits in dyslexic children. *Child Development, 61,* 1728–1743.

Shaywitz, B. A., Holford, T. R., Holahan, J. M., Fletcher, J. M., Stuebing, K. K., Francis, D. J., & Shaywitz, S. E. (1995). A Matthew effect for IQ but not for reading: Results from a longitudinal study. *Reading Research Quarterly, 30*(4), 894–906.

Shaywitz, B., Pugh, K. R., Jenner, A., Fulbright, R. K., Fletcher, J. M., Gore, J. C., & Shaywitz, S. (2000). The neurobiology of reading and reading disability (dyslexia). In M. Kamil, P. Mosenthal, P. Pearson, & R. Barr (Eds.), *Handbook of reading research* (Vol. 3, pp. 229–249). Mahwah, NJ: Erlbaum.

Shaywitz, B. A., Shaywitz, S. E., Pugh, K. R., Mencl, W. E., Fullbright, R. K., Skudlarski, P.,

Constable, R. T., Marchione, K. M., Fletcher, J. M., Lyon, G. R., & Gore, J. C. (2002). Disruption of posterior brain systems for reading in children with developmental dyslexia. *Biological Psychiatry, 52*(2), 101–110.

Shaywitz, S. (1998). Current concepts: Dyslexia. *The New England Journal of Medicine, 338*(5), 307–312.

Shaywitz, S., & Shaywitz, B. (1999). Dyslexia. In K. Swaiman & S. Ashwal (Eds.), *Pediatric neurology: Principles and practice* (3rd ed., Vol. 1, pp. 576–584). St. Louis, MO: Mosby.

Shaywitz, S. E., Escobar, M. D., Shaywitz, B. A., Fletcher, J. M., & Makuch, R. (1992). Evidence that dyslexia may represent the lower tail of a normal distribution of reading ability. *New England Journal of Medicine, 326*(3), 145–150.

Shaywitz, S. E., Fletcher, J. M., Holahan, J. M., Shneider, A. E., Marchione, K. E., Stuebing, K. K., Francis, D. J., Pugh, K. R., & Shaywitz, B. A. (1999). Persistence of dyslexia: The Connecticut Longitudinal Study at adolescence. *Pediatrics, 104,* 1351–1359.

Shaywitz, S. E., Shaywitz, B. A., Fletcher, J. M., & Escobar, M. D. (1990). Prevalence of reading disability in boys and girls: Results of the Connecticut Longitudinal Study. *Journal of the American Medical Association, 264*(8), 998–1002.

Shaywitz, S. E., Shaywitz, B. A., Pugh, K. R., Fulbright, R. K., Constable, R. T., Mencl, W. E., Shankweiler, D. P., Liberman, A. M., Skudlarski, P., Fletcher, J. M., Katz, L., Marchione, K. E., Lacadie, C., Gatenby, C., & Gore, J. C. (1998). Functional disruption in the organization of the brain for reading in dyslexia. *Proceedings of the National Academy of Science USA, 95,* 2636–2641.

Shaywitz, S., Shaywitz, B., Pugh, K., Fulbright, R., Mencl, W., Constable, R., Skudlarski, P., Fletcher, J., Lyon, G., & Gore, J. (in press). The neuropsychology of dyslexia. In S. Segalowitz & I. Rapin (Eds.), Handbook of neuropsychology (2nd ed., Vol. 7). Amsterdam: Elsevier.

Simos, P., Breier, J., Fletcher, J., Bergman, E., & Papanicolaou, A. (2000). Cerebral mechanisms involved in word reading in dyslexic children: A magnetic source imaging approach. *Cerebral Cortex, 10,* 809–816.

Stanovich, K. E., & Siegel, L. S. (1994). Phenotypic performance profile of children with reading disabilities: A regression-based test of the phonological-core variable-difference model. *Journal of Educational Psychology, 86*(1), 24–53.

Torgesen, J. K., Wagner, R., & Rashotte, C. (1999). *Test of Word Reading Efficiency.* Austin, TX: PRO-ED.

Wadsworth, S. J., DeFries, J. C., Stevenson, J., Gilger, J. W., & Pennington, B. F. (1992). Gender ratios among reading-disabled children and their siblings as a function of parental impairment. *Journal of Child Psychology and Psychiatry, 33*(7), 1229–1239.

Wagner, R., Torgesen, J. K., & Rashotte, C. (1999). *Comprehensive Test of Phonological Processing.* Austin, TX: PRO-ED.

Wiederholt, J. L., & Bryant, B. R. (1991). *Gray Oral Reading Tests–Fourth Edition.* Austin, TX: PRO-ED.

Woodcock, R. W. (1998). *Woodcock Reading Mastery Test–Revised–Normative Update.* Circle Pines, MN: American Guidance Service.

Woodcock, R. W., & Johnson, M. B. (1989). *Woodcock-Johnson Psycho-Educational Battery–Revised.* Allen, TX: Developmental Learning Materials.

# CHAPTER 25

# School-Based Violence Prevention

Hill M. Walker, Jeffrey R. Sprague,
and Herbert H. Severson

ncreasing numbers of behaviorally at-risk children and youth are following destructive pathways toward later health risk outcomes in adolescence and young adulthood (Hawkins, Catalano, Kosterman, Abbott,
& Hill, 1999). This well-traveled trajectory usually begins early in a
child's life and often ends tragically in prison. This pathway sometimes is
associated with violent acts but more often results in dysfunctional outcomes such as school failure; delinquency; substance abuse; frequent bullying, harassment, and aggression toward others; and social rejection by
peers, teachers, and even primary caregivers during adolescence (see
Loeber & Farrington, 1998; Patterson, Reid, & Dishion, 1992). The social
and economic costs of these preventable outcomes are extraordinary and
are increasingly viewed as unacceptable by society. This chapter describes
essential information that educators need to have regarding child and
adolescent violence, including youth behavioral characteristics, causal
factors and influences, developmental pathways, trends in youth violence, and solutions that can be implemented primarily within school
contexts but in collaboration with families, law enforcement, courts, and
social service agencies (i.e., mental health), as appropriate. We believe
that schools and school personnel can and should be major players in the
development of solutions to youth violence and the antisocial behavior
patterns that provide a fertile breeding ground for violent acts. During
the past decade, schools have become unfortunate targets for the rage of
very disturbed students who seek to redress their grievances through acts
of violence directed against innocent students and educators.

# VIOLENCE DEFINED

Youth violence has emerged in the past decade as one of the most pressing public health problems confronting our society (American Psychological Association, 1993; Satcher, 2001). It has spilled over into school systems in the most unfortunate manner imaginable and now ranks as a significant component of domestic terrorism. Violent acts are much like sudden natural disasters (e.g., an earthquake or tornado) that appear to come out of nowhere, account for incredible damage in a matter of minutes, and require long periods for recovery. Individuals and society are victimized not only by the actual occurrence of violent acts, but also by the fear of them. The threat of violence requires enhanced vigilance and reduces overall quality of life. If individuals are required to alter their routines or lifestyle because of the possibility of violence, then the victimization is palpable and real (Crowe, 1995).

Violence is defined by law enforcement as involving one or more of the following acts: robbery, rape, aggravated assault, and murder. Although a broad range of acts are referred to in the media and popular culture as violent, they often represent the precursors or antecedents of violent behavior rather than what is defined as actual violence. Among children and youth, the precursors of violence are antisocial acts that can involve extreme forms of aggression, bullying, intimidation, and harassment directed toward others, especially peers (Loeber & Farrington, 1998; Patterson et al., 1992; Walker, Colvin, & Ramsey, 1995). For the most severely involved at-risk youth, it is not unusual for adults, who are in positions of authority with them (e.g., teachers), to be targets of antisocial acts as well.

# BEHAVIORAL CHARACTERISTICS OF ANTISOCIAL YOUTH

Antisocial youth, many of whom engage in the precursors of violence and some of whom become violent, are challenging to their families, teachers, and social networks due to the highly aversive, confronting nature of their behavioral styles. They can be demanding, impulsive, overly active, oppositional–defiant, disruptive, and extremely aggressive. These youth are generally successful in resisting adult influence strategies designed to change their behavior but are often open to the negative influences of deviant peers, which further socializes them toward delinquent and violent lifestyles (Patterson et al., 1992). The two following vignettes illustrate how many antisocial youth are socialized to view their social environs and their respective roles in those environs.

Some years ago, the senior author and his colleagues were developing an intervention for dealing with aggressive children in Grades K through 3 (Walker, Hops, & Greenwood, 1988) who teased and bullied others during school recess. Ritchie, a second grader, was referred by his school counselor and homeroom teacher for possible inclusion in this intervention. During a playground recess period, an observer recorded his social behavior to determine if he was an appropriate candidate for this program. Ritchie impulsively attacked a kindergarten boy in the presence of the observer, playground supervisor, and program consultant. He knocked the smaller boy to the ground and was seriously choking him, with an apparent attempt to cause bodily harm and inflict pain. The playground supervisor intervened and called the principal and school counselor, who escorted Ritchie into the school to call his parents. Ritchie was asked, "Can you tell us why you were choking Jason like that?" Ritchie seemed surprised and responded with, "Well, it was recess!"

Sarah, a fourth grader, was commonly regarded as a holy terror by her teachers and peers. Sarah was passively aggressive, smart, a natural leader, and skilled in manipulating others. Billie Webb was a school psychologist who served Sarah's school part time, along with two others, and visited the school several times weekly. As a general rule, Sarah was a regular client of Billie's each time she visited the school; Billie and Sarah were on a first-name basis. During one of Billie's visits, the school's principal and counselor told Billie the latest things Sarah had done on the playground. Billie called Sarah into a conference to hear her side of things. The following exchange ensued: "Sarah, I understand you've been having problems on the playground, again." Sarah just stared at Billie and said nothing. While attempting to engage Sarah in a problem-solving process, Billie asked another question. "What do you think people will say about that, Sarah?" Sarah thought a minute, looked at Billie, and said, "Well, Billie, some people might say *you're* not doing your job!"

These actual scenarios graphically illustrate how many antisocial youth see themselves and the world around them. These youth are frequently egotistical, self-absorbed, and insensitive to the feelings and needs of others.

Their personal behavioral standards are qualitatively divergent from those of others. Children like Ritchie and Sarah are heavily into denial and often refuse to assume responsibility for their actions (Walker et al., 1995). By adolescence, approximately half of antisocial youth are also committing *covert* antisocial forms of behavior, such as vandalism, fire setting, shoplifting, property destruction, and substance abuse (Patterson et al., 1992). In the classroom setting, covert antisocial behavior is usually expressed as lying, cheating, and stealing, three forms of student behavior that teachers broadly view as among the most objectionable (see Walker, 1986).

These behavioral characteristics are dysfunctional in the extreme and set up behaviorally at-risk youth for destructive outcomes and health risk behaviors over the long term. Longitudinal studies of this population conducted over the past three decades in Australia, New Zealand, Canada, the United States, the British Isles, and Western Europe converge in documenting the following outcomes in late adolescence and young adulthood: substance abuse, heavy drinking, delinquency, severe depression, school failure, chronic disciplinary problems, dependence on welfare and social service systems, dishonorable military discharges, criminal offenses and arrests, and higher hospitalization and mortality rates (see Kazdin, 1985; Loeber & Farrington, 1998; Patterson et al., 1992; Walker et al., 1995).

The issue of comorbidity, or mixed syndromes, has emerged in the last decade as a most important development in defining the severity and long-term developmental course of behaviorally at-risk youth (see Gresham, Lane, & Lambros, 2002). For example, Seeley, Rohde, Lewinsohn, and Clarke (2002) noted that, when conduct disorder is combined or mixed with severe depression among at-risk youth, the adolescent suicide attempt rate increases from approximately 13% for adolescents in general to about 40% for this subpopulation. Similarly, Lynam (1996) reviewed extensive research on the relationship between attention-deficit/hyperactivity disorder (ADHD) and conduct disorder. Lynam developed a compelling and elegant conceptual model regarding the comorbidity of ADHD and CD, which argues that this "mixture" provides the foundation for the later development of severe psychopathology. Significant numbers of antisocial youth may be vulnerable to having this mixture, as well as others (e.g., conduct disorder with severe learning disabilities). It is essential that behaviorally at-risk youth be assessed for the presence of comorbid conditions and attempts made to divert them from this likelihood as early as possible in their lives and school careers.

# CAUSAL FACTORS AND INFLUENCES

The toxic conditions and negative forces of our society are producing thousands of children like Ritchie and Sarah who come from highly at-risk backgrounds. Dysfunctional families, drug and alcohol abuse by caregivers, poverty, neglect, weak parenting skills, deteriorating neighborhoods, association with deviant peers, and portrayals of media violence are but a few of the risks to which increasing numbers of our children and youth are being exposed. Reid (1993) noted that the more of these risks to which one is exposed and the longer such exposure lasts, the greater the likelihood that destructive outcomes will occur in the lives of behaviorally at-risk youth.

In its seminal report on youth violence, the American Psychological Association (1993) identified four causal factors for youth violence that act as accelerators along the pathway that propels at-risk youth toward destructive outcomes:

1. early involvement with drugs and alcohol
2. easy access to weapons, especially handguns
3. depiction of violent acts in the media
4. association with antisocial groups

These risk factors form a toxic mixture and are more likely to come into play in preadolescence and adolescence than earlier in a child's development. At-risk children are commonly made vulnerable to these causal influences through the risks they have previously experienced (e.g., weak parenting, dysfunctional families).

Moffitt (1994) made an important distinction between early and later starters in the development of antisocial behavior patterns. Early starters are socialized to this lifestyle by their family situations, whereas later starters are socialized to it by peers. Early starters experience a host of risk factors, and few protective factors, from the moment of birth and are likely to manifest antisocial forms of behavior over their life course. Later starters, on the other hand, have many more advantages and generally engage in "adolescent-limited" antisocial behavior, which often reduces after several years and typically does not emerge until the late elementary grades. It is essential that early starters receive appropriate screening, evaluation, and interventions as soon as possible in their lives and school careers.

Predicting future violent acts *on a case-by-case basis* is difficult to impossible given the state of our current knowledge and the limited tools available to us for this purpose. The U.S. Surgeon General's 2001 report on youth violence (Satcher, 2001), for example, correctly notes that it is nearly impossible to predict at an individual level which highly aggressive young children (i.e., early starters) will become violent in adolescence. Patterson et al. (1992) found that the following profile of antisocial youth was predictive of later, violent acts among a sample of severely at-risk adolescents: (a) the first arrest occurred early in the youth's life (i.e., at age 10 or younger); (b) the first arrest was for a serious offense; and (c) by age 12, the youth had three or more arrests and was considered a chronic offender. It is important to note, however, that although it is possible to identify and profile such high-risk groups, determining in advance *which* group members will commit a later violent act is still extremely difficult. Thus, prediction of future violent acts *at the individual child or youth level* remains extremely problematic.

## The Role of Risk and Protective Factors

In the psychological literature on antisocial behavior and youth violence, it is quite common to see causal factors and influences arrayed in terms of risk and protective factors. *Risk factors* are identifiable conditions and influences that increase the likelihood of destructive outcomes; *protective factors* are positive influences operating in a youth's life that can buffer or offset the negative impact of risk exposure. For example, a dysfunctional family is a commonly occurring risk factor, but having access to a caring adult in one's life is a protective factor that can attenuate the damaging impact of such a family environment. Both risk and protective factors have been shown to operate at five different levels: individual, family, school, peer group, and societal. Two of the strongest risk factors for youth violence early in a child's life are (a) an early pattern of general, repeat offending and (b) substance use and abuse. In adolescence, the most powerful risks in this regard are (a) having weak social ties; (b) having antisocial, delinquent peers; and (c) gang membership. Protective factors that can buffer and offset these risks are (a) having an intolerant attitude toward deviance, (b) having a high IQ, (c) being female, (d) having a positive social orientation, and (e) understanding the relationship between transgressions and sanctions (see Satcher, 2001). Appendix 25.A contains a more elaborate listing of risk and protective factors related to shared vulnerability for both delinquency and violence.

It is difficult to impossible for schools and educators to have an impact on many of the risk factors (e.g., poverty, dysfunctional families, weak parenting, neglect) that impinge directly on children's lives and impair their school performance. It is possible, however, for them to enhance and develop offsetting protective factors that will have a positive influence in children's lives. Typically, school personnel do not investigate or assess the types of risk and protective factors that operate in a student's life. We think that this practice is a shortcoming and that, if such information were available on a systematic basis, educators would be better able both to understand problematic student behavior in the school setting and to reduce or replace it.

The recent adoption of the Functional Based Assessment (FBA) approach to assessment by many school personnel (e.g., behavioral specialists, school psychologists) is an attempt to understand and identify the causal factors that account for a student's problem behavior within school contexts (O'Neill et al., 1997). In this method, hypotheses or notions are developed that may help explain what accounts for a student's problem behavior (e.g., seeking attention, avoidance of aversive tasks, seeking to establish dominance or control). Assessments are then conducted to verify or reject these hunches. However, although FBA approaches are useful in better understanding a student's behavior within a specific school setting, such as the classroom or playground, to more fully understand and account for a student's overall school behavior, it is also necessary to conduct a thorough risk and protective factor analysis (see Walker & Sprague, 1999a, for a discussion of FBA vs. risk and protective assessment issues).

## Assessing Risk and Protective Factors in the School Setting

Along with the work of Najaka, Gottfredson, and Wilson (2001), the research of Vance, Fernandez, and their colleagues ranks as some of the most important research conducted to date on assessing and analyzing risk-protective factors as they impact educational achievement and behavioral adjustment within school settings (see Vance, Fernandez, & Biber, 1998). Recently, Vance, Bowen, Fernandez, and Thompson (2002) reported a predictive study of the role of risk and protective factors as predictors of longitudinal outcomes among adolescents having serious psychiatric disorders and aggression. The study involved 337 adolescents enrolled in a treatment program for youth with severe aggression and emotional disturbance in

North Carolina. Historical and current psychosocial risk-protective factors, along with "baseline" ratings of the severity of psychiatric symptoms, were used to predict problematic outcomes (risk-taking, self-injurious, threatening, and assaultive behavior) 1 year later. These authors reported that 11 risk and protective factors predicted outcomes, whereas none of the psychiatric symptom ratings did. These findings are important in documenting the invaluable role that the assessment and analysis of risk-protective factors can play in understanding and accounting for problematic youth behavior in the context of schooling.

The Gottfredsons and their associates have developed a number of measures and batteries to assess the social ecology of school settings, including risk-protective factors. Their self-report measure of risk and resiliency factors is a highly recommended tool for use by educators in assessing student characteristics. This instrument, called *What About You?* (WAY), has three different forms that also take into account student reading levels. The WAY spans Grades 5 through 12 and provides a standardized and validated method of gathering information to identify problems, set goals and objectives, plan interventions, and evaluate progress. The WAY also provides objective measures of risk factors for problem behavior and drug use, as well as protective factors for social integration and self-esteem. G. Gottfredson and Gottfredson (1999) describe the psychometric features and technical development of this instrument.

# DEVELOPMENTAL PATHWAYS

Walker and Severson (2002) discussed the developmental pathways through which behaviorally at-risk children and youth come to acquire violent and delinquent lifestyles. The research of Patterson et al. (1992), Eddy, Reid, and Curry (2002), and Loeber and Farrington (1998) has been instrumental in illuminating the nature and etiology of these pathways, as well as the behavioral processes that operate across developmental stages within them. Through longitudinal studies of antisocial children and youth and their families, there are now strong and clearly established links between exposure to the previously mentioned risk factors, the maladaptive behavioral manifestations that result from them, the short-term negative outcomes that accrue to the at-risk child associated with these behavioral manifestations over time, and the costly and socially destructive long-term outcomes that

(a) typically complete this developmental progression and (b) prove to be very destructive to the at-risk child or youth, family members, friends, peers, and the larger society (see Vance et al., 2002). Figure 25.1 shows the connecting links in this developmental trajectory that defines a well-traveled pathway from early exposure, to experiencing serious conditions of risk, and to the later development of destructive outcomes and health risk behaviors that can reduce dramatically one's life chances and quality of life.

More and more young children are experiencing a plethora of risk factors from the moment of birth, with few offsetting protective factors. As a consequence, we are seeing many youth who are following this unfortunate path that too often ends in school failure and dropout, delinquency, adult crime, and sometimes violence. Hawkins et al. (1999) reported an impressive 12-year longitudinal intervention study where the role of school bonding, engagement, and attachment was examined as a protective factor in preventing health risk outcomes for an at-risk sample in adolescence. These researchers found that through early intervention in Grades 1 through 4 with the target child, teachers and parents had a powerful impact in preventing health risk outcomes at age 18. They concluded that the key prevention variable in their study was the protective influence of school engagement, bonding, and attachment, which was targeted by their intervention at the point of school entry. School bonding seems to be emerging in a number of experimental studies and reviews as a strong factor in predicting adolescent outcomes of this nature (see Najaka et al., 2001). We believe that assisting behaviorally at-risk children in getting off to the best start possible in their school careers enhances school bonding and attachment and thus engages the protective influences of the schooling process (Shinn, Walker, & Stoner, 2002).

## TRENDS IN YOUTH VIOLENCE

In the decade from 1983 to 1993, U.S. society experienced an epidemic of youth violence, as indicated by arrests for violent crimes (see Satcher, 2001). This epidemic was largely fueled by the crack cocaine surge of the 1980s and by large numbers of youth who had access to and carried firearms, especially handguns, during this period. Figure 25.2 provides graphic illustrations of youth violence arrests for robbery, rape, aggravated assault, and murder from 1980 to 1999. These trends show dramatic accelerations for

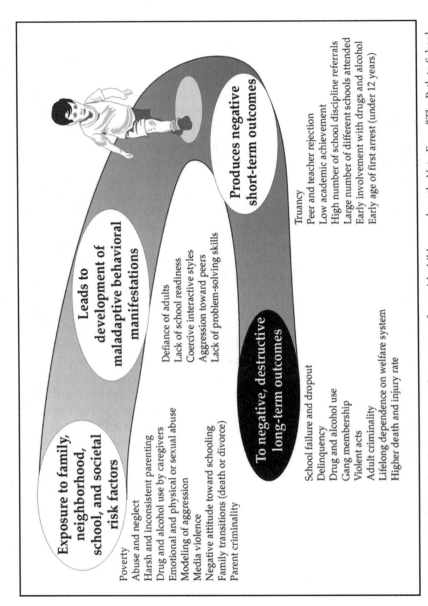

**FIGURE 25.1.** The path to long-term negative outcomes for at-risk children and youth. *Note.* From "The Path to School Failure, Delinquency, and Violence: Causal Factors and Some Potential Solutions," by H. M. Walker and J. R. Sprague, 1999, *Intervention in School and Clinic, 35,* p. 68. Copyright 1999 by PRO-ED, Inc. Reprinted with permission.

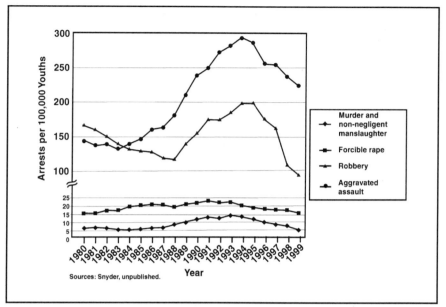

**FIGURE 25.2.** Arrest rates of youths ages 10 to 17 for serious violent crime, by type of crime, 1980–1999. *Note.* From *Youth Violence: A Report of the Surgeon General,* by D. Satcher, 2001, Washington, DC: Department of Health and Human Services, U.S. Public Health Service.

aggravated assault and robbery and more gradual increases for rape and murder during the period from the mid-1980s to the mid-1990s. During the decade of the 1990s, each of these indices returned to their preepidemic levels, and below in some cases, except aggravated assault, which continued at levels well above the beginning of its acceleration.

A true picture of a youth's criminal behavior is not provided by arrest indices alone. Youth self-reports of illegal activities that do not result in arrests are also an important index of criminal behavior, and they do not always agree with arrest data. This is true in the case of youth violence. Around 1983, for example, both arrests for violent acts and youth self-reports of violent behavior showed acceleration; however, although youth violence arrests dropped off in the mid-1990s, youth self-reports of violent activity in annual confidential reports continued at high levels through 1999. This development is of concern to policymakers, legislators, and law enforcement personnel because confidential annual surveys of adolescents' self-reported activities consistently show that (a) many youths hold attitudes and beliefs that support aggressive, violent behavior and (b) relatively large proportions (i.e., 30% and up) of responding youth report committing violent acts that could have resulted in serious injury or even death.

These findings call for systematic actions to teach all children and youth the attitudes, beliefs, and skills that support nonviolent behavior and the peaceful resolution of interpersonal conflicts, which otherwise might escalate into destructive results and sometimes dangerous situations. Schools have a key role to play in addressing this problem and are ideally positioned to do so effectively. The schools' role in this regard is discussed in the next section.

In the face of the toxic changes that have occurred in U.S. society over the past two to three decades, policymakers and legislators are confronted with the critical question of how to reduce and offset the damaging effects of the conditions of risk to which more and more of our youth are being subjected. As a starting point, we believe there is an urgent need to address as many of these risks as possible. Thousands of families are currently in crisis because of the stressors to which they are exposed daily (e.g., domestic violence, poverty, divorce, drug abuse). In a real sense, the problems our society has experienced in this domain begin and end with the family. As a society, we must recommit ourselves to raising our children safely and effectively. We seem to have lost our capacity to do so on a broad scale (Walker et al., 1995).

Next to families, perhaps the most important institutional influence on child and youth development is the school and the socializing experiences and skill development opportunities it provides. As noted previously, *effective* schooling is likely one of the most important protective influences in the lives of youth—but only if they fully engage and bond with the schooling experience (see Hawkins et al., 1999). The school is also a major source of mental health support for school-age students. Hoagwood and Erwin (1997), for example, indicate that approximately 75% of all mental health services are delivered within the context of schooling.

## THE ROLE OF SCHOOLS IN REDUCING VIOLENCE

If schools are to be significant players in developing solutions to the youth violence problems of U.S. society, some key assumptions, in our view, must be in evidence for them to be effective:

1. School systems must become far more collaborative with families and other agencies in forging and implementing promising strategies.

2. School personnel from the top down must own the problem of youth violence and resist the temptation to displace it to other sectors of society.

3. Schools must engage all students and ensure that they are connected to and bonded with the schooling process.

Public schools have an unfortunate history of making themselves unwelcome places for marginalized students and their families. For instance, the common practice of pressuring at-risk students, who do not easily accommodate the demands of schooling, to leave school early is one of the worst strategies imaginable and merely displaces this social problem to other sectors of our society, where it is even more difficult to solve. At-risk youth who leave school early and join the street culture have their overall risk status literally skyrocket. Many such youth then come into contact with social forces that rapidly propel them toward delinquency, violence, and other toxic conditions. Schools and school systems need to increase their holding power for all students and to reduce the unacceptably high dropout rates (25% and above), which result in future generations of unskilled workers who must struggle to earn a living wage.

We believe there are three groups of at-risk students for whom schools are responsible and who can benefit from the services, supports, opportunities, and experiences that effective schooling offers. These groups are (a) early starters, (b) later starters, and (c) school violence perpetrators. Early starters bring a well-developed pattern of antisocial behavior to the process of schooling and are desperately in need of interventions and supports provided at the point of school entry and continuing as needed throughout their school careers. Later starters, in contrast, begin their antisocial careers later on in the schooling process (usually around Grade 4 or 5), and engage in a period of adolescent-limited delinquency that lasts 3 to 5 years (see Moffitt, 1994). The student who commits violent acts against students or school staff with the intent to kill or injure is a special case and represents a form of terrorism. Such students can be characterized as *internalizing aggressors* who, as a rule, tend to internalize their problems and direct them inwardly rather than outwardly toward the social environment. However, some at-risk internalizing students are capable of extraordinary aggression in the process of settling their grievances—real or imagined—against others. Kip Kindel in Springfield, Oregon, and Eric Harris and Dylan Klebold at Columbine High School in Littleton, Colorado, are classic examples of such students. These three individuals are responsible for the deaths of 15 fellow students and three adults (two parents and a teacher) plus injuries to more than 30 other students.

The U.S. Secret Service (Stephens, 2000) and the Federal Bureau of Investigation (O'Toole, 2000) have conducted exhaustive analyses of the histories and characteristics of the school shooters of the past decade. Their research finds two common themes among these students: (a) fully two thirds were bullied, teased, and harassed by their fellow students and (b) they did not feel connected to school and saw no one in the school whom they believed actually cared about them. These findings speak volumes about the need to address the often coarse, cruel nature of the peer culture in schools and the importance of taking concrete steps to assist students in fully engaging schooling and to help them be successful in the process so bonding and attachment to schooling can occur.

The remainder of this chapter describes proven and promising strategies for enhancing the safety and security of the school setting, integrating and coordinating prevention-based interventions that address the needs of *all* students in the school setting, and improving the classroom teacher's ability to teach and manage all students, including those with very antisocial tendencies.

## Enhancing School Security

During the 1990s, the landscape of school safety and the expression of youth violence changed substantially. As noted, the overall rate of youth violence reached its peak in approximately 1992 and thereafter began a slow decline. However, the incidence of school-violence tragedies dramatically ramped up in this same year and continued into the latter part of the decade. The following are some assumptions about the associated characteristics of this trend and some potential causal factors:

1. Although the prevalence of school tragedies has declined since 1992, the number of deaths and injuries per tragedy has increased substantially.

2. Much larger numbers of planned school tragedies have been detected and averted in recent years, primarily because of peers revealing these plans to school authorities and parents in advance of their planned occurrence.

3. Each school tragedy now produces an immediate number of copycat incidents, suggesting that these events have been planned and contemplated for some time rather than that they spontaneously arise in connection with a tragedy.

4. The public and parents generally have moved beyond expressing concern for troubled youth who commit these tragedies to outrage about them and making demands for ensuring that schools become safer for all children and youth.

5. Schools, students, and parents are now increasingly victimized by fears about the possibility of a tragedy occurring in their particular setting, which lowers overall quality of life and reduces a student's ability to get the most out of the schooling process.

6. Our society is largely to blame for the spate of school-shooting tragedies that have occurred during the 1990s; the societal forces that spill over into the schooling process and are associated with these tragedies include dysfunctional families, incivility, substance abuse, child neglect and abuse, the coarsening of our culture, the flood of media violence, the anger and social fragmentation that is pervasive in our society, and so on. These forces have been a long time in developing and will not change or go away in the near term.

7. A major concern in relation to school tragedies is today's peer culture, which has absorbed the darker sides of our society's unfortunate changes of the past three decades; increasingly, our youth are immersed in a peer culture that is coarse, crude, cruel, uncaring, and often destructive to an individual's self-esteem.

8. Bullying, mean-spirited teasing, and the humiliation of certain peers are normative processes in many school settings and poison their climates; these destructive processes are often encouraged and supported by the presence and attention of peer bystanders. (Approximately 160,000 students miss school every day in the United States because of bullying and threats of intimidation.)

9. It is remarkable that so many of today's youth are willing to write off the rest of their lives by settling their grievances through violence against their peers and adults in the school setting; many of these same youth are very likely to be suicidal, extremely depressed, and in urgent need of mental health services and care.

We believe that the following strategic approaches, when used in combination, can move schools in the direction of greater safety and will reduce the likelihood over time of a school tragedy occurring: secure the school; address the peer culture and its problems; involve parents in making the school safer; create a positive, inclusive school culture; and develop a written school-safety and crisis-response plan. The more at risk a school is perceived to be, the more important these topical areas become for ensuring school safety and security; correspondingly, the greater is the investment that should be made in them. The importance and relevance of these strategies increase as one moves from elementary to middle to high school. The knowledge base on making schools safer does not indicate that a school must be turned into a fortress-like structure to achieve acceptable levels of security.

## Secure the School

The most immediate and direct method of addressing school safety issues is to secure the school. The three primary approaches to seriously consider in this regard are (a) the appropriate use of school security technology, (b) employment of school resource officers, and (c) use of Crime Prevention Through Environmental Design principles and techniques (see Appendix 25.B for resources that provide information on school safety). When used in combination, these three approaches can be effective in reducing the likelihood or probability of a school shooting tragedy.

Considerable progress has been made in the development and appropriate use of security technology to make schools safer while preserving their effectiveness and positive climate. This technology is being used increasingly within schools across the country. An excellent resource on this topic has been developed and published by the U.S. Office of Juvenile Justice and Delinquency Prevention (Green, 1999). School administrators should be aware of the status, advantages, and limitations of this technology when considering implementation of school safety options and strategies.

## Address the Peer Culture and Its Problems

The primary target for our efforts promoting violence prevention and safer schools should be the peer culture. The norms, actions, beliefs, and values within broad sectors of today's peer culture are socially destructive and demeaning. Many youth experience a trial by fire in negotiating the complex and difficult social tasks involved in finding one's place in this peer culture.

Far too many fail this critical test, become lost within it, and wander aimlessly while seeking acceptance that is generally not forthcoming. They become homeless persons within the larger peer group and their lack of fit is well known among peers. This process forces many marginalized youth to affiliate with atypical or deviant peer groups, which can prove destructive for them.

Transforming this destructive peer culture is perhaps our most formidable task in the area of school safety. This culture is not of the schools' making, but schools are perhaps the only social institution, excluding the family, that is capable of addressing it effectively. Five strategies are recommended for consideration in this regard.

- 1. Adopt and implement the Ribbon of Promise school violence prevention programs: *ByKids, ForKids* and *Not My Friends, Not My School* (see Appendix 25.B). These programs are designed to transform peer attitudes and beliefs about the risks to school safety that emerge from the peer culture. They promote ownership by peers of the tasks involved in preventing school tragedies and are highly recommended as a first strategy for enlisting a school's peer culture in this effort. The Ribbon of Promise videos have been widely distributed nationally and are now available to all public schools.

- 2. Bully-proof the school setting by adopting effective, anti-bullying and antiharassment programs, such as *Bully Proofing Your School* and *Steps to Respect* (see Appendix 25.B). The best disinfectant for bullying, mean-spirited teasing and harassment is sunlight. These events need to be defined as clearly unacceptable in the school by everyone—administrators, teachers, other school staff, students, and parents—and made public when they do occur. Students should be given strategies for reporting and resisting them in an adaptive, confidential manner. The reporting to school authorities of those who commit these acts should be made normative and widely acceptable. The above-cited programs incorporate these principles and strategies.

- 3. Teach anger management and conflict-resolution techniques as part of regular curricular content. The *Second Step Violence Prevention Program*, developed by the Committee for Children in Seattle (see Appendix 25.B), is one of the best means available for creating a positive peer culture of caring and civility and also for teaching specific strategies that work in controlling and managing one's anger and resolving conflicts without resorting to coercion or violence. This program was recently rated as *the* most effective of all those currently available for creating safe and positive schools by an expert panel of the Safe and Drug Free Schools Division of the U.S. Department of Education.

- 4. **Refer troubled, agitated, and depressed youth to mental health services and ensure that they receive the professional attention they need.** Youth with serious mental health problems and disorders, who are alienated, socially rejected, and taunted by peers, can be dangerous to themselves and others. These students are often known to peers and staff in the school and should be given the appropriate professional and parental attention, access to services, and social supports. When mental health problems are combined with being the target of severe bullying and taunting by peers, the result is often a dangerous combination in the context of school safety.

- 5. **Ask students to sign a pledge not to tease, bully, or put down others.** Reports from schools that have tried this tactic indicate that it makes a difference in the number of incidents that occur and in the overall school climate.

## Involve Parents in Making the School Safer

With each new school shooting tragedy, parents of school-age children and youth seek greater assurances that their child's school is safe and often ask for a voice and role in helping the school attain this goal. Recently, a prosecuting attorney, the mother of four children, described a plan for creating a parent-based advocacy group on school safety that would rate the safety of schools and make this information broadly available to all parents. Parents have much to offer schools as a resource in this regard and can be a powerful force in creating greater safety and a sense of security in the school setting. Four strategies are recommended for facilitating parent involvement.

- 1. **At each school, create a parent advisory-planning group devoted to school-safety issues for that school.** Such an advisory group would bring invaluable knowledge, experience, and advocacy to the process of dealing with local school-safety challenges. It could also serve as a forum for reacting to district- and state-level policy directives in this area.

●	2.	**Advocate for parents to teach their children adaptive, nonviolent methods of responding to bullying, teasing, and harassment at school and to avoid encouraging them to fight back.** In the vast majority of cases, fighting back will not be effective and may escalate the situation to dangerous levels. It will more likely increase the likelihood of the offensive behavior occurring again, rather than reducing it. An antibullying program at school, with parent and educator support and active involvement, will be much more effective.

●	3.	**Advocate (a) for the securing of weapons at home and (b) to access gun safety instruction for all family members.** Given the society in which we live and the number of guns in U.S. homes, it is becoming imperative that everyone have some understanding of the dangers involved in handling guns and being in proximity to those who are doing so. Trigger locks and secured gun cases (with secured keys) are essential elements for storing weapons in the home. The National Rifle Association (http://www.nra.org) has developed some excellent information on gun safety that can be accessed by anyone. In connection with these efforts, young children need to be taught a golden rule about the sanctity of life and that guns are deadly, life-ending instruments.

●	4.	**Make available to parents solid information on effective parenting practices and provide access to those parents who seek training and support in more effective parenting.** Five generic parenting practices are instrumental in determining how children develop: (a) discipline, (b) monitoring and supervision, (c) parent involvement in children's lives, (d) positive family management techniques, and (e) crisis intervention and problem solving. Appendix 25.C explains these techniques in some detail, and this information can be shared with parents as a handout or included in a school's newsletter. A large number of available parent training programs address these practices.

## Create a Positive, Inclusive School Climate and Culture

Solid evidence indicates that effective schools are safer schools and vice versa. The research of D. C. Gottfredson and her colleagues (Najaka et al., 2001), along with that of others, shows that a school climate that is positive, inclusive, and accepting is a key component of an effective school. Three recommended strategies are described for addressing this component of school safety.

- 1. **Create and promote a set of school-based positive values about how individuals should treat others that include *civility, caring,* and *respecting the rights of others.*** It is unfortunate that schools have to teach civility in addition to everything else they do, but such is now the case. Children and youth are exposed daily to very poor models of behavior toward others by adult society. Making civility a core value of the school's culture may help reduce some of the coarseness of the peer culture that has become such a problem in our schools and society.

- 2. **Teach all students how to separate from their own lives the exaggerated media images of interpersonal violence, disrespect, and incivility to which they are exposed daily.** School curricula exist that teach media literacy relative to interpersonal violence. It is especially important that young children learn how to make the disconnect between media displays of violence and their own behavior and actions.

- 3. **Establish schoolwide rules and behavioral expectations, and set specific applications of same.** Universal intervention programs designed for schoolwide application are an excellent and proven vehicle for accomplishing this goal. Examples of such intervention programs are Building Effective Schools Together and Effective Behavioral Support (see Appendix 25.B). These programs are being implemented in local districts across the country. These are highly recommended approaches for schools to use in creating orderly, positive, and well-managed school environments.

## Develop a Written School-Safety and Crisis-Response Plan

The state of Oregon recently enacted a new law requiring each school to develop a written school-safety and crisis-response plan. In today's environment, it is essential that each school go through a planning process designed to reduce the likelihood of a school tragedy and to manage a crisis when it occurs. The key elements that should be addressed in a comprehensive school-safety plan are as follows:

1. School-safety audits that evaluate school-safety and violence vulnerabilities due to structural characteristics of the building and patterns of building usage

2. A crisis-intervention plan that allows school personnel to respond to and control crises that carry potential implications for violence or reduced school safety

3. A schoolwide curricular program that teaches social skills instrumental in violence prevention (anger management, conflict resolution, empathy, and impulse control)

4. A well-established communication plan that provides interactive linkages between school personnel, public safety, and parents

These four elements are essential to improving the safety and security of any school building and surrounding grounds. Well-developed procedures exist for assessing a school's degree of risk and for implementing each of the listed components.

## School-Based Prevention Applications

Schools need to make their role in the prevention of disruptive, antisocial behavior patterns an effective reality. Educators tend to give lip service to prevention strategies but are often unwilling to invest in the strategies at the necessary levels because of suspicions about their effectiveness and worries about their long-term costs. However, the trauma of the school-shooting tragedies of the 1990s has shocked a majority of school personnel into advocating a prevention agenda and searching for intervention approaches that are proven and promising.

Table 25.1 provides some general guidelines about what does and does not work in the area of school crime prevention. These guidelines and recommendations should be considered carefully by school administrators, as they are derived from numerous and comprehensive analyses of school environments as developed through the seminal work of G. Gottfredson and Gottfredson (1999).

Walker and Sprague (1999b) recently described the key elements and components of a comprehensive approach for use by schools in addressing the mental health and behavioral needs of *all* students within a school. This approach is based on an integrated, service delivery model contributed originally by Walker et al. (1996) for the prevention of antisocial behavior patterns. It is based on the U.S. Public Health Service's classification system that involves primary, secondary, and tertiary forms of prevention. For example, primary prevention strategies rely on universal interventions, such as schoolwide discipline and behavior management systems, grade-level teaching of violence prevention skills, and effective instruction, all of which are designed to keep problems from emerging. Secondary prevention strategies, which are more costly and intensive, are designed for addressing the problems and skill deficits of children and youth who are already showing clear signs of being at risk. Primary prevention strategies are not of sufficient intensity or strength to effectively solve the problems of children and youth who require secondary prevention strategies due to the intractability or severity of their problems. Finally, tertiary prevention strategies are designed for the most severely at-risk children and youth whom schools must attempt to accommodate. Generally, their problems demand resources, supports, interventions, and services that cannot be provided by schools alone. Wraparound services and interagency partnerships are necessary to accommodate the needs of these students and their families.

Figure 25.3 illustrates these three prevention approaches and the approximate proportion of the student population that will require and likely respond to each type of prevention. There is currently a pipeline literally filled with at-risk students who are experiencing traumatic behavioral events and outcomes as they progress through it. If schools respond only reactively and rely exclusively upon secondary and tertiary strategies applied after these destructive events and outcomes are in evidence, larger and larger amounts of resources will be invested in return for weaker and weaker therapeutic effects and outcomes. There will always be students who come to school with such severe behavioral involvements that secondary and even tertiary supports and interventions will be necessary from the beginnings of their school careers. That said, however, much greater and more effective use

# TABLE 25.1
## Scientific Conclusions Regarding What's Effective in School Crime Prevention

**What Works?**

Strategies for which at least two different studies on crime and delinquency have found positive effects on measures of problem behavior and for which the preponderance of evidence is positive follow:

- Programs aimed at building school capacity to initiate and sustain innovation.

- Programs aimed at clarifying and communicating norms about behaviors—by establishing school rules, improving the consistency of their enforcement (particularly when they emphasize positive reinforcement of appropriate behavior), or communicating norms through school-wide campaigns (e.g., anti-bullying campaigns) or ceremonies.

- Comprehensive instructional programs that focus on a range of social competency skills (e.g., developing self-control, stress-management, responsible decision-making, social problem-solving, and communication skills) and that are delivered over a long period of time to continually reinforce skills.

**What Does Not Work?**

Strategies for which at least two different studies have found no positive effects on measures of problem behavior and for which the preponderance of evidence is not positive are as follows:

- Counseling students, particularly in a peer-group context, does not reduce delinquency or substance abuse.

- Offering youths alternative activities such as recreation and community service activities in the absence of more potent prevention programming does not reduce substance abuse.

- Instructional programs focusing on information dissemination, fear arousal, moral appeal, and affective education are ineffective for reducing substance abuse.

**What Is Promising?**

Several strategies have been shown in only one rigorous study to reduce delinquency or substance use. If the preponderance of evidence for these strategies is positive, they are regarded as promising until replication confirms the effect. These strategies are as follows:

- Programs that group youth into smaller "schools-within-schools" to create smaller units, more supportive interactions, or greater flexibility in instruction.

- Behavior modification programs that teach "thinking skills" to high-risk youths.

- Programs aimed at building school capacity to initiate and sustain innovation.

- Programs that improve classroom management and that use effective instructional techniques.

*Note.* Based on "School-Based Crime Prevention," by D. C. Gottfredson, 1997, in *Preventing Crime: What Works, What Doesn't, What's Promising: A Report to the United States Congress* (pp. 5-1 to 5-74), by L. Sherman et al. (Eds.), Washington, DC: U.S. Department of Justice Office of Justice Programs; and on "School-Based Crime Prevention," by D. C. Gottfredson, D. B. Wilson, and S. S. Najaka, 2002, in *Evidence-Based Crime Prevention*, L. W. Sherman, D. P. Farrington, B. C. Welsh, and D. L. MacKenzie (Eds.), London: Routledge.

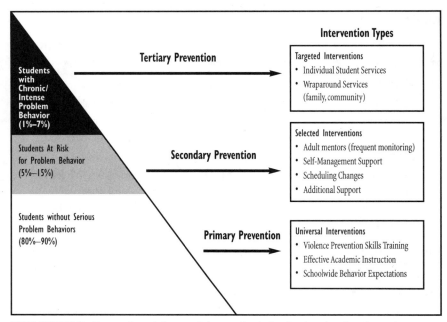

**FIGURE 25.3.** Preventing violent and destructive behavior in schools using primary, secondary, and tertiary systems of intervention. *Note.* From "The Path to School Failure, Delinquency, and Violence: Causal Factors and Some Potential Solutions," by H. M. Walker and J. R. Sprague, 1999, *Intervention in School and Clinic, 35,* p. 71. Copyright 1999 by PRO-ED, Inc. Reprinted with permission.

of primary prevention strategies in the school setting can be made than traditionally has been the case.

As noted, universal interventions are used for achieving primary prevention goals. It is estimated that 80% to 90% of a school's student population will respond positively, at some level, to these universal intervention strategies. Those who do not respond to primary prevention approaches—anywhere from 5% to 15% of the school's population—select themselves out as candidates needing additional secondary or tertiary prevention strategies and approaches. However, for those students who require the most intensive, individualized interventions—approximately 1% to 7% of all students—the existence of a well-designed and carefully implemented primary prevention base in the school setting provides a powerful context for their effective application.

## Developing Academic Competence

As noted previously, academic failure and especially difficulties in reading are strong correlates of delinquency in adolescence (Maguin & Loeber, 1996). The evidence is overwhelming as to the existence and consistency of this relationship. An intense focus on developing the academic skills of at-risk youth is an essential part of any comprehensive strategy to address their needs and to divert them from the path that leads to antisocial behavior and often later delinquency. All students and especially at-risk students should be taught to read as well as they possibly can in the primary grades. It is difficult to underestimate its importance in forging a successful school career.

## Collaborative Interagency Prevention Approaches

In our view, a primary goal is to create full-service schools that (a) have an expanded capacity to address the complex needs of today's school population and (b) can address true prevention goals through effective collaborations forged between schools, families, and communities. Several key elements are necessary to create such full-service schools and to address prevention goals, strategies, and outcomes in a manner that will be sufficient to arrest and turn around the rising tide of at-risk children and youth who appear at the schoolhouse door. They include the following critical elements: early intervention services; proactive family support systems; mental health, public health, and social services; and transition supports and services to postschooling environs. Effective partnerships need to be built between families, schools, social service systems, public safety agencies, churches, and other agencies to create the socializing experiences that will give all youth a chance to develop along positive lines.

Metzler et al. (1998) described the elements of a comprehensive approach to the prevention of child and adolescent behavior problems that integrates family and community-based approaches to strengthening the application of universal, as well as individually targeted, behavior management programs in schools. Researchers need to carefully examine prevention models of this type and learn how to scale them up so they can be adopted and implemented on a broad basis in a cost-effective manner by school systems.

## Managing Interactions with Difficult Students at the Classroom Level

Teachers today are confronted with more challenges in teaching and managing students than at any previous point in history. Today's students are more diverse, more challenging, and more powerfully influenced by negative social forces (e.g., media violence, societal fragmentation, poor anger control by adult models) that negatively impact their school performance and behavior. Teachers at all levels are more likely to encounter in their normal teaching routines antisocial students who are disrespectful and unresponsive to traditional behavior management strategies and tactics of adult social influence. Many of these students are early starters who come to the schooling experience from highly chaotic and dysfunctional family situations. They typically have developed coercive behavioral repertoires that are based on confrontation and escalation as generic strategies for dealing with interpersonal processes and negotiating social tasks. Teachers find them to be difficult in the extreme and frequently become engaged in hostile exchanges with them. Figure 25.4 contains a conceptual model developed by Colvin (1992) that illustrates the escalating and destructive properties of these unfortunate interactions.

A teacher often inadvertently becomes locked into hostile, escalating interactions with antisocial students that are very public, very damaging to the teacher–student relationship, and very difficult to extricate oneself from. These students are masters at engaging teachers both prior to and during this interaction. As long as the teacher is willing to keep responding to the student's questions and provocations, the teacher is not in control of the interaction—the student is. The longer the interaction goes on and the more hostile it becomes, the greater the likelihood of an undesirable ending and ensuing damage to the teacher's ability to teach and manage all students in the class. In this scenario, the student is generally the professional and the teacher is the amateur.

The solution is for the teacher not to play the escalation game in which the antisocial student is so accomplished. These interactions should be avoided and also stopped soon after they begin in order to prevent the resulting and inevitable damage. The teacher stops these interactions by refusing to continue the interaction. It may be necessary to prearrange the front office support necessary to remove and discipline the antisocial student whenever these events occur. After the student has settled down, the teacher can quietly approach and debrief the student about how the situa-

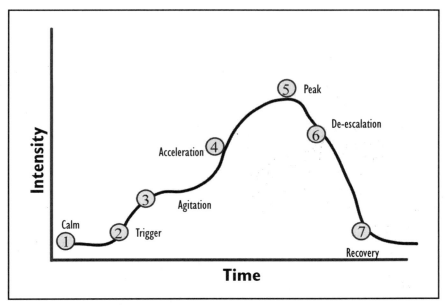

**FIGURE 25.4.** Phases of escalating behavior. *Note.* From *Managing Acting-Out Behavior: A Staff Development Program To Prevent and Manage Acting-Out Behavior* (p. 4), by Colvin, 1992, Eugene, OR: Behavior Associates. Copyright 1992 by Behavior Associates. Reprinted with permission.

tion that prompted the hostile exchange could have been handled differently and avoided.

The senior author has written extensively on the issues of managing difficult students, on classroom ecology, and on preventing behavioral episodes through the judicious use of teacher requests, demands, and commands. Perhaps a majority of hostile exchanges and difficult situations with behaviorally at-risk students could be avoided through the careful application of known behavioral principles in this context. Appendix 25.D contains a listing of suggestions for teachers to use in preventing and defusing oppositional–aggressive student behavior among at-risk student populations. See Walker (1995) for a thorough treatment of this topic.

Teaching today is qualitatively different than heretofore, primarily because of sharp changes in the student population and to our society's disinvestment in its children and youth, particularly in the realm of schooling. Teachers need strong administrative support and access to mental health specialists for managing severely involved students. The threat of school violence is always present, but teachers can play critical roles in (a) referring troubled students promptly to appropriate mental health support systems; (b) teaching all students the violence prevention skills, such as empathy, conflict resolution, impulse control, and anger management, that will assist them in avoiding violent solutions to interpersonal conflicts; and (c) demonstrating a sense of caring and concern for each and every student. If applied with conviction, these actions can be effective in helping students bond with and connect to the schooling process.

## CONCLUSION

The United States has a violent history as a country, and many experts argue that U.S. culture, by nature, is violent. Far more children and youth die each year in America through gun violence than in any other developed country (see Osofsky, 1997). As a society, we should hold up a mirror and examine ourselves in this regard so as to take a close look at what we have become, how we got here, and how we might change for the better. Grossman (1995) makes a compelling case that the United States is now the most violent developed society in the world. The tragic spate of school shootings during the decade of the 1990s offers grim testimony as to how the destructive influences and violent images that pervade our daily lives are registering their negative effects upon our children and youth (Walker & Sprague, 1999b).

Policy generally lags well behind the research that validates evidence-based approaches that can inform and guide policy decisions and practices based on them. This is especially true in the area of school safety and youth violence prevention. The pressures and demands of the moment force school administrators into making decisions about school safety strategy and tactics that may appear promising but are not, as yet, proven through the research process. Thus, educators have been left with basing many decisions on practices that appear promising, relying on experience and best judgment. However, the scientific and empirical knowledge base on school safety is rapidly expanding, and effective, proven approaches are now becoming available for implementation. It is incumbent upon school leaders and administrators to stay on top of this emerging body of knowledge. The action recommendations contained in this chapter represent what is known about these complex issues at present. We believe that schools can be made measurably safer and that behaviorally at-risk youth can be far better served by implementing well that which currently is known.

# APPENDIX 25.A

# Risk-Protective Factors Associated with Youth Violence and Delinquency

## Factors Associated with Elevated Risk for Violence and Delinquency

1. Poor social skills
2. Poor school engagement
3. Family with one or more of the following characteristics: lack of parental supervision, mother or father ever arrested, evidence of child abuse or neglect, at least one family transition such as divorce or remarriage
4. Predelinquent problem behaviors, such as bullying and annoying others, fighting, being stubborn and defiant, and telling lies
5. Early drug and alcohol use
6. Early age of onset of delinquent activity
7. A high level of "daily hassles" (minor stressors)
8. Attention-deficit/hyperactivity disorder
9. Learning disabilities
10. Low IQ, especially verbal ability
11. Poor school performance, especially poor grades in high school
12. Delinquent peers
13. Having multiple risk factors (The cumulative effect of several family and child risk variables has been found to be a better predictor of delinquency than any single variable alone.)

## Factors that Buffer Against the Risk of Developing Violent or Destructive Behavior

1. Family stability
2. Positive temperament
3. Academic success
4. Positive school experiences
5. Positive work or work training experiences
6. High self-esteem
7. Structure in the environment (school and home)

8. A good relationiship with a parent or other adult
9. Advanced self-help and problem-solving skills
10. Internal locus of control (anger management, limit setting, goal setting)
11. Identified network of family and friends who are available for support in times of crisis
12. High engagement in positive activities (e.g., sports, hobbies, art, community service)

# APPENDIX 25.B

# Recommended Resource Materials on School Safety

## Books

Gottfredson, D. (1997). School-based crime prevention. In L. Sherman, D. Gottfredson, D. MacKenzie, J. Eck, P. Ruter, & S. Bushway (Eds.), *Preventing crime: What works, what doesn't, what's promising: A report to the U.S. Congress* (pp. 1–74). Washington, DC: U.S. Department of Justice, Office of Justice Programs.

Green, M. (1999). *The appropriate and effective use of security technologies in U.S. schools.* (Available from U.S. Department of Justice, Office of Justice Programs, 810 Seventh Street NW, Washington, DC 20531)

Poland, S. (2000). *Take back your school: Empower your students to prevent violence (Grades 6–12).* Longmont, CO: Sopris West.

Poland, S., & McCormick, J. (1999). *Coping with crisis: Lessons learned.* Longmont, CO: Sopris West.

Schneider, T., Walker, H. M., & Sprague, J. R. (2000). *Safe school design.* Eugene: Educational Resources Information Clearinghouse (ERIC), University of Oregon.

Walker, H. M., & Epstein, M. H. (2000). *Making schools safer and violence free.* Austin, TX: PRO-ED.

## Reports

Citizen's Crime Commission. (2000). *Kids intervention investment delinquency solutions.* (Available from the Citizens Crime Commission, Portland Chamber of Commerce, 221 NW Second Avenue, Portland, OR 97209-3999; 503/228-9736; http://www.kiids .org)

*Early warning/timely response: A guide to safe schools.* (Available from http://www.ed.gov/ offices/OSERS/OSEP/earlywrn.html)

Oregon School Safety Coalition. (2001). *How safe are Oregon schools?* Salem: State of Oregon Attorney General's Office. (Available from http://darkwing.uoregon.edu/~ivdb/ index.html)

*Safeguarding our children: An action guide.* (Available from http://www.ed.gov/offices/ OSERS/OSEP/Action Guide)

# Articles

Hawkins, D., Catalano, R., Kosterman, R., Abbott, R., & Hill, K. (1999, March). Preventing adolescent health-risk behaviors by strengthening protection during childhood. *Archives of Pediatrics & Adolescent Medicine, 153,* 226–234.

Sprague, J. R., & Walker, H. M. (2000). Early identification and intervention for youth with antisocial and violent behavior. *Exceptional Children, 66,* 367–379.

Walker, H. M., & Walker, J. E. (2000, March). Key questions about school safety: Critical issues and recommended solutions. *NASSP Bulletin,* pp. 46–55.

# Recommended Programs for Preventing Violence and Bullying or Harassment

*Bully Proofing Your School.* (Available from Sopris West, Inc., P.O. Box 1890, Longmont, CO 80502-1809; 800/547-6747)

*Second Step Violence Prevention Program.* (Available from the Committee for Children, Seattle, WA; 800/634-4449; http://www.cfchildren.org)

*Steps to Respect* (antibullying program). (Available from the Committee for Children, Seattle, WA; 800/634-4449; http://www.cfchildren.org)

# Recommended Institute on Violence and Destructive Behavior Programs for Making Schools Safer, Effective, and Positive

*Building Effective Schools Together.* Contact Jeff Sprague at 541/346-3592; http://darkwing .uoregon.edu/~ivdb/index.html

*Effective Behavioral Support.* Contact George Sugai at 541/346-1642 or Rob Horner at 541/346-2460; http://darkwing.uoregon.edu/~ivdb/index.html

*Ribbon of Promise Programs* (*ByKids, ForKids* and *Not My Friends, Not My School*). Contact Cindy Brown at 541/726-0512; www.ribbonofpromise.org

# Safe Schools Organizational Resources

*The National School Safety Center*—Ron Stephens, Director; 141 Duesenberg Drive, Suite 11, Westlake Village, CA 91362; 805/373-9977; www.nsscl.org

*National Resource Center for Safe Schools*—Carlos Sundermann, Director; 101 SW Main Street, Suite 500, Portland, OR 97204; 800/547-6339

# APPENDIX 25.C

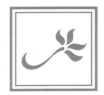

# Tips for Parents on Effective Family Management Techniques

Research has identified five key parenting practices that are very important in the upbringing of well-adjusted children. Each of these practices is briefly discussed below.

1. **Discipline.** Parental discipline needs to be fair, consistent, and predictable. It should *never* be harsh or punitive. There should be a logical relationship between child behavior and the consequences that are applied to it.

2. **Monitoring.** Careful parental monitoring of a child's activities, whereabouts, and friendships and peer associations is one of the single most important things that parents can do to ensure that their children grow up healthy, well adjusted, and safe.

3. **Parent Involvement.** This practice involves simply spending time with your child in either structured or unstructured activities. The parent–child contact is the important thing, and the activity chosen is usually incidental to the time spent together and the positive interactions that occur.

4. **Positive Parenting Techniques.** Positive parenting means being supportive and encouraging of your child. It is important to establish a warm, caring relationship between you that involves mutual respect and affection. In this way, you will be better able to influence your child in the right directions using techniques like social interest, praise and approval, persuasion, and logical thinking, without resorting to punishment and other negative methods of behavioral control.

5. **Problem Solving/Conflict Resolution/Crisis Intervention.** During their upbringing, children experience many minor crises that, nevertheless, loom very large in their lives. When they bring problems to their parents for assistance, it is very important that they be responded to immediately and completely. Alternatives should be developed for them to consider in

solving the problem and they should be encouraged to choose one that is acceptable and that works for them. Children should always have the confidence that such problems will receive a fair hearing and that they will have access to your assistance as needed.

Adherence to these simple, yet critically important practices in your parenting efforts will have a powerful, positive impact on your child and your relationship with him or her. Further, they will contribute to a much more positive set of family dynamics.

The following rules are offered for your consideration in parenting your child. They can be very helpful in the prevention of adjustment problems later on in your child's life.

1. Set up a daily debriefing time for reviewing the child's day. Ask questions such as these to encourage the child to talk: "What did you do today?" "What did you do that was fun or interesting?" "Who did you play or talk with?" "Did anything happen that was a problem or that you didn't like?" Why should you debrief? First, it tells the child you care for him or her and are concerned about what happens in his or her life. Also, it is an excellent method for screening to detect problems in the child's life that you might not discover otherwise. Once the child starts schooling, it is extremely important to conduct a daily debriefing of this type.

2. Monitor your child's activities, behavior, schedules, whereabouts, friendships, and associations very carefully. It is important to provide such monitoring in a positive, caring manner, and in a way that is not smothering or unpleasant. Careful monitoring of this type can be a very powerful protective factor in the child's life. As your child grows and matures, such monitoring may have to change form and become more subtle and less direct. However, it is extremely important that it occur, especially as your child enters adolescence, when the potential for problems is so much greater.

3. Children should be taught positive attitudes toward school, and shown that you consider schooling to be a highly valued activity. A pattern of cooperative, prosocial behavior will do a great deal to foster a good start in school that will ensure both academic achievement and social development over the long term.

4. The most important skill you can teach your child prior to entering school is to listen as you read to him or her. Your child should see the

material you are reading and associate the sounds of the words with their symbols on the page. This activity is an important precondition for developing a child who is a good reader and who is interested in reading. It is one of the best things that can be done to prevent later school failure and to help ensure academic success.

# APPENDIX 25.D

# Suggestions for Preventing and Defusing Oppositional–Aggressive Student Behavior

The following suggestions will lead to a lower frequency of oppositional–aggressive student behavior over time and across situations. The teacher should do the following:

1. Establish an ecology for the classroom setting that is positive, inclusive, and supportive of *all* students, regardless of their behavioral and academic characteristics.

2. Be aware that adults can unconsciously form and behaviorally express negative impressions of low-performing, uncooperative students to which such students are quite sensitive. The teacher should carefully monitor his or her impressions, keep them as neutral as possible, communicate a positive regard for the students, and give them the benefit of the doubt whenever possible.

3. Establish and communicate high expectations in achievement and behavior for *all* students.

4. Create a structured learning environment in which students know what is expected of them and where they can access needed assistance in completing academic tasks.

5. Allow sharp demarcation to occur between academic periods, but hold transition times between periods to a minimum.

6. Consider using cooperative learning strategies that allow diverse groups of students to interact, problem solve, and develop skills in working together.

7. Systematically teach social skills curricula that incorporate instruction in anger management and conflict resolution strategies.

8. Be sure that academic programming and task difficulty are commensurate with the skill levels of low-performing students. Acting-out students,

in particular, tend to have weak academic skills and may react negatively to academic tasks or demands that they feel are too difficult for them. These situations very often lead to hostile teacher–student interactions.

9. Teach students how to be assertive in an appropriate manner (e.g., to disagree or resist the demands of others without being hostile).

10. Use difficult situations as "teaching opportunities" for developing student skills in responding to such situations without being angry, aggressive, or coercive.

11. Be sure to find ways to praise and encourage low-performing students at the same or a higher rate than that for higher performing students.

12. Find ways to communicate a genuine interest in the progress of low-performing students and support them as they struggle to meet the complex demands of schooling.

13. Maximize the performance of low-performing students through the use of individualized instruction, cues, prompting, the breaking down of academic tasks, debriefing, coaching, and providing positive incentives (e.g., praise, free time, home privileges).

14. Try to avoid criticizing, ridiculing, verbally punishing, or arguing with any student, especially low-performing or acting-out students.

# REFERENCES

American Psychological Association. (1993). *Violence and youth: Psychology's response. Volume 1: Summary report of the American Psychological Association Commission on Violence and Youth.* Washington, DC: Author.

Colvin, G. (1992). *Managing acting-out behavior: A staff development program to prevent and manage acting-out behavior.* Eugene, OR: Behavior Associates.

Crowe, T. (1995, January). *Youth crime and community safety.* Keynote address to the Eugene City Club, Eugene, OR.

Eddy, M., Reid, J., & Curry, V. (2002). The etiology of youth antisocial behavior, delinquency, and violence and a public health approach to prevention. In M. Shinn, H. M. Walker, & G. Stoner (Eds.), *Interventions for academic and behavior problems II: Preventive and remedial approaches* (pp. 27–52). Bethesda, MD: National Association of School Psychologists.

Gottfredson, D. C. (1997). School-based crime prevention. In L. W. Sherman, D. C. Gottfredson, D. MacKenzie, J. Eck, P. Reuter, & S. Bushway (Eds.), *Preventing crime: What works, what doesn't, what's promising: A report to the United States Congress* (pp. 5-1 to 5-74). Washington, DC: U.S. Department of Justice Office of Justice Programs.

Gottfredson, G., & Gottfredson, D. (1999). *Development and applications of theoretical measures for evaluating drug and delinquency prevention programs* (Technical Manual for Research Editions of *What About You? WAY*). (Available from Gottfredson Associates, 3239-B Corporate Court, Ellicott City, MD 21042)

Gottfredson, D. C., Wilson, D. B., & Najaka, S. S. (2002). School-based crime prevention. In L. W. Sherman, D. P. Farrington, B. C. Welsh, & D. L. MacKenzie (Eds.), *Evidence-based crime prevention.* London: Routledge.

Green, M. (1999). *The appropriate and effective use of security technologies in U.S. schools: A guide for schools and law enforcement agencies.* (Available from U.S. Department of Justice, Office of Justice Programs, 810 Seventh Street NW, Washington, DC 20531)

Gresham, F. M., Lane, K. L., & Lambros, K. L. (2002). Comorbidity of conduct problems and ADHD: Identification of "fledging psychopaths." *Journal of Emotional and Behavioral Disorders, 8,* 83–93.

Grossman, D. (1995). *On killing.* Boston: Little Brown.

Hawkins, J. D., Catalano, R. F., Kosterman, R., Abbott, R., & Hill, K. G. (1999). Preventing adolescent health-risk behaviors by strengthening protection during childhood. *Archives of Pediatrics and Adolescent Medicine, 153,* 226–234.

Hoagwood, K., & Erwin, H. (1997). Effectiveness of school based mental health services for children: A 10 year research review. *Journal of Child and Family Studies, 1,* 129–140.

Kazdin, A. E. (Ed.). (1985). *Treatment of antisocial behavior in children and adolescents.* Homewood, IL: Dorsey Press.

Loeber, R., & Farrington, D. P. (Eds.). (1998). *Serious and violent juvenile offenders: Risk factors and successful interventions.* Thousand Oaks, CA: Sage.

Lynam, D. (1996). Early identification of chronic offenders: Who is the fledgling psychopath? *Psychological Bulletin, 120,* 209–234.

Maguin, E., & Loeber, R. (1996). Academic performance and delinquency. In M. Tonry (Ed.), *Crime and justice: A review of research* (Vol. 20, pp. 145–264). Chicago: University of Chicago Press.

Metzler, C., Taylor, T., Gunn, B., Fowler, R., Biglan, T., & Ary, D. (1998). A comprehensive approach to the prevention of behavior problems: Integrating family- and community-based approaches to strengthen behavior management programs in schools. *Effective School Practices, 17*(2), 8–24.

Moffitt, T. (1994). Adolescence-limited and life-course–persistent antisocial behavior: A developmental taxonomy. *Psychological Review, 100*(4), 674–701.

Najaka, S., Gottfredson, D. C., & Wilson, D. (2001). A meta-analytic inquiry into the relationship between selected risk factors and problem behavior. *Prevention Science, 2*(4), 257–271.

O'Neill, R., Horner, R. H., Albin, R. W., Sprague, J. R., Newton, S., & Storey, K. (1997). *Functional assessment and program development for problem behavior: A practical handbook* (2nd ed.). Pacific Grove, CA: Brookes/Cole.

Osofsky, J. D. (1997). *Children in a violent society.* New York: Guilford Press.

O'Toole, M. E. (2000). *The school shooter: A threat assessment perspective.* Quantico, VA: National Center for the Analysis of Violent Crime, the FBI Academy.

Patterson, G. R., Reid, J. B., & Dishion, T. J. (1992). *Antisocial boys.* Eugene, OR: Castalia Press.

Reid, J. (1993). Prevention of conduct disorder before and after school entry: Relating interventions to developmental findings. *Development and Psychopathology, 5,* 243–262.

Satcher, D. (2001). *Youth violence: A report of the Surgeon General.* Washington, DC: Department of Health and Human Services, U.S. Public Health Service.

Seeley, J., Rohde, P., Lewinhsohn, P., & Clarke, G. (2002). Depression in youth: Epidemiology, identification, and intervention. In M. Shinn, H. M. Walker, & G. Stoner (Eds.), *Interventions for academic and behavior problems II: Preventive and remedial approaches* (pp. 885–912). Bethesda, MD: National Association of School Psychologists.

Shinn, M., Walker, H. M., & Stoner, G. (2002). *Interventions for academic and behavior problems II: Preventive and remedial approaches.* Bethesda, MD: National Association of School Psychologists.

Stephens, R. (2000, December). School safety update: Secret Service study of school shootings focuses on "targeted violence." *Newsletter of the National School Safety Center,* pp. 1–4.

Vance, J., Bowen, N., Fernandez, G., & Thompson, S. (2002). Risk and protective factors as predictors of outcome in adolescents with psychiatric disorder and aggression. *Journal of the American Academy of Child and Adolescent Psychiatry, 41,* 36–43.

Vance, J., Fernandez, G., & Biber, M. (1998). Educational progress in a population of youth with aggression and emotional disturbance: The role of risk and protective factors. *Journal of Emotional and Behavioral Disorders, 6,* 214–221.

Walker, H. M. (1986). The AIMS (Assessments for Integration into Mainstream Settings) assessment system: Rationale, instruments, procedures and outcomes. *Journal of Clinical Child Psychology, 15,* 55–63.

Walker, H. M. (1995). *The acting out child.* Longmont, CO: Sopris West.

Walker, H. M., Colvin, G., & Ramsey, E. (1995). *Antisocial behavior in schools: Strategies and best practices.* Pacific Grove, CA: Brooks/Cole.

Walker, H. M., Hops, H., & Greenwood, C. R. (1988). *RECESS: Reprogramming environmental contingencies for effective social skills.* Seattle: Educational Achievement Systems.

Walker, H. M., Horner, R. H., Sugai, G., Bullis, M., Sprague, J. R., Bricker, D., & Kaufman, M. J. (1996). Integrated approaches to preventing antisocial behavior patterns among school-age children and youth. *Journal of Emotional and Behavioral Disorders, 4,* 193–256.

Walker, H. M., & Severson, H. H. (2002). Developmental prevention of at-risk outcomes for vulnerable antisocial children and youth. In K. L. Lane, F. M. Gresham, & T. E. O'Shaughnessy (Eds.), *Interventions for children with or at risk for emotional and behavioral disorders* (pp. 175–191). Boston: Allyn & Bacon.

Walker, H. M., & Sprague, J. R. (1999a). Longitudinal research and functional behavioral assessment issues. *Behavioral Disorders, 24,* 335–337.

Walker, H. M., & Sprague, J. R. (1999b). The path to school failure, delinquency, and violence: Causal factors and some potential solutions. *Intervention in School and Clinic, 35,* 67–73.

# Glossary

**Abduct.** To draw away from the median plane.

**Abortifacient.** An agent that causes abortion.

**Abscess.** A cavity filled with pus.

**Acetone.** A colorless liquid found in the urine of diabetic patients who are poorly controlled.

**Achondroplasia.** A type of dwarfism characterized by short limbs.

**Acquired.** Nongenetic, produced by external forces or influences.

**Acuity.** Keenness of vision or hearing.

**Acute pancreatitis.** Acute inflammation of the pancreas.

**Adduct.** To draw toward the median plane.

**Adipose.** Of or relating to fat.

**Adrenaline (epinephrine).** Secreted by the adrenal medulla and a powerful stimulant of the sympathetic nervous system.

**Aerosolized.** The process of dispersing in a fine mist.

**Air studies.** The introduction of air into the cerebrospinal fluid spaces for evaluation of brain anatomy.

**Alexia.** Loss of the ability to understand written language as the result of a cerebral lesion.

**Allele.** One or more contrasting characters transmitted by alternative genes.

**Alpha-fetoprotein.** A protein produced by the fetal liver that is markedly elevated in the amniotic fluid when the fetus has spina bifida or an open defect of the central nervous system.

**Amblyopia.** Decreased vision without apparent change in the eye structures.

**Ambulation.** The act of walking or moving about.

**Amenorrhea.** Absence or abnormal stoppage of the menses.

**Amnesia.** Loss of memory.

**Amniocentesis.** Surgical transabdominal perforation of the uterus to obtain amniotic fluid.

**Amphetamine.** A drug that acts as a central nervous system stimulant.

**Amplification.** Increase of auditory stimulus by the use of hearing aids.

**Analgesic.** A class of drugs used for the relief of pain.

**Ancillary.** Supplementary, additional.

**Anemia.** A condition in which blood is deficient in the quantity of hemoglobin or the number of red blood cells or both.

**Anencephaly.** Absence of the cerebral hemispheres and cranial vault in the brain.

**Anomaly.** A variance from the normal.

**Anorexia.** Loss of appetite for food.

**Anorexia nervosa.** Severe and prolonged inability or refusal to eat, sometimes associated with vomiting.

**Anoxia.** A severe reduction in the normal concentration of oxygen within the body.

**Antacid.** A drug that counteracts or relieves gastric (stomach) acidity.

**Antenatal.** Occurring before birth.

**Anterior.** Situated before or toward the front.

**Anthropometric.** Relating to the study of human body measurements, especially on a comparative basis.

**Antibiotic.** A chemical that inhibits the growth of or kills microorganisms.

**Anticholinergic.** An agent that blocks the parasympathetic nerves.

**Anticonvulsant.** A drug used to treat and prevent convulsions.

**Antidepressant.** A drug used to elevate the mood of a depressed individual.

**Aortic stenosis.** Obstruction of the aortic artery.

**Aphasia.** Defect or loss of the power to use words in speech or writing due to disease or injury of the brain.

**Arnold Chiari malformation.** A congenital malformation of the brain where the cerebellum and medulla protrude downward into the spinal cord.

**Arteriosclerosis.** Thickening and loss of elasticity of the arterial walls.

**Arteriovenous malformation.** An abnormal relationship between arteries and veins.

**Arthritis.** Inflammation of the joints due to infectious, metabolic, or constitutional causes.

**Articular.** Joint surface.

**Articulator.** A device for effecting a jointlike union.

**Asphyxia.** Lack of oxygen leading to cessation of life.

**Assay.** A biologic analysis to measure the quantity or purity of a substance.

**Astigmatism.** Unequal curvature of the eye resulting in a distorted image on the retina.

**Asymptomatic.** Presenting no subjective evidence of disease.

**Ataxia.** Incoordination of movement.

**Atonia.** Deficient muscular tone often associated with chorea.

**Atherosclerotic.** A form of arteriosclerosis with yellow plaques containing cholesterol and lipids deposited within the walls of the arteries.

**Auditory nerve.** Eighth cranial nerve, the hearing nerve.

**Aura.** A subjective sensation of phenomenon that precedes a seizure.

**Autistic.** A severe disorder of communication and behavior characterized by self-absorption, withdrawal from contact with people, and preoccupation with inanimate objects.

**Autoimmune.** Directed against the body's own tissue.

**Automatism.** The performance of nonreflex acts without conscious volition.

**Axon.** That process of a neuron by which nerve impulses travel away from the cell body.

**Bacteremia.** The presence of bacteria in the blood.

**Barbiturate.** A drug that depresses the function of the central nervous system; a useful anticonvulsant.

**Basal ganglia.** These include the caudate nucleus, putamen, and globus pallidus and serve to coordinate movement.

**Belladonna.** A plant containing various anticholinergic alkaloids, including atropine.

**Benign.** Nonmalignant, nonrecurrent.

**Benzodiazepine.** Anticonvulsant drugs including diazepam (Valium) and Klonopin.

**Bilateral.** Affecting both sides.

**Bilirubin.** Bile pigment formed by the disintegration of red blood cells.

**Binge.** An unrestrained indulgence.

**Binocular.** Relating to the use of both eyes.

**Bone mineral density.** Assessment of the compactness of bone.

**Bradycardia.** Slowness of the heart rate.

**Braille.** A system of writing and printing for the blind by means of tangible points or dots.

**Brain morphometry.** Measuring the volume and size of the brain by neuroimaging techniques.

**Brain stem.** That section of the brain that includes the vital centers for heart and respiratory rate as well as the control of consciousness.

**Bronchial.** Any of the larger air passages of the lung.

**Bronchitis.** An inflammation of the larger air passages of the lung.

**Bronchodilators.** An agent that causes dilation of the lumina of the air passages of the lungs.

**Carbohydrate.** Sugar, starch, or cellulose.

**Carcinoma.** A malignant new growth or cancer.

**Cardiomyopathy.** Disease of the heart muscle.

**Caries.** Tooth cavities.

**Cataract.** An opacity or density of the eye lens.

**Cellulitis.** Infection of the skin.

**Cerebrospinal fluid (CSF).** The fluid that surrounds and bathes the brain and spinal cord.

**Cervix.** The lower and narrow end of the uterus.

**Charcot-Marie-Tooth disease.** Congenital weakness and wasting of the extremities, particularly the legs.

**Chemotherapy.** The treatment of a disease by chemicals or drugs.

**Choreoathetosis.** Movement characterized by chorea and athetosis.

**Chorionic gonadotrophin.** A substance formed in the placenta that stimulates the gonads.

**Choriovillus.** Fetal tissue that can be biopsied for a genetic diagnosis.

**Chromosome.** A rod-shaped body within the cell nucleus that contains the DNA that transmits hereditary characteristics.

**Chronic.** Marked by long duration or frequent recurrence.

**Chronological age.** The actual age of the individual.

**Circumscribed.** Restricted to a limited space.

**Climacteric.** Menopause.

**Clitoris.** A small, erectile body situated in the anterior angle of the external genitalia in the female.

**Coarctation.** A localized stricture.

**Cognition.** The act or process of knowing, including both awareness and judgment.

**Coitus.** Sexual intercourse.

**Colostomy.** Surgical opening between the colon (large bowel) and the surface of the body.

**Comatose.** A state of unconsciousness.

**Compliance.** The act or process of following a drug treatment or weight reduction program.

**Conception.** The act of becoming pregnant; the state of being conceived.

**Concordance.** The occurrence of a given trait in both members of a twin pair.

**Condom.** A sheath or cover for the penis.

**Congenital.** Existing at or dating from birth.

**Congestive heart failure.** The heart cannot produce the output required to sustain the metabolic needs of the body.

**Conical.** Cone shaped.

**Conjunctiva.** The delicate membrane that lines the eyelids and covers the surface of the eye.

**Constitutional.** Relating to the entire body rather than a particular organ.

**Contracture.** Fixation of a joint due to fibrosis of a muscle.

**Cornea.** The transparent structure forming the anterior part of the eye.

**Corpus callosum.** Neural pathways that connect the cerebral hemispheres.

**Cortex.** The outer or external layer of the brain; gray matter.

**Cortical sulcal enlargement.** An increase in the size of the depressions (i.e., a groove, trench, or furrow) on the outer layer of the brain.

**Craniosynostosis.** Premature closure of the sutures of the skull.

**Cyanosis.** A bluish discoloration of the skin resulting from poor oxygenation.

**Cycloplegia.** The loss of the eye's ability to constrict the pupil.

**Cystic fibrosis.** An inherited disease characterized by fibrosis of the lungs and absence of digestive enzymes in the pancreas gland.

**Cytoplasm.** The protoplasm of a cell exclusive of that of the nucleus.

**Decibel.** A unit for expressing relative intensity of sound; zero is the average least perceptible sound and 130 is the average pain level.

**Decongestant.** An agent that reduces congestion or swelling.

**Degradation.** The act of reducing a chemical or compound to smaller units.

**Dehydration.** The condition that results from excessive loss of body water and electrolytes.

**Delirium tremens.** Alcoholic withdrawal characterized by anxiety, trembling, hallucinations, and excessive agitation.

**Dermatologic.** Affecting the skin.

**Detoxification.** Treatment designed to free an addict from his or her drug habit.

**Diffusion tensor MRI.** An imaging method that is sensitive to the molecular movement of water, which indicates cellular integrity and pathology; this technique can provide a structural analysis of specific tracts within the central nervous system.

**Dilatation.** The condition of being dilated or stretched beyond normal dimensions.

**Diplegia.** Weakness or paralysis of the legs.

**Diploid.** Double in appearance or arrangement, especially of the basic chromosome number.

**Diplopia.** Double vision due to weakness or paralysis of the eye muscles.

**Distal.** At the end of an extremity or organ.

**Diuretic.** An agent that promotes the excretion of urine.

**Dopamine.** An intermediate product in the synthesis of norepinephrine; acts as a neurotransmitter in the central nervous system.

**Dorsiflexion.** Backward flexion or bending of the hand or foot.

**Dura.** Thick, membranous protective covering of the brain.

**Dwarfism.** A condition characterized by short stature, less than average height.

**Dysarthria.** Imperfect articulation of speech due to a disturbance of motor control.

**Dyscalculia.** Impairment of the ability to do mathematical problems.

**Dysesthesia.** Impairment of any sense, especially touch.

**Dysgraphia.** Inability to write properly, sometimes as a part of a language disorder.

**Dyskinesia.** Fragmentary incomplete movements.

**Dyslexia.** An inability to read with understanding at age and grade level.

**Dysmorphic.** An abnormality in development.

**Dysphagia.** Difficulty in swallowing.

**Dysplastic.** Referring to abnormal development or growth.

**Dyspraxia.** Partial loss of ability to perform coordinated tasks.

**Dystonia.** Disordered tonicity of muscle.

**Echolalia.** The repetition of words or sentences by an individual, often without understanding.

**Ectopic.** Out of place or position.

**Eczema.** A skin disorder affecting the face, scalp, arms, and legs.

**Edema.** Swelling; collection of abnormally excessive amounts of fluid.

**Ejaculation.** Sudden expulsion of semen.

**Electroencephalogram (EEG).** The recording of electrical currents originating in the brain by means of electrodes placed on the scalp.

**Electrolytes.** Ions in the blood, including chloride, potassium, and sodium.

**Electrophoresis.** The movement of charged particles suspended in a liquid under the influence of an applied electric field.

**Emaciation.** A wasted or malnourished state.

**Embryo.** The developing organism from 2 weeks following fertilization to the end of the 8th week.

**Embryogenesis.** The development of a new organism by means of sexual reproduction.

**Encephalitis.** Infection of the brain.

**Encephalocele.** Hernia of the brain through a congenital or traumatic opening of the skull.

**Encephalopathy.** A process that damages or interferes with brain function.

**Endometrium.** The inner mucous membrane of the uterus.

**End organ.** The organ responsible for a particular function.

**Enteritis.** Inflammation of the small intestine.

**Enucleation.** The surgical removal of an organ (e.g., the eye).

**Enzyme.** A substance that accelerates or catalyzes specific chemical reactions within the organism.

**Epicanthus.** A vertical fold of skin on either side of the nose that covers the innermost portion of the eye.

**Epidemic.** A disease affecting many people in any region at the same time.

**Epidemiologic.** Pertaining to the incidence, distribution, and control of disease.

**Epidermis.** The outermost and nonvascular layer of skin.

**Epiglottitis.** A serious life-threatening infection of tissue covering the entrance to the larynx.

**Epiphyseal.** The end of a long bone.

**Epiphysis.** The end of a bone where the majority of growth takes place.

**Ergot.** A drug used for the treatment of migraine headaches.

**Esophagus.** The musculomembranous passage extending from the mouth to the stomach.

**Esotropia.** Deviation of the eye toward the nose.

**Etiology.** The cause of a disorder or condition.

**Euphoric.** A feeling of well-being or elation.

**Evoked response potential.** An electrical response (averaged on a computer) that follows stimulation of the central nervous system by a specific stimulus of the visual, auditory, or sensory system.

**Exchange system.** A diabetic diet that allows the trading of one item of food for another (e.g., a slice of bread for a serving of potatoes).

**Exogenous.** Outside the body or organ.

**Exophoria.** Outward deviation of the eye.

**Exophthalmos.** Abnormal protrusion of the eyeball.

**Extrapyramidal.** Outside the pyramidal tracts.

**Fallopian tubes.** Pair of tubes connecting the ovary to the uterus.

**Femur.** The bone that extends from the pelvis to the knee.

**Fertilization.** The act of rendering gametes fertile or capable of further development.

**Fetus.** A developing vertebrate organism; in the human, the period after the 3rd month of intrauterine development.

**Flaccid.** Weak, soft, or loose.

**Flora.** Bacteria normally residing in the mouth and intestine.

**Focal neurologic signs.** Neurologic abnormalities restricted to one portion of the body.

**Footcandle.** The amount of illumination produced by a standard candle at a distance of 1 ft.

**Fovea (of the retina).** A small pit in the retina that provides the clearest vision because of the concentration of a group of nerve cells called cones.

**Fricatives.** The sounds produced by a voiceless breath escaping through the larnyx or vocal tract.

**Friedreich's ataxia.** An inherited disease that begins in childhood, is characterized by progressive loss of gait and speech impairment, and often results in sudden death because of cardiac arrhythmias.

**Frontal lobe.** The most anterior portion of the brain that controls many activities, including executive function.

**Gangrene.** Death of tissue usually associated with a loss of blood supply and followed by bacterial invasion.

**Gastric.** Relating to the stomach.

**Gastroenteritis.** Inflammation of stomach and intestines.

**Generic.** Characteristic of an entire group or class.

**Germ cell.** The cell of origin that develops into the primitive embryo.

**Gestation.** The period of pregnancy.

**Glaucoma.** An eye disease characterized by increased pressure within the eye.

**Global.** Universal, comprehensive.

**Glucose.** A sugar.

**Goiter.** A visibly enlarged thyroid gland.

**Gonad.** The ovary or testes.

**Gonadal dysgenesis.** Defective development of the testes or ovary.

**Gray matter.** Neural tissue, especially of the brain and spinal cord, that contains cell bodies as well as nerve fibers, and forms most of the cortex and nuclei of the brain, the columns of the spinal cord, and the bodies of ganglia.

**Gustatory.** Pertaining to the sense of taste.

**Guttural.** Articulated in the throat.

**Habilitation.** The process of enhancing an individual's capabilities to the greatest potential.

**Halitosis.** Offensive breath.

**Half-life.** The time required to metabolize half of a drug or isotope.

**Hallucination.** A sense perception not founded upon objective reality.

**Hallucinogen.** A drug or chemical that produces hallucinations.

**Hamstring.** Muscle at the back of the thigh.

**Heart murmur.** A sound produced due to the abnormal flow of blood, usually the result of a heart defect.

**Helical.** Having the form of a helix.

**Hematocrit.** A measure of the volume of red blood cells.

**Hematologic disturbances.** Disturbances in the blood.

**Hemiplegia.** Paralysis on one side of the body.

**Hemoglobin.** The oxygen-carrying component in the red blood cells.

**Hepatitis.** Inflammation of the liver.

**Hereditary.** Genetically transmitted from parent to offspring.

**Heterosexual.** One who is sexually attracted to persons of the opposite sex.

**Hormone.** A chemical substance formed in one part of the body that has a specific action on an organ located in another site.

**Huntington's chorea.** A rare hereditary disease characterized by progressive uncontrolled movements of the extremities and mental deterioration.

**Hydrocephalus.** An enlargement of the head due to an abnormal collection of cerebrospinal fluid.

**Hyperkinesia.** Abnormally increased activity.

**Hyperopia.** Farsightedness.

**Hypertelorism.** Abnormally increased distance between the eyes.

**Hypertension.** High arterial blood pressure.

**Hyperthyroidism.** Excessive activity of the thyroid gland.

**Hypertrophy.** The enlargement of an organ.

**Hyperventilation.** Deep breathing.

**Hypochondriasis.** Overconcern about one's health.

**Hypoglycemia.** An abnormally low blood glucose level.

**Hypogonadal.** Pertaining to the decreased function of the sex glands.

**Hyposensitization.** The process of decreasing sensitivity, usually by providing the patient with gradually increasing quantities of the offending substance.

**Hypothalamic–pituitary.** The anterior lobe secretes several important hormones that regulate the functioning of the thyroids, gonads, adrenal cortex, and other endocrine organs; the cells of the posterior lobe serve as a reservoir for hormones having antidiuretic and oxytocic action.

**Hypothalamus.** The portion of the brain that includes the optic chiasm, mamillary bodies, infundibulum, and hypophysis, which integrate peripheral autonomic mechanisms, endocrine activity, and many somatic functions.

**Hypothyroidism.** Deficiency of thyroid activity.

**Hypotonia.** Decreased muscle tone.

**Hypoxia.** Reduction of oxygen supply to tissues.

**Hysterectomy.** Surgical removal of the uterus (womb).

**Iatrogenic.** Induced by the physician.

**Ileostomy.** Surgical creation of an opening from the surface of the abdominal wall into the small bowel.

**Immunity.** The ability to resist a certain disease or infection.

**Immunoglobulin.** A protein synthesized by lymphocyte and plasma cells that are responsible for the humoral aspects of immunity.

**Impotence.** Lack of ability to initiate an erection or to maintain an erection until ejaculation.

**Incest.** Sexual activity between close relatives (e.g., father and daughter; brother and sister).

**Incidence.** An expression of the rate at which a certain event occurs (e.g., number of new cases of a specific disease occurring during a certain period).

**Incisors.** Any of the four front teeth.

**Infarction.** Tissue destruction resulting from obstruction of circulation to the area.

**Insomnia.** Inability to sleep.

**Insulin-dependent diabetes mellitus.** A disease in which the body's cells cannot use glucose (sugar) properly for lack of or resistance to the hormone insulin, produced by the pancreas.

**Intestinal motility.** The ability of the intestine to move spontaneously.

**Intracranial.** Situated within the skull.

**Intramuscular.** Within the substance of a muscle.

**In utero.** Within the uterus.

**Ipecac.** A medication used to induce vomiting.

**Ischemia.** Deficiency of blood flow to a region of the body.

**Jaundice.** Abnormal deposition of bile pigment in the skin, resulting in a yellowish appearance.

**Karyotype.** The chromosome number and composition.

**Keratoconus.** A conical protrusion of the cornea.

**Kernicterus.** Excessive serum levels of bilirubin, resulting in brain damage.

**Ketone.** The substances acetone, acetoacetic acid, and $\beta$-hydroxybutyric acid.

**Kinesthesia.** The sense by which movement, weight, and position are perceived.

**Labia.** An elongated fold running downward and backward from the mons pubis of the female.

**Lacrimation.** The secretion of tears.

**Lactation.** The secretion of milk.

**Larynx.** The portion of the trachea that contains the vocal cords.

**Lesion.** A pathologic disruption of tissue or a loss of a part.

**Lethal.** Deadly, fatal.

**Leukomalacia.** Softening or destruction of the white matter.

**Leukopenia.** Decrease in white blood cells in the blood.

**Limbic system.** A highly complex, phylogenetically old portion of the brain that is thought to be involved with control of emotion.

**Lingual.** Pertaining to or toward the tongue.

**Lissencephaly.** Malformations of the brain due to abnormal convulsions of the cerebral cortex.

**Locomotor.** Pertaining to movement or locomotion.

**Lupus erythematosis.** A generalized connective tissue disorder.

**Macro-orchidism.** Enlarged testes.

**Macula.** The anatomic area of the retina that provides the clearest vision.

**Malabsorption.** Impaired intestinal absorption of nutrients.

**Malady.** An illness, usually of a chronic type.

**Malaise.** A vague sensation of discomfort.

**Malar.** Relating to the cheek or the side of the head.

**Malignancy.** Cancer, a tumor with invasive properties.

**Malingerer.** One who feigns an illness.

**Mallory-Weiss tears.** Mucosal tears and bleeding at the junction of the stomach and esophagus caused by violent vomiting.

**Malocclusion.** Improper closure of the teeth.

**Mastoid.** The bony prominence located behind each ear.

**Maturation.** The process of becoming fully developed.

**Maxilla.** The upper jaw.

**Medial.** Toward the middle.

**Megavitamins.** Extremely high doses of vitamins, sometimes used to treat autism and a wide range of developmental disorders.

**Menarche.** The onset of menstruation.

**Meningitis.** Infection of the brain and its covering membranes.

**Meningomyelocele.** Hernial protrusion of a part of the meninges and substance of the spinal cord through a defect in the bony spinal column.

**Menses.** The monthly flow of blood from the female genital tract.

**Metabolic rate.** The rate at which food is transformed into energy, which is then used for the maintenance of respiration, circulation, peristalsis, muscle tonus, body temperature, glandular activity, and other vegetative functions of the body.

**Metabolism.** The sum of chemical and physical activity that creates and destroys cells.

**Metalinguistics.** A branch of linguistics that deals with the relation between language and other cultural factors in a society.

**Methylphenidate.** Trade name Ritalin, the most commonly used stimulant medication for the treatment of attention-deficit/hyperactivity disorder.

**Microcephaly.** Abnormal smallness of the head, usually associated with mental retardation.

**Milestone.** A significant point or event in development.

**Mites.** Minute animals related to the spider.

**Mitochondrial.** Organelles in the cell cytoplasm that generate energy in the form of ATP (adenosine triphosphate).

**Mitotic cell.** A method of indirect division of a cell in which two daughter nuclei receive identical complements of the number of chromosomes characteristic of the somatic cells of the species.

**Mitral valve.** A bicuspid valve in the heart between the ventricle and the atrium.

**Mitral valve prolapse.** The downward displacement of the mitral valve, which is found between the two left chambers of the heart.

**Monoarticular.** Limited to one joint.

**Monogamy.** The practice of marrying only once during a lifetime.

**Morbidity.** The condition of being diseased or unwell.

**Morphogenesis.** The development and establishment of form.

**Mortality rate.** The ratio of deaths to a total population in a given time or place.

**Mucosa.** A mucous membrane (e.g., vaginal, urethral).

**Multidisciplinary.** Pertaining to the cooperative participation by several professional groups.

**Multifactorial.** Arising through the interaction of many factors.

**Musculoskeletal.** Referring to muscles and the bony skeleton.

**Mutagen.** A chemical or physical agent that induces genetic mutations.

**Myasthenia gravis.** Muscle weakness due to a disorder of acetylcholine receptors at the neuromuscular junction.

**Myelin.** A fatlike substance that envelops certain nerve fibers or tracts.

**Myopia.** Nearsightedness.

**Myotonic dystrophy.** An inherited form of muscular dystrophy characterized by progressive weakness, baldness, cataracts, and a peculiar stiffness of certain muscles.

**Nasogastric tube.** A soft tube inserted through a nostril into the stomach.

**Neonatal.** Pertaining to the initial month of life.

**Neoplasm.** Any new and abnormal growth of any tissue in the body.

**Nephrosis.** A disease of the kidneys characterized by loss of protein in the urine and generalized edema.

**Neural tube.** The primitive nervous system.

**Neuromuscular.** Pertaining to the peripheral nerves and muscles.

**Neuron.** Any of the conducting cells of the nervous system.

**Neurotic.** Pertaining to a functional nervous disorder without demonstrable physical lesion; pertaining to an emotionally unstable individual.

**Neurulation.** Formation of the neural plate in the embryo.

**Neurotransmitter.** A substance that is released from an axon and that inhibits or excites a target cell.

**Noradrenaline.** A catecholamine that is the principal neurotransmitter of adrenergic neurons.

**Nystagmus.** Abnormal, jerky eye movements.

**Obesity.** An excessive accumulation of body fat.

**Occipital.** Pertaining to the back or posterior part of the head.

**Ocular.** Pertaining to the eye.

**Olfactory.** Pertaining to the sense of smell.

**Ontogeny.** The development of the individual organism.

**Optic chiasm.** The crossing of the optic nerves.

**Optic nerve.** The visual nerve.

**Organ.** A part of the body with specialized function (e.g., digestion, respiration).

**Organic.** Originating within the body and affecting the function of the individual.

**Orgasm.** The apex and culmination of sexual excitement.

**Orthodontics.** The dental specialty that is concerned with malocclusion of the teeth.

**Orthographic.** The representation of the sounds of a language by written or printed symbols.

**Orthoptics.** The prescription of eye movement exercises for the treatment of various visual defects, including muscular imbalance.

**Orthotic.** A supportive device to support, align, or correct deformities, or to improve the function of movable parts of the body.

**Osmoregulation.** Concerned with the regulation and maintenance of constant osmotic pressure.

**Ossification.** The formation of bone.

**Osteoarthritis.** Degenerative joint disease characterized by pain and stiffness, particularly after prolonged activity.

**Osteogenesis imperfecta.** An inherited condition in which the bones are abnormally brittle and subject to recurrent fractures.

**Osteopenia.** Decrease in bone mass.

**Osteoporosis.** Abnormal density of bones.

**Osteotomy.** The cutting of a bone by a surgeon.

**Ototoxic.** A drug that damages the hearing mechanism, resulting in deafness.

**Ovulation.** The discharge of an egg from a vesicular follicle of the ovary.

**Ovum.** The female reproductive cell, the egg.

**Pallor.** Paleness.

**Palpebral.** Eyelid.

**Palpitations.** A subjective sensation of an unduly rapid or irregular heartbeat.

**Pancreas.** A gland that lies behind the stomach; it produces digestive enzymes and insulin.

**Parkinson disease.** A neurological disease characterized by tremor, muscle rigidity, and decreased muscle movements due to a deficiency of dopamine in the central nervous system.

**Parotid gland.** Salivary gland, located in front of the ear.

**Parturition.** The act or process of giving birth to a child.

**Pathogen.** A disease-producing microorganism.

**Pathogenesis.** The sequence of events leading to the development of a disease.

**Pathognomonic.** Specifically distinctive or characteristic of a disease or pathologic condition.

**Pathology.** The study of structural changes within the body caused by disease.

**Patterning.** A system of physical therapy for the treatment of cerebral palsy, learning disorders, and a variety of other neurological disorders. Proponents have made controversial claims that this approach is an effective therapy for these disorders.

**Pedodontics.** The branch of dentistry concerned with conditions of the teeth and mouth in children.

**Pedophilia.** Sexual activity between adults and children.

**Peptic.** Related to the action of gastric juices.

**Peptide.** The constituent part of a protein; some peptides act as hormones.

**Perinatal.** The period beginning the 28th week of gestation and ending 7 to 28 days after birth.

**Periodontal.** Situated or occurring around a tooth.

**Periventricular.** The area surrounding the ventricles of the brain.

**Phallus.** The penis or clitoris.

**Phenotype.** The visible properties of an individual that are produced by the interaction of the genotype and the environment.

**Phenytoin.** An anticonvulsant (Dilantin) effective in the management of generalized seizures.

**Philtrum.** The vertical groove in the median portion of the upper lip.

**Phobia.** Excessive fear.

**Phoneme.** A member of the set of the smallest units of speech that serve to distinguish one utterance from another.

**Photophobia.** Abnormal intolerance of light.

**Physiology.** The study of body and organ function.

**Pituitary.** A gland situated in the base of the skull that secretes several important hormones.

**Placebo.** An inactive substance or preparation used in controlled studies to determine the efficacy of medicinal substances.

**Placenta.** The organ that unites the fetus to the uterus for the provision of various nutrients.

**Plaque.** A mass adhering to the enamel surface of the tooth.

**Poliomyelitis.** An acute viral disease that may involve the motor cells in the spinal cord; it can be prevented by a specific vaccine.

**Polygenic.** Pertaining to or determined by the action of several different genes.

**Posterior.** Situated in back of or behind.

**Postnatal.** Pertaining to the time following birth.

**Postural drainage.** The process by which the patient is assisted in clearing sputum and secretions from the lungs by positioning first on one side and then the other.

**Pragmatics.** The relation between signs or linguistic expressions and their users.

**Premorbid.** The state of appearance prior to the onset of disease.

**Prenatal.** Pertaining to the period before birth.

**Prepubertal.** Preceding puberty.

**Presbyopia.** Farsightedness.

**Prevalence.** The total number of cases of a disease in existence at a certain time in a designated area.

**Primordial.** Original or primitive.

**Progeny.** Offspring, children.

**Prognosis.** A forecast as to the eventual outcome of a disease.

**Prophylactic.** Pertaining to the prevention of or warding off of a disorder.

**Prostaglandins.** A group of naturally occurring fatty acids that have the ability to lower blood pressure, regulate acid secretion of the stomach, regulate body temperature, and control inflammation and vascular permeability.

**Prostate.** A gland in the male that surrounds the neck of the bladder and the urethra. The prostate contributes fluid to the seminal secretion.

**Prosthesis.** An artificial device to replace an absent portion of the body.

**Proximal.** Nearest to the center.

**Psychoactive.** A stimulant of the central nervous system.

**Psychometric.** The measurement of intelligence.

**Psychopathology.** The branch of medicine that deals with the causes and nature of mental disorders.

**Psychopharmacologic agents.** The use of drugs to modify psychological functions and states.

**Psychosis.** Mental illness.

**Psychosomatic.** Involving both mind and body.

**Psychotropic.** Drugs that modify the intensity of feelings or alter certain behaviors or experiences.

**Ptosis.** Drooping of the upper eyelid.

**Pubescence.** Arriving at the age of puberty.

**Purging.** To cause evacuation from the bowels by the use of a laxative.

**Purulent.** Pus.

**Quadriceps.** The groups of muscles on the upper or anterior surface of the thigh.

**Quadriplegia.** Paralysis of all four extremities.

**Radiologic.** Relating to the use of X-rays for diagnosis or use of radiation in treatment.

**Recombinant DNA.** DNA that has been artificially introduced into a cell so that it alters the genotype and phenotype of the cell and is replicated along with the natural DNA.

**Refractive errors.** The imperfect deviation of light by the eye so that the image is distorted by the time it reaches the retina.

**Regional enteritis.** A localized area of inflammation within the small intestine.

**Regression.** Progressive decline or loss of skills.

**Renal.** Pertaining to the kidney.

**Reticular activating system.** The portion of the brain that is concerned with the level of consciousness.

**Retina.** The innermost membrane of the eye; it is the perceptive structure of the eye and is connected to the brain by the optic nerve.

**Rhinitis (allergic).** Inflammation of the nose caused by an allergy.

**Rhinorrhea.** Discharge from the nose.

**Rhizotomy.** Surgical interruption of the roots of spinal nerves within the spinal canal.

**Rickets.** A bone-deforming disease of children caused by a deficiency of Vitamin D.

**Rooting reflex.** The infant's primitive instinct to seek a nipple or food source.

**Rote.** Memorization with little comprehension.

**Rubella.** German measles.

**Rumination.** The regurgitation of food following a meal.

**Salicylates.** Aspirin.

**Salivation.** Excessive flow or production of saliva.

**Schizencephaly.** A congenital malformation of the brain with abnormal clefts.

**Schizophrenia.** A psychotic disorder characterized by flights of ideas, disordered thought processes, and a loss of reality reasoning.

**Scoliosis.** Curvature of the spine.

**Scurvy.** Vitamin C deficiency resulting in weakness, anemia, bleeding tendency, and spongy gums.

**Sebaceous glands.** Glands that secrete a greasy, lubricating substance called sebum.

**Secondary amenorrhea.** Cessation of menstruation after it has been established at puberty.

**Secondary sexual characteristics.** Sexual features unrelated to the genitalia, such as the beard in a male.

**Semantics.** The study of changes in the signification of words.

**Sensorineural hearing loss.** Hearing loss caused by injury to the auditory nerve.

**Sensorium.** The level or state of alertness or consciousness.

**Sensory.** Conveying nerve impulses from the sense organs to the brain.

**Sequelae.** The permanent consequences of an injury or disease.

**Serotonin.** Released by blood platelets and acts as a neurotransmitter in the central nervous system.

**Serotonin reuptake inhibitors.** These medicines are used mainly in the treatment of depression. They also are used to treat obsessive–compulsive disorder, panic disorder, and bulimia nervosa. These medicines affect the chemicals that nerves in the brain use to send messages to one another. These chemical messengers, called neurotransmitters, are released by one nerve and taken up by other nerves. These medicines work by inhibiting the reuptake of serotonin, an action that allows more serotonin to be available to be taken up by other nerves.

**Shunt.** The bypassing of an obstruction within the brain by redirecting the cerebrospinal fluid into the heart or peritoneal cavity through a plastic tube.

**Sibilants.** The *s, z, ch, zh,* or *j* sounds.

**Sicca cell therapy.** Implantation by injection of fetal sheep brain cells to promote brain growth and improve intelligence.

**Sign.** Objective evidence of a disease.

**Sinusitis.** An infection of the sinus, the air cavities within the cranial bones.

**Skinfold thickness.** A technique to measure the nutrition of an individual.

**Slough.** Shed or cast off.

**Smokeless tobacco.** "Snuff" or chewing tobacco.

**Soft neurological signs.** Abnormalities that are usually developmentally related, such as mirror movements of the hands (the opposite hand makes similar movements to the performing hand) and unusual posturing of the hands and arms when the upper extremities are extended. Soft signs do not contribute to the localization of central nervous system lesions, but rather reflect a more generalized immaturity of the brain such as occurs in learning disorders and mental retardation.

**Somatic.** Relating to the body.

**Spasticity.** Increased tone and stiffness of the muscles.

**Spermatogenesis.** The first stage of formation of sperm cells.

**Sphincter.** A ring of muscle that serves to open and close an orifice.

**Spina bifida.** A developmental anomaly characterized by defective closure of the bony encasement of the spinal cord, through which the cord and meninges may protrude.

**Squint.** Crossing of the eyes.

**Station.** The position assumed while standing.

**Stereopsis.** The perception of objects in relief and not as all in one plane.

**Stereotactic.** Precise spatial positioning of a neurosurgical instrument within discrete areas of the brain that control specific functions.

**Stimulant.** An agent or remedy that produces stimulation.

**Strabismus.** Imbalance of the muscles of the eyeball, resulting in a squint.

**Stupor.** Partial loss of consciousness, near coma.

**Subclinical.** Pertaining to a condition not detectable by the usual tests.

**Subcutaneous.** Beneath the skin.

**Subscapular.** Under the scapula, the triangular bone in the back of the shoulder.

**Substrate.** A substance acted upon by an enzyme.

**Sucrose.** A disaccharide obtained from sugar cane.

**Symptom.** The patient's perception of a change from a normal condition, which may indicate the presence of disease.

**Syndrome.** A set of symptoms that occur together.

**Synovitis.** Inflammation of the synovial membrane, the lining of the joint cavities.

**Syntax.** The way that words are put together to form phrases, clauses, or sentences.

**Synthesis.** The production of a substance.

**Systemic.** Affecting the entire body.

**Taxonomy.** Classification.

**Tay-Sachs disease.** A lethal degenerative disease of the central nervous system, particularly among Ashkenazi Jewish children.

**Teratogenic.** Tending to produce anomalies of formation.

**Tetanus.** An acute disease that causes severe spasms and rigidity in certain muscles (lockjaw).

**Thalidomide.** A sedative drug that causes serious congenital anomalies in the fetus (amelia and phocomelia) when taken by a woman during early pregnancy.

**Thermoregulation.** Heat regulation.

**Thrombocytopenia.** Decreased platelets in the blood.

**Tibial tubercle.** Bony prominence on the tibia bone.

**Titer.** The highest dilution of a serum that causes clumping of microorganisms or other particulate antigens.

**Topical.** Pertaining to a drug or substance that is applied to the skin.

**Tracheostomy.** A surgical opening into the trachea.

**Transplantation.** The transfer of an organ or tissue from one person (or place within the body) to another.

**Tremor.** Shaking, shivering, or trembling.

**Triceps.** The muscle along the back of the upper arm.

**Trichobezoar.** Hairball.

**Trimester.** A period of 3 months.

**Turner syndrome.** A form of abnormal development of the female gonads marked by short stature, undifferentiated (streak) gonads, and variable abnormalities, which may include webbing of the neck, low posterior hair line, increased carrying angle of elbow, cubitus valgus, and cardiac defects.

**Ultrasound.** The visualization of deep structures of the body by recording the reflections of pulses of ultrasonic waves directed into the tissues.

**Umbilical.** Relating to the navel.

**Unilateral.** One-sided.

**Urethra.** The canal conveying urine from the bladder to the exterior of the body.

**Urinalysis.** Physical, chemical, and microscopic examination of the urine.

**Vasectomy.** Sterilization in the male by surgical excision of the vas deferens (the tube connecting the testis and ejaculatory duct).

**Vasopressin.** A hormone that causes contraction of vascular tissue of capillaries.

**Ventricular.** A small cavity as in the brain or heart.

**Ventricular arrhythmia.** Variation from the normal rhythm of the heartbeat.

**Virus.** An infective agent responsible for a great number of diseases, including the common cold. The virus is smaller than most bacteria and is capable of multiplication only within a living cell.

**Void.** To urinate or empty the bladder.

**Volatile.** Tending to evaporate quickly.

**Voluntary muscles.** Muscle activity that is controlled by an individual.

**Vulva.** The region of the external genital organs of the female.

**White matter.** A neural tissue that consists largely of myelinated nerve fibers, has a whitish color, and underlies the gray matter of the brain and spinal cord or is gathered into nerves. White matter carries information between the nerve cells in the brain and the spinal cord.

# Index

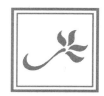

# About the Editors

**Robert H. A. Haslam,** MD, FAAP, FRCPC, is a graduate of the University of Saskatchewan School of Medicine. Following an internship and a year of family medicine, he completed pediatric training at the Johns Hopkins School of Medicine, followed by child neurology training at the University of Kentucky in Lexington. In 1970, Haslam was appointed as director of the John F. Kennedy Institute in Baltimore, and as an associate professor of pediatrics and neurology at the Johns Hopkins University School of Medicine. Haslam was named professor and chair of the department of pediatrics at the University of Calgary and director of research at the Alberta Children's Hospital in 1975. In 1986, Haslam became professor and chair of the department of pediatrics, and professor of medicine (neurology) at the University of Toronto and pediatrician-in-chief of pediatrics at the Hospital for Sick Children in Toronto. As a child neurologist, Haslam's clinical and research interests have focused on children with developmental disabilities. He has published over 150 papers and book chapters and is a frequent invited speaker and visiting professor at national and international meetings. At present, Haslam is a child neurologist at the Alberta Children's Hospital and the vice president of education for the Royal College of Physicians and Surgeons of Canada.

**Peter James Valletutti,** EdD, has an earned doctorate in special education from Columbia Teachers College, New York. He has been a teacher and principal in the schools of New York State, and professor and chair of special education at Coppin State College in Baltimore, and Virginia State University in Petersburg. He was an assistant professor in pediatrics at the Johns Hopkins School of Medicine. He was a former dean of education and graduate studies at Coppin State College. Valletutti has served as a consultant in special education and in the medical problems of children at the local, national, and international levels. The author of 24 texts in special education and rehabilitation, he is currently enjoying his retirement while working on several new writing projects.